Rapid Assessment

A flowchart guide to evaluating signs and symptoms

Rapid Assessment

A flowchart guide to evaluating signs and symptoms

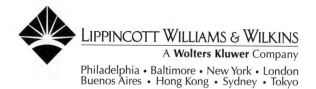

LIPPINCOTT WILLIAMS & WILKINS
A **Wolters Kluwer** Company

Philadelphia • Baltimore • New York • London
Buenos Aires • Hong Kong • Sydney • Tokyo

STAFF

Executive Publisher
Judith A. Schilling McCann, RN, MSN

Editorial Director
H. Nancy Holmes

Clinical Director
Joan M. Robinson, RN, MSN

Senior Art Director
Arlene Putterman

Editorial Project Manager
William Welsh (associate editor)

Editor
Stacey Ann Follin

Clinical Editors
Marguerite S. Ambrose, RN, DNSc, APRN,BC;
Kate McGovern, RN, MSN, CCRN

Copy Editors
Kimberly Bilotta (supervisor), Tom DeZego, Amy Furman,
Catherine Kirby, Judith Orioli, Dorothy P. Terry, Pamela Wingrod

Designer
Debra Moloshok (book design and design project manager)

Digital Composition Services
Diane Paluba (manager), Joyce Rossi Biletz (senior desktop
assistant), Donna S. Morris (senior desktop assistant)

Manufacturing
Patricia K. Dorshaw (senior manager), Beth Janae Orr
(book production coordinator)

Editorial Assistants
Megan L. Aldinger, Tara L. Carter-Bell, Arlene Claffee,
Linda K. Ruhf

Librarian
Wani Z. Larsen

The clinical treatments described and recommended in this publication are based on research and consultation with nursing, medical, and legal authorities. To the best of our knowledge, these procedures reflect currently accepted practice. Nevertheless, they can't be considered absolute and universal recommendations. For individual applications, all recommendations must be considered in light of the patient's clinical condition and, before administration of new or infrequently used drugs, in light of the latest package insert information. The authors and publisher disclaim any responsibility for any adverse effects resulting from the suggested procedures, from any undetected errors, or from the reader's misunderstanding of the text.

RA –D N O
05 04 03   10 9 8 7 6 5 4 3 2 1

Library of Congress Cataloging-in-Publication Data
Rapid assessment : a flowchart guide to evaluating signs and
symptoms.
        p. ; cm.
Includes bibliographical references and index.
    1. Nursing assessment—Handbooks, manuals, etc. 2. Flow
charts—Handbooks, manuals, etc.
    [DNLM: 1. Nursing Assessment—methods.
WY 100.4 R218 2004] I. Lippincott Williams & Wilkins.
    RT48.R364 2004
    616.07'5 — dc22
ISBN 1-58255-272-X (alk. paper)   2003014532

Contents

Contributors and consultants

Christine Clayton, RN, MS, CNP
Nurse Practitioner
Sioux Valley Clinic – Heart Partners
Sioux Falls, S. Dak.

Mary A. Helming, APRN, BC, MSN, FNP
Assistant Professor of Nursing
Quinnipiac University School of Nursing
Hamden, Conn.

Julia Anne Isen, RN, BSN, MS, FNPC
Nurse Practitioner
Veterans Affairs Medical Center
San Francisco
Assistant Clinical Professor
University of California, San Francisco

Scharalda G. Jeanfreau, MN, FNP-BC
Instructor in Nursing
Louisiana State University Health Sciences Center
School of Nursing
New Orleans

Christy R. Johnson, RN, MSN, CRNFA, FNP-C
Assistant Professor of Nursing
Gordon College
Barnesville, Ga.

Rhonda Johnston, PHD, BC-ANP, BC-FNP, CNS
Nursing Department Chair
Colorado State University
Pueblo
Director School-based Wellness Center
Parkview Medical Center
Pueblo, Colo.

Priscilla A. Lee, BSN, MN, FNP
Instructor in Nursing
Moorpark (Calif.) College

Lynda A. Mackin, RN, MS, CS, CNS, ANP
Assistant Clinical Professor
University of California, San Francisco

Alyssa Jo Solimene, MSN, APN-C
Family Nurse Practitioner
North Hunterdon Physician Associates
Hampton, N.J.

Maryellen Stahley-Brown, CRNP
Nurse Practitioner
Concentra Medical Center
Baltimore

Kathleen Tusaie, RNCS, PHD
Assistant Professor
University of Akron (Ohio)
Advance Practice Nurse
William Beckett & Assoc.
Akron, Ohio

Gail A. Viergutz, RN-C, MS, ANP-C
Nurse Practitioner
St. Michael's Hospital
Stevens Point, Wisc.

Foreword

As the health care environment becomes increasingly complex, the demand on nurses and other health care professionals to deliver the highest quality care in the most efficient, cost-effective manner possible is paramount. This challenge is daunting, but a foundation built on quick and accurate patient assessment — a basic yet vitally important step in the nursing process — can help provide the proper starting point.

Nurses know that by quickly assessing signs and symptoms, accurately analyzing and synthesizing findings, and promptly developing and modifying treatment plans to target changing patient needs, they help themselves achieve exceptional patient outcomes. However, the assessment process isn't always clear-cut. Tools that assist in this critical process are needed.

Rapid Assessment: A Flowchart Guide to Evaluating Signs and Symptoms is a unique reference that was designed with all of the above in mind. Easy to use, this guide provides the nurse with key information to assure that each patient assessment she performs is targeted toward understanding the patient's underlying condition. You won't find a more innovative approach to this important subject matter anywhere.

Each of the more than 200 signs and symptoms, arranged alphabetically, adheres to a standard format that begins with a key description of the presenting problem and continues with guidelines on how to obtain a proper patient history and conduct a thorough physical examination. Special considerations that every nurse should be aware of and additional information on patient counseling are also provided to round out the overview.

Each sign or symptom is accompanied by at least one flowchart that can be used to further direct the patient assessment. Beginning with a common sign or symptom, each flowchart guides you step-by-step through key assessment data leading to a possible diagnosis. Appropriate diagnostic tests, treatments, and related care are outlined to provide a guidepost for further interventions.

There's more. Liberal use of tables and illustrations bring clarity to concepts, and key points are highlighted by the variety of graphic icons and sidebars that are found throughout the various entries. Multiple appendices bring crucial reference material to immediate use, including cardiac arrhythmias, laboratory values, and medical abbreviations. Resources for professionals, patients, and caregivers are provided for those looking for further information.

Rapid Assessment: A Flowchart Guide to Evaluating Signs and Symptoms is an ingenious, innovative title. Within its pages, nurses will find the information needed to assure that each patient assessment is as thorough and accurate as possible. I highly recommend making it a part of your reference library.

Susan E. Appling, RN, MS, CRNP
Assistant Professor
Johns Hopkins School of Nursing
Baltimore

Signs and symptoms

A Abdominal distention

Abdominal distention refers to increased abdominal girth — the result of increased intra-abdominal pressure forcing the abdominal wall outward. Distention may be mild or severe, depending on the amount of pressure. It may be localized or diffuse and may occur gradually or suddenly. Acute abdominal distention may signal life-threatening peritonitis or acute bowel obstruction.

Abdominal distention may result from fat, flatus, an intra-abdominal mass, or fluid. Fluid and gas are normally present in the GI tract but not in the peritoneal cavity. However, if fluid and gas can't pass freely through the GI tract, abdominal distention occurs. In the peritoneal cavity, distention may reflect acute bleeding, accumulation of ascitic fluid, or air from perforation of an abdominal organ.

HISTORY
- Ask the patient about onset, duration, and associated signs and symptoms, such as pressure, fullness, difficulty breathing deeply or lying flat, and inability to bend at the waist.
- Ask the patient about abdominal pain, fever, nausea, vomiting, anorexia, altered bowel habits, and weight gain or loss.
- Review the patient's medical history for recent surgery and GI or biliary disorders that could cause peritonitis or ascites.
- Ask the patient about recent accidents, even minor ones such as a fall from a stepladder.

PHYSICAL ASSESSMENT
- Stand at the foot of the bed, and observe the recumbent patient for abdominal symmetry to determine if distention is localized or generalized.
- Inspect the patient for tense, glistening skin and bulging flanks, which may indicate ascites.
- Observe the umbilicus. An everted umbilicus may indicate ascites or umbilical hernia. An inverted umbilicus may indicate distention from gas and is also common in obese patients.
- Inspect the abdomen for signs of inguinal or femoral hernia and for incisions that may point to adhesions.
- Auscultate for bowel sounds, abdominal friction rubs (indicating peritoneal inflammation), and bruits (indicating an aneurysm).
- Percuss the abdomen to determine if distention results from air, fluid, or both.
- Palpate the abdomen for tenderness, noting whether it's localized or generalized.
- Watch for peritoneal signs and symptoms, such as rebound tenderness, guarding, or rigidity. Note any masses.

- Measure abdominal girth for a baseline value. Mark the flanks with a felt-tipped pen; use the markings as a reference for subsequent measurements.

SPECIAL CONSIDERATIONS
Obesity causes a large abdomen without shifting dullness, prominent tympany, or palpable bowel or other masses, with generalized rather then localized dullness. Also, overeating and constipation can cause distention.

A PEDIATRIC POINTERS
- *Ascites in older children usually results from heart failure, cirrhosis, or nephrosis.*
- *A hernia may cause abdominal distention if it produces an intestinal obstruction.*
- *When percussing a child's abdomen, remember that children normally swallow air when eating and crying, resulting in louder-than-normal tympany. Minimal tympany with abdominal distention may result from fluid accumulation or solid masses.*

PATIENT COUNSELING
If the patient has an obstruction or ascites, explain food and fluid restrictions.

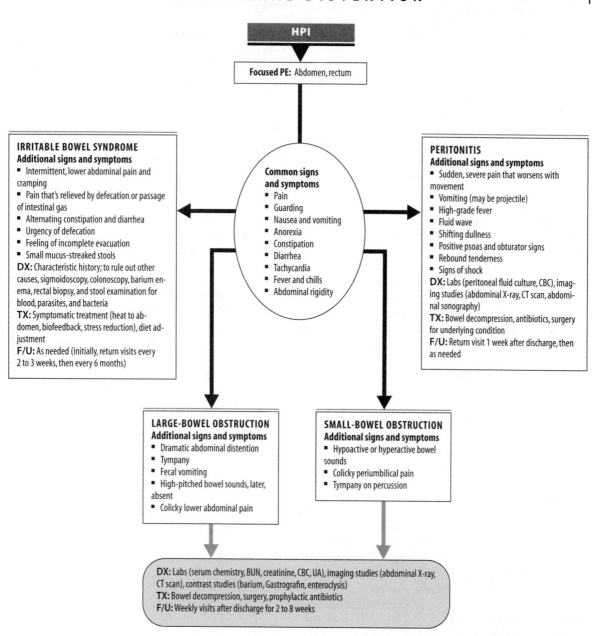

HPI

Focused PE: Abdomen, rectum

Common signs and symptoms
- Pain
- Guarding
- Nausea and vomiting
- Anorexia
- Constipation
- Diarrhea
- Tachycardia
- Fever and chills
- Abdominal rigidity

IRRITABLE BOWEL SYNDROME
Additional signs and symptoms
- Intermittent, lower abdominal pain and cramping
- Pain that's relieved by defecation or passage of intestinal gas
- Alternating constipation and diarrhea
- Urgency of defecation
- Feeling of incomplete evacuation
- Small mucus-streaked stools

DX: Characteristic history; to rule out other causes, sigmoidoscopy, colonoscopy, barium enema, rectal biopsy, and stool examination for blood, parasites, and bacteria
TX: Symptomatic treatment (heat to abdomen, biofeedback, stress reduction), diet adjustment
F/U: As needed (initially, return visits every 2 to 3 weeks, then every 6 months)

PERITONITIS
Additional signs and symptoms
- Sudden, severe pain that worsens with movement
- Vomiting (may be projectile)
- High-grade fever
- Fluid wave
- Shifting dullness
- Positive psoas and obturator signs
- Rebound tenderness
- Signs of shock

DX: Labs (peritoneal fluid culture, CBC), imaging studies (abdominal X-ray, CT scan, abdominal sonography)
TX: Bowel decompression, antibiotics, surgery for underlying condition
F/U: Return visit 1 week after discharge, then as needed

LARGE-BOWEL OBSTRUCTION
Additional signs and symptoms
- Dramatic abdominal distention
- Tympany
- Fecal vomiting
- High-pitched bowel sounds, later, absent
- Colicky lower abdominal pain

SMALL-BOWEL OBSTRUCTION
Additional signs and symptoms
- Hypoactive or hyperactive bowel sounds
- Colicky periumbilical pain
- Tympany on percussion

DX: Labs (serum chemistry, BUN, creatinine, CBC, UA), imaging studies (abdominal X-ray, CT scan), contrast studies (barium, Gastrografin, enteroclysis)
TX: Bowel decompression, surgery, prophylactic antibiotics
F/U: Weekly visits after discharge for 2 to 8 weeks

Additional differential diagnoses: abdominal cancer ▪ abdominal trauma ▪ abdominal tumor ▪ cirrhosis ▪ heart failure ▪ mesenteric artery occlusion ▪ nephrotic syndrome ▪ paralytic ileus ▪ toxic megacolon

Other causes: ascites ▪ bladder distention ▪ gastric dilation

Abdominal mass

Commonly detected on routine physical assessment, an abdominal mass is a localized swelling in an abdominal quadrant. This sign typically develops insidiously and may represent an enlarged organ, neoplasm, abscess, vascular defect, or a fecal mass.

Distinguishing an abdominal mass from a normal structure requires skillful palpation. At times, palpation must be repeated with the patient in a different position or performed by a second examiner to verify initial findings. A palpable abdominal mass is an important clinical sign and usually represents a serious and, perhaps, life-threatening disorder.

ALERT

If the patient presents with symptoms that suggest an abdominal aortic aneurysm, such as a pulsating midabdominal mass and severe abdominal or back pain:

- *quickly take his vital signs*
- *withhold food and fluids in case of emergent surgery*
- *obtain routine preoperative tests*
- *prepare the patient for angiography, if appropriate*
- *be alert for signs of shock, such as tachycardia, hypotension, and cool, clammy skin, which may indicate significant blood loss.*

If the patient's abdominal mass doesn't suggest an aortic aneurysm, perform a focused assessment.

HISTORY

- Ask the patient if the mass is painful. If so, ask if the pain is constant or if it occurs only on palpation. Is the pain localized or generalized? Determine if the patient was already aware of the mass. If he was, find out if he noticed any change in its size or location.
- Review the patient's medical history, noting especially GI disorders.
- Ask the patient about GI signs and symptoms, such as constipation, diarrhea, rectal bleeding, abnormally colored stools, and vomiting. Has the patient noticed a change in his appetite?
- If the patient is female, ask whether her menstrual cycles are regular. Also, ask her when the first day of her last menses was.

PHYSICAL ASSESSMENT

- Auscultate for bowel sounds, bruits, and friction rubs in each quadrant.
- Lightly palpate the abdomen, assessing painful or suspicious areas last; then perform deep palpation. Be sure to note the patient's position when you locate the mass.
- Determine the shape, contour, and consistency of the mass.
- Percuss the mass. A dull sound indicates a fluid-filled mass; a tympanic sound, an air-filled mass.
- Determine if the mass moves when you palpate it or if it moves in response to respiration.

SPECIAL CONSIDERATIONS

If an abdominal mass causes bowel obstruction, watch for symptoms of peritonitis, such as abdominal pain and rebound tenderness, and for signs of shock, such as tachycardia and hypotension.

[A] PEDIATRIC POINTERS

In older infants and children, enlarged organs, such as the liver and spleen, usually cause abdominal masses. Other common causes include Wilms' tumor, neuroblastoma, intussusception, volvulus, Hirschsprung's disease, pyloric stenosis, and abdominal abscess.

AGING ISSUES

Ultrasonography should be used to evaluate a prominent midepigastric mass in thin, elderly patients.

PATIENT COUNSELING

Instruct the patient on what to expect from diagnostic testing, which may include blood and urine studies, abdominal X-rays, barium enema, computed tomography scan, and gastroscopy or sigmoidoscopy. A pelvic or rectal examination is usually indicated.

ABDOMINAL MASS

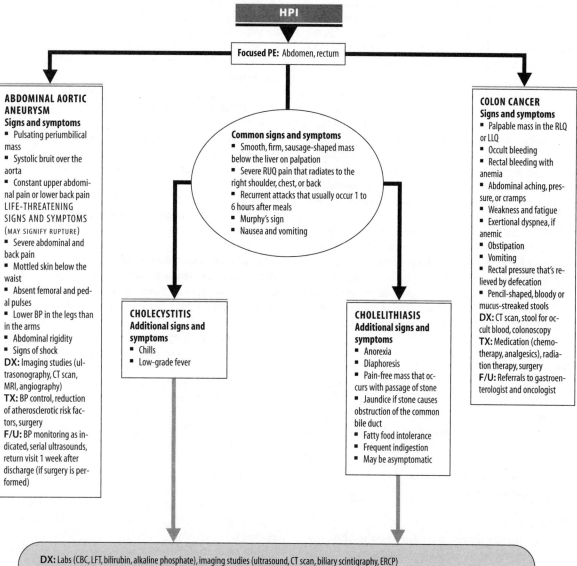

HPI

Focused PE: Abdomen, rectum

ABDOMINAL AORTIC ANEURYSM
Signs and symptoms
- Pulsating periumbilical mass
- Systolic bruit over the aorta
- Constant upper abdominal pain or lower back pain
LIFE-THREATENING SIGNS AND SYMPTOMS (MAY SIGNIFY RUPTURE)
- Severe abdominal and back pain
- Mottled skin below the waist
- Absent femoral and pedal pulses
- Lower BP in the legs than in the arms
- Abdominal rigidity
- Signs of shock
DX: Imaging studies (ultrasonography, CT scan, MRI, angiography)
TX: BP control, reduction of atherosclerotic risk factors, surgery
F/U: BP monitoring as indicated, serial ultrasounds, return visit 1 week after discharge (if surgery is performed)

Common signs and symptoms
- Smooth, firm, sausage-shaped mass below the liver on palpation
- Severe RUQ pain that radiates to the right shoulder, chest, or back
- Recurrent attacks that usually occur 1 to 6 hours after meals
- Murphy's sign
- Nausea and vomiting

CHOLECYSTITIS
Additional signs and symptoms
- Chills
- Low-grade fever

CHOLELITHIASIS
Additional signs and symptoms
- Anorexia
- Diaphoresis
- Pain-free mass that occurs with passage of stone
- Jaundice if stone causes obstruction of the common bile duct
- Fatty food intolerance
- Frequent indigestion
- May be asymptomatic

COLON CANCER
Signs and symptoms
- Palpable mass in the RLQ or LLQ
- Occult bleeding
- Rectal bleeding with anemia
- Abdominal aching, pressure, or cramps
- Weakness and fatigue
- Exertional dyspnea, if anemic
- Obstipation
- Vomiting
- Rectal pressure that's relieved by defecation
- Pencil-shaped, bloody or mucus-streaked stools
DX: CT scan, stool for occult blood, colonoscopy
TX: Medication (chemotherapy, analgesics), radiation therapy, surgery
F/U: Referrals to gastroenterologist and oncologist

DX: Labs (CBC, LFT, bilirubin, alkaline phosphate), imaging studies (ultrasound, CT scan, biliary scintigraphy, ERCP)
TX: Low-fat diet, gallstone solubilizing agent, surgery
F/U: Liver enzyme tests, serum cholesterol, imaging studies (if on medication), return visit 1 week after procedure or discharge (if surgery is performed)

Additional differential diagnoses: Crohn's disease ▪ diverticulitis ▪ gallbladder cancer ▪ gastric cancer ▪ hepatic cancer ▪ hernia (inguinal or ventral) ▪ hydronephrosis ▪ ovarian cyst ▪ pancreatic abscess ▪ pancreatic pseudocysts ▪ renal cell carcinoma ▪ splenomegaly ▪ uterine leiomyoma

Other causes: hepatomegaly

Abdominal pain

Although abdominal pain usually results from a GI disorder, it can also be caused by a reproductive, genitourinary (GU), musculoskeletal, or vascular disorder; drug use; or ingestion of toxins. At times, this symptom signals life-threatening complications.

Abdominal pain arises from the abdominopelvic viscera, the parietal peritoneum, or the capsules of the liver, kidney, or spleen. It may be acute or chronic, diffuse or localized. Visceral pain develops slowly into a deep, dull, aching pain that's poorly localized in the epigastric, periumbilical, or lower midabdominal (hypogastric) region. In contrast, somatic (parietal, peritoneal) pain produces a sharp, more intense, and well-localized discomfort that rapidly follows the insult. Movement or coughing aggravates this pain.

Pain may also be referred to the abdomen from another site with the same or a similar nerve supply. This sharp, well-localized, referred pain is felt in skin or deeper tissues and may coexist with skin hyperesthesia and muscle hyperalgesia.

Mechanisms that produce abdominal pain include stretching or tension of the gut wall, traction on the peritoneum or mesentery, vigorous intestinal contraction, inflammation, ischemia, and sensory nerve irritation.

➤ ALERT

If the patient is experiencing sudden, severe abdominal pain:
- *quickly take his vital signs*
- *palpate for pulses below the waist*
- *be alert for signs of hypovolemic shock, such as tachycardia and hypotension*
- *prepare him for emergency surgery, if necessary.*

If the patient has no life-threatening signs or symptoms, perform a focused assessment.

HISTORY

- Ask the patient if the pain is constant or intermittent, and ask when the pain began. Determine the duration of a typical episode.
- Ask the patient where the pain is located and whether it radiates to other areas. Find out if movement, coughing, exertion, vomiting, eating, elimination, or walking worsen or relieve the pain.
- Review the patient's medical history for vascular, GI, GU, or reproductive disorders.
- When appropriate, ask the female patient about the date of her last menses, changes in her menstrual pattern, or dyspareunia.
- Ask the patient about appetite changes, or onset and frequency of nausea or vomiting.

- Ask the patient about changes in bowel habits, such as constipation, diarrhea, or changes in stool consistency. When was the patient's last bowel movement?
- Ask the patient about urinary frequency, urgency, or pain. Is the urine cloudy or pink?
- Obtain a drug history, including prescription and over-the-counter drugs, herbal remedies, and recreational drugs. Also, ask the patient about alcohol intake.

PHYSICAL ASSESSMENT

- Take the patient's vital signs.
- Assess skin turgor and mucous membranes.
- Inspect the abdomen for distention or visible peristaltic waves and, if indicated, measure his abdominal girth.
- Auscultate for bowel sounds, and characterize their motility.
- Percuss all quadrants, carefully noting the percussion sounds.
- Palpate the entire abdomen for masses, rigidity, and tenderness. Note guarding.

SPECIAL CONSIDERATIONS

Withhold analgesics from the patient until a diagnosis is determined because they may mask symptoms. Also withhold food and fluids until it's decided that surgery is unnecessary.

🅰 PEDIATRIC POINTERS

- *Remember that a parent's description of a child's complaints is a subjective interpretation of what the parent believes is wrong.*
- *In children, abdominal pain can signal a disorder with greater severity or with different associated signs than are common in adults.*
- *Acute pyelonephritis may cause abdominal pain, vomiting, and diarrhea but not the classic urologic signs found in adults.*
- *Peptic ulcer, which is becoming increasingly common in teenagers, causes nocturnal pain and colic that, unlike peptic ulcer in adults, may not be relieved by food.*
- *Abdominal pain in children can also result from lactose intolerance, allergic-tension-fatigue syndrome, volvulus, Meckel's diverticulum, intussusception, mesenteric adenitis, diabetes mellitus, juvenile rheumatoid arthritis, or an uncommon disorder such as heavy metal poisoning.*

🕯 AGING ISSUES

Advanced age may decrease the signs and symptoms of acute abdominal disease. Pain may be less severe, fever less pronounced, and signs of peritoneal inflammation diminished or absent.

PATIENT COUNSELING

Instruct the patient on what to expect from diagnostic testing, which may include pelvic and rectal examination; blood, urine, and stool tests; X-rays; barium studies; ultrasonography; endoscopy; and biopsy. If surgery is needed, perform preoperative teaching.

ABDOMINAL PAIN (ACUTE)

HPI

Focused PE: Abdomen, rectum

ABDOMINAL AORTIC ANEURYSM
Signs and symptoms
- Pulsating periumbilical mass
- Systolic bruit over the aorta
- Constant upper abdominal pain or lower back pain

LIFE-THREATENING SIGNS AND SYMPTOMS
(MAY SIGNIFY RUPTURE)
- Severe abdominal and back pain
- Mottled skin below the waist
- Absent femoral and pedal pulses
- Lower BP in the legs than in the arms
- Abdominal rigidity
- Signs of shock

DX: Imaging studies (ultrasonography, CT scan, MRI, angiography)
TX: BP control, reduction of atherosclerotic risk factors, surgery
F/U: BP monitoring as indicated, serial ultrasounds, return visit 1 week after discharge (if surgery is performed)

DIVERTICULITIS (ACUTE)
Signs and symptoms
- LLQ pain
- Abdominal rigidity and guarding
- High-grade fever
- Chills
- Signs of shock

DX: Labs (CBC, UA, chemistry panel), imaging studies (abdominal upright X-ray, CT scan, ultrasonography)
TX: dietary fiber, antibiotics, surgery
F/U: Barium enema after acute episode subsides, return visit 1 week after discharge (if surgery is performed)

ECTOPIC PREGNANCY
Signs and symptoms
- Lower abdominal pain that's sharp, dull, or cramping
- Vaginal bleeding
- Nausea and vomiting
- Urinary frequency
- Tender adnexal mass
- History of amenorrhea in past 1 to 2 months

LIFE-THREATENING SIGNS AND SYMPTOMS
(MAY SIGNIFY RUPTURE)
- Sharp lower abdominal pain that radiates to the shoulders and neck and becomes extreme with cervical or adnexal palpation
- Signs of shock

DX: Labs (urine pregnancy test, serum HCG, CBC), imaging studies (vaginal and abdominal ultrasonography, CT scan, MRI, intravaginal color Doppler flow imaging)
TX: Surgery
F/U: Serial HCG levels (until 0 IU/L), follow-up imaging if retained placenta is suspected

RENAL CALCULI
Signs and symptoms
- Severe abdominal or back pain
- Severe colicky pain that travels from the costovertebral angle to the flank, suprapubic region, and external genitalia
- Pain that may be excruciating or dull and constant
- Pain-induced agitation
- Nausea and vomiting
- Abdominal distension
- Fever and chills
- Urinary frequency with hematuria and dysuria

DX: Labs (CBC, BUN, creatinine, UA), imaging studies (abdominal X-ray, I.V. urography, spinal CT scan, ultrasound)
TX: Pain relief, increased fluid intake, percutaneous chemolysis, systemic chemolysis, endourologic calculi extraction, extacorporeal shock wave lithotripsy
F/U: Urologic referral, if chronic or obstruction; weekly creatinine level until stable; continued urine straining until calculi has passed and then calculi analysis, if able

APPENDICITIS
Signs and symptoms
- Dull discomfort in the epigastric or umbilical region
- Anorexia
- Nausea and vomiting
- Localized pain at McBurney's point
- Abdominal rigidity
- Rebound tenderness
- Positive Rovsing's, psoas, and cough signs

DX: Labs (CBC, UA, amylase), imaging studies (KUB, CT scan, ultrasound)
TX: Surgery, antibiotics
F/U: Return visits at 2 and 6 weeks after discharge

...IF RUPTURED, MAY LEAD TO...

PANCREATITIS
Signs and symptoms
- Fulminating, continuous upper abdominal pain that may radiate to the flanks and back
- Nausea and vomiting
- Fever
- Pallor
- Tachycardia
- Abdominal rigidity
- Rebound tenderness
- Hypoactive bowel sounds
- Positive Turner's and Cullen's signs (indicate hemorrhagic pancreatitis)
- Jaundice

DX: Labs (amylase, lipase, CBC, bilirubin, glucose, electrolytes, LFT), imaging studies (KUB, CT scan, ultrasound)
TX: NPO, I.V. fluids, bed rest, medication (analgesics, antibiotics)
F/U: Monitoring of amylase levels until normal; if they remain elevated, repeat imaging studies

PERITONITIS
Signs and symptoms
- Sudden, severe pain that worsens with movement
- Vomiting (may be projectile)
- Constipation
- High-grade fever
- Decreased bowel sounds
- Rebound tenderness
- Abdominal rigidity and guarding
- Signs of shock

DX: Labs (peritoneal fluid culture, CBC), imaging studies (abdominal X-ray, CT scan, abdominal sonography)
TX: Bowel decompression, antibiotics, surgery for underlying condition
F/U: Return visit 1 week after discharge, then as needed

Additional differential diagnoses: abdominal cancer ▪ abdominal trauma ▪ acute cholecystitis ▪ acute cholelithiasis ▪ acute hepatitis ▪ adrenal crisis ▪ cholangitis ▪ diabetic ketoacidosis ▪ gastroenteritis ▪ heart failure ▪ hepatic abscess ▪ hepatic amebiasis ▪ hernia (inguinal or ventral) ▪ herpes zoster ▪ intestinal obstruction ▪ intestinal perforation ▪ Meckel's diverticulitis ▪ mesenteric artery ischemia ▪ MI ▪ perforated ulcer ▪ pneumonia ▪ pyelonephritis ▪ retroperitoneal bleed ▪ ruptured ovarian cyst ▪ ruptured spleen ▪ sickle cell crisis ▪ SLE

Other causes: insect toxins

ABDOMINAL PAIN (CHRONIC)

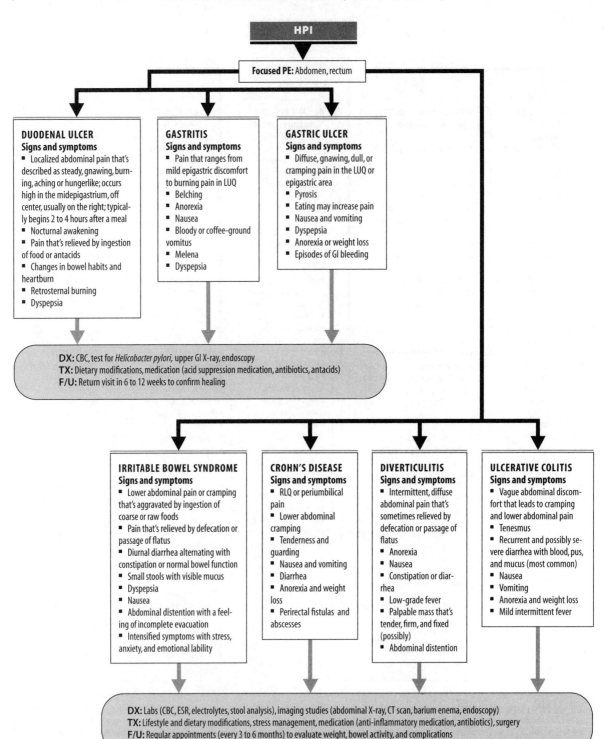

HPI

Focused PE: Abdomen, rectum

DUODENAL ULCER
Signs and symptoms
- Localized abdominal pain that's described as steady, gnawing, burning, aching or hungerlike; occurs high in the midepigastrium, off center, usually on the right; typically begins 2 to 4 hours after a meal
- Nocturnal awakening
- Pain that's relieved by ingestion of food or antacids
- Changes in bowel habits and heartburn
- Retrosternal burning
- Dyspepsia

GASTRITIS
Signs and symptoms
- Pain that ranges from mild epigastric discomfort to burning pain in LUQ
- Belching
- Anorexia
- Nausea
- Bloody or coffee-ground vomitus
- Melena
- Dyspepsia

GASTRIC ULCER
Signs and symptoms
- Diffuse, gnawing, dull, or cramping pain in the LUQ or epigastric area
- Pyrosis
- Eating may increase pain
- Nausea and vomiting
- Dyspepsia
- Anorexia or weight loss
- Episodes of GI bleeding

DX: CBC, test for *Helicobacter pylori,* upper GI X-ray, endoscopy
TX: Dietary modifications, medication (acid suppression medication, antibiotics, antacids)
F/U: Return visit in 6 to 12 weeks to confirm healing

IRRITABLE BOWEL SYNDROME
Signs and symptoms
- Lower abdominal pain or cramping that's aggravated by ingestion of coarse or raw foods
- Pain that's relieved by defecation or passage of flatus
- Diurnal diarrhea alternating with constipation or normal bowel function
- Small stools with visible mucus
- Dyspepsia
- Nausea
- Abdominal distention with a feeling of incomplete evacuation
- Intensified symptoms with stress, anxiety, and emotional lability

CROHN'S DISEASE
Signs and symptoms
- RLQ or periumbilical pain
- Lower abdominal cramping
- Tenderness and guarding
- Nausea and vomiting
- Diarrhea
- Anorexia and weight loss
- Perirectal fistulas and abscesses

DIVERTICULITIS
Signs and symptoms
- Intermittent, diffuse abdominal pain that's sometimes relieved by defecation or passage of flatus
- Anorexia
- Nausea
- Constipation or diarrhea
- Low-grade fever
- Palpable mass that's tender, firm, and fixed (possibly)
- Abdominal distention

ULCERATIVE COLITIS
Signs and symptoms
- Vague abdominal discomfort that leads to cramping and lower abdominal pain
- Tenesmus
- Recurrent and possibly severe diarrhea with blood, pus, and mucus (most common)
- Nausea
- Vomiting
- Anorexia and weight loss
- Mild intermittent fever

DX: Labs (CBC, ESR, electrolytes, stool analysis), imaging studies (abdominal X-ray, CT scan, barium enema, endoscopy)
TX: Lifestyle and dietary modifications, stress management, medication (anti-inflammatory medication, antibiotics), surgery
F/U: Regular appointments (every 3 to 6 months) to evaluate weight, bowel activity, and complications

ABDOMINAL PAIN (OTHER)

HPI

Focused PE: Abdomen, rectum, pelvis

CYSTITIS
Signs and symptoms
- Suprapubic abdominal pain
- Flank pain
- Lower back pain
- Malaise
- Urinary frequency
- Nocturia
- Dysuria
- Fever and chills

DX: Labs (UA, urine culture)
TX: Antibiotic, increased fluid intake
F/U: Reculture, if symptoms persist or recur

HEPATITIS
Signs and symptoms
- Dull pain in the RUQ
- Dark urine
- Clay-colored stools
- Nausea and vomiting
- Anorexia and weight loss
- Jaundice
- Pruritus
- Malaise

DX: Labs (serologic markers for virus, LFT, coagulation studies), possible liver biopsy to confirm type and extent of liver damage
TX: Medication (interferon alpha therapy, corticosteroids), liver transplant, lifestyle modifications
F/U: Monitoring for complications while on medication

...MAY LEAD TO...

CIRRHOSIS
Signs and symptoms
- Dull abdominal aching
- RUQ pain that worsens when the patient sits up or leans forward
- Nodular liver
- Fever
- Ascites
- Leg edema
- Weight gain
- Hepatomegaly
- Jaundice
- Severe pruritus
- Bleeding tendencies and bruising
- Palmar erythema
- Spider angiomas
- Gynecomastia and testicular atrophy

DX: LFT, imaging studies (CT scan, ultrasound), laparoscopic liver biopsy
TX: Lifestyle modifications, dietary modifications (for underlying cause)
F/U: Frequent checkups with LFT

PROSTATITIS
Signs and symptoms
- Vague lower abdominal pain
- Pain in the groin, perineum, or rectum
- Scrotal pain, penile pain, and pain on ejaculation (in chronic cases)
- Dysuria
- Urinary frequency and urgency
- Nocturia
- Fever and chills
- Tender prostate
- Lower back pain
- Myalgia
- Arthralgia

DX: Labs (fractional urine examination, urine culture), imaging studies (CT scan, transrectal ultrasound)
TX: Medication (analgesics, antibiotics, stool softener)
F/U: UA and urine culture every 30 days until infection resolves

PID
Signs and symptoms
- Pain in the RLQ or LLQ that ranges from vague discomfort to deep, severe and progressive pain
- Metrorrhagia that sometimes precedes or accompanies pain
- Cervical or adnexal palpation that causes extreme pain
- Pelvic mass (possibly)
- Fever and chills
- Nausea and vomiting
- Urinary discomfort
- Abnormal vaginal bleeding or discharge

OVARIAN CYST
Signs and symptoms
- Torsion or hemorrhage causes RLQ or LLQ pain
- Sharp and severe pain when suddenly standing or stooping
- Fever
- Anorexia
- Vomiting
- Palpable abdominal mass (possibly)
- Rupture (may cause peritonitis)

ENDOMETRIOSIS
Signs and symptoms
- Constant, severe pain in the lower abdomen that usually occurs 5 to 7 days before menstruation
- Pain that may be aggravated by defecation
- Dysmenorrhea
- Dyspareunia
- Deep sacral pain

DX: Labs (pregnancy test, CBC, ESR, serum tumor markers), imaging studies (transabdominal or transvaginal ultrasound, CT scan, MRI), laparoscopy
TX: Medication (for PID, antibiotics; for ovarian cyst, monophasic contraceptive pill; for endometriosis, gonadotropin-releasing hormone agonist), laparoscopy, or surgery
F/U: Yearly ultrasound to monitor adnexal mass (if present), varies according to symptoms

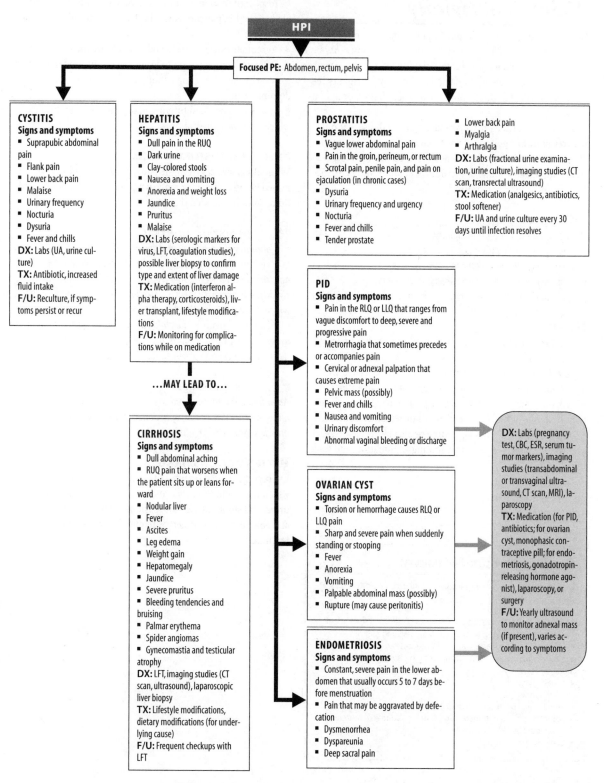

Abdominal rigidity

Detected by palpation, abdominal rigidity refers to abdominal muscle tension or inflexibility of the abdomen. Rigidity may be voluntary or involuntary. Voluntary rigidity reflects the patient's fear of or nervousness about palpation; involuntary rigidity reflects potentially life-threatening peritoneal irritation or inflammation.

Involuntary rigidity usually results from a GI disorder but may result from a pulmonary or vascular disorder or from the effects of insect toxins. It's typically accompanied by fever, nausea, vomiting, abdominal tenderness, distention, and pain. (See *Recognizing voluntary rigidity.*)

 ALERT

If the patient has abdominal rigidity:
- *quickly take his vital signs*
- *prepare him for laboratory tests and X-rays*
- *prepare him for emergency surgery, if necessary.*
  If the patient's condition permits, perform a focused assessment.

HISTORY

- Ask the patient when signs and symptoms of abdominal rigidity began.
- Ask the patient if the abdominal rigidity is associated with abdominal pain. If so, did the pain begin at the same time?
- Ask the patient if the pain is always present. Also, ask the patient if the site of the pain has changed or remained constant?
- Ask the patient about aggravating or alleviating factors, such as position changes, coughing, vomiting, elimination, and walking.

PHYSICAL ASSESSMENT

- Inspect the abdomen for peristaltic waves, which may be visible in very thin patients. Also, check for a visible distended bowel loop.
- Auscultate bowel sounds, and characterize their motility.
- Perform light palpation to locate the rigidity and determine its severity. Avoid deep palpation, which may exacerbate abdominal pain.
- Check for poor skin turgor and dry mucous membranes, which indicate dehydration.

SPECIAL CONSIDERATIONS

Withhold analgesics from the patient until a diagnosis is determined because they may mask symptoms. Withhold food and fluids until it's decided that surgery is unnecessary.

 PEDIATRIC POINTERS

- *Voluntary rigidity may be difficult to distinguish from involuntary rigidity if associated pain makes the child restless, tense, or apprehensive. However, in a child with suspected involuntary rigidity, your priority is early detection of dehydration and shock, which can rapidly become life-threatening.*
- *Abdominal rigidity in a child can stem from gastric perforation, hypertrophic pyloric stenosis, duodenal obstruction, meconium ileus, intussusception, cystic fibrosis, celiac disease, or appendicitis.*

 AGING ISSUES

Advanced age and impaired cognition decrease pain perception and intensity. Weakening of abdominal muscles may decrease muscle spasms and rigidity.

PATIENT COUNSELING

Instruct the patient on what to expect from diagnostic testing, which may include a pelvic and rectal examination; blood, urine, and stool tests; X-rays; peritoneal lavage; gastroscopy; and colonoscopy. If surgery is required, perform preoperative teaching.

RECOGNIZING VOLUNTARY RIGIDITY

Distinguishing voluntary rigidity from involuntary rigidity is essential for accurate assessment.
  Voluntary rigidity is:
- eased by relaxation techniques, such as positioning the patient comfortably and talking to him in a calm, soothing manner
- more rigid on inspiration (expiration causes muscle relaxation)
- painless when the patient sits up using his abdominal muscles alone
- usually symmetrical.
  Involuntary rigidity is:
- equally rigid on inspiration and expiration
- painful when the patient sits up using his abdominal muscles
- unaffected by relaxation techniques
- usually asymmetrical.

ABDOMINAL RIGIDITY

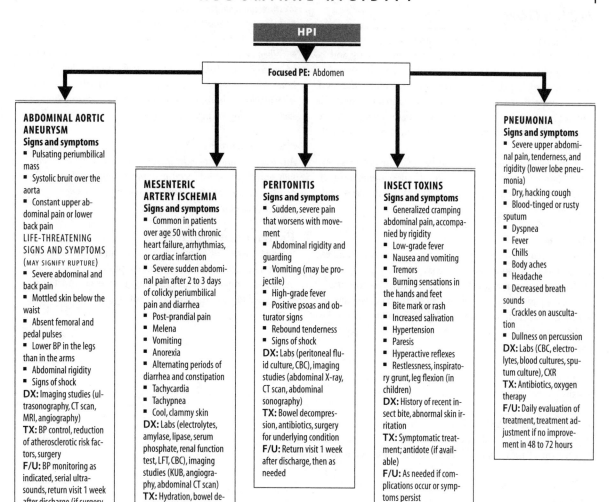

HPI

Focused PE: Abdomen

ABDOMINAL AORTIC ANEURYSM
Signs and symptoms
- Pulsating periumbilical mass
- Systolic bruit over the aorta
- Constant upper abdominal pain or lower back pain

LIFE-THREATENING SIGNS AND SYMPTOMS
(MAY SIGNIFY RUPTURE)
- Severe abdominal and back pain
- Mottled skin below the waist
- Absent femoral and pedal pulses
- Lower BP in the legs than in the arms
- Abdominal rigidity
- Signs of shock

DX: Imaging studies (ultrasonography, CT scan, MRI, angiography)
TX: BP control, reduction of atherosclerotic risk factors, surgery
F/U: BP monitoring as indicated, serial ultrasounds, return visit 1 week after discharge (if surgery is performed)

MESENTERIC ARTERY ISCHEMIA
Signs and symptoms
- Common in patients over age 50 with chronic heart failure, arrhythmias, or cardiac infarction
- Severe sudden abdominal pain after 2 to 3 days of colicky periumbilical pain and diarrhea
- Post-prandial pain
- Melena
- Vomiting
- Anorexia
- Alternating periods of diarrhea and constipation
- Tachycardia
- Tachypnea
- Cool, clammy skin

DX: Labs (electrolytes, amylase, lipase, serum phosphate, renal function test, LFT, CBC), imaging studies (KUB, angiography, abdominal CT scan)
TX: Hydration, bowel decompression, antibiotics, surgery
F/U: Return visit 1 week after discharge

PERITONITIS
Signs and symptoms
- Sudden, severe pain that worsens with movement
- Abdominal rigidity and guarding
- Vomiting (may be projectile)
- High-grade fever
- Positive psoas and obturator signs
- Rebound tenderness
- Signs of shock

DX: Labs (peritoneal fluid culture, CBC), imaging studies (abdominal X-ray, CT scan, abdominal sonography)
TX: Bowel decompression, antibiotics, surgery for underlying condition
F/U: Return visit 1 week after discharge, then as needed

INSECT TOXINS
Signs and symptoms
- Generalized cramping abdominal pain, accompanied by rigidity
- Low-grade fever
- Nausea and vomiting
- Tremors
- Burning sensations in the hands and feet
- Bite mark or rash
- Increased salivation
- Hypertension
- Paresis
- Hyperactive reflexes
- Restlessness, inspiratory grunt, leg flexion (in children)

DX: History of recent insect bite, abnormal skin irritation
TX: Symptomatic treatment; antidote (if available)
F/U: As needed if complications occur or symptoms persist

PNEUMONIA
Signs and symptoms
- Severe upper abdominal pain, tenderness, and rigidity (lower lobe pneumonia)
- Dry, hacking cough
- Blood-tinged or rusty sputum
- Dyspnea
- Fever
- Chills
- Body aches
- Headache
- Decreased breath sounds
- Crackles on auscultation
- Dullness on percussion

DX: Labs (CBC, electrolytes, blood cultures, sputum culture), CXR
TX: Antibiotics, oxygen therapy
F/U: Daily evaluation of treatment, treatment adjustment if no improvement in 48 to 72 hours

Agitation

Agitation refers to a state of hyperarousal, increased tension, and irritability that can lead to confusion, hyperactivity, and overt hostility. This common sign can result from any one of various disorders, pain, fever, anxiety, drug use and withdrawal, or a hypersensitivity reaction. It can arise gradually or suddenly and can last for minutes or months. Whether it's mild or severe, agitation worsens with increased fever, pain, stress, or external stimuli.

Agitation alone merely signals a change in the patient's condition. However, it's a useful indicator of a developing disorder when considered with the patient's history, current status, and other findings.

HISTORY

● Ask the patient specific questions to determine the number and quality of agitation-induced behaviors, such as emotional lability, confusion, memory loss, hyperactivity, and hostility.
● Ask the patient to detail his current diet and known allergies.
● Ask the patient if he's being treated for any illnesses. Has he had recent infection, trauma, stress, or changes in sleep patterns?
● Obtain a drug history, including prescription and over-the-counter drugs, herbal remedies, and recreational drugs. Also, ask the patient about alcohol intake.

PHYSICAL ASSESSMENT

● Take the patient's vital signs.
● Perform a basic neurologic assessment for future comparison.
● Check for signs of drug abuse, such as needle tracks and dilated pupils.

SPECIAL CONSIDERATIONS

Because agitation can be an early sign of many different disorders, continue to monitor the patient's vital signs and neurologic status while the cause is being determined. Eliminate stressors, which can increase agitation. Provide adequate lighting, maintain a calm environment, and allow the patient ample time to sleep. Ensure a balanced diet, and provide vitamin supplements.

Remain calm, nonjudgmental, and nonargumentative. Use restraints according to your facility's policy and only when absolutely necessary because they may increase agitation.

PEDIATRIC POINTERS

● *A common sign in children, agitation accompanies the expected childhood diseases as well as more severe disorders that can lead to brain damage, hyperbilirubinemia, phenylketonuria, vitamin A deficiency, hepatitis, frontal lobe syndrome, increased intracranial pressure, and lead poisoning.*
● *In neonates, agitation can stem from alcohol or drug withdrawal if the mother abused these substances.*
● *When evaluating an agitated child, remember to use words that he can understand and remember to look for nonverbal clues. For example, if you suspect that pain is causing agitation, ask him to tell you where it hurts, but be sure to watch for other indicators, such as wincing, crying, or moving away.*

AGING ISSUES

Any deviation from an older person's usual activities or rituals may provoke anxiety or agitation. An environmental change, such as a transfer to a nursing home or a visit from a stranger in the patient's home, may trigger agitation.

PATIENT COUNSELING

Instruct the patient on what to expect from diagnostic testing, which may include computed tomography scan, skull X-rays, magnetic resonance imaging, and blood studies, which may be performed to determine the source of agitated behavior.

AGITATION

HPI

Focused PE: Neurologic system, general physical assessment

HYPOXEMIA
Signs and symptoms
- Restlessness (at onset)
- Agitation that rapidly worsens
- Confusion
- Impaired judgment and motor coordination
- Tachycardia
- Tachypnea
- Dyspnea
- Cyanosis

DX: ABG, CXR, pulse oximetry
TX: Oxygen, treatment of underlying cause
F/U: As needed (dependent on cause)

DEMENTIA
Signs and symptoms
- Mild to severe agitation
- Decreased memory, attention span, and problem-solving abilities
- Wandering behavior
- Hallucinations
- Aphasia
- Insomnia

DX: Labs to rule out other causes (thyroid function, syphilis serology, CBC, electrolytes), imaging studies (CT scan, MRI)
TX: Patient and family support, referral to geropsychology specialist
F/U: As needed

INCREASED ICP
Signs and symptoms
- Agitation (usually the first sign)
- Headache
- Nausea and vomiting
- Cheyne-Stokes respirations
- Ataxia
- Sluggish, nonreactive pupils
- Widened pulse pressure
- Tachycardia
- Decreased LOC
- Abnormal posturing

DX: Intracranial CT scan, intracranial MRI
TX: Treatment of underlying cause, osmotic diuretics, surgery
F/U: As needed (dependent on cause)

POST-HEAD-TRAUMA SYNDROME
Signs and symptoms
- Disorientation
- Loss of concentration
- Emotional lability
- Fatigue
- Wandering behavior
- Poor judgment

DX: History of head trauma
TX: Safety precautions
F/U: Daily visits until behavior returns to baseline or stabilizes

CHRONIC RENAL FAILURE
Signs and symptoms
- Moderate to severe agitation
- Decreased urine output
- Increased BP
- Nausea and vomiting
- Anorexia
- Ammonia breath odor
- GI bleeding
- Pallor
- Dry skin
- Uremic frost
- Edema

DX: Labs (renal function studies, electrolytes, ABG), imaging studies (renal ultrasound, CT scan, MRI)
TX: Control of associated cause, diet modification, dialysis, kidney transplant
F/U: Weekly to monthly visits, depending on response to treatment

ALCOHOL WITHDRAWAL
Signs and symptoms
- Mild to severe agitation
- Hyperactivity
- Tremors
- Anxiety

LIFE-THREATENING SIGNS AND SYMPTOMS (DELIRIUM TREMENS)
- Severe agitation
- Visual hallucinations
- Insomnia
- Diaphoresis
- Tachycardia
- Depression
- Seizures
- Cardiac arrest
- Shock

DX: History of ETOH use, labs (LFT, electrolytes)
TX: Medication (benzodiazepines, barbiturates, beta-adrenergic blocker, anticonvulsant)
F/U: Referral to addiction program

Additional differential diagnoses: affective disturbance ▪ anxiety ▪ drug withdrawal syndrome ▪ endocrine disorder ▪ hepatic encephalopathy ▪ hypersensitivity reaction ▪ intracranial bleed ▪ organic brain syndrome ▪ psychotic disturbances ▪ vitamin B_6 deficiency ▪ vitamin B_{12} deficiency

Other causes: medication (famotidine, lorazepam, haloperidol) ▪ radiographic contrast media

Alopecia

Occurring most commonly on the scalp, alopecia typically develops gradually and may be diffuse or patchy. It can be classified as scarring or nonscarring. Scarring alopecia, or permanent hair loss, results from hair follicle destruction, which smoothes the skin surface, erasing follicular openings. Nonscarring alopecia, or temporary hair loss, results from hair follicle damage that spares follicular openings, allowing future hair growth. (See *Recognizing patterns of alopecia.*)

One of the most common causes of alopecia is the use of certain chemotherapeutic drugs. Alopecia may also result from the use of other drugs; radiation therapy; a skin, connective tissue, endocrine, nutritional, or psychological disorder; a neoplasm; an infection; a burn; or the effects of toxins.

HISTORY
- Ask the patient if he's receiving chemotherapeutic drug or radiation therapy. If not, ask him when he first noticed hair loss or thinning.
- Ask the patient if the hair loss is confined to the scalp or if it occurs elsewhere on the body.
- Ask the patient if itching or rashes accompany the hair loss.
- Ask the patient about recent weight change, anorexia, nausea, vomiting, and altered bowel habits.
- Ask the patient about changes in urination habits, such as hematuria or oliguria. If the patient is female, ask about menstrual irregularities and note her pregnancy history. If the patient is male, ask about sexual dysfunction, such as decreased libido or impotence.
- Ask the patient if he has been especially tired or irritable or had a cough or difficulty breathing.
- Ask the patient about joint pain or stiffness and about heat or cold intolerance.

- Ask the patient if he has been exposed to insecticides.
- Ask the patient about hair care and hair-care products.
- Check for a family history of alopecia.
- Ask the patient about nervous habits, such as pulling the hair or twirling it around a finger.

PHYSICAL ASSESSMENT
- Take the patient's vital signs.
- Assess the extent and pattern of scalp hair loss.
- Examine the skin. Note the size, color, texture, and location of lesions. Check for jaundice, edema, hyperpigmentation, pallor, or duskiness.
- Examine the nails for vertical or horizontal pitting, thickening, brittleness, or whitening.
- Observe for fine tremors in the hands, muscle weakness, and ptosis.
- Palpate for lymphadenopathy, an enlarged thyroid or salivary gland, and masses in the abdomen or chest.

SPECIAL CONSIDERATIONS
If the cause of hair loss is unknown, a skin biopsy may be performed to determine the cause.

🅰 *PEDIATRIC POINTERS*
- *Alopecia normally occurs during the first 6 months of life, as either a sudden, diffuse hair loss or a gradual thinning that's hardly noticeable. Reassure the infant's parents that this hair loss is normal and temporary.*
- *Common causes of alopecia in children include use of chemotherapeutic drugs, seborrheic dermatitis (cradle cap in infancy), alopecia mucinosa, tinea capitis, and hypopituitarism. Tinea capitis may produce a kerion lesion — a boggy, raised, tender, and hairless lesion. Trichotillomania, a psychological disorder that's more common in children than adults, may produce patchy baldness with stubby hair growth due to habitual hair pulling. Other causes of alopecia include progeria and congenital hair shaft defects such as trichorrhexis nodosa.*

🕭 *AGING ISSUES*
Aging, genetic predisposition, and hormonal changes may contribute to gradual hair thinning and hairline recession. This type of alopecia occurs in about 40% of adult men and may also occur in postmenopausal women.

PATIENT COUNSELING
When hair loss occurs because of chemotherapeutic drug use or radiation therapy, explain that this hair loss is reversible. In patients with partial baldness or alopecia areata, topical application of minoxidil (Rogaine) for several months may stimulate localized hair growth; however, hair loss may recur if the drug is discontinued.

RECOGNIZING PATTERNS OF ALOPECIA

Distinctive patterns of alopecia result from different causes.

 Alopecia areata causes expanding patches of nonscarring hair loss bordered by "exclamation point" hairs.

 Tinea capitis produces irregular bald patches with scaly red lesions.

 Trauma from habitual hair pulling or injudicious grooming habits may cause permanent peripheral alopecia.

 Chemotherapeutic medication produces diffuse temporary hair loss.

ALOPECIA

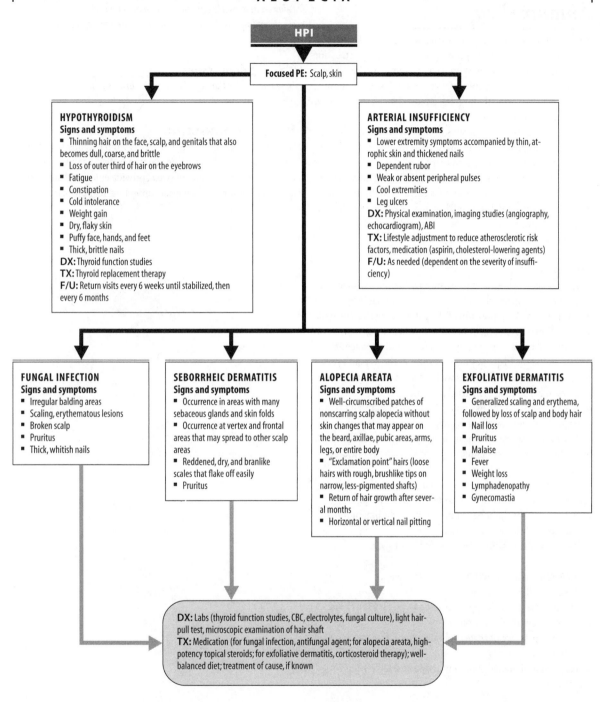

HPI

Focused PE: Scalp, skin

HYPOTHYROIDISM
Signs and symptoms
- Thinning hair on the face, scalp, and genitals that also becomes dull, coarse, and brittle
- Loss of outer third of hair on the eyebrows
- Fatigue
- Constipation
- Cold intolerance
- Weight gain
- Dry, flaky skin
- Puffy face, hands, and feet
- Thick, brittle nails

DX: Thyroid function studies
TX: Thyroid replacement therapy
F/U: Return visits every 6 weeks until stabilized, then every 6 months

ARTERIAL INSUFFICIENCY
Signs and symptoms
- Lower extremity symptoms accompanied by thin, atrophic skin and thickened nails
- Dependent rubor
- Weak or absent peripheral pulses
- Cool extremities
- Leg ulcers

DX: Physical examination, imaging studies (angiography, echocardiogram), ABI
TX: Lifestyle adjustment to reduce atherosclerotic risk factors, medication (aspirin, cholesterol-lowering agents)
F/U: As needed (dependent on the severity of insufficiency)

FUNGAL INFECTION
Signs and symptoms
- Irregular balding areas
- Scaling, erythematous lesions
- Broken scalp
- Pruritus
- Thick, whitish nails

SEBORRHEIC DERMATITIS
Signs and symptoms
- Occurrence in areas with many sebaceous glands and skin folds
- Occurrence at vertex and frontal areas that may spread to other scalp areas
- Reddened, dry, and branlike scales that flake off easily
- Pruritus

ALOPECIA AREATA
Signs and symptoms
- Well-circumscribed patches of nonscarring scalp alopecia without skin changes that may appear on the beard, axillae, pubic areas, arms, legs, or entire body
- "Exclamation point" hairs (loose hairs with rough, brushlike tips on narrow, less-pigmented shafts)
- Return of hair growth after several months
- Horizontal or vertical nail pitting

EXFOLIATIVE DERMATITIS
Signs and symptoms
- Generalized scaling and erythema, followed by loss of scalp and body hair
- Nail loss
- Pruritus
- Malaise
- Fever
- Weight loss
- Lymphadenopathy
- Gynecomastia

DX: Labs (thyroid function studies, CBC, electrolytes, fungal culture), light hair-pull test, microscopic examination of hair shaft
TX: Medication (for fungal infection, antifungal agent; for alopecia areata, high-potency topical steroids; for exfoliative dermatitis, corticosteroid therapy); well-balanced diet; treatment of cause, if known

Additional differential diagnoses: arsenic poisoning ▪ burns ▪ cutaneous T-cell lymphoma ▪ dissecting cellulitis of the scalp ▪ Hodgkin's disease ▪ hypopituitarism ▪ lichen planus ▪ myotonic dystrophy ▪ protein deficiency ▪ sarcoidosis ▪ scleroderma ▪ secondary syphilis ▪ skin metastases ▪ thallium poisoning ▪ thyrotoxicosis

Amenorrhea

Amenorrhea, the absence of menstrual flow, can be classified as primary or secondary. With primary amenorrhea, menstruation fails to begin before age 16. With secondary amenorrhea, it begins at an appropriate age but later ceases for 3 or more months in the absence of normal physiologic causes, such as pregnancy, lactation, and menopause.

Pathologic amenorrhea results from anovulation or physical obstruction to menstrual outflow, such as from an imperforate hymen, cervical stenosis, or intrauterine adhesions. Anovulation may result from hormonal imbalance, debilitating disease, stress or emotional disturbances, strenuous exercise, malnutrition, obesity, or an anatomic abnormality such as congenital absence of the ovaries or uterus. Amenorrhea may also result from drug or hormonal therapy.

HISTORY

- Ask the patient at what age her mother first menstruated because the age of menarche is fairly consistent in families.
- Form an overall impression of the patient's physical, mental, and emotional development because these factors as well as heredity and climate, may delay menarche until after age 16.
- Determine the frequency and duration of the patient's previous menstrual cycles (if any) as well as the onset and nature of changes in her normal menstrual pattern.
- Ask the patient if she has noticed associated signs and symptoms, such as breast swelling or weight changes.
- Review the patient's medical history, noting especially long-term illnesses, such as anemia, or use of hormonal contraceptives.
- Ask the patient about exercise habits, especially running, and ask whether she experiences stress on the job or at home.
- Ask the patient about her eating habits, including number and size of daily meals and snacks.
- Ask the patient about recent weight loss or gain.

PHYSICAL ASSESSMENT

- Take the patient's vital signs.
- Observe the patient's appearance for secondary sex characteristics or signs of virilization.
- Note the presence of truncal obesity, moon face, or increased pigmentation.
- Palpate the abdomen. Note any abdominal tenderness or masses.

SPECIAL CONSIDERATIONS

If the patient has secondary amenorrhea, physical and pelvic examinations must rule out pregnancy before diagnostic testing begins.

 PEDIATRIC POINTERS

Adolescent girls are especially prone to amenorrhea caused by emotional upsets, typically stemming from school, social, or family problems.

AGING ISSUES

In women older than age 50, amenorrhea usually represents the onset of menopause.

PATIENT COUNSELING

Instruct the patient on what to expect from diagnostic testing and treatment and answer her questions. Because amenorrhea can cause severe emotional stress, provide emotional support and refer her for psychological counseling, if appropriate.

AMENORRHEA

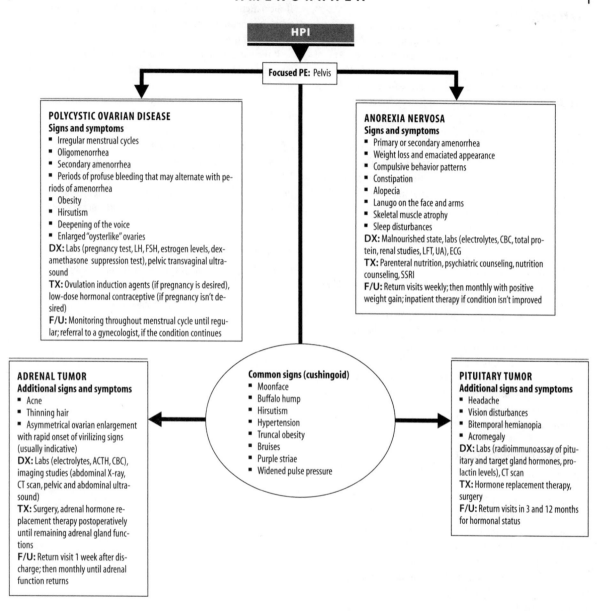

HPI

Focused PE: Pelvis

POLYCYSTIC OVARIAN DISEASE
Signs and symptoms
- Irregular menstrual cycles
- Oligomenorrhea
- Secondary amenorrhea
- Periods of profuse bleeding that may alternate with periods of amenorrhea
- Obesity
- Hirsutism
- Deepening of the voice
- Enlarged "oysterlike" ovaries

DX: Labs (pregnancy test, LH, FSH, estrogen levels, dexamethasone suppression test), pelvic transvaginal ultrasound

TX: Ovulation induction agents (if pregnancy is desired), low-dose hormonal contraceptive (if pregnancy isn't desired)

F/U: Monitoring throughout menstrual cycle until regular; referral to a gynecologist, if the condition continues

ANOREXIA NERVOSA
Signs and symptoms
- Primary or secondary amenorrhea
- Weight loss and emaciated appearance
- Compulsive behavior patterns
- Constipation
- Alopecia
- Lanugo on the face and arms
- Skeletal muscle atrophy
- Sleep disturbances

DX: Malnourished state, labs (electrolytes, CBC, total protein, renal studies, LFT, UA), ECG

TX: Parenteral nutrition, psychiatric counseling, nutrition counseling, SSRI

F/U: Return visits weekly; then monthly with positive weight gain; inpatient therapy if condition isn't improved

ADRENAL TUMOR
Additional signs and symptoms
- Acne
- Thinning hair
- Asymmetrical ovarian enlargement with rapid onset of virilizing signs (usually indicative)

DX: Labs (electrolytes, ACTH, CBC), imaging studies (abdominal X-ray, CT scan, pelvic and abdominal ultrasound)

TX: Surgery, adrenal hormone replacement therapy postoperatively until remaining adrenal gland functions

F/U: Return visit 1 week after discharge; then monthly until adrenal function returns

Common signs (cushingoid)
- Moonface
- Buffalo hump
- Hirsutism
- Hypertension
- Truncal obesity
- Bruises
- Purple striae
- Widened pulse pressure

PITUITARY TUMOR
Additional signs and symptoms
- Headache
- Vision disturbances
- Bitemporal hemianopia
- Acromegaly

DX: Labs (radioimmunoassay of pituitary and target gland hormones, prolactin levels), CT scan

TX: Hormone replacement therapy, surgery

F/U: Return visits in 3 and 12 months for hormonal status

Additional differential diagnoses: adrenocortical hyperplasia ▪ adrenocortical hypofunction ▪ amenorrhea-lactation disorders ▪ chronic renal failure ▪ congenital absence of the ovaries ▪ congenital absence of the uterus ▪ corpus luteum cysts ▪ hypothalamic tumor ▪ hypothyroidism ▪ mosaicism ▪ ovarian insensitivity to gonadotropins ▪ ovarian tumor ▪ PID ▪ physiologic delay of puberty ▪ pituitary infarction ▪ pregnancy ▪ pseudoamenorrhea ▪ pseudocyesis ▪ Sertoli-Leydig cell tumor ▪ testicular feminization ▪ thyrotoxicosis ▪ uterine hypoplasia

Amnesia

Amnesia, a disturbance in or loss of memory, may be classified as partial or complete and as anterograde or retrograde. Anterograde amnesia denotes memory loss for events that occurred after the onset of the causative trauma or disease; retrograde amnesia denotes memory loss for events that occurred before the onset. Depending on the cause, amnesia may arise suddenly or slowly and may be temporary or permanent.

Organic, or true, amnesia results from temporal lobe dysfunction, and it characteristically spares patches of memory. A common symptom among patients with seizures or head trauma, organic amnesia can also be an early indicator of Alzheimer's disease. Hysterical amnesia has a psychogenic origin and typically causes complete memory loss. Treatment-induced amnesia is usually transient.

HISTORY

Because many patients are unaware of their amnesia, you'll likely need to obtain information from the family.
● Ask the family when the amnesia first appeared and what types of things the patient can't remember. Can the patient learn and retain new information? Does the amnesia encompass a recent or remote period?
● Ask the family if the patient has a history of seizures.
● Obtain a drug history, including prescription and over-the-counter drugs, herbal remedies, and recreational drugs. Also, ask about alcohol intake.

PHYSICAL ASSESSMENT

● Note the patient's general appearance, behavior, mood, and train of thought.
● Test recent memory by asking the patient to identify and repeat three items. Retest him after 3 minutes.
● Test intermediate memory with such questions as "Who was president before the person who's currently in office?" and "What was the last type of car you bought?"
● Test remote memory with such questions as "How old are you?" and "Where were you born?"
● Take the patient's vital signs.
● Assess level of consciousness.
● Check pupils and extraocular movements.
● Test motor function by having the patient move his arms and legs through their range of motion.
● Evaluate sensory function with pinpricks on the patient's skin.

SPECIAL CONSIDERATIONS

If the patient has retrograde amnesia, provide reality orientation, and encourage his family to supply familiar photos, objects, and music.

If the patient has anterograde amnesia, adjust your patient-teaching techniques, keeping in mind that he can't acquire new information.

If the patient has severe amnesia, consider basic needs, such as safety, elimination, and nutrition.

A   PEDIATRIC POINTERS

A child who suffers seizure-induced amnesia may mistakenly be labeled as "learning disabled." To prevent mislabeling, stress the importance of adherence to the prescribed drug regimen, and discuss ways that the child, his parents, and his teachers can cope with the amnesia.

PATIENT COUNSELING

Provide the patient and his family with support. Refer them for psychological counseling if appropriate.

AMNESIA

HPI

Focused PE: Neurologic system, motor and cognitive function

ALZHEIMER'S DISEASE
Signs and symptoms
- Retrograde amnesia (initially)
- Progressive memory loss
- Agitation
- Inability to concentrate
- Disregard for personal hygiene
- Confusion, irritability, and emotional lability
- Aphasia
- Dementia
- Incontinence
- Muscle rigidity

DX: To rule out other causes, labs (CBC, electrolytes, thyroid function studies, VDRL, folate and vitamin B_{12} levels, HIV), imaging studies (CT scan, MRI, PET scan), EEG

TX: Medication (antidepressants, benzodiazepines, antipsychotics, memory-enhancing agents), lifestyle modifications, safety precautions

F/U: As needed (dependent on progression of disorder)

SEIZURES
Signs and symptoms
- Temporal lobe amnesia that occurs suddenly and lasts for several seconds to minutes
- Sensation of aura
- Irritable focus
- Verbal amnesia (left side)
- Nonverbal and graphic amnesia (right side)
- Confusion
- Visual, olfactory, and auditory hallucinations

DX: Labs (CBC, electrolytes, drug toxicity screen, serum ETOH screen), imaging studies (CT scan, MRI), EEG

TX: Anticonvulsants, surgery to remove irritable focus

F/U: Regular monitoring of anticonvulsant drug levels and adverse effects

CEREBRAL HYPOXIA
Signs and symptoms
- Total amnesia about the event
- Numbness and tingling

DX: History of carbon monoxide exposure or respiratory failure, labs (ABG, pulse oximetry), imaging studies (CT scan, MRI)

TX: Treatment of causative factor, oxygen therapy

F/U: As needed (dependent on cause and complications)

HEAD TRAUMA
Signs and symptoms
- Amnesia that may last for minutes to hours or longer
- Brief retrograde and longer anterograde amnesia
- Persistent amnesia about the event
- Possibly permanent amnesia or difficulty retaining recent memories
- Altered respirations and LOC
- Headache
- Dizziness and confusion
- Blurred or double vision

DX: History of head injury, imaging studies (CT scan, MRI)

TX: Medication (osmotic diuretic, anticonvulsant), surgery

F/U: As needed (dependent on degree of trauma and complications)

WERNICKE-KORSAKOFF SYNDROME
Signs and symptoms
- Retrograde and anterograde amnesia that may become permanent without treatment
- Apathy
- Confusion
- Inability to concentrate or sequence events
- Diplopia or ophthalmoplesia
- Decreased LOC
- Headache
- Ataxia
- Peripheral neuropathy
- Petechial hemorrhages

DX: Malnourished state, history of alcohol use, labs (electrolytes, CBC, thiamine pyrophosphate levels), imaging studies (CT scan, MRI)

TX: Thiamine

F/U: As needed (dependent on causes and complications)

Additional differential diagnoses: anoxia ▪ cerebral lesion ▪ cerebral mass ▪ dissociative disorder ▪ herpes simplex encephalitis ▪ stroke

Other causes: ECT ▪ medication (general anesthetics, barbiturates, certain benzodiazepines) ▪ temporal lobe surgery

Analgesia

Analgesia, the absence of sensitivity to pain, is an important sign of central nervous system disease that commonly indicates a specific type and location of spinal cord lesion. It always occurs with loss of temperature sensation (thermanesthesia) because these two sensory nerve impulses travel together in the spinal cord. It can also occur with other sensory deficits (such as paresthesia, loss of proprioception and vibratory sense, and tactile anesthesia) that are common in disorders involving the peripheral nerves, spinal cord, and brain. However, when accompanied only by thermanesthesia, analgesia denotes an incomplete lesion of the spinal cord.

Analgesia can be classified as partial or total below the level of the lesion and as unilateral or bilateral, depending on the cause and level of the lesion. Its onset may be slow and progressive (such as with a tumor) or abrupt (such as with trauma), and it may resolve spontaneously.

 ALERT

If the patient complains of unilateral or bilateral analgesia over a large body area that's accompanied by paralysis, suspect spinal cord injury and perform the following:

● *Immobilize the patient's spine in proper alignment, using a cervical collar and a long backboard, or keep the patient in a supine position on a flat surface and place sandbags around his head, neck, and torso.*

● *Continuously monitor respiratory rate and rhythm, and observe the patient for accessory muscle use.*

● *Have emergency equipment available.*

When you're satisfied that the patient's spine and respiratory status are stabilized — or if the analgesia isn't severe and isn't accompanied by signs of spinal cord injury — perform a focused assessment.

HISTORY

● Ask the patient when his symptoms began.
● Determine if the patient suffered recent trauma.
● Review the patient's medical history, noting especially recent trauma and incidence of cancer in the patient or his family.

PHYSICAL ASSESSMENT

● Take the patient's vital signs.
● Assess level of consciousness; pupillary, corneal, cough, and gag reflexes; speech; and ability to swallow.
● If possible, observe the patient's gait and posture, and assess his balance and coordination.
● Evaluate muscle tone and strength in all extremities.
● Thoroughly check pain sensitivity, vibration sense, and temperature sensation over all dermatomes.

SPECIAL CONSIDERATIONS

Focus your care on preventing further injury to the patient because analgesia can mask injury or developing complications.

 PEDIATRIC POINTERS

Because a child may have difficulty describing analgesia, carefully observe the patient during your assessment for nonverbal clues to pain, such as facial expressions, crying, and retraction from stimuli. Remember that infants have a high threshold for pain, so your assessment findings may be unreliable.

PATIENT COUNSELING

Discuss safety measures with the patient and his family. Advise the patient to test bath temperature using a thermometer or a body part with intact sensation to avoid injury.

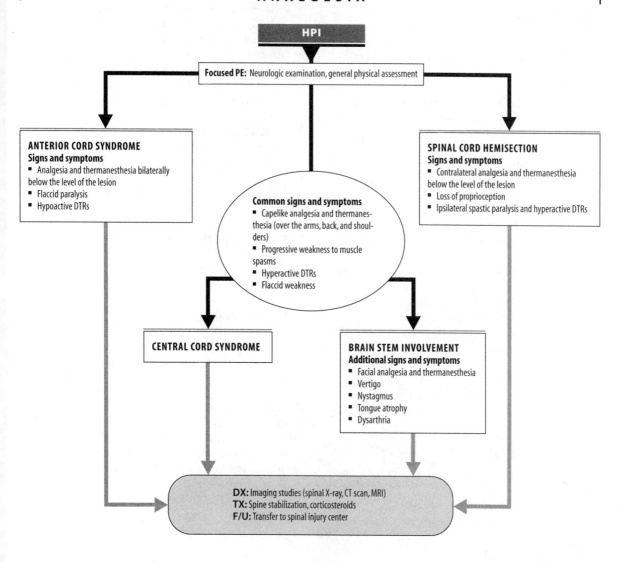

HPI

Focused PE: Neurologic examination, general physical assessment

ANTERIOR CORD SYNDROME
Signs and symptoms
- Analgesia and thermanesthesia bilaterally below the level of the lesion
- Flaccid paralysis
- Hypoactive DTRs

Common signs and symptoms
- Capelike analgesia and thermanesthesia (over the arms, back, and shoulders)
- Progressive weakness to muscle spasms
- Hyperactive DTRs
- Flaccid weakness

SPINAL CORD HEMISECTION
Signs and symptoms
- Contralateral analgesia and thermanesthesia below the level of the lesion
- Loss of proprioception
- Ipsilateral spastic paralysis and hyperactive DTRs

CENTRAL CORD SYNDROME

BRAIN STEM INVOLVEMENT
Additional signs and symptoms
- Facial analgesia and thermanesthesia
- Vertigo
- Nystagmus
- Tongue atrophy
- Dysarthria

DX: Imaging studies (spinal X-ray, CT scan, MRI)
TX: Spine stabilization, corticosteroids
F/U: Transfer to spinal injury center

Other causes: medication, such as topical and local anesthetics

Anorexia

Anorexia is a lack of appetite in the presence of a physiologic need for food. This symptom is common with GI and endocrine disorders and is characteristic of certain severe psychological disturbances such as anorexia nervosa. It can also result from such factors as anxiety, chronic pain, poor oral hygiene, increased blood temperature due to hot weather or fever, and changes in taste or smell that normally accompany aging. Anorexia can also result from drug therapy or abuse. Short-term anorexia rarely jeopardizes health, but chronic anorexia can lead to life-threatening malnutrition. (See *Common signs and symptoms of malnutrition.*)

HISTORY

- Ask the patient about previous minimum and maximum weights.
- Ask the patient about his dietary habits, such as when and what he eats, what foods he likes and dislikes, and why.
- Ask the patient about dental problems that interfere with chewing, including poorly fitting dentures.
- Ask the patient about swallowing problems and about GI disturbances after eating.

COMMON SIGNS AND SYMPTOMS OF MALNUTRITION

When assessing a patient with anorexia, check for these common signs of malnutrition:
- **abdomen** — enlarged liver and spleen
- **cardiovascular system** — heart rate greater than 100 beats/minute, arrhythmias, elevated blood pressure
- **eyes** — dull appearance; dry and pale or red membranes; triangular, shiny gray spots on the conjunctivae; red, fissured eyelid corners; bloodshot ring around the cornea
- **face** — generalized swelling, dark areas on the cheeks and under the eyes, lumpy or flaky skin around the nose and mouth, enlarged parotid glands
- **hair** — dull, dry, thin, fine, and straight; easily plucked; areas of lighter or darker spots; hair loss
- **lips** — red and swollen, especially at the corners
- **musculoskeletal system** — muscle wasting, knock-kneed or bowlegged, bumps on the ribs, swollen joints, musculoskeletal hemorrhages
- **nails** — spoon shaped, brittle, and ridged
- **neck** — swollen thyroid gland
- **nervous system** — irritability, confusion, paresthesia in the hands and feet, loss of proprioception, decreased ankle and knee reflexes
- **reproductive system** — decreased libido, amenorrhea
- **skin** — dry, flaky, and swollen; dark with lighter or darker spots, some resembling bruises; tight and drawn with poor turgor
- **teeth** — missing or emerging abnormally; visible cavities or dark spots; spongy, bleeding gums
- **tongue** — swollen, purple, and raw looking; sores or abnormal papillae.

- Ask the patient how frequently and intensely he exercises.
- Review the patient's medical history, noting especially stomach or bowel disorders and changes in bowel habits.
- Obtain a drug history, including prescription and over-the-counter drugs, herbal remedies, and recreational drugs. Also, ask the patient about alcohol intake.
- Explore psychological factors that may affect appetite, including recent loss or life change and depression.

PHYSICAL ASSESSMENT

- Take the patient's vital signs.
- Weigh the patient, and evaluate him for signs of malnutrition.
- Palpate the abdomen, noting complaints of tenderness or palpable masses.

SPECIAL CONSIDERATIONS

Because anorexia and poor nutrition increase susceptibility to infection, monitor the patient's vital signs and white blood cell count, and closely observe wounds.

 PEDIATRIC POINTERS

In children, anorexia commonly accompanies many illnesses but usually resolves promptly. However, in preadolescent and adolescent girls, be alert for the commonly subtle signs of anorexia nervosa.

PATIENT COUNSELING

Promote protein and calorie intake. Encourage supplemental nutritional support. Advise the patient to eat high-calorie snacks or frequent small meals. Refer the patient to a nutritionist for additional dietary information and for psychological counseling, if appropriate.

ANOREXIA

HPI

Focused PE: HEENT; dentition; cranial nerves; skin; abdomen; musculoskeletal, cardiovascular, neurologic, and reproductive systems

APPENDICITIS
Signs and symptoms
- Dull discomfort in the epigastric or umbilical region
- Nausea and vomiting
- Localized pain at McBurney's point
- Abdominal rigidity
- Rebound tenderness
- Positive Rovsing's, psoas, and cough signs

DX: CBC, imaging studies (KUB, CT scan, ultrasound)
TX: Surgery, antibiotics
F/U: Return visits at 2 and 6 weeks after discharge

ADRENOCORTICAL HYPOFUNCTION
Signs and symptoms
- Gradual weight loss
- Nausea and vomiting
- Abdominal pain
- Diarrhea

DX: Labs (CBC, electrolytes, BUN, creatinine, cortisol level, serum calcium, ACTH), imaging studies (CXR, CT scan)
TX: Aggressive fluid volume replacement, electrolyte correction, glucocorticoids
F/U: Referral to endocrinologist

ALCOHOLISM
Signs and symptoms
- Chronic loss of appetite
- Liver disease
- Paresthesia
- GI bleeding

DX: History of ETOH use, labs (ETOH level, LFT, electrolytes)
TX: Detoxification
F/U: Referral to detoxification support group

ANOREXIA NERVOSA
Signs and symptoms
- Loss of fatty tissue
- Distorted self-image
- Primary or secondary amenorrhea
- Weight loss and emaciated appearance
- Chronic loss of appetite
- Compulsive behavior patterns
- Constipation
- Alopecia
- Lanugo on the face and arms
- Skeletal muscle atrophy
- Sleep disturbances

DX: Malnourished state, labs (electrolytes, CBC, total protein, renal studies, LFT, UA)
TX: Parenteral nutrition, psychological counseling, nutrition counseling
F/U: Return visits weekly, then monthly with positive weight gain; inpatient therapy if condition doesn't improve

CANCER
DX: CEA, imaging studies (CT scan, MRI, bone scan)
TX: Varies (dependent on type of cancer and individual choices)
F/U: As needed (dependent on treatment), referral to oncologist

Common signs and symptoms
- Chronic anorexia
- Weight loss
- Apathy
- Cachexia
- Fatigue

AIDS
Additional signs and symptoms
- GI infection
- Pulmonary infection
- Kaposi's sarcoma
- Oral thrush
- Gingivitis

DX: Labs (ELISA, Western blot test)
TX: Nutritional counseling, medication (nucleoside reverse transcriptase inhibitors, protease inhibitors, nonnucleoside reverse transcriptase inhibitors)
F/U: As needed (dependent on stage of illness and reaction to treatment)

Additional differential diagnoses: chronic renal failure ▪ cirrhosis ▪ Crohn's disease ▪ decreased gastric emptying ▪ depressive syndrome ▪ electrolyte imbalance ▪ esophagitis ▪ gastritis ▪ hepatitis ▪ hypopituitarism ▪ hypothyroidism ▪ ketoacidosis ▪ osteoporosis ▪ pernicious anemia

Other causes: cardiomegaly ▪ constipation ▪ digoxin toxicity ▪ medication (amphetamines, chemotherapeutic agents, sympathomimetics such as ephedrine, and some antibiotics) ▪ radiation therapy ▪ TPN

Anosmia

Although it's usually an insignificant consequence of nasal congestion or obstruction, anosmia—absence of the sense of smell—occasionally heralds a serious defect. (See *Understanding the sense of smell.*) Temporary anosmia can result from any condition that irritates and causes swelling of the nasal mucosa and obstructs the olfactory area in the nose, such as heavy smoking, rhinitis, or sinusitis. Permanent anosmia usually results when the olfactory neuroepithelium, or any part of the olfactory nerve, is destroyed. Permanent or temporary anosmia can also result from inhaling irritants, such as cocaine or acid fumes, that paralyze nasal cilia. Anosmia may also be reported—without an identifiable organic cause—by patients suffering from hysteria, depression, or schizophrenia.

Anosmia is invariably perceived as bilateral; unilateral anosmia can also occur but is seldom recognized by the patient. Because combined stimulation of taste buds and olfactory cells produces the sense of taste, anosmia is usually accompanied by ageusia, loss of the sense of taste.

HISTORY

● Ask the patient about the onset and duration of anosmia and its related signs and symptoms: stuffy nose, nasal discharge or bleeding, postnasal drip, sneezing, dry or sore mouth and throat, ageusia, loss of appetite, excessive tearing, and facial or ocular pain.
● Review the patient's medical history for nasal disease, allergies, and head trauma.
● Ask the patient if he smokes and, if so, how often.
● Obtain a drug history, including prescription and over-the-counter drugs, herbal remedies, and recreational drugs. Also, ask the patient about alcohol intake.

PHYSICAL ASSESSMENT

● Inspect and palpate nasal structures for obvious injury, inflammation, deformities, and septal deviation or perforation.
● Observe the contour and color of the nasal mucosa.
● Note the source and character of nasal discharge.
● Palpate the sinus areas for tenderness and contour.

SPECIAL CONSIDERATIONS

Although permanent anosmia usually doesn't respond to treatment, vitamin A given orally or by injection occasionally provides improvement.

 PEDIATRIC POINTERS

Anosmia in children usually results from nasal obstruction by a foreign body or enlarged adenoids.

PATIENT COUNSELING

If anosmia results from nasal congestion, instruct the patient to use a local decongestant or antihistamine, along with a vaporizer or humidifier. Advise the patient to avoid excessive use of local decongestants, which can lead to rebound nasal congestion.

UNDERSTANDING THE SENSE OF SMELL

Our noses can distinguish the odors of thousands of chemicals, thanks to a highly developed complex of sensory cells. The olfactory epithelium contains olfactory receptor cells, along with olfactory glands and sustentacular cells—both of which secrete mucus to keep the epithelial surface moist. The mucus covering the olfactory cells probably traps airborne odorous molecules, which then fit into the appropriate receptors on the cell surface. In response to this stimulus, the receptor cell transmits an impulse along the olfactory nerve (cranial nerve I) to the olfactory area of the cortex, where it's interpreted. Any disruption along this transmission pathway, or any obstruction of the epithelial surface due to dryness or congestion, can cause anosmia.

ANOSMIA

HPI

Focused PE: Neurologic system, HEENT, cranial nerves, sinuses, psychological assessment

PERMANENT OR SECONDARY TO OLFACTORY NERVE DAMAGE

ASSOCIATED WITH NASAL MUCOSA CHANGES

NEOPLASMS (BRAIN, NASAL, OR SINUS)
Signs and symptoms
- Epistaxis
- Swelling and tenderness in the affected area
- Vision disturbances
- Decreased tearing
- Elevated ICP

DX: Imaging studies (CT scan, MRI), biopsy
TX: Optimization of neuro-function, vitamin A, corticosteroids
F/U: Referral to neurosurgeon

HEAD TRAUMA
Signs and symptoms
- Epistaxis
- Nausea and vomiting
- Altered LOC
- Blurred or double vision
- Raccoon eyes
- Battle's sign
- Otorrhea

DX: Imaging studies (skull radiograph, CT scan)
TX: Vitamin A, corticosteroids, LOC monitoring
F/U: As needed (dependent on extent of injury), transfer to brain injury center or rehabilitation unit

ANTERIOR CEREBRAL ARTERY OCCLUSION
Signs and symptoms
- Contralateral weakness and numbness (especially in the lower extremities)
- Confusion
- Impaired motor and sensory functions

DX: Imaging studies (CT scan, angiogram)
TX: ASA, surgery
F/U: Referral to vascular surgeon

Common signs and symptoms
- Nasal congestion or stuffiness
- Sneezing
- Watery or purulent nasal discharge
- Red, swollen nasal mucosa
- Dryness or tickling sensation in nasopharynx

LEAD POISONING
Signs and symptoms
- Nasal mucosa erosion
- Abdominal pain
- Weakness
- Headache
- Nausea and vomiting
- Constipation
- Wristdrop or footdrop
- Lead line on the gums
- Metallic taste
- Seizures
- Delirium

DX: Serum lead level, abdominal X-ray
TX: Medication (chelating agent, vitamin A), removal of lead-based paints and paint chips, low-fat diet
F/U: Monitoring of lead level in 7 to 10 days, biweekly, or monthly; then every 3 months until level is decreased

SEPTAL FRACTURE
Signs and symptoms
- Septal deviation
- Nasal mucosal swelling
- Epistaxis
- Hematoma
- Nasal congestion
- Ecchymosis

DX: History of facial trauma, facial X-ray
TX: Reduction and immobilization, cold therapy, NSAIDs
F/U: Return visit if swelling continues or complications occur

NASAL POLYPS
Signs and symptoms
- Smooth, pale, grapelike clusters
- Chronic allergic rhinitis
- Nasal obstruction
- Mouth breathing
- Watery mucus discharge
- Feeling of fullness

DX: Inspection, imaging studies (sinus X-ray, CT scan)
TX: Treatment of underlying cause, medication (inhaled corticosteroids, local astringent), surgery
F/U: Symptomatic monitoring, return visit 1 week after procedure (if surgery is performed)

RHINITIS

SINUSITIS
Additional signs and symptoms
- Sinus pain
- Sinus tenderness and swelling
- Severe headache
- Inflamed throat
- Postnasal drip
- Inflamed turbinates
- Malaise
- Low-grade fever
- Chills

DX: Inspection that's positive for sinus transillumination, imaging studies (sinus X-ray, CT scan)
TX: Medication (analgesics, decongestants, antihistamines, antibiotics)
F/U: Evaluation 48 to 72 hours after treatment is initiated, then until condition clinically clears

---

Additional differential diagnoses: diabetes mellitus ▪ frontal lobe brain tumor ▪ lethal midline granulomas ▪ nasal polyps ▪ optic chiasm ▪ pernicious anemia ▪ septal hematoma

Other causes: medication (prolonged use of nasal decongestants, naphazoline, reserpine and, less commonly, amphetamines, phenothiazines, and estrogen) ▪ radiation therapy ▪ surgery

Anuria

Clinically defined as urine output of less than 75 ml daily, anuria indicates either urinary tract obstruction or renal failure due to various mechanisms. (See *Major causes of acute renal failure.*) Fortunately, anuria is rare; even in those with renal failure, the kidneys usually produce at least 75 ml of urine daily.

Because urine output is easily measured, anuria rarely goes undetected. However, without immediate treatment, it can rapidly cause uremia and other complications of urine retention.

HISTORY

- Ask the patient about changes in his voiding pattern.
- Determine the amount of fluid normally ingested each day, the amount of fluid ingested in the past 24 to 48 hours, and the time and amount of the patient's last urination.
- Review the patient's medical history, noting especially previous kidney disease, urinary tract obstruction or infection, prostate enlargement, renal calculi, neurogenic bladder, congenital abnormalities, and abdominal, renal, or urinary tract surgery.
- Obtain a drug history, including prescription and over-the-counter drugs, herbal remedies, and recreational drugs. Also, ask the patient about alcohol intake.

PHYSICAL ASSESSMENT

- Take the patient's vital signs.

- Inspect and palpate the abdomen for asymmetry, distention, or bulging.
- Inspect the flank area for edema or erythema, and percuss and palpate the bladder.
- Assess a urine sample for cloudiness and foul odor.

ALERT

After detecting anuria, determine if urine formation is occurring and:
- *catheterize the patient to relieve a lower urinary tract obstruction or to check for residual urine*
- *obtain kidney function studies*
- *assess the patient for signs of fluid overload.*

SPECIAL CONSIDERATIONS

Restrict the patient's fluid intake until the cause of anuria is determined. Monitor vital signs, intake and output, and kidney function studies. If anuria is caused by an obstruction, prepare the patient for surgery.

PEDIATRIC POINTERS

- *Anuria in neonates is defined as the absence of urine output for 24 hours. It can be classified as primary or secondary. Primary anuria results from bilateral renal agenesis, aplasia, or multicystic dysplasia. Secondary anuria, which is associated with edema or dehydration, results from renal ischemia, renal vein thrombosis, or congenital anomalies of the genitourinary tract.*
- *Anuria in children commonly results from loss of renal function.*

AGING ISSUES

In elderly patients, anuria is commonly a gradual manifestation of an underlying pathology. A hospitalized or bedridden elderly patient may be unable to generate the pressure necessary to void if he remains in the supine position.

PATIENT COUNSELING

If the patient requires immediate surgery or dialysis, provide him with support. Instruct the patient on what to expect from diagnostic testing and treatment, and answer questions.

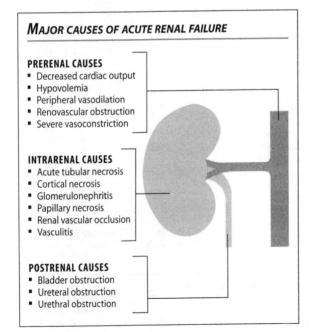

MAJOR CAUSES OF ACUTE RENAL FAILURE

PRERENAL CAUSES
- Decreased cardiac output
- Hypovolemia
- Peripheral vasodilation
- Renovascular obstruction
- Severe vasoconstriction

INTRARENAL CAUSES
- Acute tubular necrosis
- Cortical necrosis
- Glomerulonephritis
- Papillary necrosis
- Renal vascular occlusion
- Vasculitis

POSTRENAL CAUSES
- Bladder obstruction
- Ureteral obstruction
- Urethral obstruction

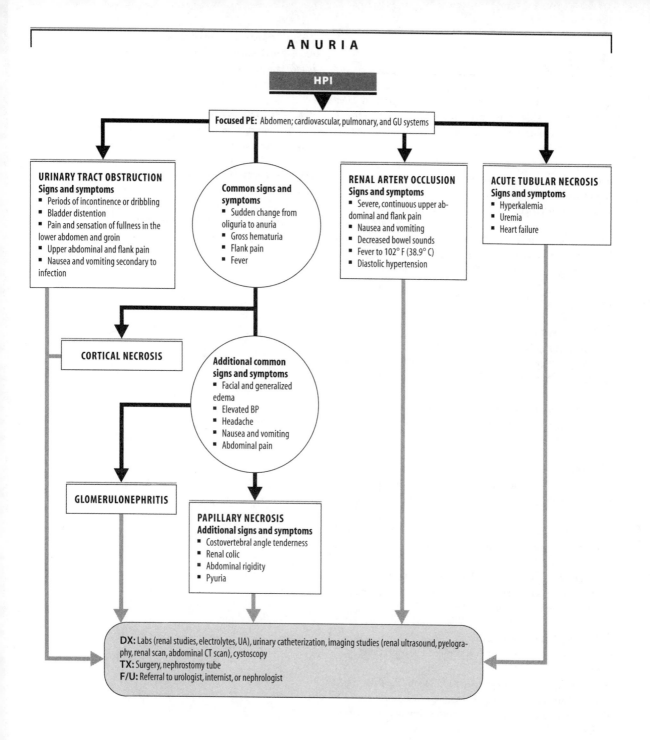

HPI

Focused PE: Abdomen; cardiovascular, pulmonary, and GU systems

URINARY TRACT OBSTRUCTION
Signs and symptoms
- Periods of incontinence or dribbling
- Bladder distention
- Pain and sensation of fullness in the lower abdomen and groin
- Upper abdominal and flank pain
- Nausea and vomiting secondary to infection

Common signs and symptoms
- Sudden change from oliguria to anuria
- Gross hematuria
- Flank pain
- Fever

RENAL ARTERY OCCLUSION
Signs and symptoms
- Severe, continuous upper abdominal and flank pain
- Nausea and vomiting
- Decreased bowel sounds
- Fever to 102° F (38.9° C)
- Diastolic hypertension

ACUTE TUBULAR NECROSIS
Signs and symptoms
- Hyperkalemia
- Uremia
- Heart failure

CORTICAL NECROSIS

Additional common signs and symptoms
- Facial and generalized edema
- Elevated BP
- Headache
- Nausea and vomiting
- Abdominal pain

GLOMERULONEPHRITIS

PAPILLARY NECROSIS
Additional signs and symptoms
- Costovertebral angle tenderness
- Renal colic
- Abdominal rigidity
- Pyuria

DX: Labs (renal studies, electrolytes, UA), urinary catheterization, imaging studies (renal ultrasound, pyelography, renal scan, abdominal CT scan), cystoscopy
TX: Surgery, nephrostomy tube
F/U: Referral to urologist, internist, or nephrologist

Additional differential diagnoses: burns ▪ crush injury ▪ hemolytic-uremic syndrome ▪ hepatic renal syndrome ▪ renal artery or vein occlusion ▪ vasculitis

Other causes: contrast dye for imaging studies ▪ medication (antibiotics, especially aminoglycosides; anesthetics; heavy metals; ethyl alcohol; adrenergics; anticholinergics; NSAIDs; ACE inhibitors; amphotericin B; ASA; methotrexate)

Anxiety

A subjective reaction to a real or imagined threat, anxiety is a nonspecific feeling of uneasiness or dread. It may be mild, moderate, or severe. Mild anxiety may cause slight physical or psychological discomfort. Severe anxiety may be incapacitating or even life-threatening.

Everyone experiences anxiety from time to time—it's a normal response to actual danger, prompting the body (through stimulation of the sympathetic and parasympathetic nervous systems) to purposeful action. It's also a normal response to physical and emotional stress, which can be produced by virtually any illness. Anxiety can also be precipitated or exacerbated by many nonpathologic factors, including lack of sleep, poor diet, and excessive intake of caffeine or other stimulants. However, excessive, unwarranted anxiety may indicate an underlying psychological problem.

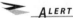 *ALERT*

If the patient displays acute, severe anxiety:
- *quickly take his vital signs, and determine his reason for seeking care (this will serve as a guide for how to proceed)*
- *try to keep him as calm as possible; suggest relaxation techniques and talk in a reassuring, soothing voice.*

If the patient displays mild or moderate anxiety, perform a focused assessment.

HISTORY
- Ask the patient about the duration of his anxiety. Is the anxiety constant or sporadic? Did he notice any precipitating factors?
- Ask the patient if the anxiety is exacerbated by stress, lack of sleep, or excessive caffeine intake. Does rest, exercise, or a tranquilizer alleviate it?
- Obtain a drug history, including prescription and over-the-counter drugs, herbal remedies, and recreational drugs. Also, ask the patient about alcohol intake.

PHYSICAL ASSESSMENT
- Focus on complaints that may trigger or be aggravated by anxiety.
- If significant physical signs don't accompany the patient's anxiety, suspect a psychological basis.
- Determine the patient's level of consciousness, and observe his behavior.

SPECIAL CONSIDERATIONS
Many drugs cause anxiety, especially sympathomimetics and central nervous system stimulants, and many antidepressants cause paradoxical anxiety.

 PEDIATRIC POINTERS

Anxiety in children usually results from painful physical illness or inadequate oxygenation. Its autonomic signs tend to be more common and dramatic than in adults.

 AGING ISSUES

In elderly patients, distractions from the patient's ritual activity may provoke anxiety or agitation.

PATIENT COUNSELING
Supportive care can help relieve anxiety. Provide a calm, quiet atmosphere, and make the patient comfortable. Encourage him to express his feelings and concerns freely.

ANXIETY

HPI

Focused PE: Systems involved in symptom complaints, psychological assessment

Common signs and symptoms
- Sharp, crushing substernal or anterior chest pain
- SOB
- Tachycardia

ANGINA PECTORIS

Additional common signs and symptoms
- Worsening or prolonged chest pain
- Diaphoresis
- Pain that radiates to the arm, jaw, or back
- Nausea and vomiting

MI

CARDIOGENIC SHOCK
Additional signs and symptoms
- Hypotension
- Hemodynamic instability
- Bradycardia
- Cool, clammy skin
- Heart failure
- Pulmonary edema

PANIC DISORDER
Signs and symptoms
- Tachycardia
- Dyspnea
- Diaphoresis
- Choking sensation
- Paresthesia
- Flushing

GENERALIZED ANXIETY DISORDER
Signs and symptoms
- Restlessness
- Fatigue
- Irritability
- Autonomic hyperactivity
- Difficulty sleeping and concentrating

DX: History, ruling out of serious medical condition, labs (CBC, electrolytes, serum and urine screens for medication)
TX: Medication (dependent on psychological cause of anxiety), distraction and relaxation techniques
F/U: Referral to psychiatrist, advanced practice psychiatric nurse, or psychologist

Common signs and symptoms
- SOB
- Wheezing
- Poor gas exchange

ASTHMA

ARDS
Signs and symptoms
- Respiratory distress
- Tachycardia
- Mental sluggishness
- Hypotension

ANAPHYLACTIC SHOCK
Additional signs and symptoms
- Respiratory distress
- Urticaria
- Angioedema
- Hypotension
- Tachycardia

DX: Physical examination, ABG, CXR
TX: Airway maintenance, oxygen therapy, medication (epinephrine, corticosteroids, beta-agonists)
F/U: As needed (dependent on response to treatment and complications)

DX: ECG, labs (cardiac enzymes, troponin I and T levels, C-reactive protein)
TX: Medication (aspirin, vasodilator, analgesic, thrombolytic, anticoagulant), cardiac catheterization, PCI
F/U: Referral to cardiologist, cardiac rehabilitation

Additional differential diagnoses: alcohol withdrawal ▪ autonomic hyperreflexia ▪ COPD ▪ depression ▪ hyperthyroidism ▪ hyperventilation syndrome ▪ hypoglycemia ▪ mitral valve prolapse ▪ obsessive-compulsive disorder ▪ pheochromocytoma ▪ phobias ▪ pneumonia ▪ pneumothorax ▪ postconcussion syndrome ▪ posttraumatic stress disorder ▪ pulmonary embolism ▪ rabies ▪ somatoform disorder

Other causes: antidepressants ▪ CNS stimulants ▪ sympathomimetics

Aphasia

Aphasia is the impaired expression or comprehension of written or spoken language and reflects disease or injury of the brain's language centers. Depending on its severity, aphasia may slightly impede communication, or it may make speech impossible. It can be classified as Broca's, Wernicke's, anomic, or global aphasia. Anomic aphasia eventually resolves in more than 50% of patients, but global aphasia is usually irreversible. (See *Identifying types of aphasia*.)

➤ **ALERT**

If the patient is experiencing aphasia:
- *look for signs of increased intracranial pressure, such as pupillary changes, decreased level of consciousness (LOC), vomiting, seizures, bradycardia, widening pulse pressure, and irregular respirations*
- *assess for signs of stroke*
- *have emergency equipment nearby*
- *prepare the patient for surgery, if appropriate.*

If the patient doesn't display signs of increased intracranial pressure or stroke, or if his aphasia has developed gradually, perform a focused assessment.

IDENTIFYING TYPES OF APHASIA

TYPE	CLINICAL FINDINGS
Broca's aphasia (expressive aphasia)	• Ability to understand written and spoken language intact • Nonfluent speech, evidenced by difficulty finding words, use of jargon, paraphasia, limited vocabulary, and simple sentence construction • Inability to repeat words or phrases
Wernicke's aphasia (receptive aphasia)	• Difficulty understanding written and spoken language • Inability to repeat words or phrases or follow directions • Fluent speech but may be rapid and rambling with paraphasia • Difficulty naming objects (anomia) • Lack of awareness of speech errors
Anomic aphasia	• Ability to understand written and spoken language intact • Fluent speech but lacks meaningful content • Difficulty finding words and circumlocution • Paraphasia (rarely)
Global aphasia	• Profoundly impaired receptive and expressive aphasia ability • Inability to repeat words or phrases or follow directions • Speech marked by paraphasia or jargon

HISTORY

Because of the patient's impairment, you'll likely need to obtain information from his family.
- Ask the family about the patient's history of headaches, hypertension, seizure disorders, and drug use.
- Ask the family about the patient's ability to communicate and to perform routine activities before the aphasia began.

PHYSICAL ASSESSMENT

- Check for obvious signs of neurologic deficit, such as paresis or altered LOC.
- Take the patient's vital signs.
- Assess pupillary response, eye movements, and motor function, especially his mouth and tongue movement, swallowing ability, and spontaneous movements and gestures.

SPECIAL CONSIDERATIONS

When speaking to the patient, don't assume that he understands you. He may simply be interpreting subtle clues to meaning, such as social context, facial expressions, and gestures. To help avoid misunderstanding, use nonverbal techniques, speak to him in simple phrases, and use demonstration to clarify your verbal directions.

Ⓐ **PEDIATRIC POINTERS**

- *Recognize that the term* childhood aphasia *is sometimes mistakenly applied to children who fail to develop normal language skills but who aren't considered mentally retarded or developmentally delayed. Aphasia refers solely to loss of previously developed communication skills.*
- *Brain damage associated with aphasia in children most commonly follows anoxia—the result of near drowning or airway obstruction.*

PATIENT COUNSELING

Make sure the patient has necessary aids, such as eyeglasses or dentures, to facilitate communication. Refer the patient to a speech pathologist to help him cope with his aphasia.

APHASIA

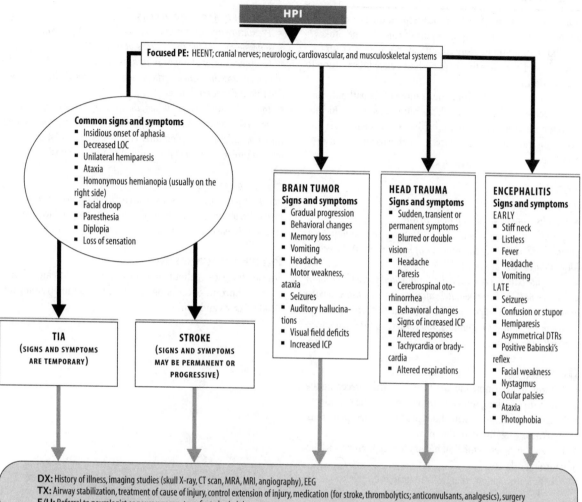

HPI

Focused PE: HEENT; cranial nerves; neurologic, cardiovascular, and musculoskeletal systems

Common signs and symptoms
- Insidious onset of aphasia
- Decreased LOC
- Unilateral hemiparesis
- Ataxia
- Homonymous hemianopia (usually on the right side)
- Facial droop
- Paresthesia
- Diplopia
- Loss of sensation

TIA
(SIGNS AND SYMPTOMS ARE TEMPORARY)

STROKE
(SIGNS AND SYMPTOMS MAY BE PERMANENT OR PROGRESSIVE)

BRAIN TUMOR
Signs and symptoms
- Gradual progression
- Behavioral changes
- Memory loss
- Vomiting
- Headache
- Motor weakness, ataxia
- Seizures
- Auditory hallucinations
- Visual field deficits
- Increased ICP

HEAD TRAUMA
Signs and symptoms
- Sudden, transient or permanent symptoms
- Blurred or double vision
- Headache
- Paresis
- Cerebrospinal oto-rhinorrhea
- Behavioral changes
- Signs of increased ICP
- Altered responses
- Tachycardia or brady-cardia
- Altered respirations

ENCEPHALITIS
Signs and symptoms
EARLY
- Stiff neck
- Listless
- Fever
- Headache
- Vomiting
LATE
- Seizures
- Confusion or stupor
- Hemiparesis
- Asymmetrical DTRs
- Positive Babinski's reflex
- Facial weakness
- Nystagmus
- Ocular palsies
- Ataxia
- Photophobia

DX: History of illness, imaging studies (skull X-ray, CT scan, MRA, MRI, angiography), EEG
TX: Airway stabilization, treatment of cause of injury, control extension of injury, medication (for stroke, thrombolytics; anticonvulsants, analgesics), surgery
F/U: Referral to neurologist or neurosurgeon, transfer to brain injury center

Additional differential diagnoses: Alzheimer's disease ▪ brain abscess ▪ Creutzfeldt-Jakob disease

Apnea

Apnea, the cessation of spontaneous respiration, is occasionally temporary and self-limiting, as occurs during Cheyne-Stokes and Biot's respirations. More commonly, however, it's a life-threatening emergency that requires immediate intervention to prevent death.

Apnea usually results from one or more of six pathophysiologic mechanisms, each of which has numerous causes. Its most common causes include trauma, cardiac arrest, neurologic disease, aspiration of a foreign object, bronchospasm, and drug overdose.

 ALERT

If you detect apnea:
● establish and maintain a patent airway
● quickly look, listen, and feel for spontaneous respiration; if it's absent, begin artificial ventilation until it occurs or until mechanical ventilation can be initiated
● assess the patient's carotid pulse (or brachial pulse if he's an infant or a small child) immediately after you've established a patent airway. If you can't palpate a pulse, begin cardiac compressions.

When the patient's respiratory and cardiac status are stable, perform a focused assessment.

HISTORY
● Attempt to determine the events immediately preceding the apneic event by asking someone who witnessed the episode.
● When able, ask the patient about headache, chest pain, muscle weakness, sore throat, or dyspnea.
● Review the patient's medical history for respiratory, cardiac, or neurologic disease.
● Ask the patient about allergies and drug use.

PHYSICAL ASSESSMENT
● Inspect the patient's head, face, neck, and trunk for soft-tissue injury, hemorrhage, or skeletal deformity.
● Auscultate the lungs for adventitious breath sounds, particularly crackles and rhonchi.
● Percuss the lung fields for increased dullness or hyperresonance.
● Auscultate the heart for murmurs, pericardial friction rub, and arrhythmias.
● Check for cyanosis, pallor, jugular vein distention, and edema.

SPECIAL CONSIDERATIONS
Central nervous system (CNS) depressants can cause hypoventilation and apnea. Benzodiazepines can cause respiratory depression and apnea when given I.V. with other CNS depressants to elderly or acutely ill patients.

 PEDIATRIC POINTERS
● Premature infants are especially susceptible to periodic apneic episodes because of the immaturity of their CNS.
● Common causes of apnea in infants include sepsis, intraventricular or subarachnoid hemorrhage, seizures, bronchiolitis, and sudden infant death syndrome.
● In toddlers and older children, the primary cause of apnea is acute airway obstruction from aspiration of a foreign object. Other causes include acute epiglottiditis, croup, asthma, and such systemic disorders as muscular dystrophy and cystic fibrosis.

AGING ISSUES
In elderly patients, increased sensitivity to analgesics, sedative-hypnotics, or any combination of these drugs can produce apnea, even within normal dosage ranges.

PATIENT COUNSELING
Educate the patient about safety measures related to ingestion of drugs. Encourage cardiopulmonary resuscitation training for all adolescents and adults.

APNEA

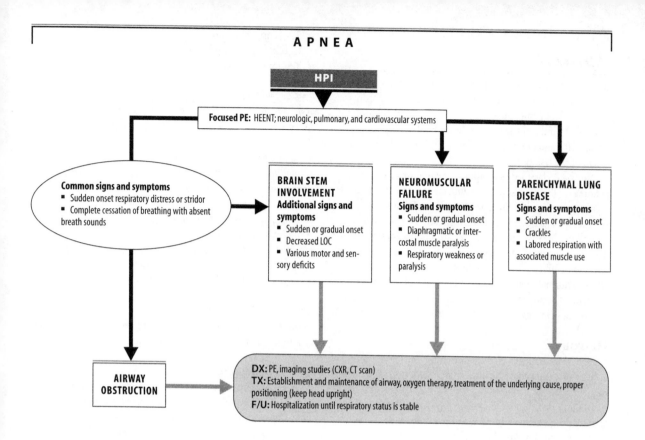

HPI

Focused PE: HEENT; neurologic, pulmonary, and cardiovascular systems

Common signs and symptoms
- Sudden onset respiratory distress or stridor
- Complete cessation of breathing with absent breath sounds

BRAIN STEM INVOLVEMENT
Additional signs and symptoms
- Sudden or gradual onset
- Decreased LOC
- Various motor and sensory deficits

NEUROMUSCULAR FAILURE
Signs and symptoms
- Sudden or gradual onset
- Diaphragmatic or intercostal muscle paralysis
- Respiratory weakness or paralysis

PARENCHYMAL LUNG DISEASE
Signs and symptoms
- Sudden or gradual onset
- Crackles
- Labored respiration with associated muscle use

AIRWAY OBSTRUCTION

DX: PE, imaging studies (CXR, CT scan)
TX: Establishment and maintenance of airway, oxygen therapy, treatment of the underlying cause, proper positioning (keep head upright)
F/U: Hospitalization until respiratory status is stable

Additional differential diagnoses: drug overdose ▪ head injury ▪ stroke

Apraxia

Apraxia is the inability to perform purposeful movements in the absence of significant weakness, sensory loss, poor coordination, or lack of comprehension or motivation. This neurologic sign usually indicates a lesion in the cerebral hemisphere. Its onset, severity, and duration vary, depending on the location and extent of the lesion.

Apraxia is classified as ideational, ideomotor, or kinetic, depending on the stage at which voluntary movement is impaired. It can also be classified by type of motor or skill impairment. For example, facial and gait apraxia involve specific motor groups and are easily perceived. Constructional apraxia refers to inability to copy simple drawings or patterns. Dressing apraxia refers to inability to dress oneself correctly. Callosal apraxia refers to normal motor function on one side of the body accompanied by an inability to reproduce movements on the other side. (See *How apraxia interferes with purposeful movement.*)

HISTORY

- Review the patient's medical history for neurologic, cerebrovascular, and neoplastic disease; atherosclerosis; and infection.
- Obtain a drug history, including prescription and over-the-counter drugs, herbal remedies, and recreational drugs. Also, ask the patient about alcohol intake.
- Ask the patient about recent headaches or dizziness.

PHYSICAL ASSESSMENT

- Take the patient's vital signs.
- Assess level of consciousness, keeping alert for evidence of aphasia or dysarthria.
- Test motor function, observing for weakness and tremors.

- Test sensory function.
- Check deep tendon reflexes for quality and symmetry.
- Test for visual field deficits.

ALERT

If the patient displays signs and symptoms of increased intracranial pressure, such as headache and vomiting, during your assessment:
- *elevate the head of the bed 30 degrees*
- *monitor him closely for altered pupil size and reactivity, bradycardia, widened pulse pressure, and irregular respirations*
- *have emergency resuscitation equipment nearby.*
  If the patient is having seizures:
- *maintain airway patency and safety*
- *help him to a lying position, loosen tight clothing, and place a pillow or other soft object beneath his head*
- *turn his head to provide an open airway.*

SPECIAL CONSIDERATIONS

Because weakness, sensory deficits, confusion, and seizures may accompany apraxia, take measures to ensure safety.

PEDIATRIC POINTERS

- *In many cases, detecting apraxia in children is difficult. However, any sudden inability to perform a previously accomplished movement warrants prompt neurologic evaluation because a brain tumor—the most common cause of apraxia in children—can be treated effectively if detected early.*
- *Brain damage in a young child may cause developmental apraxia, which interferes with the ability to learn activities that require sequential movement, such as hopping, jumping, hitting or kicking a ball, and dancing.*
- *When caring for a child with apraxia, be aware of his limitations but provide an environment that's conducive to rehabilitation. Provide emotional support because playmates will often tease a child who can't perform normal physical activities.*

PATIENT COUNSELING

Explain the patient's apraxia to him, and encourage his participation in normal activities. Avoid giving complex directions, and teach the family to participate in rehabilitation. Refer the patient to a physical or occupational therapist.

HOW APRAXIA INTERFERES WITH PURPOSEFUL MOVEMENT

TYPE OF APRAXIA	DESCRIPTION
Ideational apraxia	The patient can physically perform the steps required to complete a task but fails to remember the sequence in which they're performed.
Ideomotor apraxia	The patient understands and can physically perform the steps required to complete the task but can't formulate a plan to carry them out.
Kinetic apraxia	The patient understands the task and formulates a plan but fails to set the proper muscles in motion.

APRAXIA

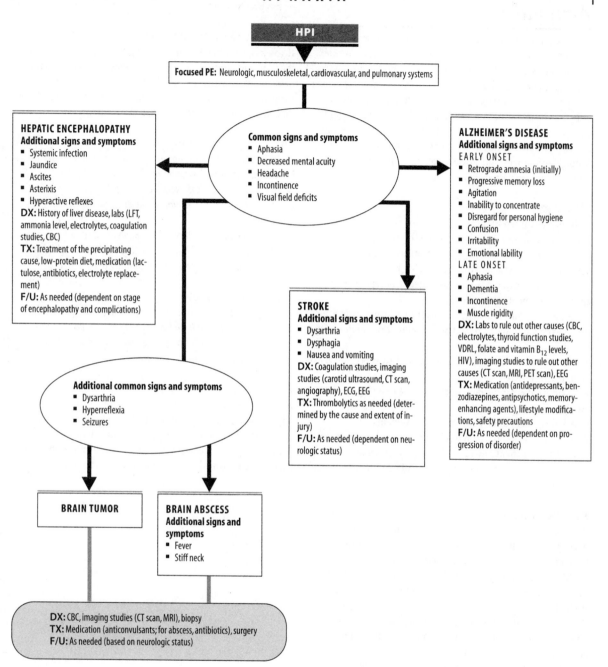

HPI

Focused PE: Neurologic, musculoskeletal, cardiovascular, and pulmonary systems

Common signs and symptoms
- Aphasia
- Decreased mental acuity
- Headache
- Incontinence
- Visual field deficits

HEPATIC ENCEPHALOPATHY
Additional signs and symptoms
- Systemic infection
- Jaundice
- Ascites
- Asterixis
- Hyperactive reflexes

DX: History of liver disease, labs (LFT, ammonia level, electrolytes, coagulation studies, CBC)
TX: Treatment of the precipitating cause, low-protein diet, medication (lactulose, antibiotics, electrolyte replacement)
F/U: As needed (dependent on stage of encephalopathy and complications)

ALZHEIMER'S DISEASE
Additional signs and symptoms
EARLY ONSET
- Retrograde amnesia (initially)
- Progressive memory loss
- Agitation
- Inability to concentrate
- Disregard for personal hygiene
- Confusion
- Irritability
- Emotional lability
LATE ONSET
- Aphasia
- Dementia
- Incontinence
- Muscle rigidity

DX: Labs to rule out other causes (CBC, electrolytes, thyroid function studies, VDRL, folate and vitamin B_{12} levels, HIV), imaging studies to rule out other causes (CT scan, MRI, PET scan), EEG
TX: Medication (antidepressants, benzodiazepines, antipsychotics, memory-enhancing agents), lifestyle modifications, safety precautions
F/U: As needed (dependent on progression of disorder)

STROKE
Additional signs and symptoms
- Dysarthria
- Dysphagia
- Nausea and vomiting

DX: Coagulation studies, imaging studies (carotid ultrasound, CT scan, angiography), ECG, EEG
TX: Thrombolytics as needed (determined by the cause and extent of injury)
F/U: As needed (dependent on neurologic status)

Additional common signs and symptoms
- Dysarthria
- Hyperreflexia
- Seizures

BRAIN TUMOR

BRAIN ABSCESS
Additional signs and symptoms
- Fever
- Stiff neck

DX: CBC, imaging studies (CT scan, MRI), biopsy
TX: Medication (anticonvulsants; for abscess, antibiotics), surgery
F/U: As needed (based on neurologic status)

Arm pain

Arm pain usually results from a musculoskeletal disorder, but it can also stem from a neurovascular or cardiovascular disorder. In some cases, it may be referred pain from another area, such as the chest, neck, or abdomen. Its location, onset, and character provide clues to its cause. The pain may affect the entire arm or only the upper arm or forearm. It may arise suddenly or gradually and be constant or intermittent. Arm pain can be described as sharp or dull, burning or numbing, and shooting or penetrating. Diffuse arm pain, however, may be difficult to describe, especially if it isn't associated with injury.

HISTORY

● If the patient reports arm pain after an injury, take a brief history of the injury from the patient or his family.
● If the patient reports continuous or intermittent arm pain, ask him to describe it, and find out when it began.
● Ask the patient if the pain is associated with repetitive or specific movements or positions.
● Ask the patient about activities that he performs during the day at work and if the arm pain prevents him from performing his job.
● Ask the patient to point out other painful areas because arm pain may be referred.
● Ask the patient if the pain worsens in the morning or in the evening.
● Ask the patient if the pain restricts movements.
● Ask the patient if the pain is relieved by heat, rest, or drugs.
● Review the patient's medical history for preexisting illnesses.
● Ask the patient about a family history of gout or arthritis and current drug therapy.

PHYSICAL ASSESSMENT

● Observe the way the patient walks, sits, and holds his arm.
● Inspect the entire arm, comparing it with the opposite arm for symmetry, movement, and muscle atrophy.
● Palpate the entire arm for swelling, nodules, and tender areas. In both arms, compare active range of motion, muscle strength, and reflexes.
● Examine the neck for pain on motion, point tenderness, muscle spasms, or arm pain when the neck is extended with the head toward the involved side.
● If the patient reports numbness or tingling, check his sensation to vibration, temperature, and pinprick; then compare bilateral hand grasps and shoulder strength to detect weakness.
● If the patient has a cast, splint, or restrictive dressing, check his arm for circulation, sensation, and mobility distal to the dressing; then ask him if he has experienced edema and if the pain has worsened in the last 24 hours as well as which activities he has been performing.

SPECIAL CONSIDERATIONS

If you suspect a fracture, apply a sling or a splint to immobilize the arm, and monitor the patient for worsening pain, numbness, or decreased circulation distal to the injury site. Promote the patient's comfort by elevating his arm and applying ice until diagnostic testing and treatment is administered.

Ⓐ PEDIATRIC POINTERS

● *In children, arm pain commonly results from a fracture, a muscle sprain, muscular dystrophy, or rheumatoid arthritis.*
● *In young children, the exact location of the pain may be difficult to establish. Watch for nonverbal clues, such as wincing or guarding.*
● *If the child has a fracture or sprain, obtain a complete account of the injury. Closely observe interactions between the child and his family, and don't rule out the possibility of child abuse.*

AGING ISSUES

Elderly patients with osteoporosis may experience fractures from simple trauma or even from heavy lifting or unexpected movements. They're also prone to degenerative joint disease that can involve several joints in the arm or neck.

PATIENT COUNSELING

Advise a patient with a cast to notify his physician if he detects any worsening swelling, purple discoloration of fingers, or numbness or tingling. Advise patients with angina that arm pain, usually left-sided, may represent an ischemic event, especially if accompanied by diaphoresis, nausea, vomiting, and anxiety.

ARM PAIN (ELBOW)

HPI

Focused PE: Pain; musculoskeletal, neurovascular, and cardiovascular systems

Common signs and symptoms
- Decreased motion
- Pain on movement
- Tenderness at olecranon process and epicondyles

Common signs and symptoms
- Decreased motion
- Deformity
- Edema
- Possible impaired circulation
- Possible paresthesia

ARTHRITIS
Signs and symptoms
- Warmth at site
- Boggy, soft, or fluctuant swelling
- Tenderness

DX: Arm X-ray
TX: Medication (ASA, NSAIDs, analgesics), physical therapy
F/U: As needed (dependent on symptoms)

TENDINITIS

Additional common signs and symptoms
- Swelling, erythema, and inflammation superficial to the olecranon bursa

LATERAL EPICONDYLITIS
Additional signs and symptoms
- Muscle weakness
- Pain and tenderness at the lateral epicondyle
- Increased pain with wrist extension on resistance

BURSITIS

FRACTURE
Additional signs and symptoms
- Crepitus
- Ecchymosis
- Impaired circulation
- Paresthesia

DISLOCATION

DX: PE, elbow X-ray
TX: Rest and elevation, ice, compression, physical therapy, medication (NSAIDs, analgesics)
F/U: Return visit 48 to 72 hours after treatment, then later if symptoms recur

DX: Arm X-ray
TX: Arm cast, rest and elevation, medication (NSAIDs, analgesics)
F/U: Referral to orthopedic surgeon

Additional differential diagnoses: angina ▪ ankylosis ▪ biceps rupture ▪ cellulitis ▪ compartment syndrome ▪ medical epicondylitis ▪ MI ▪ muscle contusion ▪ neoplasm of the arm ▪ osteomyelitis

ARM PAIN (SHOULDER)

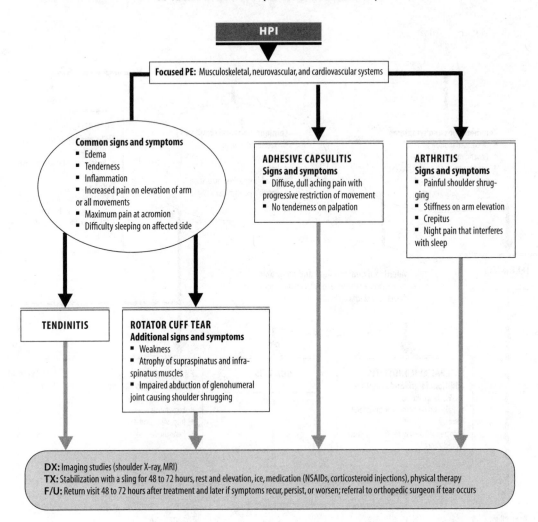

HPI

Focused PE: Musculoskeletal, neurovascular, and cardiovascular systems

Common signs and symptoms
- Edema
- Tenderness
- Inflammation
- Increased pain on elevation of arm or all movements
- Maximum pain at acromion
- Difficulty sleeping on affected side

ADHESIVE CAPSULITIS
Signs and symptoms
- Diffuse, dull aching pain with progressive restriction of movement
- No tenderness on palpation

ARTHRITIS
Signs and symptoms
- Painful shoulder shrugging
- Stiffness on arm elevation
- Crepitus
- Night pain that interferes with sleep

TENDINITIS

ROTATOR CUFF TEAR
Additional signs and symptoms
- Weakness
- Atrophy of supraspinatus and infraspinatus muscles
- Impaired abduction of glenohumeral joint causing shoulder shrugging

DX: Imaging studies (shoulder X-ray, MRI)
TX: Stabilization with a sling for 48 to 72 hours, rest and elevation, ice, medication (NSAIDs, corticosteroid injections), physical therapy
F/U: Return visit 48 to 72 hours after treatment and later if symptoms recur, persist, or worsen; referral to orthopedic surgeon if tear occurs

---

Additional differential diagnoses: acromioclavicular separation ▪ acute pancreatitis ▪ angina pectoris ▪ bursitis ▪ cellulitis ▪ cervical nerve root compression ▪ cholecystitis ▪ cholelithiasis ▪ clavicle fracture ▪ diaphragmatic pleurisy ▪ dislocation ▪ dissecting aortic aneurysm ▪ gastritis ▪ humeral neck fracture ▪ infection ▪ MI ▪ muscle contusion ▪ neoplasm of the arm ▪ osteomyelitis ▪ Pancoast's syndrome ▪ pneumothorax ▪ ruptured spleen ▪ shoulder-hand syndrome ▪ subphrenic abscess ▪ thoracic outlet syndrome

Other causes: laparoscopy

ARM PAIN (WRIST)

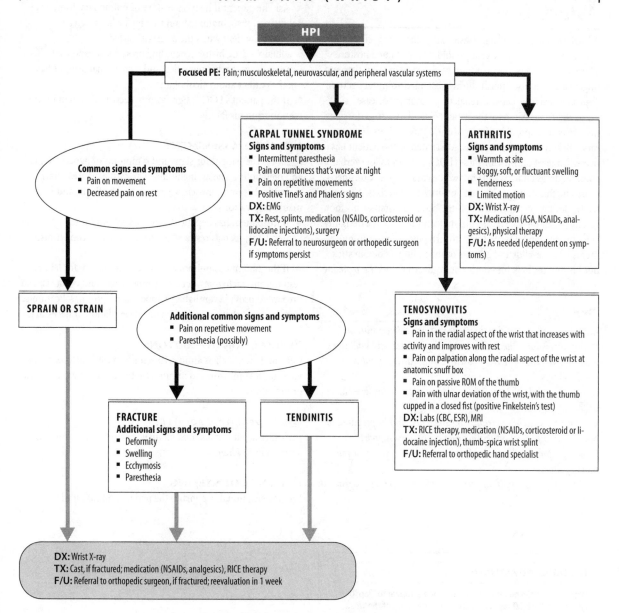

HPI

Focused PE: Pain; musculoskeletal, neurovascular, and peripheral vascular systems

Common signs and symptoms
- Pain on movement
- Decreased pain on rest

SPRAIN OR STRAIN

CARPAL TUNNEL SYNDROME
Signs and symptoms
- Intermittent paresthesia
- Pain or numbness that's worse at night
- Pain on repetitive movements
- Positive Tinel's and Phalen's signs

DX: EMG
TX: Rest, splints, medication (NSAIDs, corticosteroid or lidocaine injections), surgery
F/U: Referral to neurosurgeon or orthopedic surgeon if symptoms persist

ARTHRITIS
Signs and symptoms
- Warmth at site
- Boggy, soft, or fluctuant swelling
- Tenderness
- Limited motion

DX: Wrist X-ray
TX: Medication (ASA, NSAIDs, analgesics), physical therapy
F/U: As needed (dependent on symptoms)

Additional common signs and symptoms
- Pain on repetitive movement
- Paresthesia (possibly)

FRACTURE
Additional signs and symptoms
- Deformity
- Swelling
- Ecchymosis
- Paresthesia

TENDINITIS

TENOSYNOVITIS
Signs and symptoms
- Pain in the radial aspect of the wrist that increases with activity and improves with rest
- Pain on palpation along the radial aspect of the wrist at anatomic snuff box
- Pain on passive ROM of the thumb
- Pain with ulnar deviation of the wrist, with the thumb cupped in a closed fist (positive Finkelstein's test)

DX: Labs (CBC, ESR), MRI
TX: RICE therapy, medication (NSAIDs, corticosteroid or lidocaine injection), thumb-spica wrist splint
F/U: Referral to orthopedic hand specialist

DX: Wrist X-ray
TX: Cast, if fractured; medication (NSAIDs, analgesics), RICE therapy
F/U: Referral to orthopedic surgeon, if fractured; reevaluation in 1 week

---

Additional differential diagnoses: biceps rupture ▪ cellulitis ▪ compartment syndrome ▪ ganglion cyst ▪ Kienböck's disease ▪ muscle contusion ▪ neoplasm of the arm ▪ osteomyelitis

Asterixis

A bilateral, coarse movement, asterixis is characterized by sudden relaxation of muscle groups holding a sustained posture. This elicited sign is most commonly observed in the wrists and fingers but may also appear during sustained voluntary action. Typically, it signals hepatic, renal, or pulmonary disease.

To elicit asterixis, have the patient extend his arms, dorsiflex his wrists, and spread his fingers (or do this for him, if necessary). Briefly watch for asterixis. Alternately, if the patient has a decreased level of consciousness (LOC) but can follow verbal commands, ask him to squeeze two of your fingers. Consider rapid clutching and unclutching positive for asterixis. Alternatively, elevate the patient's leg off the bed and dorsiflex his foot. Briefly watch for asterixis in the ankle. If the patient can tightly close his eyes and mouth, watch for irregular tremulous movements of the eyelids and corners of the mouth. If he can stick out his tongue, look for continuous quivering. (See *Recognizing asterixis.*)

 ALERT

Because asterixis may signal serious metabolic deterioration:
- *quickly evaluate the patient's neurologic status and vital signs; then compare the data to his baseline, and watch carefully for acute changes*
- *continue to closely monitor neurologic status, vital signs, and urine output*
- *watch for signs of respiratory insufficiency, and be prepared to provide endotracheal intubation and ventilatory support*
- *be alert for complications of end-stage hepatic, renal, or pulmonary disease.*

If the patient's condition permits, perform a focused assessment.

HISTORY

- Ask the patient if he has a history of pulmonary, liver, or renal disease. If so, inquire about therapy he has received.
- Ask the patient when the asterixis started.
- Obtain a drug history, including prescription and over-the-counter drugs, herbal remedies, and recreational drugs. Also, ask the patient about alcohol intake.
- If the patient's LOC is significantly decreased, obtain information from his family.

PHYSICAL ASSESSMENT

- Assess the patient for signs and symptoms of hyperkalemia and metabolic acidosis, including tachycardia, nausea, diarrhea, abdominal cramps, muscle weakness, hyperreflexia, and Kussmaul's respirations.
- If the patient has hepatic disease, assess him for early signs of hemorrhage, such as restlessness, tachypnea, and cool, moist, pale skin.
- If the patient has pulmonary disease, assess him for labored respirations, tachypnea, accessory muscle use, and cyanosis, and prepare to provide ventilatory support through a nasal cannula, a mask, or intubation and mechanical ventilation, if necessary.

SPECIAL CONSIDERATIONS

Certain drugs, such as anticonvulsants, can cause asterixis. Provide comfort measures to minimize fatigue and relieve dyspnea or orthopnea.

 PEDIATRIC POINTERS

End-stage hepatic, renal, and pulmonary disease may also cause asterixis in children.

PATIENT COUNSELING

Provide emotional support to the patient and his family.

RECOGNIZING ASTERIXIS

With asterixis, the patient's wrists and fingers appear to "flap" because there's a brief, rapid relaxation of dorsiflexion of the wrist.

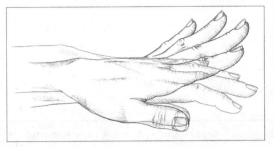

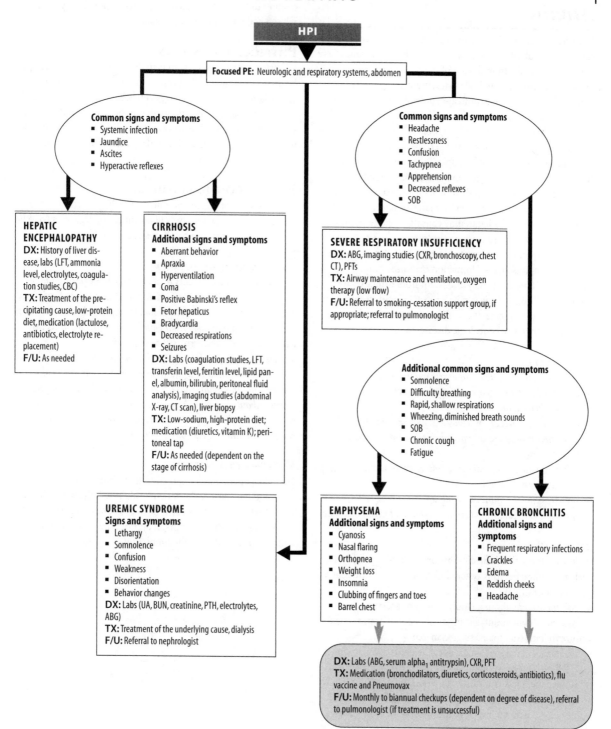

HPI

Focused PE: Neurologic and respiratory systems, abdomen

Common signs and symptoms
- Systemic infection
- Jaundice
- Ascites
- Hyperactive reflexes

Common signs and symptoms
- Headache
- Restlessness
- Confusion
- Tachypnea
- Apprehension
- Decreased reflexes
- SOB

HEPATIC ENCEPHALOPATHY
DX: History of liver disease, labs (LFT, ammonia level, electrolytes, coagulation studies, CBC)
TX: Treatment of the precipitating cause, low-protein diet, medication (lactulose, antibiotics, electrolyte replacement)
F/U: As needed

CIRRHOSIS
Additional signs and symptoms
- Aberrant behavior
- Apraxia
- Hyperventilation
- Coma
- Positive Babinski's reflex
- Fetor hepaticus
- Bradycardia
- Decreased respirations
- Seizures
DX: Labs (coagulation studies, LFT, transferin level, ferritin level, lipid panel, albumin, bilirubin, peritoneal fluid analysis), imaging studies (abdominal X-ray, CT scan), liver biopsy
TX: Low-sodium, high-protein diet; medication (diuretics, vitamin K); peritoneal tap
F/U: As needed (dependent on the stage of cirrhosis)

SEVERE RESPIRATORY INSUFFICIENCY
DX: ABG, imaging studies (CXR, bronchoscopy, chest CT), PFTs
TX: Airway maintenance and ventilation, oxygen therapy (low flow)
F/U: Referral to smoking-cessation support group, if appropriate; referral to pulmonologist

Additional common signs and symptoms
- Somnolence
- Difficulty breathing
- Rapid, shallow respirations
- Wheezing, diminished breath sounds
- SOB
- Chronic cough
- Fatigue

UREMIC SYNDROME
Signs and symptoms
- Lethargy
- Somnolence
- Confusion
- Weakness
- Disorientation
- Behavior changes
DX: Labs (UA, BUN, creatinine, PTH, electrolytes, ABG)
TX: Treatment of the underlying cause, dialysis
F/U: Referral to nephrologist

EMPHYSEMA
Additional signs and symptoms
- Cyanosis
- Nasal flaring
- Orthopnea
- Weight loss
- Insomnia
- Clubbing of fingers and toes
- Barrel chest

CHRONIC BRONCHITIS
Additional signs and symptoms
- Frequent respiratory infections
- Crackles
- Edema
- Reddish cheeks
- Headache

DX: Labs (ABG, serum alpha$_1$ antitrypsin), CXR, PFT
TX: Medication (bronchodilators, diuretics, corticosteroids, antibiotics), flu vaccine and Pneumovax
F/U: Monthly to biannual checkups (dependent on degree of disease), referral to pulmonologist (if treatment is unsuccessful)

Other causes: medication such as phenytoin

Ataxia

Classified as cerebellar or sensory, ataxia refers to incoordination and irregularity of voluntary, purposeful movements. Cerebellar ataxia results from disease of the cerebellum and its pathways to and from the cerebral cortex, brain stem, and spinal cord. It causes gait, trunk, limb and, possibly, speech disorders. Sensory ataxia, which can cause gait disorders, typically results from impaired position sense (proprioception) due to interruption of afferent nerve fibers in the peripheral nerves, posterior roots, posterior columns of the spinal cord, or medial lemnisci. It may also be caused by a lesion in either parietal lobe.

Ataxia occurs in acute and chronic forms. Acute ataxia may result from stroke, hemorrhage, or a large tumor in the posterior fossa. With this life-threatening condition, the cerebellum may herniate downward through the foramen magnum behind the cervical spinal cord or upward through the tentorium on the cerebral hemispheres. Herniation may also compress the brain stem. Acute ataxia may also result from drug toxicity or poisoning. Chronic ataxia can be progressive and, at times, can result from acute disease. It can also occur in metabolic and chronic degenerative neurologic disease.

➤ ALERT

If the patient suddenly develops ataxic movements:
- *examine him for signs of increased intracranial pressure and impending herniation*
- *determine his level of consciousness, and be alert for pupillary changes, motor weakness or paralysis, neck stiffness or pain, and vomiting*
- *check his vital signs (Make sure emergency resuscitation equipment is readily available.)*
- *prepare him for computed tomography scanning or surgery.*
  If the patient's condition permits, perform a focused assessment.

HISTORY

- Review the patient's medical history for multiple sclerosis, diabetes, central nervous system infection, neoplastic disease, and previous stroke.
- Ask the patient about a family history of ataxia.
- Ask the patient about chronic alcohol abuse or prolonged exposure to industrial toxins such as mercury.
- If the patient has gait ataxia, ask if he tends to fall to one side or if falling is more common at night.
- If the patient has truncal ataxia, remember that his inability to walk or stand, combined with the absence of other signs while he's lying down, may give the impression of hysteria or drug or alcohol intoxication.

- Obtain a drug history, including prescription and over-the-counter drugs, herbal remedies, and recreational drugs. Also, ask the patient about alcohol intake.

PHYSICAL ASSESSMENT

- Perform Romberg's test to help distinguish between cerebellar and sensory ataxia. Test results may indicate normal posture and balance (minimal swaying), cerebellar ataxia (swaying and inability to maintain balance with eyes open or closed), or sensory ataxia (increased swaying and inability to maintain balance with eyes closed). Stand close to the patient during this test to prevent him from falling.

SPECIAL CONSIDERATIONS

Toxic levels of an anticonvulsant, especially phenytoin, may result in gait ataxia. Toxic levels of an anticholinergic or a tricyclic antidepressant may also result in ataxia.

 PEDIATRIC POINTERS

- *In children, ataxia occurs in acute and chronic forms and results from congenital or acquired disease. Acute ataxia may stem from febrile infection, a brain tumor, mumps, and other disorders. Chronic ataxia may stem from Gaucher's disease, Refsum's disease, and other inborn errors of metabolism.*
- *When assessing a child for ataxia, consider his motor-skill level and emotional state. Your examination may be limited to observing the child in spontaneous activity and carefully questioning his parents about changes in his motor activity, such as increased unsteadiness or falling. If you suspect ataxia, refer the child for a neurologic evaluation to rule out a brain tumor.*

PATIENT COUNSELING

Help the patient adapt to his condition. Promote rehabilitation goals and help ensure the patient's safety. Ask the patient's family to check the home for hazards, such as uneven surfaces or the absence of handrails on stairs. If appropriate, refer the patient with progressive disease for counseling.

ATAXIA

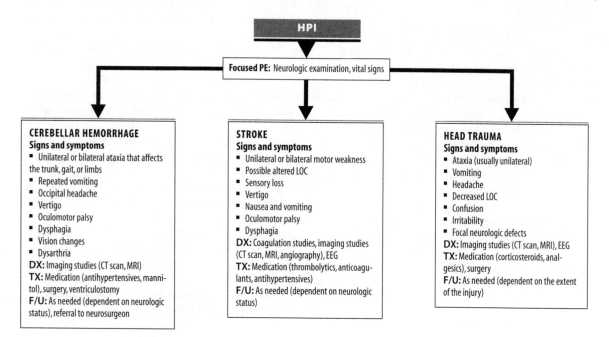

HPI

Focused PE: Neurologic examination, vital signs

CEREBELLAR HEMORRHAGE
Signs and symptoms
- Unilateral or bilateral ataxia that affects the trunk, gait, or limbs
- Repeated vomiting
- Occipital headache
- Vertigo
- Oculomotor palsy
- Dysphagia
- Vision changes
- Dysarthria

DX: Imaging studies (CT scan, MRI)
TX: Medication (antihypertensives, mannitol), surgery, ventriculostomy
F/U: As needed (dependent on neurologic status), referral to neurosurgeon

STROKE
Signs and symptoms
- Unilateral or bilateral motor weakness
- Possible altered LOC
- Sensory loss
- Vertigo
- Nausea and vomiting
- Oculomotor palsy
- Dysphagia

DX: Coagulation studies, imaging studies (CT scan, MRI, angiography), EEG
TX: Medication (thrombolytics, anticoagulants, antihypertensives)
F/U: As needed (dependent on neurologic status)

HEAD TRAUMA
Signs and symptoms
- Ataxia (usually unilateral)
- Vomiting
- Headache
- Decreased LOC
- Confusion
- Irritability
- Focal neurologic defects

DX: Imaging studies (CT scan, MRI), EEG
TX: Medication (corticosteroids, analgesics), surgery
F/U: As needed (dependent on the extent of the injury)

Additional differential diagnoses: cerebellar abscess ▪ Creutzfeldt-Jakob disease ▪ diabetic neuropathy ▪ diphtheria ▪ encephalomyelitis ▪ Friedreich's ataxia ▪ Guillain-Barré syndrome ▪ hepatocerebral degeneration ▪ hyperthermia ▪ metastatic cancer ▪ multiple sclerosis ▪ olivopontocerebellar atrophy ▪ poisoning ▪ polyarteritis nodosa ▪ polyneuropathy ▪ porphyria ▪ posterior fossa tumor ▪ spinocerebellar ataxia ▪ syringomyelia ▪ Wernicke's disease

Other causes: aminoglutethimide ▪ anticholinergics ▪ anticonvulsants (phenytoin) ▪ tricyclic antidepressants

Athetosis

Athetosis, an extrapyramidal sign, is characterized by slow, continuous, twisting, involuntary movements. Typically, these movements involve the face, neck, and distal extremities, such as the forearm, wrist, and hand. Facial grimaces, jaw and tongue movements, and occasional phonation are associated with neck movements. Athetosis worsens during stress and voluntary activity, may subside during relaxation, and disappears during sleep. Commonly a lifelong affliction, athetosis is sometimes difficult to distinguish from chorea (hence the term choreoathetosis). Typically, however, athetoid movements are slower than choreiform movements.

Athetosis usually begins during childhood, resulting from hypoxia at birth, kernicterus, or a genetic disorder. In adults, athetosis usually results from a vascular or neoplastic lesion, a degenerative disease, drug toxicity, or hypoxia. (See *Distinguishing athetosis from chorea*.)

DISTINGUISHING ATHETOSIS FROM CHOREA

With *athetosis*, movements are typically slow, twisting, and writhing. They're associated with spasticity and most commonly involve the face, neck, and distal extremities.

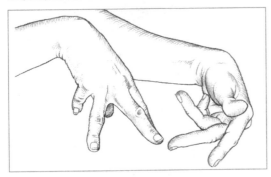

With *chorea*, movements are brief, rapid, jerky, and unpredictable. They can occur at rest or during normal movement. Typically, they involve the hands, lower arm, face, and head.

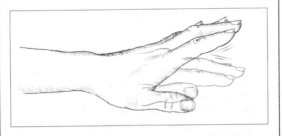

HISTORY

● Take a comprehensive prenatal and postnatal history, covering maternal and child health, labor and delivery, and possible trauma.
● Obtain a family health history because many genetic disorders can cause athetosis.
● Ask the patient about current drug therapy.
● Ask the patient about the decline in his functional abilities: When was he last able to roll over, sit up, or carry out daily activities?
● Ask the patient what problem — uncontrollable movements, mental deterioration, or a speech impediment — prompted him to seek medical help.
● Ask the patient about the effects of rest, stress, and routine activity on his symptoms.

PHYSICAL ASSESSMENT

● Test muscle strength and tone, range of motion, fine muscle movements, and ability to perform rapidly alternating movements.
● Observe the limb muscles during voluntary movements, noting the rhythm and duration of contraction and relaxation.

SPECIAL CONSIDERATIONS

Occasionally, athetosis can be prevented or treated by decreasing body copper stores in Wilson's disease or by adjusting drug dosages. Typically, though, it has a lifelong impact on the patient's ability to carry out even routine activities.

Ⓐ PEDIATRIC POINTERS

Childhood athetosis may be acquired or inherited. It can result from hypoxia at birth, which causes an athetoid cerebral palsy, kernicterus, Sydenham's chorea (in school-age children), and paroxysmal choreoathetosis. Inherited causes of athetosis include Lesch-Nyhan syndrome, Tay-Sachs disease, and phenylketonuria.

PATIENT COUNSELING

Help the patient develop self-esteem and a positive self-image. Encourage him and his family to set realistic goals. As appropriate, refer the patient to special education services, rehabilitation centers, and support services and groups. Provide him with emotional support during the frequent medical evaluations he'll be required to undergo.

ATHETOSIS

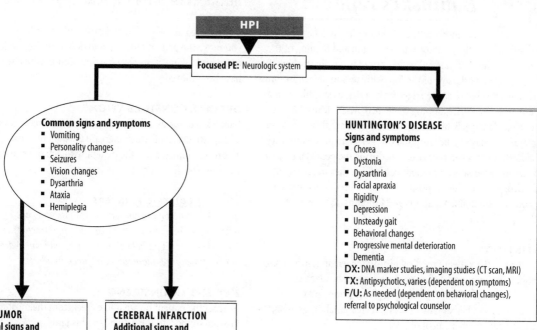

HPI

Focused PE: Neurologic system

Common signs and symptoms
- Vomiting
- Personality changes
- Seizures
- Vision changes
- Dysarthria
- Ataxia
- Hemiplegia

HUNTINGTON'S DISEASE
Signs and symptoms
- Chorea
- Dystonia
- Dysarthria
- Facial apraxia
- Rigidity
- Depression
- Unsteady gait
- Behavioral changes
- Progressive mental deterioration
- Dementia

DX: DNA marker studies, imaging studies (CT scan, MRI)
TX: Antipsychotics, varies (dependent on symptoms)
F/U: As needed (dependent on behavioral changes), referral to psychological counselor

BRAIN TUMOR
Additional signs and symptoms (vary with type of tumor and degree of invasion)
- Contralateral choreoathetosis and dystonia
- Headache
- Malaise

DX: Imaging studies (CT scan, MRI, angiography), CT guided biopsy
TX: Medication (chemotherapy, corticosteroids, osmotic diuretics, anticonvulsants, analgesics), surgery, radiation therapy
F/U: As needed (dependent on neurologic status), referrals to oncologist and neurosurgeon

CEREBRAL INFARCTION
Additional signs and symptoms
- Contralateral athetosis
- Altered LOC
- Contralateral paralysis of the face or limbs
- Weakness
- Language difficulties
- Memory loss
- Dysphagia

DX: Imaging studies (CT scan, MRI, carotid ultrasound)
TX: Medication (anticoagulant, antihypertensives), surgery
F/U: As needed (dependent on neurologic status), referral to neurologist

---

Additional differential diagnoses: calcification of the basal ganglia ▪ hepatic encephalopathy ▪ Wilson's disease

Other causes: levodopa ▪ phenothiazines and other antipsychotics ▪ phenytoin

B Babinski's reflex

Babinski's reflex (extensor plantar reflex) involves dorsiflexion of the great toe with extension and fanning of the other toes. It's an abnormal reflex elicited by firmly stroking the lateral aspect of the sole of the foot with a blunt object. In some patients, this reflex can be triggered by noxious stimuli, such as pain, noise, or even bumping of the bed. An indicator of corticospinal damage, Babinski's reflex may occur unilaterally or bilaterally. It may also be temporary or permanent. A temporary Babinski's reflex commonly occurs during the postictal phase of a seizure, whereas a permanent Babinski's reflex occurs with corticospinal damage. A positive Babinski's reflex is normal in neonates and in infants up to age 24 months. (See *Positive Babinski's reflex.*)

HISTORY
- Review the patient's medical history for seizures, incoordination, muscle spasms, difficulty speaking, and headache.
- Obtain a drug history, including prescription and over-the-counter drugs, herbal remedies, and recreational drugs. Also, ask the patient about alcohol intake.
- Ask the patient if he has experienced nausea, vomiting, fever, or neck pain.
- Ask the patient if he has suffered recent head trauma.

PHYSICAL ASSESSMENT
- Evaluate muscle strength in each extremity by asking the patient to push or pull against your resistance.
- Check for evidence of incoordination by asking the patient to perform a repetitive activity.

- Test deep tendon reflexes in the patient's elbow, antecubital area, wrist, knee, and ankle by striking the tendon with a reflex hammer.
- Evaluate pain sensation and proprioception in the feet. As you move the patient's toes up and down, ask him to identify (without looking at his feet) the direction in which the toes have been moved.

SPECIAL CONSIDERATIONS
Babinski's reflex usually occurs with incoordination, weakness, and spasticity, all of which increase the patient's risk of injury. To prevent injury, assist the patient with activity and keep his environment free from obstructions.

Ⓐ PEDIATRIC POINTERS
Babinski's reflex occurs normally in infants up to age 24 months, reflecting the immaturity of the corticospinal tract. After age 2, Babinski's reflex is pathologic and may result from hydrocephalus or one of the causes more commonly seen in adults.

PATIENT COUNSELING
Instruct the patient on what to expect from diagnostic testing. Provide support to the patient and his family.

POSITIVE BABINSKI'S REFLEX

With a positive Babinski's reflex, the great toe dorsiflexes and the other toes fan out, as shown below right.

NORMAL TOE FLEXION

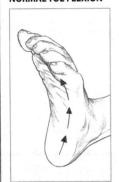

POSITIVE BABINSKI'S REFLEX

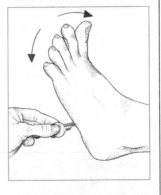

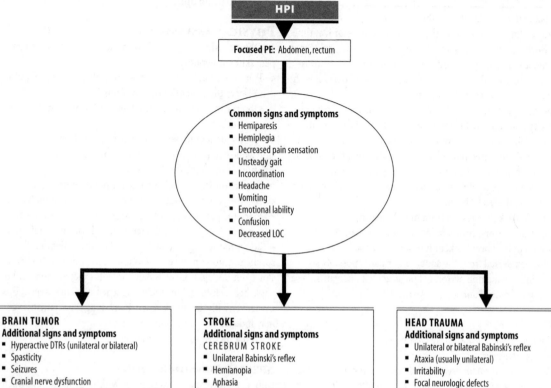

HPI

Focused PE: Abdomen, rectum

Common signs and symptoms
- Hemiparesis
- Hemiplegia
- Decreased pain sensation
- Unsteady gait
- Incoordination
- Headache
- Vomiting
- Emotional lability
- Confusion
- Decreased LOC

BRAIN TUMOR
Additional signs and symptoms
- Hyperactive DTRs (unilateral or bilateral)
- Spasticity
- Seizures
- Cranial nerve dysfunction

DX: Imaging studies (CT scan, MRI, angiography), CT guided biopsy
TX: Medication (chemotherapy, corticosteroids, osmotic diuretics, anticonvulsants, analgesics), surgery, radiation therapy
F/U: As needed (dependent on neurologic status), referrals to oncologist and neurosurgeon

STROKE
Additional signs and symptoms
CEREBRUM STROKE
- Unilateral Babinski's reflex
- Hemianopia
- Aphasia
BRAINSTEM STROKE
- Bilateral Babinski's reflex
- Cranial nerve dysfunction

DX: Imaging studies (CT scan, MRI, angiography)
TX: Medication (thrombolytics; if embolic, anticoagulants; antihypertensives), surgery for hemorrhagic stroke
F/U: As needed (dependent on neurologic status), referral to neurologist

HEAD TRAUMA
Additional signs and symptoms
- Unilateral or bilateral Babinski's reflex
- Ataxia (usually unilateral)
- Irritability
- Focal neurologic defects
- Hyperactive DTRs
- Spasticity
- Weakness

DX: Imaging studies (CT scan, MRI), EEG
TX: Medication (corticosteroids, analgesics), surgery
F/U: As needed (dependent on extent of injury)

Additional differential diagnoses: ALS ▪ cervical lesion ▪ cervical stenosis ▪ familial spastic paraparesis ▪ Friedreich's ataxia ▪ hepatic encephalopathy ▪ meningitis ▪ multiple sclerosis ▪ pernicious anemia ▪ rabies ▪ spinal cord injury ▪ spinal cord tumor ▪ spinal paralytic poliomyelitis ▪ spinal tuberculosis ▪ syringomyelia

Back pain

Back pain affects about 80% of the U.S. population, and it's the second-leading reason — after the common cold — for lost time from work. Although this symptom may herald a spondylogenic disorder, it may also result from a genitourinary, GI, cardiovascular, or neoplastic disorder. Postural imbalance associated with pregnancy may also cause back pain.

The onset, location, and distribution of pain and its response to activity and rest provide important clues about the causative disorder. Pain may be acute or chronic, constant or intermittent. It may remain localized in the back or radiate along the spine or down one or both legs. Pain may be exacerbated by activity — usually, bending, stooping, or lifting — and alleviated by rest, or it may be unaffected by both.

Intrinsic back pain results from muscle spasm, nerve root irritation, fracture, or a combination of these mechanisms. It usually occurs in the lower back, or lumbosacral area. Back pain may also be referred from the abdomen or flank, possibly signaling a life-threatening perforated ulcer, acute pancreatitis, or a dissecting abdominal aortic aneurysm.

ALERT

If the patient reports acute, severe back pain:
- *take his vital signs*
- *ask him when the pain began and if he can relate it to a cause.*
 If the patient describes deep lumbar pain unaffected by activity:
- *palpate for a pulsating epigastric mass; if this sign is present, suspect dissecting abdominal aortic aneurysm.*
 If the patient describes severe epigastric pain that radiates through the abdomen to the back:
- *assess him for absent bowel sounds and for abdominal rigidity and tenderness; if these occur, suspect a perforated ulcer or acute pancreatitis.*
 If life-threatening causes of acute back pain are ruled out, perform a focused assessment.

HISTORY
- Review the patient's medical history for past injuries and illnesses, and ask the patient for a family history.
- Ask the patient about activities that may affect the back.
- Obtain a drug history, including prescription and over-the-counter drugs, herbal remedies, and recreational drugs. Also, ask the patient about alcohol intake.
- Ask the patient to describe the pain. Is it burning, stabbing, throbbing, or aching? Is it constant or intermittent? Does it radiate to the buttocks or legs? Any leg weakness? Or does the pain seem to originate in the abdomen and radiate to the back?
- Ask the patient about unusual sensations in his legs, such as numbness and tingling.
- Ask the patient if he has had pain like this before.
- Ask the patient if anything makes it better or worse. Is it affected by activity or rest? Is it worse in the morning or evening? Does it wake him up?

PHYSICAL ASSESSMENT
- Observe skin color, especially in the patient's legs, and palpate skin temperature.
- Palpate femoral, popliteal, posterior tibial, and pedal pulses.
- Observe the patient's posture, if possible.
- Observe the level of the shoulders and pelvis and the curvature of the back.
- Ask the patient to bend forward, backward, and from side to side while you palpate for paravertebral muscle spasms. Note rotation of the spine on the trunk.
- Palpate the dorsolumbar spine for point tenderness.
- Ask the patient to walk — first on his heels, then on his toes.
- Place the patient in a sitting position to evaluate and compare patellar tendon, Achilles tendon, and Babinski's reflexes.
- To reproduce leg and back pain, place the patient in the supine position on the examination table. Grasp his heel and slowly lift his leg. If he feels pain, note its exact location and the angle between the table and his leg when it occurs. Repeat this maneuver with the opposite leg. Pain along the sciatic nerve may indicate disk herniation or sciatica.
- Note range of motion of the hip and knee.

SPECIAL CONSIDERATIONS
Until a tentative diagnosis is made, withhold analgesics, which may mask symptoms. Also withhold food and fluids in case surgery is necessary.

Be aware that back pain is notoriously associated with malingering.

PEDIATRIC POINTERS
- *Because a child may have difficulty describing back pain, be alert for nonverbal clues, such as wincing or refusing to walk.*
- *While taking the patient's history, closely observe family dynamics for clues suggesting child abuse.*
- *Back pain in a child may stem from intervertebral disk inflammation (diskitis), a neoplasm, idiopathic juvenile osteoporosis, or spondylolisthesis.*

AGING ISSUES
Suspect metastatic cancer, especially of the prostate, if the patient is older than age 55 with a recent onset of back pain that usually isn't relieved by rest and worsens at night.

PATIENT COUNSELING
Teach the patient pain-relief measures as an alternative to taking an analgesic. Refer the patient to physical therapy, occupational therapy, a psychologist, or support groups, as appropriate.

BACK PAIN

HPI

Focused PE: Neurovascular and musculoskeletal systems

ABDOMINAL AORTIC ANEURYSM (DISSECTING)
Signs and symptoms
- Lower back pain or dull abdominal pain (initially)
- Constant upper abdominal pain (more common)
- Pulsating abdominal mass in the epigastrium (no longer pulsates after rupture)
- Mottled skin below the waist
- Absent femoral and pedal pulses
- Lower BP in the legs than in the arms
- Mild to moderate tenderness with guarding and abdominal rigidity
- Signs of shock

DX: CBC, imaging studies (abdominal X-ray, CT scan, MRI, angiography)
TX: Maintenance of stable hemodynamic status, medication (antihypertensives, analgesics), surgery
F/U: Referral to vascular surgeon

Common signs and symptoms
- Gradual or sudden lower back pain with or without leg pain
- Pain that's exacerbated by activity, coughing, and sneezing
- Pain that's relieved by rest
- Stiffness

ANKYLOSING SPONDYLITIS
Signs and symptoms
- Sacroiliac pain that travels up the spine and is aggravated by lateral pressure on the pelvis
- Pain that's most severe in the morning or after inactivity
- Pain that's unrelieved by rest
- Local tenderness
- Fatigue
- Fever
- Anorexia
- Weight loss
- Iritis (occasional)

DX: Labs (histocompatibility antigens, HLA-B27, ESR, CBC), imaging studies (spinal and pelvic X-rays)
TX: NSAIDs, physical therapy, surgery (for severe joint damage and pain)
F/U: Return visit in 6 to 12 months for evaluation of posture and ROM

LUMBOSACRAL SPRAIN
Additional sign
- History of recent back injury

INTERVERTEBRAL DISK DISORDER
Additional signs and symptoms
- Positive sciatic scratch test
- Positive cross straight-leg raising sign
- Paresthesia

DX: Imaging studies (spinal X-ray, CT scan, MRI, myelogram), EMG, nerve conduction velocity test
TX: Bed rest, medication (analgesics, NSAIDs, muscle relaxants), surgery (for disk disorder), physical therapy
F/U: Reevaluation 10 days after treatment, then again in 2 months; referral to neurosurgeon

---

Additional differential diagnoses: acute cauda equina ▪ appendicitis ▪ cholecystitis ▪ chordoma ▪ endometriosis ▪ metastatic tumors ▪ myeloma ▪ pancreatitis (acute) ▪ perforated ulcer ▪ prostate cancer ▪ pyelonephritis (acute) ▪ Reiter's syndrome ▪ renal calculi ▪ sacroiliac strain ▪ spinal neoplasm (benign) ▪ spinal stenosis ▪ spondylolisthesis ▪ transverse process fracture ▪ vertebral compression fracture ▪ vertebral osteomyelitis ▪ vertebral osteoporosis

Other causes: neurologic tests, such as lumbar puncture and myelography

Barrel chest

With barrel chest, the normal elliptical configuration of the chest is replaced by a rounded one in which the anteroposterior diameter enlarges to approximate the transverse diameter. The diaphragm is depressed and the sternum is pushed forward with the ribs attached in a horizontal, not angular, fashion. As a result, the chest appears continuously in the inspiratory position. (See *Recognizing barrel chest.*)

Typically a late sign of chronic obstructive pulmonary disease (COPD), barrel chest results from augmented lung volumes due to chronic airflow obstruction. The patient may not notice it because it develops gradually.

RECOGNIZING BARREL CHEST

For a normal adult chest, the ratio of anteroposterior to transverse (or lateral) diameter is 1:2. For a patient with barrel chest, the ratio approaches 1:1 as the anteroposterior diameter enlarges.

NORMAL CHEST   **BARREL CHEST**

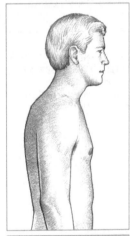
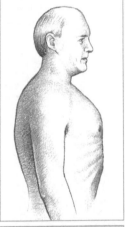
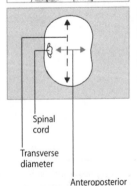
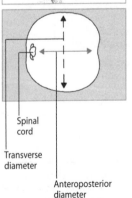

Spinal cord

Transverse diameter

Anteroposterior diameter

Spinal cord

Transverse diameter

Anteroposterior diameter

HISTORY
- Ask the patient about a history of pulmonary disease. Note chronic exposure to environmental irritants such as asbestos.
- Ask the patient if he smokes. If so, find out how much.
- Ask the patient if he has a cough. Is it productive or nonproductive? If it's productive, have him describe the sputum color, amount, and consistency.
- Ask the patient if he experiences shortness of breath. Is it related to activity?

PHYSICAL ASSESSMENT
- Observe the patient's general appearance. Look for central cyanosis in the cheeks, nose, and mucosa inside the lips. Also look for peripheral cyanosis in the nail beds. Note clubbing, a late sign of COPD.
- Observe the patient for accessory muscle use, intercostal retractions, and tachypnea.
- Auscultate for abnormal breath sounds, such as crackles and wheezes.
- Percuss the chest; hyperresonant sounds indicate trapped air, whereas dull or flat sounds indicate mucus buildup.

SPECIAL CONSIDERATIONS
To ease breathing, have the patient sit and lean forward, resting his hands on his knees to support the upper torso (tripod position).

🅰 PEDIATRIC POINTERS
- *In infants, the ratio of anteroposterior to transverse diameter normally approximates 1:1. As the child grows, this ratio gradually changes, reaching 1:2 by ages 5 and 6.*
- *Cystic fibrosis and chronic asthma may cause barrel chest in a child.*

AGING ISSUES
In elderly patients, senile kyphosis of the thoracic spine may be mistaken for barrel chest. However, unlike barrel chest, patients with senile kyphosis lack signs of pulmonary disease.

PATIENT COUNSELING
Advise the patient to avoid bronchial irritants, especially smoking, which may exacerbate COPD. Tell him to report purulent sputum production. Instruct him to space his activities to help minimize exertional dyspnea.

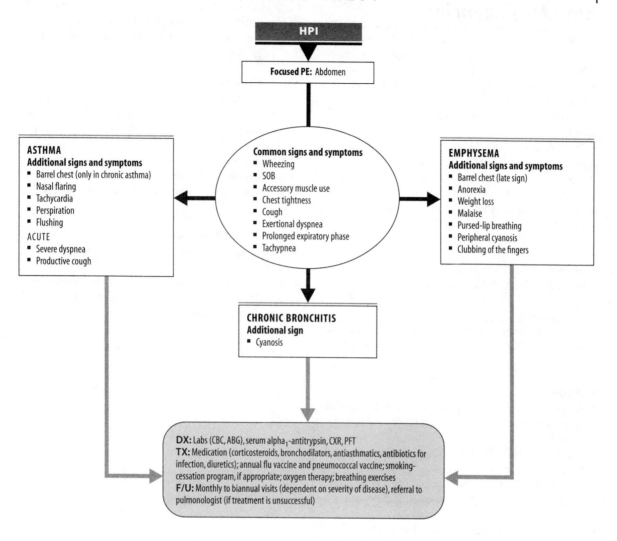

HPI

Focused PE: Abdomen

Common signs and symptoms
- Wheezing
- SOB
- Accessory muscle use
- Chest tightness
- Cough
- Exertional dyspnea
- Prolonged expiratory phase
- Tachypnea

ASTHMA
Additional signs and symptoms
- Barrel chest (only in chronic asthma)
- Nasal flaring
- Tachycardia
- Perspiration
- Flushing

ACUTE
- Severe dyspnea
- Productive cough

EMPHYSEMA
Additional signs and symptoms
- Barrel chest (late sign)
- Anorexia
- Weight loss
- Malaise
- Pursed-lip breathing
- Peripheral cyanosis
- Clubbing of the fingers

CHRONIC BRONCHITIS
Additional sign
- Cyanosis

DX: Labs (CBC, ABG), serum alpha$_1$-antitrypsin, CXR, PFT
TX: Medication (corticosteroids, bronchodilators, antiasthmatics, antibiotics for infection, diuretics); annual flu vaccine and pneumococcal vaccine; smoking-cessation program, if appropriate; oxygen therapy; breathing exercises
F/U: Monthly to biannual visits (dependent on severity of disease), referral to pulmonologist (if treatment is unsuccessful)

Bladder distention

Bladder distention—abnormal enlargement of the bladder—results from an inability to excrete urine, leading to its accumulation. Distention can be caused by mechanical or anatomic obstruction, a neuromuscular disorder, or the use of certain drugs. Relatively common in all ages and in both sexes, it's most common in older men with prostate disorders that cause urine retention.

Bladder distention usually develops gradually, but occasionally its onset is sudden. Gradual distention usually remains asymptomatic until stretching of the bladder produces discomfort. Acute distention produces suprapubic fullness, pressure, and pain. If severe distention isn't corrected promptly by catheterization or massage, the bladder rises within the abdomen, its walls become thin, and renal function can be impaired.

Bladder distention is aggravated by intake of caffeine, alcohol, large quantities of fluid, and diuretics.

➤ ALERT

If bladder distention is severe, immediately arrange for bladder catheterization. If bladder distention isn't severe, perform a focused assessment.

HISTORY

- Review the patient's voiding patterns. Ask him if he has difficulty urinating. Does he use Valsalva's or Credé's maneuver to initiate urination?
- Ask the patient if he has urinary urgency or frequency. Is urination painful or irritating?
- Ask the patient about the force and continuity of his urine stream and whether he feels that his bladder is empty after voiding.
- Review the patient's medical history for urinary tract obstruction or infections; venereal disease; neurologic, intestinal, or pelvic surgery; lower abdominal or urinary tract trauma; and systemic or neurologic disorders.
- Obtain a drug history, including prescription and over-the-counter drugs, herbal remedies, and recreational drugs. Also, ask the patient about alcohol intake.

PHYSICAL ASSESSMENT

- Take the patient's vital signs.
- Percuss and palpate the bladder.
- Inspect the urethral meatus. Describe the appearance and amount of discharge.

SPECIAL CONSIDERATIONS

Use of an indwelling catheter can result in urine retention and bladder distention if the tubing is kinked or occluded.

If interventions fail to relieve bladder distention or obstruction, the patient will need surgical intervention.

PEDIATRIC POINTERS

- *Look for urine retention and bladder distention in any infant who fails to void normal amounts. (In the first 48 hours of life, a neonate excretes about 60 ml of urine; during the next week, he excretes about 300 ml of urine daily.)*
- *In males, posterior urethral valves, meatal stenosis, phimosis, spinal cord anomalies, bladder diverticula, and other congenital defects can cause urinary obstruction and resultant bladder distention.*

PATIENT COUNSELING

Provide privacy to the patient to help him assume a normal voiding position. Teach him to perform Credé's maneuver, stroke or apply ice to the inner thigh, or relax in a warm tub or sitz bath. Use the power of suggestion to stimulate voiding, such as tapes of aquatic sounds.

BLADDER DISTENTION

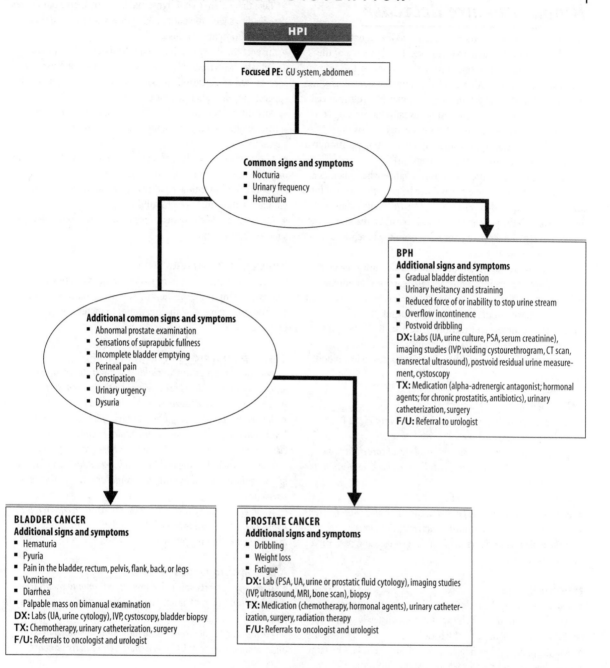

HPI

Focused PE: GU system, abdomen

Common signs and symptoms
- Nocturia
- Urinary frequency
- Hematuria

BPH
Additional signs and symptoms
- Gradual bladder distention
- Urinary hesitancy and straining
- Reduced force of or inability to stop urine stream
- Overflow incontinence
- Postvoid dribbling

DX: Labs (UA, urine culture, PSA, serum creatinine), imaging studies (IVP, voiding cystourethrogram, CT scan, transrectal ultrasound), postvoid residual urine measurement, cystoscopy
TX: Medication (alpha-adrenergic antagonist; hormonal agents; for chronic prostatitis, antibiotics), urinary catheterization, surgery
F/U: Referral to urologist

Additional common signs and symptoms
- Abnormal prostate examination
- Sensations of suprapubic fullness
- Incomplete bladder emptying
- Perineal pain
- Constipation
- Urinary urgency
- Dysuria

BLADDER CANCER
Additional signs and symptoms
- Hematuria
- Pyuria
- Pain in the bladder, rectum, pelvis, flank, back, or legs
- Vomiting
- Diarrhea
- Palpable mass on bimanual examination

DX: Labs (UA, urine cytology), IVP, cystoscopy, bladder biopsy
TX: Chemotherapy, urinary catheterization, surgery
F/U: Referrals to oncologist and urologist

PROSTATE CANCER
Additional signs and symptoms
- Dribbling
- Weight loss
- Fatigue

DX: Lab (PSA, UA, urine or prostatic fluid cytology), imaging studies (IVP, ultrasound, MRI, bone scan), biopsy
TX: Medication (chemotherapy, hormonal agents), urinary catheterization, surgery, radiation therapy
F/U: Referrals to oncologist and urologist

Additional differential diagnoses: bladder calculi ▪ multiple sclerosis ▪ prostatitis ▪ spinal neoplasms ▪ urethral calculi ▪ urethral stricture

Other causes: anesthetics ▪ anticholinergics ▪ catheterization ▪ ganglionic blockers ▪ opiates ▪ parasympatholytics ▪ sedatives

Blood pressure decrease

Low blood pressure (hypotension) refers to inadequate intravascular pressure to maintain the oxygen requirements of the body's tissues. Although commonly linked to shock, this sign may also result from cardiovascular, respiratory, neurologic, and metabolic disorders. Low blood pressure may be drug-induced or may accompany diagnostic tests — usually, those using contrast media. It may stem from stress or change of position — specifically, rising abruptly from a supine or sitting position to a standing position (orthostatic hypotension).

Normal blood pressure varies considerably; what qualifies as low blood pressure for one person may be perfectly normal for another. Consequently, every blood pressure reading must be compared with the patient's baseline. Typically, a reading below 90/60 mm Hg or a drop of 30 mm Hg from the baseline is considered low blood pressure.

Low blood pressure can reflect an expanded intravascular space (as with severe infections, allergic reactions, or adrenal insufficiency), reduced intravascular volume (as with dehydration and hemorrhage), or decreased cardiac output (as with impaired cardiac muscle contractility). Because the body's pressure-regulating mechanisms are complex and interrelated, a combination of these factors usually contributes to low blood pressure.

 ALERT

If the patient's systolic pressure is less than 80 mm Hg or is 30 mm Hg below his baseline:
- *quickly evaluate him for a decreased level of consciousness*
- *check the apical pulse for tachycardia and check respirations for tachypnea*
- *inspect for cool, clammy skin*
- *elevate his legs above the level of his heart or place him in Trendelenburg's position and institute emergency measures.*

If the patient's blood pressure isn't dangerously low, perform a focused assessment.

HISTORY
- Ask the patient if he feels unusually weak or fatigued.
- Ask the patient if he has blurred vision, unsteady gait, chest or abdominal pain, or difficulty breathing.
- Ask the patient if he's had episodes of dizziness. Has he fainted? Do these episodes occur when he stands up suddenly?
- Obtain a drug history, including prescription and over-the-counter drugs, herbal remedies, and recreational drugs. Also, ask the patient about alcohol intake.

PHYSICAL ASSESSMENT
- Take the patient's vital signs, making sure to take blood pressure readings with the patient lying down, sitting, and then standing. Compare readings.
- Inspect the skin for pallor, diaphoresis, and clamminess.
- Palpate the peripheral pulses. Note paradoxical pulse — an accentuated fall in systolic pressure during inspiration, which suggests pericardial tamponade.
- Auscultate for abnormal heart sounds, rate, or rhythm.
- Auscultate the lungs for abnormal breath sounds, rate, or rhythm.
- Look for signs of hemorrhage, including visible bleeding and palpable masses, bruising, and tenderness.
- Check for abdominal rigidity and rebound tenderness; auscultate for abnormal bowel sounds.
- Carefully assess the patient for possible sources of infection such as open wounds.

SPECIAL CONSIDERATIONS
Check the patient's vital signs to determine if low blood pressure is constant or intermittent. The patient may need drug therapy (for example, with dopamine) to increase his blood pressure.

 PEDIATRIC POINTERS
- *Normal blood pressure for children is lower than that for adults. Because accidents are common with children, suspect trauma or shock first as a possible cause of low blood pressure.*
- *Remember that low blood pressure typically doesn't accompany head injury in adults because intracranial hemorrhage is insufficient to cause hypovolemia. However, it does accompany head injury in infants and young children; their expandable cranial vaults allow significant blood loss into the cranial space, resulting in hypovolemia.*
- *Another common cause of low blood pressure in children is dehydration, which results from failure to thrive or from persistent diarrhea and vomiting for as little as 24 hours.*

 AGING ISSUES
- *In elderly patients, low blood pressure commonly results from using multiple drugs that have low blood pressure as an adverse effect.*
- *Orthostatic hypotension due to autonomic dysfunction is another common cause of low blood pressure in elderly patients.*

PATIENT COUNSELING
If the patient has orthostatic hypotension, instruct him to stand up slowly. If the patient has vasovagal syncope, advise him to avoid situations that trigger episodes. Evaluate the patient's need for a cane or walker.

BLOOD PRESSURE DECREASE

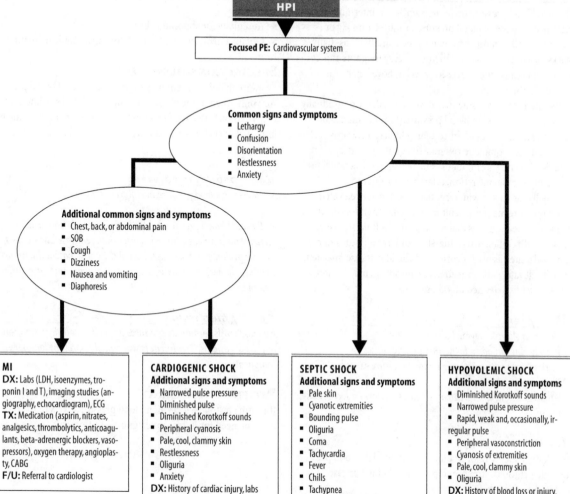

HPI

Focused PE: Cardiovascular system

Common signs and symptoms
- Lethargy
- Confusion
- Disorientation
- Restlessness
- Anxiety

Additional common signs and symptoms
- Chest, back, or abdominal pain
- SOB
- Cough
- Dizziness
- Nausea and vomiting
- Diaphoresis

MI
DX: Labs (LDH, isoenzymes, troponin I and T), imaging studies (angiography, echocardiogram), ECG
TX: Medication (aspirin, nitrates, analgesics, thrombolytics, anticoagulants, beta-adrenergic blockers, vasopressors), oxygen therapy, angioplasty, CABG
F/U: Referral to cardiologist

CARDIOGENIC SHOCK
Additional signs and symptoms
- Narrowed pulse pressure
- Diminished pulse
- Diminished Korotkoff sounds
- Peripheral cyanosis
- Pale, cool, clammy skin
- Restlessness
- Oliguria
- Anxiety
DX: History of cardiac injury, labs (ABG, cardiac markers), imaging studies (echocardiogram, angiography, nuclear scan), pulmonary artery catheterization
TX: Medication (vasopressors, inotropics), oxygen therapy, I.V. fluids, IABP
F/U: Referral to cardiologist

SEPTIC SHOCK
Additional signs and symptoms
- Pale skin
- Cyanotic extremities
- Bounding pulse
- Oliguria
- Coma
- Tachycardia
- Fever
- Chills
- Tachypnea
- Narrowed pulse pressure
DX: Labs (ABG, blood cultures), pulmonary artery catheterization
TX: Medication (vasopressors, antibiotics), oxygen therapy, I.V. fluids
F/U: Return visit 1 week after discharge from hospital

HYPOVOLEMIC SHOCK
Additional signs and symptoms
- Diminished Korotkoff sounds
- Narrowed pulse pressure
- Rapid, weak and, occasionally, irregular pulse
- Peripheral vasoconstriction
- Cyanosis of extremities
- Pale, cool, clammy skin
- Oliguria
DX: History of blood loss or injury, CBC, imaging studies (CT scan, MRI, X-rays of suspected areas)
TX: I.V. fluids, blood products, medication (vasopressors, inotropics)
F/U: Return visit 1 week after discharge from hospital

Additional differential diagnoses: acute adrenal insufficiency ▪ alcohol toxicity ▪ anaphylactic shock ▪ cardiac arrhythmias ▪ cardiac contusion ▪ cardiac tamponade ▪ cardiomyopathy ▪ diabetic ketoacidosis ▪ heart failure ▪ hyperosmolar hyperglycemic nonketotic coma ▪ hypoxemia ▪ MI ▪ neurogenic shock ▪ pulmonary embolism ▪ vasovagal syncope

Other causes: alpha- and beta-adrenergic blockers ▪ antianxiety agents such as benzodiazepines ▪ calcium channel blockers ▪ diuretics ▪ gastric acid stimulation test with histamine ▪ general anesthetics ▪ MAO inhibitors ▪ most I.V. antiarrhythmics ▪ opioid analgesic ▪ tranquilizers ▪ vasodilators ▪ X-ray studies with contrast media

Blood pressure increase

Elevated blood pressure (hypertension)—an intermittent or sustained increase in blood pressure to 140/90 mm Hg or greater—strikes more men than women and twice as many blacks as whites. For many patients, it's easy to ignore this common sign because they can't see or feel it; however, its causes can be life-threatening.

Elevated blood pressure may develop suddenly or gradually. A sudden, severe rise in blood pressure (to more than 200/120 mm Hg) indicates life-threatening hypertensive crisis. However, even a less-dramatic rise may be equally significant if it heralds dissecting aortic aneurysm, increased intracranial pressure, a myocardial infarction, eclampsia, or thyrotoxicosis.

Usually associated with essential hypertension, elevated blood pressure may also result from a renal or endocrine disorder; a treatment, such as dialysis, that affects fluid status; or therapy with certain drugs. Ingestion of large amounts of certain foods, such as black licorice and cheddar cheese, may temporarily elevate blood pressure. Serial readings may be necessary to establish elevated blood pressure.

 ALERT

If you detect sharply elevated blood pressure:
- *quickly rule out possible life-threatening causes*
- *initiate emergency measures if blood pressure exceeds 200/120 mm Hg.*

After ruling out life-threatening causes, perform a focused assessment.

HISTORY
- Ask the patient about a family history of high blood pressure, pheochromocytoma, and polycystic kidney disease.
- Ask the patient his age.
- Ask the patient if he has experienced headache, palpitations, blurred vision, or sweating.
- Ask the patient if he has experienced punch-colored urine or decreased urine output.
- Obtain a drug history, including prescription and over-the-counter drugs (especially decongestants), herbal remedies, and recreational drugs. Also, ask the patient about alcohol intake.
- If the patient is already taking an antihypertensive, determine how well he complies with the regime.

PHYSICAL ASSESSMENT
- Take the patient's blood pressure while he's lying in a supine position, sitting, and standing.
- Check for carotid bruits and neck vein distention.
- Assess skin color, temperature, and turgor.
- Palpate peripheral pulses.

- Auscultate for abnormal heart sounds, rate, and rhythm.
- Auscultate for abnormal breath sounds, rate, and rhythm.
- Palpate the abdomen for tenderness, masses, or liver enlargement.
- Auscultate for abdominal bruits.
- Obtain a urine sample to check for microscopic hematuria.

SPECIAL CONSIDERATIONS
Be aware that the patient may experience elevated blood pressure only when in the physician's office (known as "white coat" hypertension). Twenty-four-hour blood pressure monitoring is indicated in such cases to confirm elevated readings in other settings.

 PEDIATRIC POINTERS
- *Normally, blood pressure in children is lower than that in adults.*
- *Elevated blood pressure in children may result from lead or mercury poisoning, essential hypertension, renovascular stenosis, chronic pyelonephritis, coarctation of the aorta, patent ductus arteriosus, glomerulonephritis, adrenogenital syndrome, or neuroblastoma.*

AGING ISSUES
Atherosclerosis commonly produces isolated systolic hypertension in elderly patients. Treatment is warranted to prevent long-term complications.

PATIENT COUNSELING
If routine testing detects high blood pressure, stress to the patient the need for follow-up diagnostic testing.

BLOOD PRESSURE INCREASE

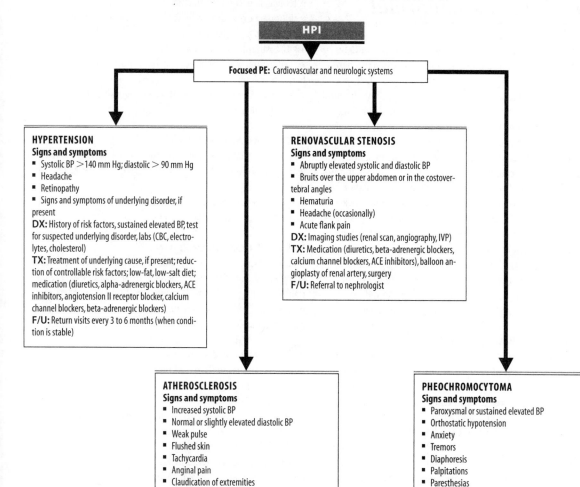

HPI

Focused PE: Cardiovascular and neurologic systems

HYPERTENSION
Signs and symptoms
- Systolic BP >140 mm Hg; diastolic > 90 mm Hg
- Headache
- Retinopathy
- Signs and symptoms of underlying disorder, if present

DX: History of risk factors, sustained elevated BP, test for suspected underlying disorder, labs (CBC, electrolytes, cholesterol)

TX: Treatment of underlying cause, if present; reduction of controllable risk factors; low-fat, low-salt diet; medication (diuretics, alpha-adrenergic blockers, ACE inhibitors, angiotension II receptor blocker, calcium channel blockers, beta-adrenergic blockers)

F/U: Return visits every 3 to 6 months (when condition is stable)

RENOVASCULAR STENOSIS
Signs and symptoms
- Abruptly elevated systolic and diastolic BP
- Bruits over the upper abdomen or in the costovertebral angles
- Hematuria
- Headache (occasionally)
- Acute flank pain

DX: Imaging studies (renal scan, angiography, IVP)

TX: Medication (diuretics, beta-adrenergic blockers, calcium channel blockers, ACE inhibitors), balloon angioplasty of renal artery, surgery

F/U: Referral to nephrologist

ATHEROSCLEROSIS
Signs and symptoms
- Increased systolic BP
- Normal or slightly elevated diastolic BP
- Weak pulse
- Flushed skin
- Tachycardia
- Anginal pain
- Claudication of extremities

DX: Labs (cholesterol level, LDL, HDL), imaging studies (ultrasound of affected area, arteriography of affected area)

TX: Treatment of affected area; medication (aspirin, antilipemic agents); low-fat, low-cholesterol, low-salt diet; exercise program

F/U: As needed (dependent on symptoms)

PHEOCHROMOCYTOMA
Signs and symptoms
- Paroxysmal or sustained elevated BP
- Orthostatic hypotension
- Anxiety
- Tremors
- Diaphoresis
- Palpitations
- Paresthesias
- Nausea
- Weight loss
- Headache
- Vision disturbances

DX: Labs (urine metanephrine, urine catecholamines), imaging studies (MRI, MIBG scintiscan), adrenal biopsy

TX: Combined alpha- and beta-adrenergic blockers (preoperatively), surgery

F/U: Daily BP monitoring preoperatively, urine catecholamine level 2 weeks postoperatively

---

Additional differential diagnoses: aldosteronism (primary) ▪ anemia ▪ aortic aneurysm (dissecting) ▪ Cushing's syndrome ▪ eclampsia ▪ essential hypertension ▪ increased ICP ▪ malignant hypertension ▪ MI ▪ polycystic kidney disease ▪ preeclampsia ▪ thyrotoxicosis

Other causes: alcohol use (heavy) ▪ ephedra ▪ ginseng ▪ licorice ▪ medication (CNS stimulants [such as amphetamines], sympathomimetics, corticosteroids, hormonal contraceptives, MAO inhibitors, cocaine) ▪ St. John's wort ▪ treatments (kidney dialysis and transplantation)

Bowel sounds, abnormal

Absent bowel sounds refers to an inability to hear bowel sounds through a stethoscope after listening for at least 5 minutes in each abdominal quadrant. Bowel sounds cease when mechanical or vascular obstruction or neurogenic inhibition halts peristalsis. When peristalsis stops, gas from bowel contents and fluid secreted from the intestinal walls accumulate and distend the lumen, leading to life-threatening complications, such as perforation, peritonitis and sepsis, or hypovolemic shock.

Simple mechanical obstruction—resulting from adhesions, hernia, or tumor—causes loss of fluids and electrolytes and induces dehydration. Vascular obstruction cuts off circulation to the intestinal walls, leading to ischemia, necrosis, and shock. Neurogenic inhibition, affecting innervation of the intestinal wall, may result from infection, bowel distention, or trauma.

Abrupt cessation of bowel sounds—when accompanied by abdominal pain, rigidity, and distention—signals a life-threatening crisis requiring immediate intervention. Absent bowel sounds following a period of hyperactive sounds are equally ominous and may indicate strangulation of a mechanically obstructed bowel.

Sometimes audible without a stethoscope, hyperactive bowel sounds reflect increased intestinal motility (peristalsis). They're commonly characterized as rapid, rushing, gurgling waves of sounds. They may stem from life-threatening bowel obstruction or GI hemorrhage as well as from GI infection, inflammatory bowel disease, food allergies, and stress.

Hypoactive bowel sounds, detected by auscultation, are diminished in regularity, tone, and loudness from normal bowel sounds. Hypoactive bowel sounds result from decreased peristalsis, which can result from a developing bowel obstruction.

➤ ALERT
- If you fail to detect bowel sounds, assess the patient for abdominal pain and cramping or abdominal distention.
- If you detect hyperactive bowel sounds, quickly check the patient's vital signs, and ask the patient about abdominal pain, vomiting, and diarrhea.

If the patient's pain isn't severe or accompanied by other life-threatening signs, perform a focused assessment.

HISTORY
- Ask the patient if he's experiencing abdominal pain. If so, when did it start?
- Ask the patient about a sensation of bloating and about flatulence. What was the time and nature of his last stool?
- Review the patient's medical history, noting especially surgeries, abdominal trauma, acute pancreatitis, diverticulitis, toxic

conditions such as uremia, spinal cord injury, and, if the patient is female, gynecologic infection.
- Obtain a drug history, including prescription and over-the-counter drugs, herbal remedies, and recreational drugs. Also, ask the patient about alcohol intake.
- Determine whether stress may have contributed to the patient's problem.
- Ask about food allergies and recent ingestion of unusual foods or fluids.

PHYSICAL ASSESSMENT
- Check the patient's vital signs. Note the presence of fever.
- Inspect abdominal contour to detect localized or generalized distention.
- Gently percuss and palpate the abdomen. Palpate for abdominal rigidity and guarding.

SPECIAL CONSIDERATIONS
If a nasogastric tube is inserted, restrict the patient's oral intake, elevate the head of the bed at least 30 degrees, and turn the patient to facilitate drainage. If an intestinal tube is inserted, refrain from securing the tube to the patient's face, and turn the patient to facilitate passage of the tube through the GI tract.

[A] PEDIATRIC POINTERS
- *Absent bowel sounds in children may result from Hirschsprung's disease or intussusception, both of which can lead to life-threatening obstructions.*
- *Hyperactive bowel sounds in children usually result from gastroenteritis, erratic eating habits, excessive ingestion of certain foods (such as unripened fruit), or food allergy.*
- *Hypoactive bowel sounds in a child may simply be due to bowel distention from excessive swallowing of air while the child was eating or crying.*

PATIENT COUNSELING
Instruct the patient on what to expect from diagnostic testing. Explain prescribed dietary changes that may be necessary.

BOWEL SOUNDS (ABSENT)

HPI

Focused PE: Vital signs, abdomen, rectum, pelvis

Common signs and symptoms
- Abdominal distention
- Constipation
- Nausea and vomiting
- Fever

Additional common signs and symptoms
- Dehydration
- Acute, colicky, abdominal pain that may radiate to the flank or lumbar area
- Rebound tenderness
- Abdominal rigidity
- Signs of shock (possibly)

STRANGULATED BOWEL
Additional signs and symptoms
- Absent bowel sounds with a period of hyperactive bowel sounds

COMPLETE MECHANICAL OBSTRUCTION

MESENTERIC ARTERY OCCLUSION
Additional signs and symptoms
- Absent bowel sounds with a period of hyperactive bowel sounds
- Sudden, severe epigastric or periumbilical pain
- Bruits (possibly)
- Abdominal rigidity
- Signs of shock (possibly)

PARALYTIC ILEUS
Additional signs and symptoms
- Generalized discomfort
- Small, liquid stools (possibly)
- Abdominal pain (possibly)

DX: Labs (CBC with differential, UA, HCG, electrolytes), imaging studies (CT scan, abdominal X-ray)
TX: NG tube, I.V. fluids, medication (electrolyte replacement, analgesics), surgery
F/U: Referral to surgeon

Other causes: abdominal surgery

BOWEL SOUNDS (HYPERACTIVE)

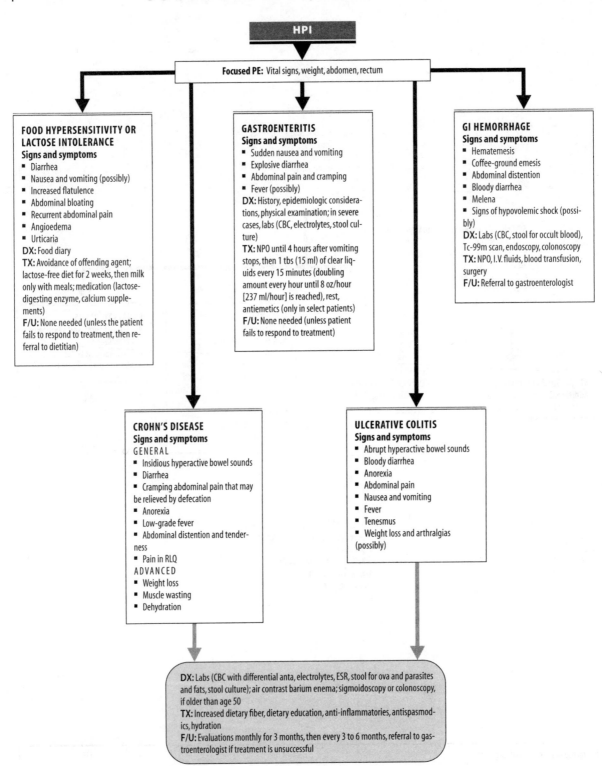

HPI

Focused PE: Vital signs, weight, abdomen, rectum

FOOD HYPERSENSITIVITY OR LACTOSE INTOLERANCE
Signs and symptoms
- Diarrhea
- Nausea and vomiting (possibly)
- Increased flatulence
- Abdominal bloating
- Recurrent abdominal pain
- Angioedema
- Urticaria

DX: Food diary
TX: Avoidance of offending agent; lactose-free diet for 2 weeks, then milk only with meals; medication (lactose-digesting enzyme, calcium supplements)
F/U: None needed (unless the patient fails to respond to treatment, then referral to dietitian)

GASTROENTERITIS
Signs and symptoms
- Sudden nausea and vomiting
- Explosive diarrhea
- Abdominal pain and cramping
- Fever (possibly)

DX: History, epidemiologic considerations, physical examination; in severe cases, labs (CBC, electrolytes, stool culture)
TX: NPO until 4 hours after vomiting stops, then 1 tbs (15 ml) of clear liquids every 15 minutes (doubling amount every hour until 8 oz/hour [237 ml/hour] is reached), rest, antiemetics (only in select patients)
F/U: None needed (unless patient fails to respond to treatment)

GI HEMORRHAGE
Signs and symptoms
- Hematemesis
- Coffee-ground emesis
- Abdominal distention
- Bloody diarrhea
- Melena
- Signs of hypovolemic shock (possibly)

DX: Labs (CBC, stool for occult blood), Tc-99m scan, endoscopy, colonoscopy
TX: NPO, I.V. fluids, blood transfusion, surgery
F/U: Referral to gastroenterologist

CROHN'S DISEASE
Signs and symptoms
GENERAL
- Insidious hyperactive bowel sounds
- Diarrhea
- Cramping abdominal pain that may be relieved by defecation
- Anorexia
- Low-grade fever
- Abdominal distention and tenderness
- Pain in RLQ
ADVANCED
- Weight loss
- Muscle wasting
- Dehydration

ULCERATIVE COLITIS
Signs and symptoms
- Abrupt hyperactive bowel sounds
- Bloody diarrhea
- Anorexia
- Abdominal pain
- Nausea and vomiting
- Fever
- Tenesmus
- Weight loss and arthralgias (possibly)

DX: Labs (CBC with differential anta, electrolytes, ESR, stool for ova and parasites and fats, stool culture); air contrast barium enema; sigmoidoscopy or colonoscopy, if older than age 50
TX: Increased dietary fiber, dietary education, anti-inflammatories, antispasmodics, hydration
F/U: Evaluations monthly for 3 months, then every 3 to 6 months, referral to gastroenterologist if treatment is unsuccessful

BOWEL SOUNDS (HYPOACTIVE)

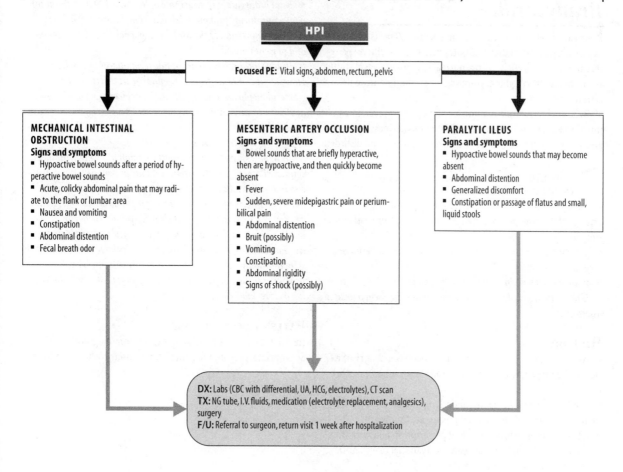

HPI

Focused PE: Vital signs, abdomen, rectum, pelvis

MECHANICAL INTESTINAL OBSTRUCTION
Signs and symptoms
- Hypoactive bowel sounds after a period of hyperactive bowel sounds
- Acute, colicky abdominal pain that may radiate to the flank or lumbar area
- Nausea and vomiting
- Constipation
- Abdominal distention
- Fecal breath odor

MESENTERIC ARTERY OCCLUSION
Signs and symptoms
- Bowel sounds that are briefly hyperactive, then are hypoactive, and then quickly become absent
- Fever
- Sudden, severe midepigastric pain or periumbilical pain
- Abdominal distention
- Bruit (possibly)
- Vomiting
- Constipation
- Abdominal rigidity
- Signs of shock (possibly)

PARALYTIC ILEUS
Signs and symptoms
- Hypoactive bowel sounds that may become absent
- Abdominal distention
- Generalized discomfort
- Constipation or passage of flatus and small, liquid stools

DX: Labs (CBC with differential, UA, HCG, electrolytes), CT scan
TX: NG tube, I.V. fluids, medication (electrolyte replacement, analgesics), surgery
F/U: Referral to surgeon, return visit 1 week after hospitalization

Other causes: anticholinergics such as propantheline bromide ▪ opiates such as codeine ▪ phenothiazines such as chlorpromazine ▪ radiation therapy ▪ surgery ▪ vinca alkaloids such as vincristine

Bradycardia

Bradycardia refers to a heart rate of less than 60 beats/minute. It occurs normally in young adults, trained athletes, elderly people, and during sleep. It's also a normal response to vagal stimulation caused by coughing, vomiting, or straining during defecation.

By itself, bradycardia is a nonspecific sign. However, in conjunction with such symptoms as chest pain, dizziness, syncope, and shortness of breath, it can signal a life-threatening disorder.

◤ ALERT

After detecting bradycardia:
* *check for other symptoms, such as chest pain, dizziness, shortness of breath, syncope, prolonged exposure to cold, or head or neck trauma*
* *place the patient on a cardiac monitor, or obtain an echocardiogram*
* *initiate emergency measures, if appropriate.*

If the patient's bradycardia is asymptomatic, perform a focused assessment.

HISTORY

* Ask the patient if he or a family member has a history of a slow pulse rate because bradycardia may be an inherited condition.
* Ask the patient if he has an underlying metabolic disorder such as hypothyroidism that can precipitate bradycardia.
* Obtain a drug history, including prescription and over-the-counter drugs, herbal remedies, and recreational drugs. Also, ask the patient about alcohol intake.

PHYSICAL ASSESSMENT

* Take the patient's vital signs.
* Inspect the skin for pallor, diaphoresis, and clamminess.
* Palpate the peripheral pulses. Note paradoxical pulse — an accentuated fall in systolic pressure during inspiration that suggests pericardial tamponade.
* Auscultate for abnormal heart sounds, rate, and rhythm.
* Look for indications of hemorrhage, including visible bleeding and palpable masses, bruising, and tenderness.
* Assess the patient for abdominal rigidity and rebound tenderness; auscultate for abnormal bowel sounds.

SPECIAL CONSIDERATIONS

Suctioning can induce hypoxia and vagal stimulation, causing bradycardia. Continue to frequently monitor vital signs.

 PEDIATRIC POINTERS

* *Fetal bradycardia (a heart rate of less than 120 beats/minute) may occur during prolonged labor or complications of delivery, such as compression of the umbilicus, partial abruptio placentae, and placenta previa.*
* *Bradycardia rarely occurs in full-term infants or children. However, it can result from congenital heart defects, acute glomerulonephritis, and transient or complete heart block associated with cardiac catheterization or cardiac surgery.*

 AGING ISSUES

Sinus node dysfunction is the most common bradyarrhythmia encountered among elderly patients. It may present as fatigue, exercise intolerance, dizziness, or syncope. If the patient is asymptomatic, no intervention is necessary. Symptomatic patients, however, require careful scrutiny of their medications. Beta-adrenergic blockers, verapamil, diazepam, sympatholytic and antihypertensive medications, and some antiarrhythmics have been implicated; symptoms may clear when these drugs are discontinued. Pacing is usually indicated in patients with symptomatic bradycardia lacking a correctable cause.

PATIENT COUNSELING

Instruct the patient on what to expect from diagnostic testing. If appropriate, prepare the patient for 24-hour Holter monitoring.

HPI

Focused PE: Vital signs; thyroid; cardiovascular, neurologic, and pulmonary systems

CARDIAC ARRHYTHMIA
Signs and symptoms
- Bradycardia (transient or sustained)
- Hypotension
- Palpitations
- Dizziness or syncope
- Nausea
- Weakness or fatigue
- Pallor

DX: Labs (ABG, CBC, cardiac enzymes, electrolytes, glucose), ECG, 24-hour Holter monitoring
TX: Medication (antiarrhythmic, vagolytic), pacemaker
F/U: Referral to cardiologist

CARDIOMYOPATHY
Signs and symptoms
- Bradycardia (transient or sustained)
- Dizziness or syncope
- Edema
- JVD
- Fatigue
- Orthopnea
- Dyspnea
- Peripheral cyanosis
- Chest pain

DX: Drug screen, electrolytes, imaging studies (CXR, echocardiogram), ECG, cardiac catheterization
TX: Medication (antiarrhythmics, diuretics, ACE inhibitors); oxygen therapy; limited activity; low-fat, low-salt diet
F/U: Referral to cardiologist

CERVICAL SPINE INJURY
Signs and symptoms
- Bradycardia (transient or sustained)
- Hypotension
- Hypothermia
- Slowed peristalsis
- Leg paralysis
- Partial arm paralysis

DX: History of trauma, imaging studies (CT scan, spine MRI)
TX: Spine stabilization, corticosteroids
F/U: Transfer to spinal injury center

HYPOTHYROIDISM
Signs and symptoms
- Fatigue
- Constipation
- Weight gain
- Cold sensitivity
- Cool, dry, thick skin
- Sparse, dry hair
- Alopecia
- Facial swelling
- Periorbital edema
- Thick, brittle nails
- Neck swelling
- Goiter

DX: Thyroid studies, ECG
TX: Thyroid hormone replacement
F/U: Return visits every 4 to 6 weeks until TSH is normal, then every 6 months

MI
Signs and symptoms
- Chest, back, or abdominal pain
- SOB
- Cough
- Dizziness
- Nausea and vomiting
- Diaphoresis
- Anxiety

DX: Labs (LDH, isoenzymes, troponin I and T), imaging studies (angiography, echocardiogram), ECG, cardiac catheterization
TX: Medication (aspirin, nitrates, analgesics, thrombolytics, anticoagulants, beta-adrenergic blockers, vasopressors), oxygen therapy, angioplasty, CABG
F/U: Referral to cardiologist; return visit 3 to 6 weeks after hospitalization, then every 3 months

HYPOTHERMIA
Signs and symptoms
- Temperature below 89.6° F (32° C)
- Shivering
- Peripheral cyanosis
- Muscle rigidity
- Bradypnea
- Confusion and stupor

DX: Temperature, ECG
TX: Establishment of ABCs, temperature monitoring, warm I.V. fluids, warming blanket, treatment of the underlying cause (if physiologic)
F/U: Return visit 2 weeks after hospitalization

INTRACRANIAL HYPERTENSION
Signs and symptoms
- Bradypnea or tachypnea
- Widened pulse pressure
- Persistent headache
- Projectile vomiting
- Fixed, unequal, or dilated pupils
- Decreased LOC

DX: Imaging studies (CT scan, MRI)
TX: Treatment of underlying cause, medication (osmotic diuretics, barbiturates), ventilatory support
F/U: Referral to neurologist or neurosurgeon

Other causes: beta-adrenergic blockers ▪ cardiac glycosides ▪ cardiac surgery ▪ diagnostic tests (cardiac catheterization, electrophysiologic studies) ▪ failure to take thyroid replacements ▪ protamine sulfate ▪ quinidine and other antiarrhythmics ▪ some calcium channel blockers ▪ suctioning ▪ sympatholytics ▪ topical miotics

Bradypnea

Commonly preceding life-threatening apnea or respiratory arrest, bradypnea is a pattern of regular respirations with a rate of less than 12 breaths/minute. This sign may result from a neurologic or metabolic disorder or a drug overdose, all of which can depress the brain's respiratory control centers. (See *Understanding neurologic control of breathing.*)

▶ ALERT

If the patient with bradypnea seems excessively sleepy:
● *try to arouse him by shaking and instructing him to breathe, and then secure his airway*

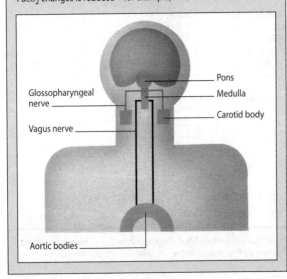

UNDERSTANDING NEUROLOGIC CONTROL OF BREATHING

The mechanical aspects of breathing are regulated by respiratory centers, groups of discrete neurons in the medulla and pons that function as a unit. In the medullary respiratory center, neurons associated with inspiration and neurons associated with expiration interact to control respiratory rate and depth. In the pons, two additional centers interact with the medullary center to regulate rhythm: The apneustic center stimulates inspiratory neurons in the medulla to precipitate inspiration; these, in turn, stimulate the pneumotaxic center to inhibit inspiration, allowing passive expiration to occur.

Normally, the breathing mechanism is stimulated by increased carbon dioxide levels and decreased oxygen levels in the blood. Chemoreceptors in the medulla and in the carotid and aortic bodies respond to changes in partial pressure of arterial carbon dioxide, partial pressure of arterial oxygen, and pH, signaling respiratory centers to adjust respiratory rate and depth. Respiratory depression occurs when decreased cerebral perfusion inactivates respiratory center neurons, when changes in $Paco_2$ and arterial blood pH affect chemoreceptor responsiveness, or when neuron responsiveness to $Paco_2$ changes is reduced—for example, with narcotic overdose.

Pons

Glossopharyngeal nerve

Medulla

Vagus nerve

Carotid body

Aortic bodies

● *quickly take his vital signs*
● *assess his neurologic status by checking his pupil size and reactions and by evaluating his level of consciousness (LOC) and his ability to move his extremities*
● *be prepared to institute emergency measures.*

If the bradypnea is asymptomatic, perform a focused assessment.

HISTORY

● Ask the patient or whoever accompanied him to the hospital if he may be having a drug overdose. If so, try to determine which drugs he used, how much, when, and by what route.
● Review the patient's medical history for diabetes; liver, renal, or brain tumor; neurologic infection; stroke, pulmonary disease, and recent head trauma.
● Review with the patient all drugs and dosages taken during the past 24 hours.

PHYSICAL ASSESSMENT

● Take the patient's vital signs.
● Inspect the skin for cyanosis or pallor. Administer oxygen at an appropriate rate.
● Inspect the head for signs of trauma.
● Check the arms for possible signs of drug abuse.
● Check neurologic status, including pupil size, LOC, and motor function.
● Auscultate the lungs for abnormal sounds.

SPECIAL CONSIDERATIONS

Because the patient with bradypnea may develop apnea, frequently check his respiratory status and be prepared to offer ventilatory support, if necessary.

 PEDIATRIC POINTERS

Because respiratory rates are higher in children than adults, bradypnea in children is defined according to age.

 AGING ISSUES

Elderly patients who are prescribed drugs have a higher risk of developing bradypnea secondary to drug toxicity because they often take several drugs that can potentiate this effect, and they typically have other conditions that predispose them to it. Warn your patient about this potentially life-threatening complication.

PATIENT COUNSELING

Patients taking narcotics regularly, such as patients with advanced cancer or sickle cell anemia, should be alerted to bradypnea as a serious complication and be taught to recognize early signs of toxicity, such as nausea and vomiting.

BRADYPNEA

HPI

Focused PE: Vital signs; skin; pulmonary, neurologic, and cardiovascular systems

DIABETIC KETOACIDOSIS
Signs and symptoms
- Kussmaul's respirations
- Decreased LOC
- Fatigue and weakness
- Fruity breath odor
- Oliguria or polyuria
- Polydipsia
- Weight loss

DX: Labs (glucose, electrolytes, ABG)
TX: I.V. fluids, medication (insulin, electrolyte replacement), nutritional education
F/U: Return visit 1 week after hospitalization

END-STAGE HEPATIC FAILURE
Signs and symptoms
- Coma
- Hyperreactive reflexes
- Asterixis
- Positive Babinski's reflex
- Fetor hepaticus

DX: Labs (CBC, LFT, serum ammonia), liver ultrasound
TX: Medication (lactulose, thiazide diuretic), bed rest, sodium and fluid restriction, protein restriction
F/U: Referral to hepatologist or gastroenterologist, return visit 1 week after hospitalization

Common signs and symptoms
- Decreased LOC
- Deteriorating motor function
- Fixed, dilated pupils
- Papilledema

SEVERE INTRACRANIAL HYPERTENSION

LATE MEDULLARY STRANGULATION
Additional signs and symptoms
- Widened pulse pressure
- Bradycardia
- Hypertension

DX: Imaging studies (CT scan, MRI)
TX: Medication (osmotic diuretics, barbiturates), ventilatory support, ICP monitoring
F/U: Referral to neurologist or neurosurgeon

END-STAGE RENAL FAILURE
Signs and symptoms
- Seizures
- Decreased LOC
- GI bleeding
- Hypotension or hypertension
- Uremic frost
- Nausea and vomiting
- Weakness, fatigue
- Weight loss or gain
- Coma

DX: Labs (BUN, creatinine, electrolytes, UA, ABG), imaging studies (ultrasound, IVP)
TX: Dialysis, medication (electrolytes, antihypertensives)
F/U: Referral to nephrologist

END-STAGE RESPIRATORY FAILURE
Signs and symptoms
- Cyanosis
- Diminished breath sounds
- Tachycardia
- Decreased LOC

DX: ABG, CXR, PFT
TX: Maintenance of airway, ventilation management, oxygen therapy, medication (beta-agonist, corticosteroids)
F/U: Referral to pulmonologist

Other causes: overdose of narcotic analgesics or, less commonly, sedatives, barbiturates, phenothiazines, or other CNS depressants (use of any of these medications with alcohol can also cause bradypnea)

Breast nodule

A frequently reported gynecologic sign, a breast nodule has two chief causes: benign breast disease and cancer. Benign breast disease, the leading cause of nodules, can stem from cyst formation in obstructed and dilated lactiferous ducts, hypertrophy or tumor formation in the ductal system, inflammation, or infection.

Although fewer than 20% of breast nodules are malignant, the signs and symptoms of breast cancer aren't easily distinguished from those of benign breast disease. Breast cancer is a leading cause of death among women but also occasionally occurs in men, with signs and symptoms mimicking those found in women. Thus, breast nodules in both sexes should always be evaluated.

A woman who performs monthly breast self-examinations can detect a nodule 5 mm or less in size, considerably smaller than the 1-cm nodule that's readily detectable by an experienced examiner. However, a woman may fail to report a nodule because of fear of breast cancer.

HISTORY
- Ask the patient how and when the breast nodule was discovered.
- Ask the patient if the lump varies in size and tenderness with her menstrual cycle.
- Ask the patient to describe pain or tenderness associated with the lump. Is the pain in one breast only? Has she sustained recent trauma to the breast?
- Ask the patient if the lump has changed since she first noticed it. Is there any change in breast shape, size, or contour? Does she have nipple discharge?
- Ask the patient if she's lactating.
- Ask the patient about fever, chills, fatigue, and other flulike signs and symptoms.
- Review the patient's medical history for factors that increase her risk of breast cancer. Also, ask the patient for a family history.

PHYSICAL ASSESSMENT
- Carefully palpate a suspected breast nodule, noting its location, shape, size, consistency, mobility, and delineation. Note whether you feel one nodule or several small ones.
- Inspect and palpate the skin over the nodule for warmth, redness, and edema.
- Palpate the lymph nodes of the breast and axilla for enlargement.
- Observe the contour of the breasts, looking for asymmetry and irregularities. Be alert for signs of retraction, such as skin dimpling and nipple deviation, retraction, or flattening.

- Be alert for a nipple discharge that's spontaneous, unilateral, and nonmilky (serous, bloody, or purulent). Be careful not to confuse it with the grayish discharge that can commonly be elicited from the nipples of a woman who has been pregnant.

SPECIAL CONSIDERATIONS
Postpone teaching the patient how to perform breast self-examination until she overcomes her initial anxiety over discovering a nodule.

A PEDIATRIC POINTERS
- *Most nodules in children and adolescents reflect the normal response of breast tissue to hormonal fluctuations. For instance, the breasts of young teenage girls may normally contain cordlike nodules that become tender just before menstruation.*
- *A transient breast nodule in young boys (as well as women between ages 20 and 30) may result from juvenile mastitis, which usually affects one breast. Signs of inflammation are present in a firm mass beneath the nipple.*

AGING ISSUES
In women age 70 and older, three-quarters of all breast lumps are malignant.

PATIENT COUNSELING
If the patient is lactating and has mastitis, advise her to pump her breasts to prevent further milk stasis, to discard the milk, and to substitute formula until the infection responds to an antibiotic. When teaching a patient how to perform breast self-examination, advise her to do the examination 5 to 7 days after the first day of her last menstrual period.

BREAST NODULE

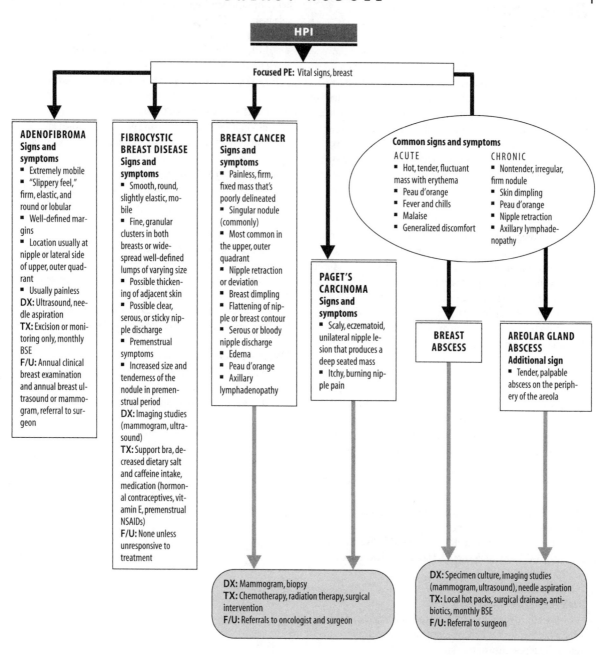

HPI

Focused PE: Vital signs, breast

ADENOFIBROMA
Signs and symptoms
- Extremely mobile
- "Slippery feel," firm, elastic, and round or lobular
- Well-defined margins
- Location usually at nipple or lateral side of upper, outer quadrant
- Usually painless

DX: Ultrasound, needle aspiration
TX: Excision or monitoring only, monthly BSE
F/U: Annual clinical breast examination and annual breast ultrasound or mammogram, referral to surgeon

FIBROCYSTIC BREAST DISEASE
Signs and symptoms
- Smooth, round, slightly elastic, mobile
- Fine, granular clusters in both breasts or widespread well-defined lumps of varying size
- Possible thickening of adjacent skin
- Possible clear, serous, or sticky nipple discharge
- Premenstrual symptoms
- Increased size and tenderness of the nodule in premenstrual period

DX: Imaging studies (mammogram, ultrasound)
TX: Support bra, decreased dietary salt and caffeine intake, medication (hormonal contraceptives, vitamin E, premenstrual NSAIDs)
F/U: None unless unresponsive to treatment

BREAST CANCER
Signs and symptoms
- Painless, firm, fixed mass that's poorly delineated
- Singular nodule (commonly)
- Most common in the upper, outer quadrant
- Nipple retraction or deviation
- Breast dimpling
- Flattening of nipple or breast contour
- Serous or bloody nipple discharge
- Edema
- Peau d'orange
- Axillary lymphadenopathy

Common signs and symptoms
ACUTE
- Hot, tender, fluctuant mass with erythema
- Peau d'orange
- Fever and chills
- Malaise
- Generalized discomfort

CHRONIC
- Nontender, irregular, firm nodule
- Skin dimpling
- Peau d'orange
- Nipple retraction
- Axillary lymphadenopathy

PAGET'S CARCINOMA
Signs and symptoms
- Scaly, eczematoid, unilateral nipple lesion that produces a deep seated mass
- Itchy, burning nipple pain

BREAST ABSCESS

AREOLAR GLAND ABSCESS
Additional sign
- Tender, palpable abscess on the periphery of the areola

DX: Mammogram, biopsy
TX: Chemotherapy, radiation therapy, surgical intervention
F/U: Referrals to oncologist and surgeon

DX: Specimen culture, imaging studies (mammogram, ultrasound), needle aspiration
TX: Local hot packs, surgical drainage, antibiotics, monthly BSE
F/U: Referral to surgeon

Additional differential diagnoses: actinomycosis ▪ hydatid cyst ▪ intraductal papilloma ▪ mastitis ▪ sebaceous cyst

Breast pain

An unreliable indicator of cancer, breast pain commonly results from benign breast disease. It may occur during rest or movement and may be aggravated by manipulation or palpation. (*Breast tenderness* refers to pain elicited by physical contact.) Breast pain may be unilateral or bilateral; cyclic, intermittent, or constant; and dull or sharp. It may result from a surface cut, a furuncle, a contusion, or a similar lesion (superficial pain); a nipple fissure or inflammation in the papillary duct or areola (severe localized pain); stromal distention in the breast parenchyma; or a tumor that affects nerve endings (severe, constant pain). Breast pain may radiate to the back, the arms, or the neck.

Breast tenderness in women may occur before menstruation and during pregnancy. Before menstruation, breast pain or tenderness stems from increased mammary blood flow due to hormonal changes. During pregnancy, breast tenderness and throbbing, tingling, or pricking sensations may occur, also from hormonal changes. In men, breast pain may stem from gynecomastia (especially during puberty and senescence), a reproductive tract anomaly, or an organic disease of the liver or the pituitary, adrenal cortex, or thyroid gland.

HISTORY

- Ask the patient about the breast pain's onset and character. Is it constant or intermittent? If it's intermittent, determine the relationship of pain to the phase of the menstrual cycle.
- Ask the patient to describe the pain. Determine if the pain affects one breast or both, and ask her to point to the painful area.
- Ask the patient if she's lactating. If not, ask her if she's experiencing nipple discharge. If so, have her describe it.
- Ask the patient if she's pregnant, uses a hormonal contraceptive, or has reached menopause.
- Ask the patient if she recently experienced flulike symptoms or a sustained injury to the breast. Has she noticed any change in breast shape or contour?

PHYSICAL ASSESSMENT

- Instruct the patient to place her arms at her sides, and then inspect her breasts. Note their size, symmetry, and contour as well as the appearance of the skin.
- Note the size, shape, and symmetry of the nipples and areolae. Do you detect ecchymosis, a rash, ulceration, or a discharge? Do the nipples point in the same direction? Do you see signs of retraction, such as skin dimpling or nipple inversion or flattening? Repeat your inspection, first with the patient's arms raised above her head and then with her hands pressed against her hips.

- Palpate the breasts, first with the patient seated and then with her lying down and a pillow placed under her shoulder on the side being examined. Note any warmth, tenderness, nodules, masses, or irregularities.
- Palpate the nipples, noting tenderness and nodules, and check for discharge.
- Palpate axillary lymph nodes, noting any enlargement.

SPECIAL CONSIDERATIONS

Provide emotional support for the patient and, when appropriate, emphasize the importance of monthly self-examination.

[A] PEDIATRIC POINTERS
Transient gynecomastia can cause breast pain in males during puberty.

AGING ISSUES
- *Breast pain secondary to benign breast disease is rare in postmenopausal women.*
- *Breast pain can result from trauma, either from falls or physical abuse.*
- *Because of decreased pain perception and decreased cognitive function, an elderly patient may not report breast pain.*

PATIENT COUNSELING

Advise the patient to wear a brassiere that cups and supports the entire breast with wide shoulder and back straps. Tell the patient that warm or cold compresses may aid pain relief.

BREAST PAIN

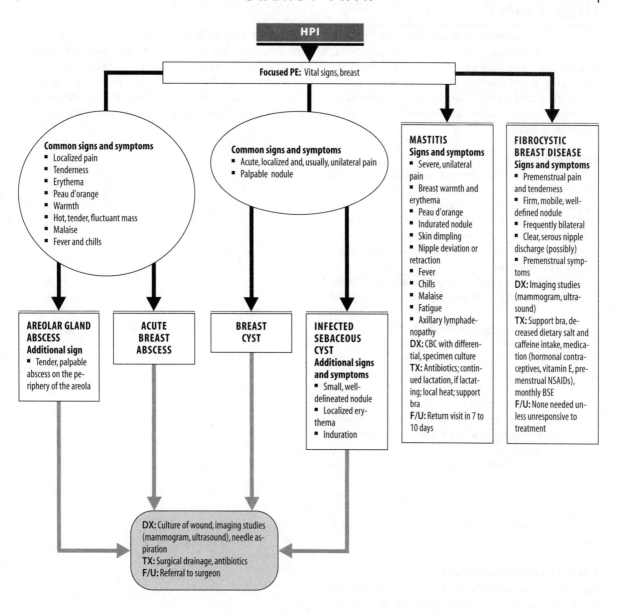

HPI

Focused PE: Vital signs, breast

Common signs and symptoms
- Localized pain
- Tenderness
- Erythema
- Peau d'orange
- Warmth
- Hot, tender, fluctuant mass
- Malaise
- Fever and chills

Common signs and symptoms
- Acute, localized and, usually, unilateral pain
- Palpable nodule

MASTITIS
Signs and symptoms
- Severe, unilateral pain
- Breast warmth and erythema
- Peau d'orange
- Indurated nodule
- Skin dimpling
- Nipple deviation or retraction
- Fever
- Chills
- Malaise
- Fatigue
- Axillary lymphadenopathy

DX: CBC with differential, specimen culture
TX: Antibiotics; continued lactation, if lactating; local heat; support bra
F/U: Return visit in 7 to 10 days

FIBROCYSTIC BREAST DISEASE
Signs and symptoms
- Premenstrual pain and tenderness
- Firm, mobile, well-defined nodule
- Frequently bilateral
- Clear, serous nipple discharge (possibly)
- Premenstrual symptoms

DX: Imaging studies (mammogram, ultrasound)
TX: Support bra, decreased dietary salt and caffeine intake, medication (hormonal contraceptives, vitamin E, premenstrual NSAIDs), monthly BSE
F/U: None needed unless unresponsive to treatment

AREOLAR GLAND ABSCESS
Additional sign
- Tender, palpable abscess on the periphery of the areola

ACUTE BREAST ABSCESS

BREAST CYST

INFECTED SEBACEOUS CYST
Additional signs and symptoms
- Small, well-delineated nodule
- Localized erythema
- Induration

DX: Culture of wound, imaging studies (mammogram, ultrasound), needle aspiration
TX: Surgical drainage, antibiotics
F/U: Referral to surgeon

Breast ulcer

Appearing on the nipple or areola or on the breast itself, an ulcer indicates destruction of the skin and subcutaneous tissue. A breast ulcer is usually a late sign of cancer, appearing well after the confirming diagnosis. However, it may be the presenting sign of breast cancer in men, who are more apt to dismiss earlier breast changes. Breast ulcers can also result from trauma, infection, or radiation.

HISTORY
- Ask the patient when she first noticed the ulcer and if it was preceded by other breast changes, such as nodules, edema, and nipple discharge, deviation, or retraction.
- Ask the patient if anything has made the ulcer better or worse. Does it cause pain or produce drainage?
- Ask the patient if she has noticed a change in breast shape. Has she had a skin rash?
- Review the patient's medical history for factors that increase the risk of breast cancer. Also, ask the patient for a family history.
- If the patient recently gave birth, ask her if she breast-feeds her infant or has recently weaned him.
- Ask the patient if she's taking an oral antibiotic or if she's diabetic.

PHYSICAL ASSESSMENT
- Inspect the breast, noting asymmetry or flattening. Look for a rash, scaling, cracking, or red excoriation on the nipple, areola, or inframammary fold.
- Check for skin changes, such as warmth, erythema, or peau d'orange.
- Palpate the breast for masses, noting any induration beneath the ulcer.
- Palpate for tenderness or nodules around the areola and the axillary lymph nodes.

SPECIAL CONSIDERATIONS
After radiation treatment, the breasts appear sunburned. Subsequently, the skin ulcerates and the surrounding area becomes red and tender.

AGING ISSUES
- *Because the risk of breast cancer is increased in this population, breast ulcers should be considered cancerous until proved otherwise.*
- *Ulcers can result from normal skin changes in elderly patients, such as thinning, decreased vascularity, and loss of elasticity as well as from poor skin hygiene.*
- *Pressure ulcers may result from tight brassieres; traumatic ulcers may result from falls or abuse.*

PATIENT COUNSELING
Because breast ulcers are easily infected, teach the patient how to apply topical antifungal ointment or cream. Instruct her to keep the ulcer dry to reduce chafing and to wear loose-fitting undergarments. If breast cancer is suspected, provide emotional support and encourage the patient to express her feelings.

BREAST ULCER

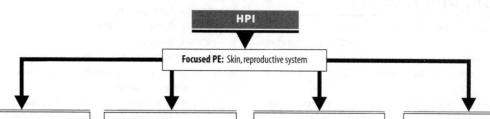

HPI

Focused PE: Skin, reproductive system

BREAST CANCER
Signs and symptoms
- Painless, firm, fixed mass that's poorly delineated
- Singular nodule (commonly)
- Most common in the upper, outer quadrant
- Nipple retraction or deviation
- Breast dimpling
- Flattening of nipple or breast contour
- Serous or bloody nipple discharge
- Edema
- Peau d'orange
- Axillary lymphadenopathy

DX: Mammogram, biopsy, breast ultrasound
TX: Chemotherapy, radiation therapy, surgery
F/U: Referrals to oncologist and surgeon

CANDIDA ALBICANS INFECTION
Signs and symptoms
- Well-defined, bright red papular patches with scaly borders
- Location in breast folds (usually)
- Occurrence in breast feeding or obese women with dry, cracked nipples
- Burning pain that penetrates the chest wall

DX: Inspection of site, labs (wound culture, blood cultures, ELISA, analgesics)
TX: Antifungals, wound care
F/U: Return visit 1 week after treatment

PAGET'S DISEASE
Signs and symptoms
- Bright red nipple excoriation that may extend to the areola
- Serous or bloody discharge
- Symptoms (usually unilateral)
- Local hyperemia
- Local edema
- Pruritus

DX: Mammography, biopsy
TX: Chemotherapy, surgery
F/U: Referrals to oncologist and surgeon

BREAST TRAUMA
Signs and symptoms
- Pain at the affected site
- Ecchymosis
- Laceration
- Abrasions
- Swelling
- Hematoma

DX: History of injury or surgery, inspection of site
TX: Varies (based on extent of injury), medication (NSAIDs; analgesics; if infection present, antibiotics), surgery
F/U: As needed (dependent on extent of injury, 7 to 10 days after treatment), referral to surgeon (if injury is extensive or isn't responding to treatment)

Other causes: radiation therapy

Breath, abnormal

Ammonia breath odor—commonly described as urinous or "fishy" breath—typically occurs in those with end-stage chronic renal failure. This sign improves slightly after hemodialysis and persists throughout the course of the disorder but isn't of great concern.

Fecal breath odor typically accompanies fecal vomiting associated with a long-standing intestinal obstruction or gastrojejunocolic fistula. It represents an important late diagnostic clue to a potentially life-threatening GI disorder because complete obstruction of any part of the bowel, if untreated, can cause death within hours from vascular collapse and shock.

Fruity breath odor results from respiratory elimination of excess acetone. This sign characteristically occurs in those with ketoacidosis—a potentially life-threatening condition that requires immediate treatment to prevent severe dehydration, irreversible coma, and death.

HISTORY

If you detect ammonia breath odor:
- Ask the patient if he has experienced a metallic taste, loss of smell, increased thirst, heartburn, difficulty swallowing, loss of appetite at the sight of food, and early-morning vomiting.
- Ask the patient about his bowel habits. Has he had melenic stools or constipation?

If you detect fecal breath odor:
- Ask the patient about previous abdominal surgery, appetite, and abdominal pain. If he's having pain, have him describe its onset, duration, and location. Is the pain intense, persistent, or spasmodic?
- Have the patient describe his normal bowel habits, especially noting constipation, diarrhea, or leakage of stool. Ask when the patient's last bowel movement occurred, and have him describe the stool's color and consistency.

If you detect a fruity breath odor:
- Ask the patient about changes in his breathing pattern.
- Ask the patient if he's experienced increased thirst, frequent urination, weight loss, fatigue, or abdominal pain.
- Ask the female patient if she has had candidal vaginitis or vaginal secretions with itching.
- If the patient has a history of diabetes mellitus, ask about stress, infections, and noncompliance with therapy.
- If the patient is suspected of having anorexia nervosa, obtain a dietary and weight history.

PHYSICAL ASSESSMENT

If you detect ammonia breath odor:
- inspect the patient's oral cavity for bleeding, swollen gums or tongue, and ulceration with drainage.

If you detect a fecal breath odor:
- take the patient's vital signs, watching for indications of hypertension; hypotension; tachycardia; tachypnea; cool, clammy skin; and altered mental status
- auscultate for bowel sounds
- inspect the abdomen, noting contour and surgical scars, and measure abdominal girth to provide baseline data for subsequent assessment of distention
- palpate for tenderness, distention, and rigidity
- percuss for tympany, indicating a gas-filled bowel, and dullness, indicating fluid.

If you detect fruity breath odor:
- check for Kussmaul's respirations
- examine the patient's level of consciousness.

SPECIAL CONSIDERATIONS

Ammonia odor is offensive to others, but the patient may become accustomed to it. Remind him to perform frequent mouth care.

A   PEDIATRIC POINTERS
- *Carefully monitor the child with fecal breath odor for fluid and electrolyte imbalance because dehydration can occur rapidly from persistent vomiting.*
- *Fruity breath odor in an infant or a child usually stems from uncontrolled diabetes mellitus. Ketoacidosis develops rapidly in this age-group because of low glycogen reserves.*

AGING ISSUES
Elderly patients may have poor oral hygiene, increased dental caries, decreased salivary function with dryness, and poor dietary intake. In addition, many of them take multiple drugs. Consider all of these factors when evaluating an elderly patient with mouth odor.

PATIENT COUNSELING

Teach the patient appropriate oral hygiene and make appropriate referrals. Involve the patient in various aspects of treatment, such as dietary and drug therapies.

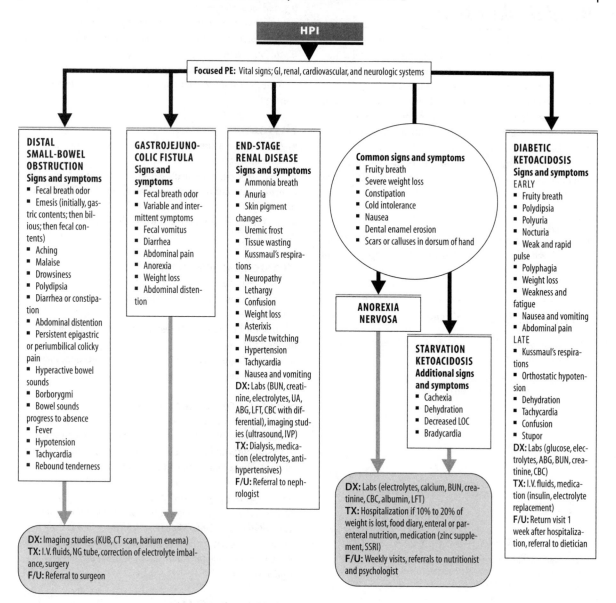

HPI

Focused PE: Vital signs; GI, renal, cardiovascular, and neurologic systems

DISTAL SMALL-BOWEL OBSTRUCTION
Signs and symptoms
- Fecal breath odor
- Emesis (initially, gastric contents; then bilious; then fecal contents)
- Aching
- Malaise
- Drowsiness
- Polydipsia
- Diarrhea or constipation
- Abdominal distention
- Persistent epigastric or periumbilical colicky pain
- Hyperactive bowel sounds
- Borborygmi
- Bowel sounds progress to absence
- Fever
- Hypotension
- Tachycardia
- Rebound tenderness

DX: Imaging studies (KUB, CT scan, barium enema)
TX: I.V. fluids, NG tube, correction of electrolyte imbalance, surgery
F/U: Referral to surgeon

GASTROJEJUNO-COLIC FISTULA
Signs and symptoms
- Fecal breath odor
- Variable and intermittent symptoms
- Fecal vomitus
- Diarrhea
- Abdominal pain
- Anorexia
- Weight loss
- Abdominal distention

END-STAGE RENAL DISEASE
Signs and symptoms
- Ammonia breath
- Anuria
- Skin pigment changes
- Uremic frost
- Tissue wasting
- Kussmaul's respirations
- Neuropathy
- Lethargy
- Confusion
- Weight loss
- Asterixis
- Muscle twitching
- Hypertension
- Tachycardia
- Nausea and vomiting

DX: Labs (BUN, creatinine, electrolytes, UA, ABG, LFT, CBC with differential), imaging studies (ultrasound, IVP)
TX: Dialysis, medication (electrolytes, antihypertensives)
F/U: Referral to nephrologist

Common signs and symptoms
- Fruity breath
- Severe weight loss
- Constipation
- Cold intolerance
- Nausea
- Dental enamel erosion
- Scars or calluses in dorsum of hand

ANOREXIA NERVOSA

STARVATION KETOACIDOSIS
Additional signs and symptoms
- Cachexia
- Dehydration
- Decreased LOC
- Bradycardia

DX: Labs (electrolytes, calcium, BUN, creatinine, CBC, albumin, LFT)
TX: Hospitalization if 10% to 20% of weight is lost, food diary, enteral or parenteral nutrition, medication (zinc supplement, SSRI)
F/U: Weekly visits, referrals to nutritionist and psychologist

DIABETIC KETOACIDOSIS
Signs and symptoms
EARLY
- Fruity breath
- Polydipsia
- Polyuria
- Nocturia
- Weak and rapid pulse
- Polyphagia
- Weight loss
- Weakness and fatigue
- Nausea and vomiting
- Abdominal pain
LATE
- Kussmaul's respirations
- Orthostatic hypotension
- Dehydration
- Tachycardia
- Confusion
- Stupor

DX: Labs (glucose, electrolytes, ABG, BUN, creatinine, CBC)
TX: I.V. fluids, medication (insulin, electrolyte replacement)
F/U: Return visit 1 week after hospitalization, referral to dietician

Other causes: fad diets (especially those encouraging little or no carbohydrate intake) ▪ medication (any drug known to cause metabolic acidosis)

Brudzinski's sign

A positive Brudzinski's sign (flexion of the hips and knees in response to passive flexion of the neck) signals meningeal irritation. Passive flexion of the neck stretches the nerve roots, causing pain and involuntary flexion of the knees and hips.

Brudzinski's sign is a common and important early indicator of life-threatening meningitis and subarachnoid hemorrhage. It can be elicited in children as well as adults, although more reliable indicators of meningeal irritation exist for infants.

Testing for Brudzinski's sign isn't part of the routine examination, unless you suspect meningeal irritation. (See *Testing for Brudzinski's sign.*)

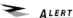

ALERT

If the patient has signs of increased intracranial pressure (ICP), such as altered level of consciousness, pupillary changes, bradycar-

dia, widened pulse pressure, irregular respiratory patterns, vomiting, and moderate fever:
- *elevate the head of the bed 30 to 60 degrees*
- *administer medication (such as an osmotic diuretic or a barbiturate), as ordered*
- *be prepared to initiate emergency measures.*
  If the patient doesn't have signs of ICP, perform a focused assessment.

HISTORY
- Ask the patient about headache, neck pain, nausea, and vision disturbances.
- Review the patient's medical history for hypertension, spinal arthritis, endocarditis, open head injury, and recent head trauma.
- Ask the patient about dental work, abscessed teeth, and I.V. drug abuse.

PHYSICAL ASSESSMENT
- Take the patient's vital signs.
- Evaluate cranial nerve function, noting motor or sensory deficits.
- Look for Kernig's sign (resistance to knee extension after flexion of the hip).
- Look for signs of central nervous system infection, such as fever and nuchal rigidity.

SPECIAL CONSIDERATIONS
Many patients with a positive Brudzinski's sign are critically ill and need constant ICP monitoring and frequent neurologic checks, along with intensive assessments and monitoring of vital signs, intake and output, and cardiopulmonary status.

A   PEDIATRIC POINTERS
Brudzinski's sign may not be the most useful indicator of meningeal irritation in infants. More reliable signs—such as bulging fontanels, weak cry, fretfulness, vomiting, and poor feeding—will commonly signal meningeal irritation before you assess for Brudzinski's sign.

PATIENT COUNSELING
Instruct the patient and family on what to expect from diagnostic testing and about emergency measures and equipment that are used. Provide emotional support.

TESTING FOR BRUDZINSKI'S SIGN

Here's how to test for Brudzinski's sign, which will help to confirm meningeal irritation.

With the patient in the supine position, place your hands behind her head and lift her head toward her chest.

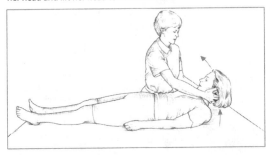

If your patient has meningeal irritation, you'll observe a positive Brudzinski's sign—the patient's hips and knees will flex in response to the passive neck flexion.

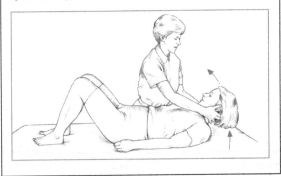

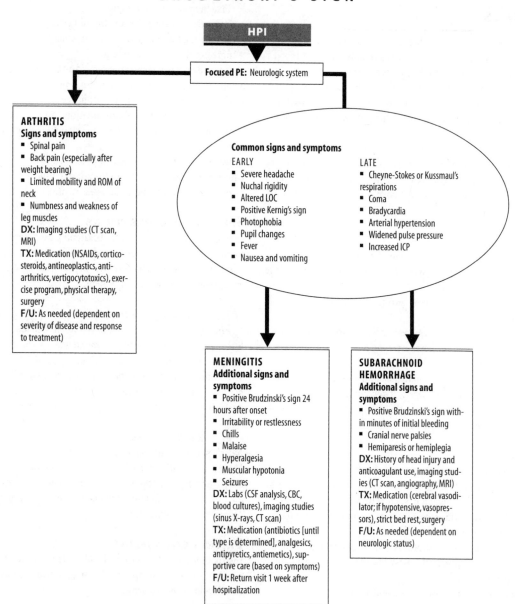

HPI

Focused PE: Neurologic system

ARTHRITIS
Signs and symptoms
- Spinal pain
- Back pain (especially after weight bearing)
- Limited mobility and ROM of neck
- Numbness and weakness of leg muscles

DX: Imaging studies (CT scan, MRI)

TX: Medication (NSAIDs, corticosteroids, antineoplastics, antiarthritics, vertigocytotoxics), exercise program, physical therapy, surgery

F/U: As needed (dependent on severity of disease and response to treatment)

Common signs and symptoms

EARLY
- Severe headache
- Nuchal rigidity
- Altered LOC
- Positive Kernig's sign
- Photophobia
- Pupil changes
- Fever
- Nausea and vomiting

LATE
- Cheyne-Stokes or Kussmaul's respirations
- Coma
- Bradycardia
- Arterial hypertension
- Widened pulse pressure
- Increased ICP

MENINGITIS
Additional signs and symptoms
- Positive Brudzinski's sign 24 hours after onset
- Irritability or restlessness
- Chills
- Malaise
- Hyperalgesia
- Muscular hypotonia
- Seizures

DX: Labs (CSF analysis, CBC, blood cultures), imaging studies (sinus X-rays, CT scan)

TX: Medication (antibiotics [until type is determined], analgesics, antipyretics, antiemetics), supportive care (based on symptoms)

F/U: Return visit 1 week after hospitalization

SUBARACHNOID HEMORRHAGE
Additional signs and symptoms
- Positive Brudzinski's sign within minutes of initial bleeding
- Cranial nerve palsies
- Hemiparesis or hemiplegia

DX: History of head injury and anticoagulant use, imaging studies (CT scan, angiography, MRI)

TX: Medication (cerebral vasodilator; if hypotensive, vasopressors), strict bed rest, surgery

F/U: As needed (dependent on neurologic status)

Bruits

Commonly an indicator of life- or limb-threatening vascular disease, bruits are swishing sounds caused by turbulent blood flow. They're characterized by location, duration, intensity, pitch, and time of onset in the cardiac cycle. Loud bruits produce intense vibration and a palpable thrill. A thrill, however, doesn't provide any further clue to the causative disorder or to its severity.

Bruits are most significant when heard over the abdominal aorta; the renal, carotid, femoral, popliteal, or subclavian artery; or the thyroid gland. They're also significant when heard consistently, despite changes in patient position and when heard during diastole.

 ALERT

If you detect bruits over the abdominal aorta:
- *check for a pulsating mass or a bluish discoloration around the umbilicus (Cullen's sign)*
- *ask the patient about severe, tearing pain in the abdomen, flank, or lower back*
- *check peripheral pulses, comparing the intensity in the upper extremities to that in the lower extremities*
- *monitor vital signs*
- *withhold food and fluids until a definitive diagnosis is made*
- *prepare the patient for surgery, if appropriate.*

If you don't detect bruits over the abdominal aorta, perform a focused assessment.

HISTORY

If you detect bruits over the thyroid gland:
- ask the patient if he has a history of hyperthyroidism or signs and symptoms that suggest it, such as nervousness, tremors, weight loss, palpitations, heat intolerance and, in female patients, amenorrhea
- watch for signs and symptoms of life-threatening thyroid storm, such as tremor, restlessness, diarrhea, abdominal pain, and hepatomegaly.

If you detect bruits over the carotid artery:
- ask the patient about signs and symptoms of a transient ischemic attack, including dizziness, diplopia, slurred speech, flashing lights, and syncope.

If you detect bruits over the femoral, popliteal, or subclavian artery:
- ask the patient if he has experienced edema, weakness, or paresthesia of the extremities
- ask the patient if he has a history of intermittent claudication.

PHYSICAL ASSESSMENT
- Take the patient's vital signs.

  If you detect bruits over the thyroid gland:
- palpate the thyroid gland for enlargement
- note exophthalmos if present.

  If you detect bruits over the carotid artery:
- observe the patient's speech, noting aphasia
- check the patient's pupils for proper reaction
- test muscle strength and coordination, noting weakness.

  If you detect bruits over the femoral, popliteal, or subclavian artery:
- watch for a sudden absence of pulse, pallor, or coolness, which may indicate a threat to the affected limb
- perform a thorough cardiac assessment.

SPECIAL CONSIDERATIONS

Because bruits can signal a life-threatening vascular disorder, frequently check the patient's vital signs and auscultate over the affected arteries. Be especially alert for bruits that become louder or develop a diastolic component.

 PEDIATRIC POINTERS
- *Although bruits are common in young children and usually of little significance—for example, cranial bruits are normal until age 4—some bruits may be significant.*
- *Because birthmarks commonly accompany congenital arteriovenous fistulas, carefully auscultate for bruits in a child with port-wine spots or cavernous or diffuse hemangiomas.*

AGING ISSUES

Elderly patients with atherosclerosis may have bruits that can be heard over several arteries. Those related to carotid artery stenosis are particularly important because of the high incidence of associated stroke. Close follow-up is mandatory as well as prompt surgical referral when indicated.

PATIENT COUNSELING

Instruct the patient to inform the physician if he develops dizziness, pain, or other symptoms that suggest stroke because his condition may be worsening.

BRUITS

HPI

Focused PE: Cardiovascular system

CAROTID ARTERY STENOSIS
Signs and symptoms
- Continuous bruits heard over one or both carotid arteries
- Dizziness and vertigo
- Headache
- Syncope
- Aphasia
- Dysarthria
- Sudden vision loss
- Hemiparesis or hemiparalysis

DX: Lipid profile, imaging studies (Doppler ultrasound, MRI, angiography)
TX: Modification of controllable risk factors, medication (antiplatelet therapy, antilipemics, antihypertensives), surgery
F/U: Return visit 1 week after surgery, then biannually if asymptomatic

Common signs and symptoms
- Diminished peripheral pulses
- Claudication
- Numbness, weakness, and pain in the lower extremities

ABDOMINAL AORTIC ANEURYSM
Additional signs and symptoms
- Systolic bruit over the aorta
- Pulsating periumbilical mass
- Constant upper abdominal pain or lower back pain

LIFE-THREATENING SIGNS AND SYMPTOMS
(MAY SIGNIFY RUPTURE)
- Severe abdominal and back pain
- Mottled skin below the waist
- Absent femoral and pedal pulses
- Lower BP in the legs than in the arms
- Abdominal rigidity
- Signs of shock

DX: Imaging studies (ultrasonography, CT scan, MRI, angiography)
TX: BP control, reduction of atherosclerotic risk factors, surgery
F/U: BP monitoring as indicated, serial ultrasounds, return visit 1 week after discharge, if surgery is performed

PERIPHERAL VASCULAR DISEASE
Additional signs and symptoms
EARLY
- Bruits over the femoral arteries and other arteries in the legs
- Cool, shiny skin and hair loss on the affected extremity
- Slow healing lower extremity ulcers

LATE SIGNS
- Mottling
- Absent pulse
- Classic five Ps — pulselessness, paralysis, paresthesia, pain, pallor

DX: Labs (lipid profile, coagulation studies), imaging studies (Doppler ultrasound, MRI, arteriography), ankle-brachial index, transcutaneous oximetry
TX: Reduction of risk factors, low-fat diet, pulse monitoring, medication (aspirin; anticoagulants, if occlusion present), surgery for occlusion
F/U: As needed (dependent on severity of disease)

RENAL ARTERY STENOSIS
Signs and symptoms
- Systolic bruits over the abdominal midline and flank of the affected side
- Hypertension
- Headache
- Palpitations
- Tachycardia
- Anxiety
- Dizziness
- Retinopathy
- Hematuria
- Mental sluggishness

DX: BP, labs (BUN, creatinine, electrolytes), imaging studies (radionuclide cystogram, ultrasound, kidney X-ray, CT scan, arteriography)
TX: Antihypertensives, balloon angioplasty, smoking-cessation program
F/U: As needed (dependent on BP and renal function), referral to nephrologist

Additional differential diagnoses: abdominal aortic atherosclerosis ▪ anemia ▪ carotid cavernous fistula ▪ peripheral arteriovenous fistula ▪ subclavian steal syndrome ▪ thyrotoxicosis

Butterfly rash

The presence of a butterfly rash is commonly a sign of systemic lupus erythematosus (SLE); however, it can also signal a dermatologic disorder. Typically, a butterfly rash appears in a malar distribution across the nose and cheeks. (See *Recognizing butterfly rash.*) Similar rashes may appear on the neck, scalp, and other areas. Butterfly rash is sometimes mistaken for sunburn because it can be provoked or aggravated by ultraviolet rays, but it has more substance, is more sharply demarcated, and has a thicker feel than surrounding skin.

HISTORY

- Ask the patient when he first noticed the butterfly rash and if he has noticed a rash elsewhere on his body.
- Ask the patient if he has recently been exposed to the sun.
- Ask the patient about recent weight or hair loss.
- Ask the patient if there's a family history of lupus.
- Obtain a drug history, including prescription and over-the-counter drugs, herbal remedies, and recreational drugs. Also, ask the patient about alcohol intake.
- Ask the patient if he has experienced malaise, fatigue, weakness, nausea, or vomiting.

PHYSICAL ASSESSMENT

- Inspect the skin for the extent of the rash. Note other areas of skin disruption.
- Observe the patient for periorbital edema, dyspnea, and weakness.
- Inspect the scalp for scaling and alopecia.
- Palpate the joints, noting pain, stiffness, or deformity.
- Palpate the lymph nodes for tenderness and enlargement.
- Inspect the scalp and hair for scaling and alopecia.
- Inspect the rash, noting macules, papules, pustules, and scaling. Is the rash edematous? Are areas of hypopigmentation or hyperpigmentation present?
- Look for blisters or ulcers in the mouth, and note inflamed lesions.
- Check for rashes elsewhere on the body.

SPECIAL CONSIDERATIONS

Be aware that hydralazine and procainamide can cause an SLE-like syndrome.

Ⓐ PEDIATRIC POINTER

Rare in pediatric patients, a butterfly rash may occur as part of an infectious disease such as erythema infectiosum, or "slapped cheek syndrome."

PATIENT COUNSELING

Instruct the patient to avoid exposure to the sun or, if he's going to be in the sun, to use sunscreen. Suggest the use of hypoallergenic makeup to help conceal facial lesions.

RECOGNIZING BUTTERFLY RASH

In classic butterfly rash, lesions appear on the cheeks and the bridge of the nose, creating a characteristic butterfly pattern. The rash may vary in severity from malar erythema to discoid lesions (plaques).

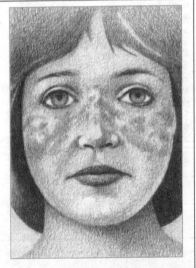

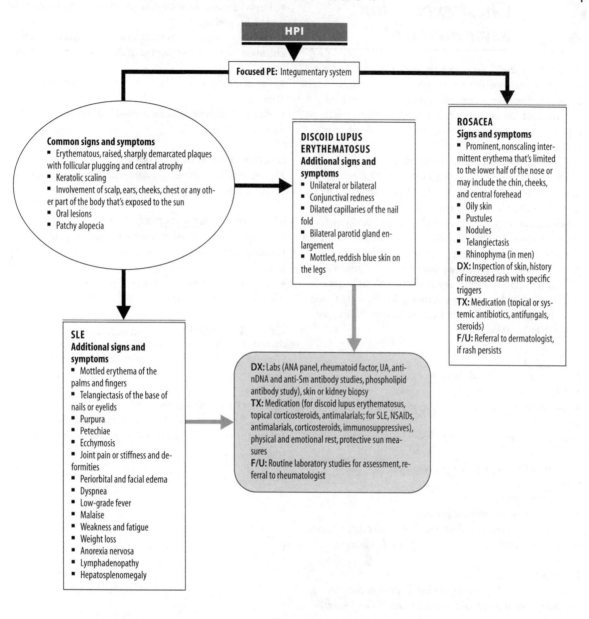

HPI

Focused PE: Integumentary system

Common signs and symptoms
- Erythematous, raised, sharply demarcated plaques with follicular plugging and central atrophy
- Keratolic scaling
- Involvement of scalp, ears, cheeks, chest or any other part of the body that's exposed to the sun
- Oral lesions
- Patchy alopecia

DISCOID LUPUS ERYTHEMATOSUS
Additional signs and symptoms
- Unilateral or bilateral
- Conjunctival redness
- Dilated capillaries of the nail fold
- Bilateral parotid gland enlargement
- Mottled, reddish blue skin on the legs

ROSACEA
Signs and symptoms
- Prominent, nonscaling intermittent erythema that's limited to the lower half of the nose or may include the chin, cheeks, and central forehead
- Oily skin
- Pustules
- Nodules
- Telangiectasis
- Rhinophyma (in men)
DX: Inspection of skin, history of increased rash with specific triggers
TX: Medication (topical or systemic antibiotics, antifungals, steroids)
F/U: Referral to dermatologist, if rash persists

SLE
Additional signs and symptoms
- Mottled erythema of the palms and fingers
- Telangiectasis of the base of nails or eyelids
- Purpura
- Petechiae
- Ecchymosis
- Joint pain or stiffness and deformities
- Periorbital and facial edema
- Dyspnea
- Low-grade fever
- Malaise
- Weakness and fatigue
- Weight loss
- Anorexia nervosa
- Lymphadenopathy
- Hepatosplenomegaly

DX: Labs (ANA panel, rheumatoid factor, UA, anti-nDNA and anti-Sm antibody studies, phospholipid antibody study), skin or kidney biopsy
TX: Medication (for discoid lupus erythematosus, topical corticosteroids, antimalarials; for SLE, NSAIDs, antimalarials, corticosteroids, immunosuppressives), physical and emotional rest, protective sun measures
F/U: Routine laboratory studies for assessment, referral to rheumatologist

---

Additional differential diagnoses: polymorphous light eruption ▪ seborrheic dermatitis

Other causes: hydralazine ▪ procainamide

C

Chest expansion, asymmetrical

Asymmetrical chest expansion is the uneven extension of portions of the chest wall during inspiration. During normal respiration, the thorax uniformly expands upward and outward and then contracts downward and inward. When this process is disrupted, breathing becomes uncoordinated, resulting in asymmetrical chest expansion.

Asymmetrical chest expansion may develop suddenly or gradually and may affect one or both sides of the chest wall. It may occur as delayed expiration (chest lag); as abnormal movement during inspiration (for example, intercostal retractions, paradoxical movement, or chest-abdomen asynchrony); or as unilateral absence of movement. This sign usually results from a pleural disorder, such as life-threatening hemothorax or tension pneumothorax. However, it can also result from a musculoskeletal or urologic disorder, airway obstruction, or trauma. Regardless of its underlying cause, asymmetrical chest expansion produces rapid and shallow or deep respirations that increase the work of breathing.

 ALERT

If you detect asymmetrical chest expansion:
- *take the patient's vital signs*
- *look for signs of acute respiratory distress, and administer oxygen*
- *use tape or sandbags to temporarily splint the unstable flail segment*
- *insert an I.V. line for fluid replacement and administration of pain medication*
- *contact the physician*
- *have emergency equipment available.*

If you don't suspect flail chest, and if the patient isn't experiencing acute respiratory distress, perform a focused assessment.

HISTORY
- Ask the patient if he's experiencing dyspnea or pain during breathing. If so, it is constant or intermittent? Does the pain worsen his feeling of breathlessness? Does repositioning, coughing, or any other activity relieve or worsen his dyspnea or pain? Is the pain more noticeable during inspiration or expiration? Can he inhale deeply?
- Review the patient's medical history for pulmonary or systemic illness, blunt or penetrating chest trauma, and thoracic surgery.
- Obtain an occupational history to find out if the patient may have inhaled toxic fumes or aspirated a toxic substance.

PHYSICAL ASSESSMENT
- Inspect the neck for ecchymosis, swelling, or hematomas and the face for swelling.
- Listen for noisy air movement. Inspect the jugular veins for distention, and gently palpate the trachea for midline positioning.
- Examine the posterior chest wall for areas of tenderness or deformity.
- Auscultate all lung fields for normal and adventitious breath sounds.

SPECIAL CONSIDERATIONS
Asymmetrical chest expansion can result from surgical removal of several ribs.

 P EDIATRIC POINTERS
- *Children develop asymmetrical chest expansion, paradoxical breathing, and retractions with acute respiratory illnesses, such as bronchiolitis, asthma, and croup.*
- *Congenital abnormalities, such as cerebral palsy or diaphragmatic hernia, can cause asymmetrical chest expansion.*

 A GING ISSUES

Asymmetrical chest expansion may be more difficult to determine in an elderly patient because of the structural deformities associated with aging.

PATIENT COUNSELING
Instruct the patient on what to expect from diagnostic testing and treatment. Provide emotional support to the patient and family.

CHEST EXPANSION, ASYMMETRICAL

HPI

Focused PE: Pulmonary and cardiovascular systems

FLAIL CHEST
Signs and symptoms
- Paradoxical movement of the chest
- Ecchymoses
- Severe localized pain
- Rapid shallow respirations
- Tachycardia
- Cyanosis

DX: History of chest injury, PE, ABG, CXR
TX: Oxygen therapy, mechanical ventilation, analgesia
F/U: Referral to pulmonologist

Additional common signs and symptoms
- Pain that may radiate to the arms, face, back, or abdomen
- Decreased tactile fremitus
- Absent breath sounds on the affected side

Common signs and symptoms
- Sudden stabbing pain
- Tachypnea
- Tachycardia
- Anxiety
- Restlessness

TENSION PNEUMOTHORAX
Additional signs and symptoms
- Cyanosis
- Hypotension
- Severe restlessness and anxiety
- Subcutaneous crepitation of the upper trunk, neck, and face
- Tracheal deviation
- Distended neck veins

PNEUMOTHORAX

HEMOTHORAX
Additional signs and symptoms
- Pain at injury site
- Dullness on percussion
- Signs of traumatic chest injury

DX: History of chest injury, ABG, CXR
TX: Aspiration of air or blood by needle thoracentesis, chest tube, surgery (if recurrent)
F/U: Return visit 1 week after hospitalization, referral to pulmonologist if symptoms recur

Additional differential diagnoses: bronchial obstruction ▪ kyphoscoliosis ▪ myasthenia gravis ▪ phrenic nerve dysfunction ▪ pleural effusion ▪ pneumonia ▪ poliomyelitis ▪ pulmonary embolism

Other causes: intubation of a mainstem bronchus ▪ pneumonectomy ▪ surgery

Chest pain

Chest pain usually results from a disorder affecting the thoracic or abdominal organs—the heart, pleurae, lungs, esophagus, rib cage, gallbladder, pancreas, or stomach. An important indicator of several acute and life-threatening cardiopulmonary and GI disorders, chest pain can also result from a musculoskeletal or hematologic disorder, anxiety, or drug therapy.

Chest pain can arise suddenly or gradually, and its cause may be difficult to ascertain initially. The pain can radiate to the arms, neck, jaw, or back. It can be steady or intermittent, mild or acute. It can range in character from a sharp shooting sensation to a dull, achy pain, a feeling of heaviness, a feeling of fullness, or even indigestion. It can occur at rest or be provoked or aggravated by stress, anxiety, physical exertion, deep breathing, or certain foods.

ALERT

When a patient complains of chest pain:
- *take his vital signs*
- *administer oxygen until the cause of the pain is determined*
- *attach the patient to a cardiac monitor*
- *have emergency equipment available.*
  If the patient's condition permits, perform a focused assessment.

HISTORY

- Ask the patient if he has experienced this type of pain in the past. Ask him to describe the pain. Did it begin suddenly or gradually? Is it more severe or frequent now than when it first started?
- Ask the patient if anything in particular seems to cause the pain.
- Ask the patient if anything makes the pain better or worse, or if it's constant or intermittent.
- Ask the patient what time of day the pain occurs.
- Ask the patient about associated symptoms, such as belching.
- Ask the patient if the pain radiates to other areas.
- Review the patient's medical history for cardiac or pulmonary disease, chest trauma, psychiatric disorders, GI disease, and sickle cell anemia.
- Obtain a drug history, including prescription and over-the-counter drugs, herbal remedies, and recreational drugs, and ask about recent dosage or schedule changes. Also, ask the patient about alcohol intake.
- Ask the patient about his smoking habits and cholesterol levels. Assess his family history for hypertension, coronary artery disease, myocardial infarction, and diabetes mellitus.

PHYSICAL ASSESSMENT

- Take the patient's vital signs, noting tachypnea, fever, tachycardia, paradoxical pulse, and hypertension or hypotension. Also, look for jugular vein distention and peripheral edema.
- Observe the patient for restlessness and anxiety.
- Observe the patient's skin color. Note diaphoresis or cool, clammy skin.
- Observe the patient's breathing pattern, and inspect his chest for asymmetrical expansion. Auscultate his lungs for pleural friction rub, crackles, rhonchi, wheezing, or diminished or absent breath sounds.
- Auscultate the chest for murmurs, clicks, gallops, or pericardial friction rub. Palpate for lifts, heaves, thrills, gallops, tactile fremitus, and abdominal mass or tenderness.

SPECIAL CONSIDERATIONS

Keep in mind that a patient with chest pain may deny his discomfort, so stress the importance of reporting symptoms so that his treatment can be adjusted accordingly.

PEDIATRIC POINTERS

- *Even children old enough to talk may have difficulty describing chest pain, so be alert for nonverbal clues, such as restlessness, facial grimaces, or holding of the painful area. Ask the child to first point to the painful area and then to point to where the pain goes. Determine the pain's severity by asking the parents if the pain interferes with the child's normal activities and behavior.*
- *A child may complain of chest pain in an attempt to get attention or to avoid attending school.*

AGING ISSUES

Because older patients are at higher risk for developing life-threatening conditions, such as a myocardial infarction, angina, or aortic dissection, carefully evaluate chest pain in an elderly patient.

PATIENT COUNSELING

If the patient has coronary artery disease, teach him about the typical features of cardiac ischemia and about the symptoms that should prompt him to seek medical attention. If the pain doesn't disappear after taking sublingual nitroglycerin, lasts more than 20 minutes, or has a different pattern than the usual angina, the patient must be evaluated immediately.

CHEST PAIN (CARDIAC)

HPI

Focused PE: Cardiovascular and pulmonary systems

Common signs and symptoms
- Chest tightness or pressure
- Pain that may radiate to the neck, shoulder, jaw, and arms
- Dyspnea
- Nausea and vomiting
- Tachycardia
- Palpitations
- Diaphoresis
- Dizziness
- Syncope
- Gallops and murmurs, S_3 or S_4

MI
Additional signs and symptoms
- Feeling of impending doom
- Pain that may escalate to crushing
- Hypotension or hypertension
- Pallor
- Clammy skin

PERICARDITIS
Signs and symptoms
- Sharp or stabbing precordial or retrosternal pain
- Pain that's aggravated by movement, inspiration, or lying supine
- Pericardial friction rub
- Low-grade fever
- Dyspnea
- Cough
- Dysphagia

DX: Imaging studies (echocardiogram, CT scan, MRI), ECG
TX: Medication (NSAIDs; if bacterial, antibiotics)
F/U: Return visit 2 weeks after treatment

Additional common signs and symptoms
- Pain that typically lasts 2 to 10 minutes
- Pain that may be provoked by exertion, heavy stress, or a big meal

ANGINA

HYPERTROPHIC CARDIOMYOPATHY
Additional signs and symptoms
- Cough
- Bradycardia associated with tachycardia
- S_4

DX: Imaging studies (CXR, echocardiogram, thallium scan, cardiac catheterization), electro-physiologic studies
TX: Avoidance of strenuous activity, medication (beta-adrenergic blockers, calcium channel blockers, antiarrhythmics), surgery
F/U: Referral to cardiologist

DX: Labs (serial cardiac enzymes, troponin, myoglobin, electrolytes, coagulation studies), imaging studies (echocardiogram, CXR, Tc-99m sestamibi scan, ECG, cardiac catheterization)
TX: Maintenance of ABCs; medication (dependent on severity of myocardial involvement and medical history — antithrombic agents, vasodilators, analgesics, beta-adrenergic agents, thrombolytics, anticoagulants, platelet aggregation inhibitors, anxiolytics, antiarrhythmics); low-fat, low-sodium diet; PCI; surgery
F/U: Referral to cardiologist

Additional differential diagnoses: aortic aneurysm (dissecting) ▪ costochondritis ▪ mediastinitis

Other causes: beta-adrenergic blockers (abrupt withdrawal can cause rebound angina in patients with coronary heart disease) ▪ Chinese restaurant syndrome ▪ cocaine use

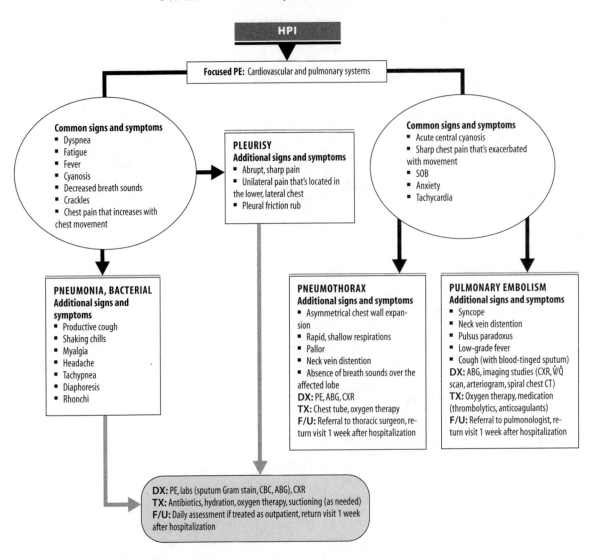

HPI

Focused PE: Cardiovascular and pulmonary systems

Common signs and symptoms
- Dyspnea
- Fatigue
- Fever
- Cyanosis
- Decreased breath sounds
- Crackles
- Chest pain that increases with chest movement

PLEURISY
Additional signs and symptoms
- Abrupt, sharp pain
- Unilateral pain that's located in the lower, lateral chest
- Pleural friction rub

Common signs and symptoms
- Acute central cyanosis
- Sharp chest pain that's exacerbated with movement
- SOB
- Anxiety
- Tachycardia

PNEUMONIA, BACTERIAL
Additional signs and symptoms
- Productive cough
- Shaking chills
- Myalgia
- Headache
- Tachypnea
- Diaphoresis
- Rhonchi

PNEUMOTHORAX
Additional signs and symptoms
- Asymmetrical chest wall expansion
- Rapid, shallow respirations
- Pallor
- Neck vein distention
- Absence of breath sounds over the affected lobe
DX: PE, ABG, CXR
TX: Chest tube, oxygen therapy
F/U: Referral to thoracic surgeon, return visit 1 week after hospitalization

PULMONARY EMBOLISM
Additional signs and symptoms
- Syncope
- Neck vein distention
- Pulsus paradoxus
- Low-grade fever
- Cough (with blood-tinged sputum)
DX: ABG, imaging studies (CXR, V̇/Q̇ scan, arteriogram, spiral chest CT)
TX: Oxygen therapy, medication (thrombolytics, anticoagulants)
F/U: Referral to pulmonologist, return visit 1 week after hospitalization

DX: PE, labs (sputum Gram stain, CBC, ABG), CXR
TX: Antibiotics, hydration, oxygen therapy, suctioning (as needed)
F/U: Daily assessment if treated as outpatient, return visit 1 week after hospitalization

Additional differential diagnoses: blastomycosis ▪ bronchitis ▪ coccidioidomycosis ▪ interstitial lung disease ▪ lung abscess ▪ lung cancer ▪ pulmonary actinomycosis ▪ pulmonary hypertension ▪ tuberculosis

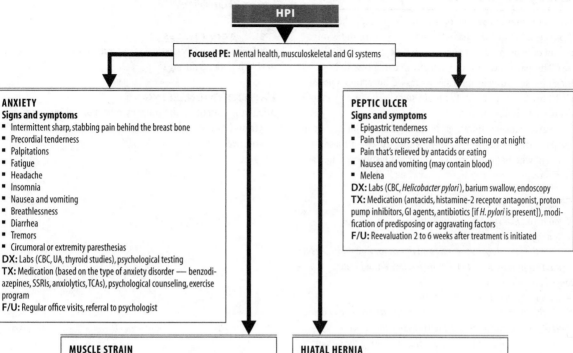

HPI

Focused PE: Mental health, musculoskeletal and GI systems

ANXIETY
Signs and symptoms
- Intermittent sharp, stabbing pain behind the breast bone
- Precordial tenderness
- Palpitations
- Fatigue
- Headache
- Insomnia
- Nausea and vomiting
- Breathlessness
- Diarrhea
- Tremors
- Circumoral or extremity paresthesias

DX: Labs (CBC, UA, thyroid studies), psychological testing
TX: Medication (based on the type of anxiety disorder — benzodiazepines, SSRIs, anxiolytics, TCAs), psychological counseling, exercise program
F/U: Regular office visits, referral to psychologist

PEPTIC ULCER
Signs and symptoms
- Epigastric tenderness
- Pain that occurs several hours after eating or at night
- Pain that's relieved by antacids or eating
- Nausea and vomiting (may contain blood)
- Melena

DX: Labs (CBC, *Helicobacter pylori*), barium swallow, endoscopy
TX: Medication (antacids, histamine-2 receptor antagonist, proton pump inhibitors, GI agents, antibiotics [if *H. pylori* is present]), modification of predisposing or aggravating factors
F/U: Reevaluation 2 to 6 weeks after treatment is initiated

MUSCLE STRAIN
Signs and symptoms
- Superficial or continuous ache or "pulling" sensation that's located in the chest
- Pain that's aggravated by lifting, pulling, or pushing heavy objects
- Pain that increases with palpation
ACUTE
- Fatigue
- Swelling of the affected area
- Weakness

DX: History of excessive muscle use, PE, ECG
TX: NSAIDs, rest or avoidance of increased muscle use
F/U: Reevaluation in 2 weeks (if pain persists or increases)

HIATAL HERNIA
Signs and symptoms
- Chest pain or pressure after meals
- Dysphagia
- Belching
- Pyrosis
- Hiccups

DX: Labs (CBC, cardiac enzymes, LFT, amylase, lipase), imaging studies (CXR, barium swallow), ECG, endoscopy
TX: Antacids, diet and activity modification, surgery (rare)
F/U: Reevaluation as needed (based on symptoms and lifestyle modifications)

Additional differential diagnoses: esophageal spasm ▪ GERD ▪ herpes zoster ▪ norcardiosis ▪ pancreatitis ▪ rib fracture ▪ sickle cell crisis ▪ thoracic outlet syndrome

Cheyne-Stokes respirations

The most common pattern of periodic breathing, Cheyne-Stokes respirations are characterized by a waxing and waning period of hyperpnea that alternates with a shorter period of apnea. This pattern can occur normally in patients with heart or lung disease. It usually indicates increased intracranial pressure (ICP) from a deep cerebral or brain stem lesion or a metabolic disturbance in the brain.

Cheyne-Stokes respirations may indicate a major change in the patient's condition — usually for the worse. For example, in a patient who has had head trauma or brain surgery, Cheyne-Stokes respirations may signal increasing ICP.

 ALERT

If you detect Cheyne-Stokes respirations:
- *quickly take the patient's vital signs*
- *time the periods of hyperpnea and apnea for 3 to 4 minutes to evaluate respirations and to obtain baseline data; be alert for prolonged periods of apnea*
- *elevate the patient's head 30 degrees*
- *check skin color and obtain a pulse oximetry reading to detect signs of hypoxemia; administer oxygen, if appropriate*
- *perform a rapid neurologic examination noting the patient's level of consciousness, pupillary reactions, and ability to move his extremities*
- *maintain airway patency, and institute emergency measures if necessary.*

If the patient's condition permits, perform a more thorough focused assessment.

HISTORY
- Review the patient's medical history for head trauma, recent brain surgery, and other brain insults.
- Obtain a drug history, including prescription and over-the-counter drugs, herbal remedies, and recreational drugs. Also, ask the patient about alcohol intake.

PHYSICAL ASSESSMENT
- In addition to the emergent examination, auscultate for abnormal breath sounds and note chest expansion during respirations.
- Monitor vital signs and neurologic status.

SPECIAL CONSIDERATIONS
When evaluating Cheyne-Stokes respirations, be careful not to mistake periods of hypoventilation or decreased tidal volume for complete apnea.

 PEDIATRIC POINTERS

Cheyne-Stokes respirations rarely occur in children, except during late-stage heart failure.

 AGING ISSUES

Subtle evidence of Cheyne-Stokes respirations can occur normally in elderly patients during sleep.

PATIENT COUNSELING
Advise the patient or his family members that sleep apnea differs from Cheyne-Stokes respirations in both causes and methods of treatment.

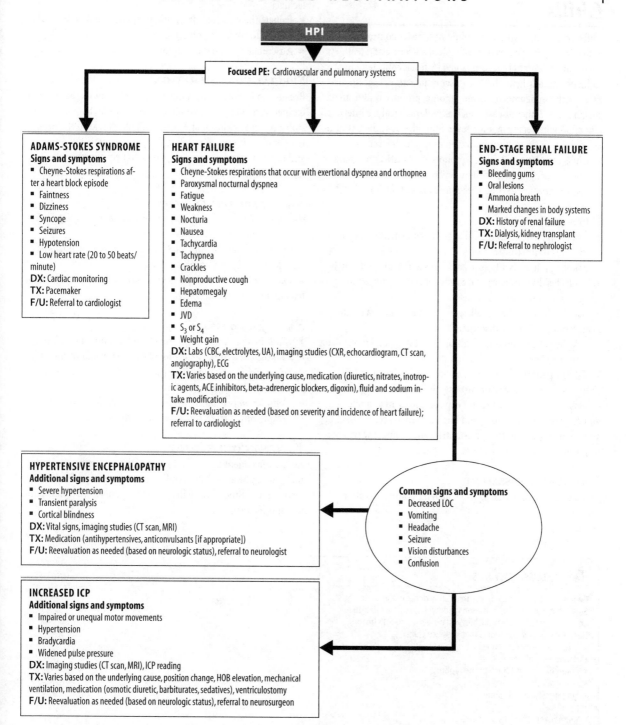

HPI

Focused PE: Cardiovascular and pulmonary systems

ADAMS-STOKES SYNDROME
Signs and symptoms
- Cheyne-Stokes respirations after a heart block episode
- Faintness
- Dizziness
- Syncope
- Seizures
- Hypotension
- Low heart rate (20 to 50 beats/minute)

DX: Cardiac monitoring
TX: Pacemaker
F/U: Referral to cardiologist

HEART FAILURE
Signs and symptoms
- Cheyne-Stokes respirations that occur with exertional dyspnea and orthopnea
- Paroxysmal nocturnal dyspnea
- Fatigue
- Weakness
- Nocturia
- Nausea
- Tachycardia
- Tachypnea
- Crackles
- Nonproductive cough
- Hepatomegaly
- Edema
- JVD
- S_3 or S_4
- Weight gain

DX: Labs (CBC, electrolytes, UA), imaging studies (CXR, echocardiogram, CT scan, angiography), ECG
TX: Varies based on the underlying cause, medication (diuretics, nitrates, inotropic agents, ACE inhibitors, beta-adrenergic blockers, digoxin), fluid and sodium intake modification
F/U: Reevaluation as needed (based on severity and incidence of heart failure); referral to cardiologist

END-STAGE RENAL FAILURE
Signs and symptoms
- Bleeding gums
- Oral lesions
- Ammonia breath
- Marked changes in body systems

DX: History of renal failure
TX: Dialysis, kidney transplant
F/U: Referral to nephrologist

HYPERTENSIVE ENCEPHALOPATHY
Additional signs and symptoms
- Severe hypertension
- Transient paralysis
- Cortical blindness

DX: Vital signs, imaging studies (CT scan, MRI)
TX: Medication (antihypertensives, anticonvulsants [if appropriate])
F/U: Reevaluation as needed (based on neurologic status), referral to neurologist

Common signs and symptoms
- Decreased LOC
- Vomiting
- Headache
- Seizure
- Vision disturbances
- Confusion

INCREASED ICP
Additional signs and symptoms
- Impaired or unequal motor movements
- Hypertension
- Bradycardia
- Widened pulse pressure

DX: Imaging studies (CT scan, MRI), ICP reading
TX: Varies based on the underlying cause, position change, HOB elevation, mechanical ventilation, medication (osmotic diuretic, barbiturates, sedatives), ventriculostomy
F/U: Reevaluation as needed (based on neurologic status), referral to neurosurgeon

Other causes: large doses of hypnotics, opioids, or barbiturates

Chills

Chills (rigors) are extreme, involuntary muscle contractions with characteristic paroxysms of violent shivering and teeth chattering. Commonly accompanied by fever, chills tend to arise suddenly, usually heralding the onset of infection. Certain diseases, such as pneumococcal pneumonia, produce only a single, shaking chill. Other diseases, such as malaria, produce intermittent chills with recurring high fever. Still others produce continuous chills for up to 1 hour, precipitating a high fever.

Chills can also result from lymphomas, transfusion reactions, and certain drugs. Chills without fever occur as a normal response to exposure to cold. (See *Rare causes of chills.*)

HISTORY

- Ask the patient when the chills began and whether they're continuous or intermittent.
- Ask the patient about associated signs and symptoms, such as headache, dysuria, diarrhea, confusion, chest pain, abdominal pain, cough, sore throat, or nausea.
- Ask the patient if he has allergies, an infection, or a recent history of an infectious disorder.
- Ask the patient about medications he's taking and if any drug has improved or worsened his symptoms.
- Ask the patient if he has received treatment (such as chemotherapy) that may predispose him to an infection.
- Ask the patient about recent exposure to farm animals, guinea pigs, hamsters, dogs, and birds as well as recent insect or animal bites, travel to foreign countries, and contact with a person who has an active infection.

PHYSICAL ASSESSMENT

- Take the patient's vital signs. Note temperature elevation, if present.
- Inspect the skin for any evidence of insect bites, rash, or petechiae.
- Palpate the lymph nodes, noting any enlargement. Inspect the throat for redness or discharge.
- Auscultate the lungs for abnormal sounds.

SPECIAL CONSIDERATIONS

Because chills are an involuntary response to an increasing body temperature set by the hypothalmic thermostat, blankets won't stop a patient's chills or shivering. Despite this, keep the room temperature as even as possible. Provide adequate hydration and nutrients, and give an antipyretic to help control fever. Irregular use of antipyretics can trigger compensatory chills.

PEDIATRIC POINTERS

- *Infants don't get chills because they have poorly developed shivering mechanisms.*
- *Most classic febrile childhood infections, such as measles and mumps, typically don't produce chills.*
- *Older children and teenagers may have chills with mycoplasma pneumonia or acute osteomyelitis.*

AGING ISSUES

- *Chills in an elderly patient usually indicate an underlying infection, such as a urinary tract infection, pneumonia (commonly associated with aspiration of gastric contents), diverticulitis, and skin breakdown in pressure areas.*
- *Consider an ischemic bowel in an elderly patient whose reason for seeking care is fever, chills, and abdominal pain.*

PATIENT COUNSELING

Advise the patient to measure his temperature with a thermometer when he experiences chills and to document the exact readings and times. This will help reveal patterns that may point to a specific diagnosis.

RARE CAUSES OF CHILLS

Chills can result from disorders that rarely occur in the United States but may be fairly common worldwide. So, remember to ask about recent foreign travel when you obtain a patient's history. Here are some rare disorders that produce chills:

- brucellosis (undulant fever)
- dengue (breakbone fever)
- epidemic typhus (louse-borne typhus)
- leptospirosis
- lymphocytic choriomeningitis
- plague
- pulmonary tularemia
- rat bite fever
- relapsing fever.

CHILLS

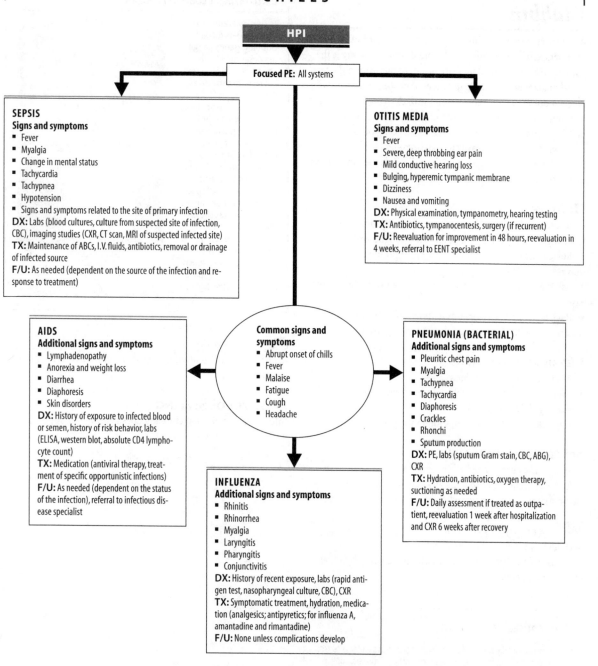

HPI

Focused PE: All systems

SEPSIS
Signs and symptoms
- Fever
- Myalgia
- Change in mental status
- Tachycardia
- Tachypnea
- Hypotension
- Signs and symptoms related to the site of primary infection

DX: Labs (blood cultures, culture from suspected site of infection, CBC), imaging studies (CXR, CT scan, MRI of suspected infected site)
TX: Maintenance of ABCs, I.V. fluids, antibiotics, removal or drainage of infected source
F/U: As needed (dependent on the source of the infection and response to treatment)

OTITIS MEDIA
Signs and symptoms
- Fever
- Severe, deep throbbing ear pain
- Mild conductive hearing loss
- Bulging, hyperemic tympanic membrane
- Dizziness
- Nausea and vomiting

DX: Physical examination, tympanometry, hearing testing
TX: Antibiotics, tympanocentesis, surgery (if recurrent)
F/U: Reevaluation for improvement in 48 hours, reevaluation in 4 weeks, referral to EENT specialist

AIDS
Additional signs and symptoms
- Lymphadenopathy
- Anorexia and weight loss
- Diarrhea
- Diaphoresis
- Skin disorders

DX: History of exposure to infected blood or semen, history of risk behavior, labs (ELISA, western blot, absolute CD4 lymphocyte count)
TX: Medication (antiviral therapy, treatment of specific opportunistic infections)
F/U: As needed (dependent on the status of the infection), referral to infectious disease specialist

Common signs and symptoms
- Abrupt onset of chills
- Fever
- Malaise
- Fatigue
- Cough
- Headache

PNEUMONIA (BACTERIAL)
Additional signs and symptoms
- Pleuritic chest pain
- Myalgia
- Tachypnea
- Tachycardia
- Diaphoresis
- Crackles
- Rhonchi
- Sputum production

DX: PE, labs (sputum Gram stain, CBC, ABG), CXR
TX: Hydration, antibiotics, oxygen therapy, suctioning as needed
F/U: Daily assessment if treated as outpatient, reevaluation 1 week after hospitalization and CXR 6 weeks after recovery

INFLUENZA
Additional signs and symptoms
- Rhinitis
- Rhinorrhea
- Myalgia
- Laryngitis
- Pharyngitis
- Conjunctivitis

DX: History of recent exposure, labs (rapid antigen test, nasopharyngeal culture, CBC), CXR
TX: Symptomatic treatment, hydration, medication (analgesics; antipyretics; for influenza A, amantadine and rimantadine)
F/U: None unless complications develop

Additional differential diagnoses: bacteremia ▪ cholangitis (gram-negative) ▪ hemolytic anemia ▪ hepatic abscess ▪ Hodgkin's disease ▪ infective endocarditis ▪ lung abscess ▪ Lyme disease ▪ lymphangitis ▪ lymphogranuloma venereum ▪ malaria ▪ miliary tuberculosis ▪ PID ▪ peritonitis ▪ puerperal or postabortal sepsis ▪ pyelonephritis ▪ renal abscess ▪ Rocky Mountain spotted fever ▪ septic arthritis ▪ sinusitis ▪ snake bite

Other causes: amphotericin B ▪ hemolytic reaction ▪ infection at I.V. insertion site ▪ I.V. bleomycin ▪ I.V. therapy ▪ nonhemolytic febrile reaction ▪ oral antipyretics ▪ phenytoin ▪ transfusion reaction

Clubbing

A nonspecific sign of pulmonary and cyanotic cardiovascular disorders, cirrhosis, colitis and thyroid disease, clubbing is the painless, usually bilateral increase in soft tissue around the terminal phalanges of the fingers or toes. (See *Rare causes of clubbing.*) It doesn't involve changes in the underlying bone. In early clubbing, the normal 160-degree angle between the nail and the nail base approximates 180 degrees. As clubbing progresses, this angle widens and the base of the nail becomes visibly swollen. In late clubbing, the angle where the nail meets the now-convex nail base extends more than halfway up the nail.

HISTORY

- Ask the patient if he has experienced hemoptysis, a productive cough, chest pain, dyspnea, anorexia, fatigue, or fever.
- Review the patient's medical history for pulmonary or cardiovascular disease.
- Ask the patient about a history of alcohol use or thyroid disease.
- Review the patient's current treatment plan because clubbing may resolve with correction of the underlying disorder.

PHYSICAL ASSESSMENT

- Take the patient's vital signs.
- Evaluate the extent of clubbing in the fingers and toes. (See *Evaluating clubbed fingers.*)
- Auscultate the patient's lungs for abnormal sounds.

SPECIAL CONSIDERATIONS

Don't mistake curved nails — a normal variation — for clubbing. Always remember that the angle between the nail and its base remains normal in curved nails but not in clubbed nails.

Ⓐ PEDIATRIC POINTERS

In children, clubbing occurs most commonly in cyanotic congenital heart disease and cystic fibrosis. Surgical correction of heart defects may reverse clubbing.

RARE CAUSES OF CLUBBING

Clubbing is typically a sign of pulmonary or cardiovascular disease, but it can also result from certain hepatic and GI disorders, such as cirrhosis, Crohn's disease, and ulcerative colitis. However, clubbing occurs only rarely with these disorders, so first check for more common signs and symptoms. For example, a patient with cirrhosis usually experiences right-upper-quadrant pain and hepatomegaly. A patient with Crohn's disease typically has abdominal cramping and tenderness. A patient with ulcerative colitis may develop diffuse abdominal pain and blood-streaked diarrhea.

EVALUATING CLUBBED FINGERS

To quickly examine a patient's fingers for early clubbing, gently palpate the bases of his nails. Normally, they feel firm; however, in early clubbing, nail bases feel springy when palpated. To evaluate late clubbing, have the patient place the first phalanges of the forefingers together, as shown. Normal nail bases are concave and create a small space when the first phalanges are opposed (as shown above right).

In late clubbing, however, the now-convex nail bases can touch without leaving a space (as shown below right).

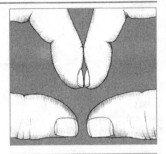

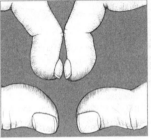

🕭 AGING ISSUES

Arthritic deformities of the fingers or toes may disguise the presence of clubbing.

PATIENT COUNSELING

Inform the patient that clubbing doesn't always disappear, even if the cause has been resolved.

CLUBBING

HPI

Focused PE: Cardiovascular and pulmonary systems

HEART FAILURE
Signs and symptoms
- Exertional dyspnea and orthopnea
- Paroxysmal nocturnal dyspnea
- Fatigue
- Nocturia
- Nausea
- Weakness
- Tachycardia
- Tachypnea
- Crackles and wheezing
- Nonproductive cough
- Hepatomegaly
- Edema
- JVD
- Weight gain
- S_3 or S_4

DX: Labs (CBC, electrolytes, UA), imaging studies (CXR, echocardiogram, CT scan, angiography), ECG
TX: Varies based on the underlying cause, medication (diuretics, nitrates, inotropic agents, ACE inhibitors, beta-adrenergic blockers, digoxin), fluid and sodium intake modification
F/U: Reevaluation based on severity and incidence of heart failure; referral to cardiologist

INTERSTITIAL LUNG DISEASE
Signs and symptoms
- Nonproductive cough
- Progressive dyspnea
- Cyanosis (late)
- Fine crackles
- Fatigue
- Variable chest pain
- Weight loss

DX: CBC, CXR, PFT, lung biopsy
TX: Removal of the source of the problem, if known; supportive therapy; medication (corticosteroids, cytotoxic drugs); single lung transplantation, oxygen therapy
F/U: Reevaluation (dependent on the severity of the disease), referral to pulmonologist

CHRONIC BRONCHITIS
Signs and symptoms
- Barrel chest
- SOB
- Productive cough
- Dyspnea on exertion
- Tachypnea
- Cyanosis
- Pursed-lip breathing
- Anorexia
- Malaise
- Coarse breath sounds
- Use of accessory muscles of respiration

DX: Labs (CBC, ABG), CXR, PFT
TX: Smoking-cessation program, medication (bronchodilators, sympathomimetics, anticholinergics, corticosteroids)
F/U: Reevaluation once per month if severe, biannually if stable

---

Additional differential diagnoses: bronchiectasis ▪ emphysema ▪ endocarditis ▪ lung abscess ▪ lung and pleural cancer

Confusion

An umbrella term for puzzling or inappropriate behavior or responses, confusion is the inability to think quickly and coherently. Depending on its cause, confusion may arise suddenly or gradually and may be temporary or irreversible. Aggravated by stress and sensory deprivation, confusion often occurs in hospitalized patients—especially elderly patients, in whom it may be mistaken for senility.

When severe confusion arises suddenly and the patient also has hallucinations and psychomotor hyperactivity, his condition is classified as delirium. Long-term, progressive confusion with deterioration of all cognitive functions is classified as dementia.

Confusion can result from a fluid and electrolyte imbalance or hypoxemia due to a pulmonary disorder. It can also have a metabolic, neurologic, cardiovascular, cerebrovascular, or nutritional origin or can result from a severe systemic infection or the effects of toxins, drugs, or alcohol. Confusion may signal worsening of an underlying and, perhaps, irreversible disease.

HISTORY

- Ask the patient to describe what's bothering him. He may not report confusion as his chief complaint but instead may complain of memory loss, persistent apprehension, or inability to concentrate.
- If the patient is unable to respond logically to direct questions, check with his family about onset and frequency of the confusion.
- Review the patient's medical history for head trauma or a cardiopulmonary, metabolic, cerebrovascular, or neurologic disorder.
- Obtain a drug history, including prescription and over-the-counter drugs, herbal remedies, and recreational drugs. Also, ask the patient about alcohol intake.
- Ask the patient about changes in eating or sleeping habits.

PHYSICAL ASSESSMENT

- Check the patient's vital signs, and assess the patient for changes in blood pressure, temperature, and pulse.
- Perform a neurologic assessment to establish the patient's level of consciousness. Also, perform a Mini–Mental Status Examination.

SPECIAL CONSIDERATIONS

Never leave a confused patient unattended; this will help prevent injury to himself and others. Keep the patient calm and quiet, and plan uninterrupted rest periods. Remember that herbal medicines, such as St. John's wort, can cause confusion, especially when taken with an antidepressant or other serotonergic drugs.

PEDIATRIC POINTERS

- Confusion can't be determined in infants and young children.
- Older children with acute febrile illnesses commonly experience transient delirium or acute confusion.

PATIENT COUNSELING

Advise the family to help orient the confused patient by keeping a large calendar and clock visible and that making a list of his activities with specific dates and times also helps.

CONFUSION

HPI

Focused PE: Neurologic system

FLUID AND ELECTROLYTE IMBALANCE
Signs and symptoms (dependent on extent of imbalance)
- Dehydration
- Lassitude
- Poor skin turgor
- Dry skin and mucus membranes
- Oliguria
- Hypotension
- Low-grade fever

DX: Electrolytes, identification of underlying disorder
TX: Electrolyte and fluid replacement, treatment of underlying disorder
F/U: Weekly evaluation of electrolytes until stable

Common signs and symptoms
- Confusion (may be intermittent)
- Headache
- Pupillary changes
- Sensory and motor deficits
- Personality disturbance
- Seizure

CEREBROVASCULAR DISORDER
Additional signs and symptoms
- Neurologic deficits (unilateral or bilateral)

HEAD TRAUMA
Additional signs and symptoms
- Swelling or laceration at the site of the injury
- Depression of skull
- Hematotympanum
- Vomiting
- Vision changes

BRAIN TUMOR
Additional signs and symptoms
- Progressive confusion
- Bizarre behavior

DX: History of injury, coagulation studies, PE, imaging studies (skull X-ray, CT scan, MRI, MRA, ultrasonography, angiography)
TX: Medication (analgesics, osmotic diuretics, anticonvulsants, thrombolytics for thrombotic stroke, chemotherapy and steroids for brain tumor), radiation therapy for brain tumor, surgery
F/U: As needed (dependent on neurologic status and extent of brain injury), referral to neurologist, neurosurgeon, or oncologist (as appropriate)

Additional differential diagnoses: decreased cerebral perfusion ▪ heatstroke ▪ heavy metal poisoning ▪ hypothermia ▪ hypoxemia ▪ metabolic encephalapathy ▪ nutritional deficiencies ▪ seizure disorders ▪ thyroid hormone disorders

Other causes: alcohol intoxication ▪ alcohol withdrawal ▪ carbon monoxide poisoning ▪ drugs ▪ herbal medicines

Conjunctival injection

A common ocular sign associated with inflammation, conjunctival injection is nonuniform redness of the conjunctiva from hyperemia. This redness can be diffuse, localized, or peripheral, or it may encircle a clear cornea.

Conjunctival injection usually results from bacterial or viral conjunctivitis, but it can also signal a severe ocular disorder that, if untreated, may lead to permanent blindness. In particular, conjunctival injection is an early sign of trachoma, a leading cause of blindness in third world countries and among Native Americans living in the southwestern United States.

Conjunctival injection can also result from minor eye irritation due to inadequate sleep, overuse of contact lenses, environmental irritants, and excessive eye rubbing.

ALERT

If the patient with conjunctival injection reports a chemical splash to the eye:
- *remove contact lenses, if appropriate*
- *irrigate the eye with copious amounts of normal saline solution*
- *evert the lids, and wipe the fornices with a cotton-tipped applicator to remove any foreign body particles and as much of the chemical as possible.*

If the patient's condition permits, perform a focused assessment.

HISTORY
- Ask the patient if he has associated pain. If so, when did the pain begin and where is it located? Is it constant or intermittent?
- Ask the patient about itching, burning, photophobia, blurred vision, halo vision, excessive tearing, or a foreign body sensation in the eye.
- Review the patient's medical history for eye disease, allergies, and trauma.

PHYSICAL ASSESSMENT
- Determine the location and severity of conjunctival injection. Is it circumoral or localized? Peripheral or diffuse? Note conjunctival or lid edema, ocular deviation, conjunctival follicles, ptosis, or exophthalmos. Also, note the type and amount of any discharge, if present.
- Test the patient's visual acuity to establish a baseline. Note if the patient has had vision changes. Is his vision blurred or his visual acuity markedly decreased?
- Test pupillary reaction to light.

SPECIAL CONSIDERATIONS
Because most forms of conjunctivitis are contagious, the infection can easily spread to the other eye or to family members. Stress the importance of hand washing and of not touching the affected eye to prevent contagion.

PEDIATRIC POINTERS
- *An infant can develop self-limiting chemical conjunctivitis at birth from ocular instillation of silver nitrate.*
- *An infant may develop bacterial conjunctivitis 2 to 5 days after birth due to contamination of the birth canal.*
- *An infant with congenital syphilis has prominent conjunctival injection and grayish pink corneas.*

PATIENT COUNSELING
If the patient complains of photophobia, tell him to keep the room dark or wear sunglasses. If the patient's visual acuity is markedly decreased, orient him to his environment to ensure his comfort and safety.

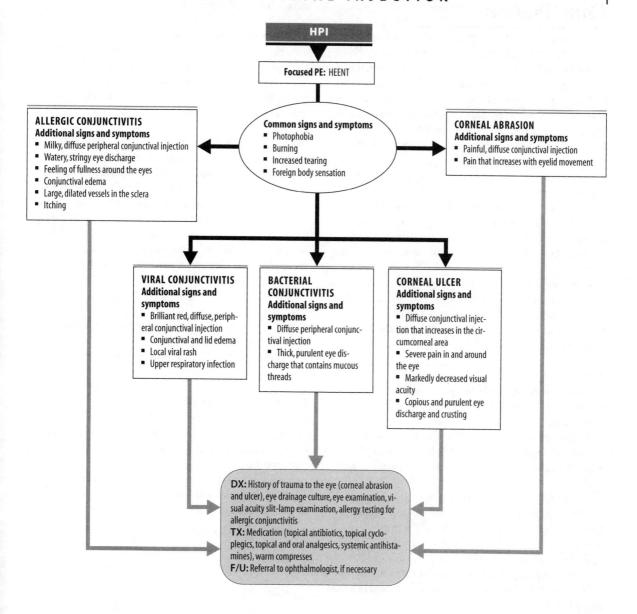

HPI

Focused PE: HEENT

Common signs and symptoms
- Photophobia
- Burning
- Increased tearing
- Foreign body sensation

ALLERGIC CONJUNCTIVITIS
Additional signs and symptoms
- Milky, diffuse peripheral conjunctival injection
- Watery, stringy eye discharge
- Feeling of fullness around the eyes
- Conjunctival edema
- Large, dilated vessels in the sclera
- Itching

CORNEAL ABRASION
Additional signs and symptoms
- Painful, diffuse conjunctival injection
- Pain that increases with eyelid movement

VIRAL CONJUNCTIVITIS
Additional signs and symptoms
- Brilliant red, diffuse, peripheral conjunctival injection
- Conjunctival and lid edema
- Local viral rash
- Upper respiratory infection

BACTERIAL CONJUNCTIVITIS
Additional signs and symptoms
- Diffuse peripheral conjunctival injection
- Thick, purulent eye discharge that contains mucous threads

CORNEAL ULCER
Additional signs and symptoms
- Diffuse conjunctival injection that increases in the circumcorneal area
- Severe pain in and around the eye
- Markedly decreased visual acuity
- Copious and purulent eye discharge and crusting

DX: History of trauma to the eye (corneal abrasion and ulcer), eye drainage culture, eye examination, visual acuity slit-lamp examination, allergy testing for allergic conjunctivitis
TX: Medication (topical antibiotics, topical cycloplegics, topical and oral analgesics, systemic antihistamines), warm compresses
F/U: Referral to ophthalmologist, if necessary

Additional differential diagnoses: blepharitis ▪ chemical burn ▪ corneal erosion ▪ dacryoadenitis ▪ episcleritis ▪ foreign body ▪ glaucoma ▪ hyphema ▪ iritis ▪ keratoconjunctivitis sicca ▪ ocular laceration ▪ ocular tumor ▪ Stevens-Johnson syndrome ▪ uveitis

Constipation

Constipation is defined as small, infrequent, or difficult bowel movements. Because normal bowel movements can vary in frequency and from individual to individual, constipation must be determined in relation to the patient's normal elimination pattern. Constipation may be a minor annoyance or, uncommonly, a sign of a life-threatening disorder such as acute intestinal obstruction. If untreated, constipation can lead to headache, anorexia, and abdominal discomfort and can adversely affect the patient's lifestyle and well-being.

Constipation most commonly occurs when the urge to defecate is suppressed and the muscles associated with bowel movements remain contracted. Because the autonomic nervous system controls bowel movements—by sensing rectal distention from fecal contents and by stimulating the external sphincter—any factor that influences this system can cause bowel dysfunction.

Acute constipation usually has an organic cause, such as an anal or rectal disorder. In a patient older than age 45, recent onset of constipation may be an early sign of colorectal cancer. Conversely, chronic constipation typically has a functional cause and may be related to stress.

HISTORY

- Ask the patient to describe the frequency of his bowel movements and the size and consistency of his stools. How long has he been constipated?
- Ask the patient if he has pain related to constipation. If so, when did he first notice the pain and where is it located?
- Ask the patient if defecation worsens or helps relieve the pain.
- Ask the patient to describe a typical day's menu. Estimate his daily fiber and fluid intake. Ask him about changes in eating habits, in drug or alcohol use, or in physical activity.
- Ask the patient if he has experienced recent emotional distress. Has constipation affected his family life or social contacts?
- Review the patient's medical history for GI, rectoanal, neurologic, or metabolic disorders; abdominal surgery; and radiation therapy.
- Obtain a drug history, including prescription and over-the-counter drugs, herbal remedies, and recreational drugs. Also, ask the patient about alcohol intake.

PHYSICAL ASSESSMENT

- Inspect the abdomen for distention or scars from previous surgery.
- Auscultate for bowel sounds, and characterize their motility.
- Percuss all four quadrants, and gently palpate for abdominal tenderness, a palpable mass, and hepatomegaly.

- Examine the rectum, and inspect for inflammation, lesions, scars, fissures, and external hemorrhoids.

SPECIAL CONSIDERATIONS

If the patient is on bed rest, reposition him frequently and help him perform active or passive exercises, as indicated. If the patient's abdominal muscles are weak, teach abdominal toning exercises. Also teach him relaxation techniques to help him reduce stress related to constipation.

 PEDIATRIC POINTERS

- *The high content of casein and calcium in cow's milk can produce hard stools and possible constipation in bottle-fed infants. Other causes of constipation in infants include inadequate fluid intake, Hirschsprung's disease, and anal fissures.*
- *In older children, constipation usually results from inadequate fiber intake and excessive intake of milk; it can also result from bowel spasm, mechanical obstruction, hypothyroidism, reluctance to stop playing for bathroom breaks, and the lack of privacy in some school bathrooms.*

AGING ISSUES

- *Acute constipation in elderly patients is usually associated with underlying structural abnormalities.*
- *Chronic constipation is chiefly caused by lifelong bowel and dietary habits and laxative use.*

PATIENT COUNSELING

Caution the patient not to strain during defecation to prevent injuring rectoanal tissue. Instruct him to avoid using laxatives or enemas. If he has been abusing these products, begin to wean him from them.

Stress the importance of a high-fiber diet, and encourage the patient to drink plenty of fluids. Also encourage him to exercise at least 1½ hours each week, if possible.

CONSTIPATION

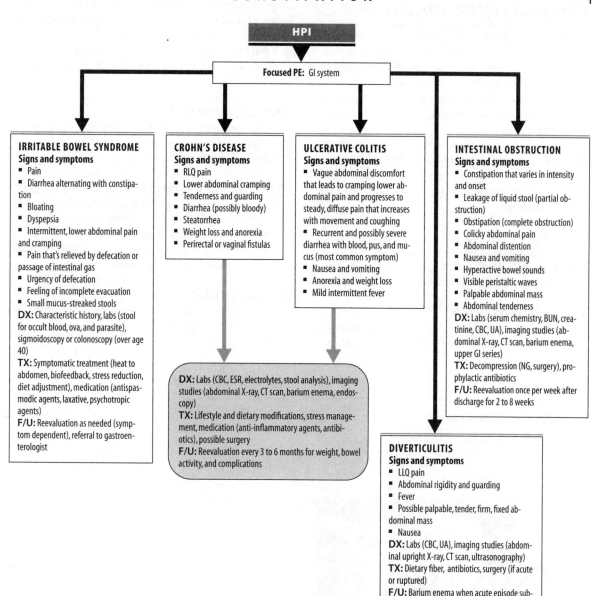

HPI

Focused PE: GI system

IRRITABLE BOWEL SYNDROME
Signs and symptoms
- Pain
- Diarrhea alternating with constipation
- Bloating
- Dyspepsia
- Intermittent, lower abdominal pain and cramping
- Pain that's relieved by defecation or passage of intestinal gas
- Urgency of defecation
- Feeling of incomplete evacuation
- Small mucus-streaked stools

DX: Characteristic history, labs (stool for occult blood, ova, and parasite), sigmoidoscopy or colonoscopy (over age 40)
TX: Symptomatic treatment (heat to abdomen, biofeedback, stress reduction, diet adjustment), medication (antispasmodic agents, laxative, psychotropic agents)
F/U: Reevaluation as needed (symptom dependent), referral to gastroenterologist

CROHN'S DISEASE
Signs and symptoms
- RLQ pain
- Lower abdominal cramping
- Tenderness and guarding
- Diarrhea (possibly bloody)
- Steatorrhea
- Weight loss and anorexia
- Perirectal or vaginal fistulas

DX: Labs (CBC, ESR, electrolytes, stool analysis), imaging studies (abdominal X-ray, CT scan, barium enema, endoscopy)
TX: Lifestyle and dietary modifications, stress management, medication (anti-inflammatory agents, antibiotics), possible surgery
F/U: Reevaluation every 3 to 6 months for weight, bowel activity, and complications

ULCERATIVE COLITIS
Signs and symptoms
- Vague abdominal discomfort that leads to cramping lower abdominal pain and progresses to steady, diffuse pain that increases with movement and coughing
- Recurrent and possibly severe diarrhea with blood, pus, and mucus (most common symptom)
- Nausea and vomiting
- Anorexia and weight loss
- Mild intermittent fever

INTESTINAL OBSTRUCTION
Signs and symptoms
- Constipation that varies in intensity and onset
- Leakage of liquid stool (partial obstruction)
- Obstipation (complete obstruction)
- Colicky abdominal pain
- Abdominal distention
- Nausea and vomiting
- Hyperactive bowel sounds
- Visible peristaltic waves
- Palpable abdominal mass
- Abdominal tenderness

DX: Labs (serum chemistry, BUN, creatinine, CBC, UA), imaging studies (abdominal X-ray, CT scan, barium enema, upper GI series)
TX: Decompression (NG, surgery), prophylactic antibiotics
F/U: Reevaluation once per week after discharge for 2 to 8 weeks

DIVERTICULITIS
Signs and symptoms
- LLQ pain
- Abdominal rigidity and guarding
- Fever
- Possible palpable, tender, firm, fixed abdominal mass
- Nausea

DX: Labs (CBC, UA), imaging studies (abdominal upright X-ray, CT scan, ultrasonography)
TX: Dietary fiber, antibiotics, surgery (if acute or ruptured)
F/U: Barium enema when acute episode subsides; if surgery was performed, reevaluation 1 week after discharge

---

Additional differential diagnoses: anal fissure ▪ anorectal abscess ▪ cirrhosis ▪ diabetic neuropathy ▪ diverticulosis ▪ hemorrhoids ▪ hepatic porphyria ▪ hypercalcemia ▪ hypothyroidism ▪ ischemia ▪ mesenteric artery ▪ multiple sclerosis ▪ paraplegia ▪ Parkinson's disease ▪ spinal cord lesion ▪ tabes dorsalis ▪ ulcerative proctitis

Other causes: barium retention (from GI study) ▪ drugs (narcotic analgesics, excessive use of laxatives or enemas) ▪ radiation therapy ▪ surgery

Corneal reflex, absent

The corneal reflex is tested bilaterally by drawing a fine-pointed wisp of sterile cotton from a corner of each eye to the cornea. Normally, even though only one eye is tested at a time, the patient blinks bilaterally each time either cornea is touched — this is the corneal reflex. When this reflex is absent, neither eyelid closes when the cornea of one eye is touched. (See *Eliciting the corneal reflex.*)

The site of the afferent fibers for this reflex is in the ophthalmic branch of the trigeminal nerve (cranial nerve V); the efferent fibers are located in the facial nerve (cranial nerve VII). Unilateral or bilateral absence of the corneal reflex may result from damage to these nerves.

HISTORY

- Ask the patient about associated symptoms, such as facial pain, dysphagia, and limb weakness.
- Ask the patient if he has noticed hearing loss or tinnitus.

PHYSICAL ASSESSMENT

- Assess the patient for signs and symptoms of increased intracranial pressure, such as decreased level of consciousness, headache, and vomiting.
- Look for other signs of trigeminal nerve dysfunction. To test the three sensory portions of the nerve, touch each side of the patient's face on the brow, cheek, and jaw with a cotton wisp and ask him to compare the sensations.
- If you suspect facial nerve involvement, note if the upper face (brow and eyes) and lower face (cheek, mouth, and chin) are weak bilaterally.

SPECIAL CONSIDERATIONS

When the corneal reflex is absent, take measures to protect the patient's affected eye from injury, such as lubricating the eye with artificial tears to prevent drying.

Ⓐ PEDIATRIC POINTERS

- *Brain stem lesions and injuries are the most common causes of absent corneal reflexes in children; Guillain-Barré syndrome and trigeminal neuralgia are less common.*
- *Infants, especially those born prematurely, may have an absent corneal reflex due to anoxic damage to the brain stem.*

PATIENT COUNSELING

Provide emotional support. The cause of the absent corneal reflex may be disfiguring and cause anxiety over body image disturbances.

ELICITING THE CORNEAL REFLEX

To elicit the corneal reflex, have the patient turn her eyes away from you to avoid involuntary blinking during the procedure. Then approach the patient from the opposite side, out of her line of vision, and brush the cornea lightly with a fine wisp of sterile cotton. Repeat the procedure on the other eye.

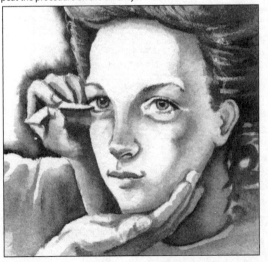

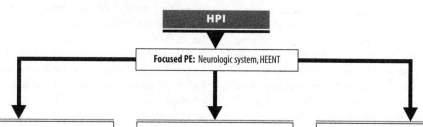

Focused PE: Neurologic system, HEENT

ACOUSTIC NEUROMA
Signs and symptoms
- Tinnitus
- Unilateral hearing impairment
- Facial palsy
- Anesthesia
- Palate weakness
- Cerebellar dysfunction
- Pain in the face
- Drooling

DX: Imaging studies (CT scan, MRI), audiology, caloric stimulation, electronystagmography, brain stem–evoked response audiometry

TX: Stereotactic radiosurgery, surgery

F/U: Reevaluation 1 week after hospitalization for neurologic evaluation and auditory testing, referral to otolaryngologist

BELL'S PALSY
Signs and symptoms
- Hemifacial weakness or paralysis
- Drooling on the affected side
- Sagging of the affected side
- Trouble shutting the eye of the affected side
- Constant tearing of the eye of the affected side

DX: PE, CT scan

TX: Medication (corticosteroids, lubricating eye drops, antiviral agents), eye patch (while sleeping if the eye can't be completely closed)

F/U: Referral to neurologist

BRAIN STEM INFARCTION OR INJURY
Signs and symptoms
- Absent or diminished corneal reflex on the side opposite the lesion
- Decreased LOC
- Dysphagia
- Dysarthria
- Contralateral limb weakness
- Early signs of increased ICP
- Respiratory changes
- Bilateral pupillary dilation or constriction with decreased responsiveness to light
- Nystagmus
- Rising systolic BP
- Widened pulse pressure
- Bradycardia
- Coma

DX: Imaging studies (skull X-ray, CT scan, MRI, angiography), EEG, ICP monitoring

TX: Medication (if embolic event, anticoagulants; antihypertensives; corticosteroids; if increased ICP, osmotic diuretics)

F/U: Referral to neurologist

Additional differential diagnoses: Guillain-Barré syndrome ▪ herpetic keratoconjunctivitis ▪ trigeminal neuralgia (tic douloureux)

Cough

Resonant, brassy, and harsh, a barking cough indicates edema of the larynx and surrounding tissue. Because children's airways are smaller in diameter than those of adults, edema can rapidly lead to airway occlusion—a life-threatening emergency.

A nonproductive cough is a noisy, forceful expulsion of air from the lungs that doesn't yield sputum or blood. A nonproductive cough not only is ineffective but can also cause damage, such as airway collapse or rupture of alveoli or blebs. A nonproductive cough that later becomes productive is a classic sign of progressive respiratory disease.

A nonproductive cough may occur in paroxysms and can worsen by becoming more frequent. An acute cough has a sudden onset and may be self-limiting; a cough that persists beyond 3 months is considered chronic and, in many cases, results from cigarette smoking.

A productive cough is a sudden, forceful, noisy expulsion of air that contains sputum, blood, or both. (The sputum's color, consistency, and odor provide important clues about the patient's condition.) Productive coughing can occur as a single cough or as paroxysmal coughing and can be voluntarily induced, although it's usually a reflexive response to stimulation of the airway mucosa.

Productive coughing commonly results from an acute or a chronic cardiovascular or respiratory infection that causes inflammation, edema, and increased mucus production in the airways. The most common cause of chronic productive coughing is cigarette smoking, which produces mucoid sputum ranging in color from clear to yellow to brown.

HISTORY

- Ask the patient when the cough began and whether body position, time of day, or specific activity affects it. Try to determine if the cough is related to smoking or an environmental irritant.
- Ask the patient to describe the cough. Is it harsh, brassy, dry, or hacking?
- Ask the patient about the frequency and intensity of coughing. If he has pain associated with coughing, breathing, or activity, when did it begin? Where is it located? If the patient is a child, ask the parents when the cough began and what signs and symptoms accompanied it. Has he had previous episodes of coughing? Did his condition improve with exposure to cold air?
- Review the patient's medical history for recent or chronic illness (especially a cardiovascular, pulmonary, or GI disorder), allergies, cancer, surgery, and trauma.
- Ask the patient about hypersensitivity to drugs, foods, pets, dust, or pollen.
- Obtain a drug history, including prescription and over-the-counter drugs, herbal remedies, and recreational drugs. Ask the patient about recent changes in schedule or dosages. Also, ask the patient about alcohol intake.
- Ask the patient about recent changes in appetite, weight, exercise tolerance, or energy level and recent exposure to irritating fumes, chemicals, smoke, or infectious persons.
- If the patient has a productive cough, ask him how much sputum he's coughing up each day, at what time of day, and if he has noticed an increase in sputum production since his coughing began. Also, ask about the color, odor, and consistency of the sputum.

PHYSICAL ASSESSMENT

- Observe the patient's general appearance and manner. Note whether he's cyanotic or has clubbed fingers or peripheral edema.
- Take the patient's vital signs. Check the depth and rhythm of his respirations, and note if wheezing or "crowing" noises occur with breathing.
- Inspect the patient's neck for distended veins and tracheal deviation, and palpate for masses or enlarged lymph nodes.
- Examine the patient's chest. Note retractions or accessory muscle use. Percuss for dullness, tympany, or flatness. Auscultate for wheezing, crackles, rhonchi, pleural friction rubs, and decreased or absent breath sounds.

SPECIAL CONSIDERATIONS

A patient with a productive cough can develop acute respiratory distress from thick or excessive secretions, bronchospasm, or fatigue, so examine him before you take his history. Avoid taking measures to suppress a productive cough because retention of sputum may interfere with alveolar aeration or impair pulmonary resistance to infection.

PEDIATRIC POINTERS

- *Sudden onset of paroxysmal nonproductive coughing may indicate aspiration of a foreign body—a common danger in children, especially those between ages 6 months and 4 years.*
- *Causes of nonproductive coughing in infants and children include asthma, bacterial pneumonia, acute bronchiolitis, acute otitis media, measles, cystic fibrosis, life-threatening pertussis, and airway hyperactivity, stress, emotional stimulation, or attention-seeking behavior.*

AGING ISSUES

Always ask an elderly patient about a cough because it may be an indication of serious acute or chronic illness.

PATIENT COUNSELING

Encourage the patient who smokes to quit. Teach the patient how to breathe deeply and cough effectively. Teach the patient and his family how to perform chest percussion to loosen secretions.

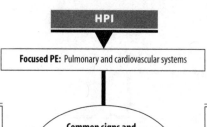

Focused PE: Pulmonary and cardiovascular systems

Common signs and symptoms
- Hoarseness
- Dyspnea
- Restlessness
- Tachycardia

EPIGLOTTIDITIS
Additional signs and symptoms
- Stridor
- High fever
- Dysphagia
- Severe respiratory distress
- Nasal flaring
- Cyanosis
- Throat pain out of proportion to throat appearance
- Copious oral secretions

DX: Labs (throat culture, blood culture, CBC), lateral neck X-ray, indirect laryngoscopy

TX: Airway protection, emergency tracheostomy (if spasm present), humidified oxygen, medication (corticosteroids, antibiotics), I.V. fluids

F/U: Reevaluation 1 week after hospitalization

SPASMODIC CROUP
Additional signs and symptoms
- Barking cough while sleeping
- Nasal flaring
- Cyanosis
- Anxious, frantic appearance
- Absence of fever
- Decreased breath sounds
- Wheezing
- Prolonged inspiration or expiration

DX: History of repeated episodes, PE

TX: Oxygen therapy, humidified air

F/U: Referral to allergist

LARYNGOTRACHEOBRONCHITIS, ACUTE
Additional signs and symptoms
- Substernal and intercostal retractions
- Barking cough
- Low-grade to moderate fever
- Runny nose
- Poor appetite
- Shallow, rapid respirations
- Decreased breath sounds
- Wheezing
- Prolonged inspiration or expiration
- Red epiglottis

DX: PE, neck X-ray

TX: Warm or cool humidified air, oxygen therapy, antibiotics

F/U: Reevaluation 1 week after the beginning of treatment (unless condition worsens) or 1 week after hospitalization

---

Additional differential diagnosis: aspiration of foreign body

COUGH (NONPRODUCTIVE)

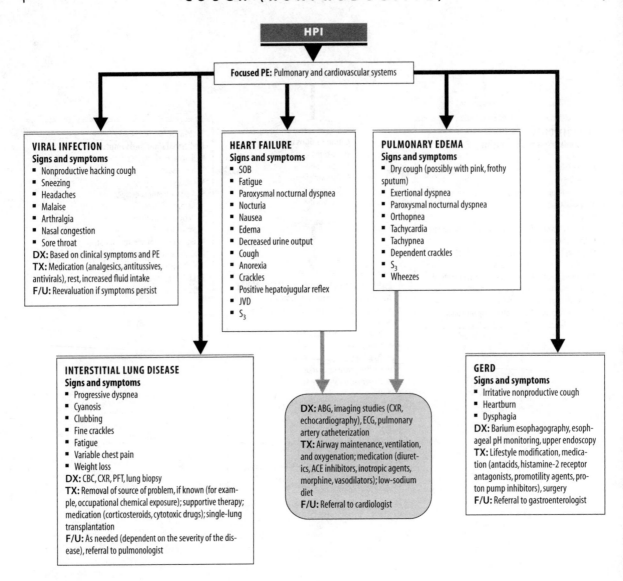

HPI

Focused PE: Pulmonary and cardiovascular systems

VIRAL INFECTION
Signs and symptoms
- Nonproductive hacking cough
- Sneezing
- Headaches
- Malaise
- Arthralgia
- Nasal congestion
- Sore throat

DX: Based on clinical symptoms and PE
TX: Medication (analgesics, antitussives, antivirals), rest, increased fluid intake
F/U: Reevaluation if symptoms persist

HEART FAILURE
Signs and symptoms
- SOB
- Fatigue
- Paroxysmal nocturnal dyspnea
- Nocturia
- Nausea
- Edema
- Decreased urine output
- Cough
- Anorexia
- Crackles
- Positive hepatojugular reflex
- JVD
- S_3

PULMONARY EDEMA
Signs and symptoms
- Dry cough (possibly with pink, frothy sputum)
- Exertional dyspnea
- Paroxysmal nocturnal dyspnea
- Orthopnea
- Tachycardia
- Tachypnea
- Dependent crackles
- S_3
- Wheezes

INTERSTITIAL LUNG DISEASE
Signs and symptoms
- Progressive dyspnea
- Cyanosis
- Clubbing
- Fine crackles
- Fatigue
- Variable chest pain
- Weight loss

DX: CBC, CXR, PFT, lung biopsy
TX: Removal of source of problem, if known (for example, occupational chemical exposure); supportive therapy; medication (corticosteroids, cytotoxic drugs); single-lung transplantation
F/U: As needed (dependent on the severity of the disease), referral to pulmonologist

DX: ABG, imaging studies (CXR, echocardiography), ECG, pulmonary artery catheterization
TX: Airway maintenance, ventilation, and oxygenation; medication (diuretics, ACE inhibitors, inotropic agents, morphine, vasodilators); low-sodium diet
F/U: Referral to cardiologist

GERD
Signs and symptoms
- Irritative nonproductive cough
- Heartburn
- Dysphagia

DX: Barium esophagography, esophageal pH monitoring, upper endoscopy
TX: Lifestyle modification, medication (antacids, histamine-2 receptor antagonists, promotility agents, proton pump inhibitors), surgery
F/U: Referral to gastroenterologist

Additional differential diagnoses: airway occlusion (partial) ▪ aortic aneurysm (thoracic) ▪ asthma ▪ atelectasis ▪ bronchogenic carcinoma ▪ Hantavirus pulmonary syndrome ▪ laryngeal tumor ▪ laryngitis ▪ Legionnaire's disease ▪ pleural effusion ▪ sarcoidosis ▪ sinusitis (chronic)

Other causes: bronchoscopy ▪ inhalants ▪ intermittent positive-pressure breathing ▪ PFTs ▪ tracheal suctioning

COUGH (PRODUCTIVE)

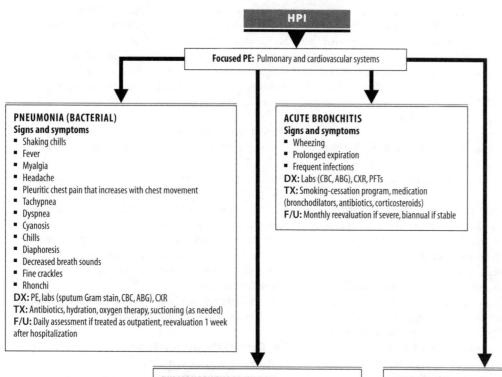

HPI

Focused PE: Pulmonary and cardiovascular systems

PNEUMONIA (BACTERIAL)
Signs and symptoms
- Shaking chills
- Fever
- Myalgia
- Headache
- Pleuritic chest pain that increases with chest movement
- Tachypnea
- Dyspnea
- Cyanosis
- Chills
- Diaphoresis
- Decreased breath sounds
- Fine crackles
- Rhonchi

DX: PE, labs (sputum Gram stain, CBC, ABG), CXR
TX: Antibiotics, hydration, oxygen therapy, suctioning (as needed)
F/U: Daily assessment if treated as outpatient, reevaluation 1 week after hospitalization

ACUTE BRONCHITIS
Signs and symptoms
- Wheezing
- Prolonged expiration
- Frequent infections

DX: Labs (CBC, ABG), CXR, PFTs
TX: Smoking-cessation program, medication (bronchodilators, antibiotics, corticosteroids)
F/U: Monthly reevaluation if severe, biannual if stable

PULMONARY TUBERCULOSIS
Signs and symptoms
- Mild to severe productive cough
- Hemoptysis
- Malaise
- Dyspnea
- Pleuritic chest pain
- Night sweats
- Weight loss
- Chest dullness on percussion

DX: Tuberculin skin test, sputum for AFB, CXR, bronchoscopy, open lung biopsy
TX: Medication (antitubercular drugs, specific drugs for resistant strains)
F/U: Referral to pulmonologist

LUNG CANCER
Signs and symptoms
- Chronic cough that produces small amounts of purulent, blood-streaked sputum (bronchogenic carcinoma)
- Cough that produces large amounts of frothy sputum (bronchoalveolar carcinoma)
- Dyspnea
- Anorexia
- Fatigue
- Weight loss
- Chest pain
- Fever
- Wheezing

DX: Imaging studies (CXR, CT scan, MRI), bronchoscopy, needle biopsy, open lung biopsy
TX: Varies (dependent on the type and stage of the cancer), medication (chemotherapy, analgesia), radiation therapy, surgery
F/U: Referral to oncologist and surgeon

Additional differential diagnoses: actinomycosis ▪ aspiration pneumonitis ▪ asthma (acute) ▪ bronchiectasis ▪ chemical pneumonitis ▪ nocardiosis ▪ psittacosis ▪ pulmonary edema ▪ silicosis

Other causes: bronchoscopy ▪ drugs (expectorants) ▪ respiratory treatments ▪ PFTs

Crackles

A common finding in certain cardiovascular and pulmonary disorders, crackles are nonmusical clicking or rattling noises heard during auscultation of breath sounds. Also known as rales or crepitations, crackles usually occur during inspiration and recur constantly from one respiratory cycle to the next. They can be unilateral or bilateral, moist or dry. They're characterized by their pitch, loudness, location, persistence, and occurrence during the respiratory cycle.

Pulmonary edema causes fine crackles at the bases of the lungs, and bronchiectasis produces moist crackles. Sickle cell anemia may produce crackles when it causes pulmonary infarction or infection.

Crackles indicate abnormal movement of air through fluid-filled airways. They can be irregularly dispersed, as in pneumonia, or localized, as in bronchiectasis. (A few basilar crackles can be heard in normal lungs after prolonged shallow breathing. These normal crackles clear with a few deep breaths.) Usually, though, crackles indicate the degree of an underlying illness. When crackles result from a generalized disorder, they usually occur in the less distended and more dependent areas of the lungs, such as the lung bases when the patient is standing. Crackles due to air passing through inflammatory exudate may not be audible if the involved portion of the lung isn't being ventilated because of shallow respirations.

◢ ALERT

If the patient with crackles shows signs of respiratory distress:
- *quickly take the patient's vital signs, and examine him for airway obstruction*
- *check the depth and rhythm of respirations, for increased accessory muscle use and chest wall motion, retractions, stridor, or nasal flaring*
- *maintain a patent airway, administer oxygen, and institute emergency measures, if necessary.*

If the patient doesn't present with signs of respiratory distress, perform a focused assessment.

HISTORY

- Review the patient's medical history for respiratory or cardiovascular problems or recent surgery, trauma, and illness.
- Ask the patient whether he smokes or drinks alcohol.
- If the patient also has a cough, ask him when it began and whether it's constant or intermittent. Find out what the cough sounds like and whether he's coughing up sputum or blood. If the cough is productive, determine the sputum's consistency, amount, odor, and color.
- Ask the patient if he has pain. If so where is it located and does it radiate to other areas? Also ask the patient if movement, coughing, or breathing worsens or helps relieve his pain.

- Ask the patient if he's experiencing hoarseness or difficulty swallowing.
- Obtain a drug history, including prescription and over-the-counter drugs, herbal remedies, and recreational drugs. Also, ask the patient about alcohol intake.
- Ask the patient about recent weight loss, anorexia, nausea, vomiting, fatigue, weakness, vertigo, and syncope.
- Ask the patient if he has been exposed to irritants, such as vapors, fumes, or smoke.

PHYSICAL ASSESSMENT

- Note the patient's position: Is he lying still or moving about restlessly?
- Examine the patient's nose and mouth for signs of infection, such as inflammation or increased secretions. Note his breath odor. Check his neck for masses, tenderness, swelling, lymphadenopathy, or venous distention.
- Inspect the chest for abnormal configuration or uneven expansion. Percuss for dullness, tympany, or flatness.
- Auscultate the lungs for other abnormal, diminished, or absent breath sounds.
- Listen to the patient's heart for abnormal sounds, and check his hands and feet for edema or clubbing.

SPECIAL CONSIDERATIONS

Plan daily uninterrupted rest periods to help the patient relax and sleep. To keep the patient's airway patent and facilitate his breathing, elevate the head of his bed.

Ⓐ PEDIATRIC POINTERS

- *Crackles in an infant or child may indicate a serious cardiovascular or respiratory disorder.*
- *Pneumonia produces diffuse, sudden crackles in children.*
- *Esophageal atresia and tracheoesophageal fistula can cause bubbling, moist crackles due to aspiration of food or secretions into the lungs—especially in neonates.*
- *Cystic fibrosis produces widespread, fine to coarse inspiratory crackles and wheezing in infants.*

◉ AGING ISSUES

- *Crackles that clear after deep breathing may indicate mild basilar atelectasis.*
- *In older patients, auscultate lung bases before and after auscultating apices.*

PATIENT COUNSELING

Teach the patient how to deep-breathe and cough effectively. Encourage him to stop smoking or using aerosols, powders, or other products that might irritate his airways. If the patient needs to restrict fluid intake, teach him how to measure fluids accurately, and instruct him on fluids that he might consider solids such as gelatin.

CRACKLES

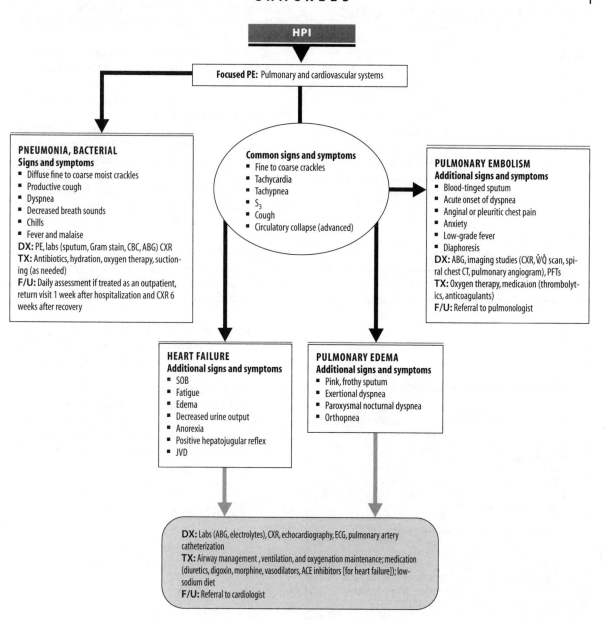

HPI

Focused PE: Pulmonary and cardiovascular systems

PNEUMONIA, BACTERIAL
Signs and symptoms
- Diffuse fine to coarse moist crackles
- Productive cough
- Dyspnea
- Decreased breath sounds
- Chills
- Fever and malaise

DX: PE, labs (sputum, Gram stain, CBC, ABG) CXR
TX: Antibiotics, hydration, oxygen therapy, suctioning (as needed)
F/U: Daily assessment if treated as an outpatient, return visit 1 week after hospitalization and CXR 6 weeks after recovery

Common signs and symptoms
- Fine to coarse crackles
- Tachycardia
- Tachypnea
- S_3
- Cough
- Circulatory collapse (advanced)

PULMONARY EMBOLISM
Additional signs and symptoms
- Blood-tinged sputum
- Acute onset of dyspnea
- Anginal or pleuritic chest pain
- Anxiety
- Low-grade fever
- Diaphoresis

DX: ABG, imaging studies (CXR, $\dot{V}/\dot{Q}$ scan, spiral chest CT, pulmonary angiogram), PFTs
TX: Oxygen therapy, medication (thrombolytics, anticoagulants)
F/U: Referral to pulmonologist

HEART FAILURE
Additional signs and symptoms
- SOB
- Fatigue
- Edema
- Decreased urine output
- Anorexia
- Positive hepatojugular reflex
- JVD

PULMONARY EDEMA
Additional signs and symptoms
- Pink, frothy sputum
- Exertional dyspnea
- Paroxysmal nocturnal dyspnea
- Orthopnea

DX: Labs (ABG, electrolytes), CXR, echocardiography, ECG, pulmonary artery catheterization
TX: Airway management , ventilation, and oxygenation maintenance; medication (diuretics, digoxin, morphine, vasodilators, ACE inhibitors [for heart failure]); low-sodium diet
F/U: Referral to cardiologist

Additional differential diagnoses: ARDS ▪ asthma (acute) ▪ bronchiectasis ▪ bronchitis (chronic) ▪ interstitial fibrosis of the lungs ▪ legionnaires' disease ▪ lung abscess ▪ pneumonia ▪ psittacosis ▪ pulmonary tuberculosis ▪ sarcoidosis ▪ silicosis ▪ tracheobronchitis

Crepitation, subcutaneous

When bubbles of air or other gases (such as carbon dioxide) are trapped in subcutaneous tissue, palpation or stroking of the skin produces a crackling sound called subcutaneous crepitation. The bubbles feel like small, unstable nodules and aren't painful, even though subcutaneous crepitation is commonly associated with painful disorders. Usually, the affected tissue is visibly edematous; this can lead to life-threatening airway occlusion if the edema affects the neck or upper chest.

The air or gas bubbles enter the tissues through open wounds, from the action of anaerobic microorganisms, or from traumatic or spontaneous rupture or perforation of pulmonary or GI organs.

 ALERT

Because subcutaneous crepitation can indicate a life-threatening disorder, you'll need to perform a rapid initial evaluation and intervene, if necessary. (See Managing subcutaneous crepitation.) If the patient's condition permits, perform a focused assessment.

HISTORY

● Ask the patient if he's experiencing pain or having difficulty breathing. If he's in pain, find out where the pain is located, how severe it is, and when it began.
● Ask the patient about recent thoracic surgery, diagnostic testing, and respiratory therapy or a history of trauma or chronic pulmonary disease.

PHYSICAL ASSESSMENT

● Palpate the affected skin to evaluate the location and extent of subcutaneous crepitation and to obtain baseline information. Repalpate frequently to determine if the subcutaneous crepitation is increasing.
● Check the patient's temperature and vital signs.
● If the patient has a wound, assess for drainage, odor, swelling, and discoloration.

SPECIAL CONSIDERATIONS

Because excessive edema from subcutaneous crepitation in the neck and upper chest can cause airway obstruction, be alert for signs of respiratory distress.

 PEDIATRIC POINTERS

Children may develop subcutaneous crepitation in the neck from ingestion of corrosive substances that perforate the esophagus.

PATIENT COUNSELING

Reassure the patient that the affected tissues will eventually absorb the air or gas bubbles, so the subcutaneous crepitation will decrease. Warn patients with asthma or chronic bronchitis to be alert for subcutaneous crepitation, which can signal pneumothorax, a dangerous complication.

MANAGING SUBCUTANEOUS CREPITATION

Subcutaneous crepitation occurs when air or gas bubbles escape into tissues. It may signal life-threatening rupture of an air-filled or gas-producing organ or a fulminating anaerobic infection.

ORGAN RUPTURE

If the patient shows signs of respiratory distress — such as severe dyspnea, tachypnea, accessory muscle use, nasal flaring, air hunger, or tachycardia — quickly test for Hamman's sign to detect trapped air bubbles in the mediastinum.

To test for Hamman's sign, help the patient assume a left-lateral recumbent position. Then place your stethoscope over the precordium. If you hear a loud crunching sound that synchronizes with his heartbeat, the patient has a positive Hamman's sign.

Depending on which organ is ruptured, be prepared for endotracheal intubation, an emergency tracheotomy, or chest tube insertion. Start administering supplemental oxygen immediately. Start an I.V. line to administer fluids and medication, and connect the patient to a cardiac monitor.

ANAEROBIC INFECTION

If the patient has an open wound with a foul odor and local swelling and discoloration, you must act quickly. Take the patient's vital signs, checking especially for fever, tachycardia, hypotension, and tachypnea. Next, start an I.V. line to administer fluids and medication, and provide supplemental oxygen.

In addition, be prepared for emergency surgery to drain and debride the wound. If the patient's condition is life-threatening, you may need to prepare him for transfer to a facility with a hyperbaric chamber.

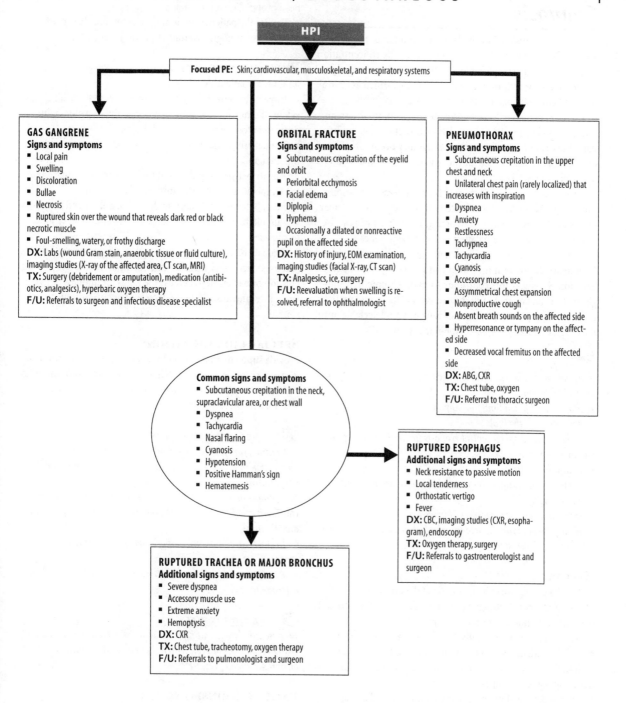

HPI

Focused PE: Skin; cardiovascular, musculoskeletal, and respiratory systems

GAS GANGRENE
Signs and symptoms
- Local pain
- Swelling
- Discoloration
- Bullae
- Necrosis
- Ruptured skin over the wound that reveals dark red or black necrotic muscle
- Foul-smelling, watery, or frothy discharge

DX: Labs (wound Gram stain, anaerobic tissue or fluid culture), imaging studies (X-ray of the affected area, CT scan, MRI)
TX: Surgery (debridement or amputation), medication (antibiotics, analgesics), hyperbaric oxygen therapy
F/U: Referrals to surgeon and infectious disease specialist

ORBITAL FRACTURE
Signs and symptoms
- Subcutaneous crepitation of the eyelid and orbit
- Periorbital ecchymosis
- Facial edema
- Diplopia
- Hyphema
- Occasionally a dilated or nonreactive pupil on the affected side

DX: History of injury, EOM examination, imaging studies (facial X-ray, CT scan)
TX: Analgesics, ice, surgery
F/U: Reevaluation when swelling is resolved, referral to ophthalmologist

PNEUMOTHORAX
Signs and symptoms
- Subcutaneous crepitation in the upper chest and neck
- Unilateral chest pain (rarely localized) that increases with inspiration
- Dyspnea
- Anxiety
- Restlessness
- Tachypnea
- Tachycardia
- Cyanosis
- Accessory muscle use
- Assymmetrical chest expansion
- Nonproductive cough
- Absent breath sounds on the affected side
- Hyperresonance or tympany on the affected side
- Decreased vocal fremitus on the affected side

DX: ABG, CXR
TX: Chest tube, oxygen
F/U: Referral to thoracic surgeon

Common signs and symptoms
- Subcutaneous crepitation in the neck, supraclavicular area, or chest wall
- Dyspnea
- Tachycardia
- Nasal flaring
- Cyanosis
- Hypotension
- Positive Hamman's sign
- Hematemesis

RUPTURED ESOPHAGUS
Additional signs and symptoms
- Neck resistance to passive motion
- Local tenderness
- Orthostatic vertigo
- Fever

DX: CBC, imaging studies (CXR, esophagram), endoscopy
TX: Oxygen therapy, surgery
F/U: Referrals to gastroenterologist and surgeon

RUPTURED TRACHEA OR MAJOR BRONCHUS
Additional signs and symptoms
- Severe dyspnea
- Accessory muscle use
- Extreme anxiety
- Hemoptysis

DX: CXR
TX: Chest tube, tracheotomy, oxygen therapy
F/U: Referrals to pulmonologist and surgeon

Other causes: bronchoscopy ▪ intermittent positive-pressure breathing ▪ mechanical ventilation ▪ respiratory treatments ▪ thoracic surgery ▪ upper GI tract endoscopy

Cyanosis

Cyanosis—a bluish or bluish black discoloration of the skin and mucous membranes—results from excessive concentration of unoxygenated hemoglobin in the blood. This common sign may develop abruptly or gradually. It can be classified as central or peripheral, although the two types may coexist.

Central cyanosis reflects inadequate oxygenation of systemic arterial blood caused by right-to-left cardiac shunting, pulmonary disease, or hematologic disorders. It may occur anywhere on the skin and also on the mucous membranes of the mouth, lips, and conjunctiva.

Peripheral cyanosis reflects sluggish peripheral circulation caused by vasoconstriction, reduced cardiac output, or vascular occlusion. It may be widespread or may occur locally in one extremity; however, it doesn't affect mucous membranes.

Although cyanosis is an important sign of cardiovascular and pulmonary disorders, it isn't always an accurate gauge of oxygenation. Several factors contribute to its development: hemoglobin level and oxygen saturation, cardiac output, and partial pressure of oxygen (PO_2). Cyanosis is usually undetectable until the oxygen saturation of hemoglobin falls below 80%.

◢ ALERT

If the patient displays sudden, localized cyanosis and other signs of arterial occlusion:
- *protect the affected limb from injury*
- *don't massage the limb.*

If the patient displays central cyanosis stemming from a pulmonary disorder or shock:
- *maintain the airway*
- *obtain a pulse oximetry or arterial blood gas analysis and administer oxygen*
- *institute emergency measures, if necessary.*

If the patient's cyanosis accompanies less-acute conditions, perform a focused assessment.

HISTORY

- Ask the patient when he first noticed the cyanosis. Does it subside and recur? Is it aggravated by cold, smoking, or stress? Is it alleviated by massage or rewarming?
- Ask the patient about headaches, dizziness, or blurred vision.
- Ask the patient about pain in the arms and legs (especially with walking) and about abnormal sensations, such as numbness, tingling, and coldness.
- Ask the patient about chest pain, its severity, and any aggravating and alleviating factors.
- Ask the patient if he has a cough. If so, is it productive? Ask the patient to describe the sputum.

- Ask the patient about sleep apnea. Does he sleep with his head propped up on pillows?
- Review the patient's medical history for a cardiac, pulmonary, or hematologic disorder or previous surgery.

PHYSICAL ASSESSMENT

- Take the patient's vital signs.
- Inspect the skin and mucous membranes to determine the extent of cyanosis. Check the skin for coolness, pallor, redness, pain, and ulceration. Also, note clubbing.
- Evaluate the patient's level of consciousness, and test his motor strength.
- Palpate peripheral pulses and test capillary refill time. Note the temperature of the extremities and any edema.
- Auscultate heart rate and rhythm, note gallops and murmurs.
- Auscultate the abdominal aorta and femoral arteries to detect bruits.
- Evaluate respiratory rate and rhythm. Check for nasal flaring and use of accessory muscles. Inspect for asymmetrical chest expansion or barrel chest. Percuss the lungs for dullness or hyperresonance, and auscultate for decreased or adventitious breath sounds.

SPECIAL CONSIDERATIONS

Provide supplemental oxygen to relieve shortness of breath and decrease cyanosis. However, deliver small doses (2 L/minute) in patients with chronic obstructive pulmonary disease (COPD), who may retain carbon dioxide.

PEDIATRIC POINTERS

- *Central cyanosis may result from cystic fibrosis, asthma, airway obstruction by a foreign body, acute laryngotracheobronchitis, or epiglottiditis.*
- *Cyanosis may result from a congenital heart defect, such as transposition of the great vessels, that cause right-to-left intracardiac shunting.*
- *In children, circumoral cyanosis may precede generalized cyanosis.*
- *Acrocyanosis may occur in infants because of excessive crying or exposure to cold.*

◢ AGING ISSUES

Because elderly patients have reduced tissue perfusion, peripheral cyanosis can present even with a slight decrease in cardiac output or systemic blood pressure.

PATIENT COUNSELING

Teach patients with chronic cardiopulmonary disease, such as heart failure or COPD, to recognize cyanosis as a sign of severe disease and to get immediate medical attention when it occurs.

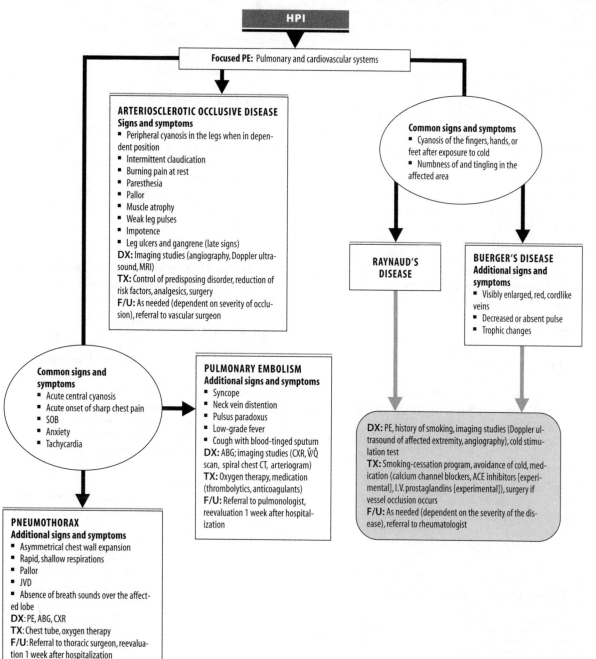

HPI

Focused PE: Pulmonary and cardiovascular systems

ARTERIOSCLEROTIC OCCLUSIVE DISEASE
Signs and symptoms
- Peripheral cyanosis in the legs when in dependent position
- Intermittent claudication
- Burning pain at rest
- Paresthesia
- Pallor
- Muscle atrophy
- Weak leg pulses
- Impotence
- Leg ulcers and gangrene (late signs)
DX: Imaging studies (angiography, Doppler ultrasound, MRI)
TX: Control of predisposing disorder, reduction of risk factors, analgesics, surgery
F/U: As needed (dependent on severity of occlusion), referral to vascular surgeon

Common signs and symptoms
- Cyanosis of the fingers, hands, or feet after exposure to cold
- Numbness of and tingling in the affected area

RAYNAUD'S DISEASE

BUERGER'S DISEASE
Additional signs and symptoms
- Visibly enlarged, red, cordlike veins
- Decreased or absent pulse
- Trophic changes

Common signs and symptoms
- Acute central cyanosis
- Acute onset of sharp chest pain
- SOB
- Anxiety
- Tachycardia

PULMONARY EMBOLISM
Additional signs and symptoms
- Syncope
- Neck vein distention
- Pulsus paradoxus
- Low-grade fever
- Cough with blood-tinged sputum
DX: ABG; imaging studies (CXR, V̇/Q̇ scan, spiral chest CT, arteriogram)
TX: Oxygen therapy, medication (thrombolytics, anticoagulants)
F/U: Referral to pulmonologist, reevaluation 1 week after hospitalization

DX: PE, history of smoking, imaging studies (Doppler ultrasound of affected extremity, angiography), cold stimulation test
TX: Smoking-cessation program, avoidance of cold, medication (calcium channel blockers, ACE inhibitors [experimental], I.V. prostaglandins [experimental]), surgery if vessel occlusion occurs
F/U: As needed (dependent on the severity of the disease), referral to rheumatologist

PNEUMOTHORAX
Additional signs and symptoms
- Asymmetrical chest wall expansion
- Rapid, shallow respirations
- Pallor
- JVD
- Absence of breath sounds over the affected lobe
DX: PE, ABG, CXR
TX: Chest tube, oxygen therapy
F/U: Referral to thoracic surgeon, reevaluation 1 week after hospitalization

---

Additional differential diagnoses: bronchiectasis ▪ COPD ▪ heart failure ▪ lung cancer ▪ lupus erythematosus ▪ peripheral arterial occlusion (acute) ▪ pneumonia ▪ polycythemia vera ▪ pulmonary edema ▪ pulmonary embolism ▪ shock

D Decerebrate posture

Decerebrate posture (decerebrate rigidity, abnormal extensor reflex) is characterized by adduction and extension of the arms, with the wrists pronated and the fingers flexed. The legs are stiffly extended, with plantar flexion of the feet. In severe cases, the back is acutely arched (opisthotonos). (See *Recognizing decerebrate posture.*) This sign indicates upper brain stem damage, which may result from primary lesions, such as infarction, hemorrhage, or tumor; metabolic encephalopathy; head injury; or brain stem compression associated with increased intracranial pressure (ICP).

Decerebrate posture may be elicited by noxious stimuli or may occur spontaneously. It may be unilateral or bilateral. With concurrent brain stem and cerebral damage, decerebrate posture may affect only the arms, with the legs remaining flaccid. Alternatively, decerebrate posture may affect one side of the body and decorticate posture the other. The two postures may also alternate as the patient's neurologic status fluctuates. Generally, the duration of each posturing episode correlates with the severity of brain stem damage.

ALERT

If you observe decerebrate posture:
- *ensure a patent airway*
- *turn the patient's head to the side to prevent aspiration (Don't disrupt spinal alignment if you suspect spinal cord injury.)*
- *examine spontaneous respirations, and institute emergency measures if necessary.*
After the patient has stabilized, perform a focused assessment.

HISTORY
- Explore the history of the patient's coma. If you can't obtain this information, look for clues to the causative disorder, such as hepatomegaly, cyanosis, diabetic skin changes, needle tracks, or obvious trauma.

- Ask the patient's family when his level of consciousness (LOC) began deteriorating. Did it occur abruptly? What did the patient complain of before he lost consciousness?
- Review the patient's medical history for diabetes, liver disease, cancer, blood clots, or aneurysm.
- Ask the patient's family about an accident or trauma that could be responsible for the coma.

PHYSICAL ASSESSMENT
- Take the patient's vital signs, and determine his LOC; use the Glasgow Coma Scale as a reference. Be alert for signs of increased ICP (such as bradycardia, increasing systolic blood pressure, and widening pulse pressure) and neurologic deterioration (such as altered respiratory pattern and abnormal temperature).
- Evaluate the pupils for size, equality, and response to light.
- Assess deep tendon and cranial nerve reflexes, and test for doll's eye sign.

SPECIAL CONSIDERATIONS
Relief of high ICP by removal of spinal fluid during a lumbar puncture may precipitate cerebral compression of the brain stem and cause decerebrate posture and coma.

A PEDIATRIC POINTERS
- *Children younger than age 2 may not display decerebrate posture because of the immaturity of their central nervous system. However, if the posture does occur, it's usually the more severe opisthotonos. In fact, opisthotonos is more common in infants and young children than in adults and is usually a terminal sign.*
- *In children, the most common cause of decerebrate posture is head injury. It also occurs with Reye's syndrome—the result of increased ICP causing brain stem compression.*

PATIENT COUNSELING
Inform the patient's family that decerebrate posture is a reflex response, not a voluntary response to pain or a sign of recovery. Offer emotional support.

RECOGNIZING DECEREBRATE POSTURE

Decerebrate posture results from damage to the upper brain stem. In this posture, the arms are adducted and extended, with the wrists pronated and the fingers flexed. The legs are stiffly extended, with plantar flexion of the feet.

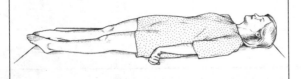

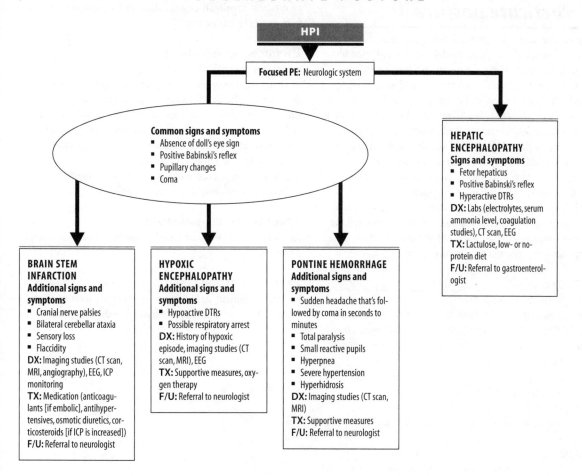

HPI

Focused PE: Neurologic system

Common signs and symptoms
- Absence of doll's eye sign
- Positive Babinski's reflex
- Pupillary changes
- Coma

BRAIN STEM INFARCTION
Additional signs and symptoms
- Cranial nerve palsies
- Bilateral cerebellar ataxia
- Sensory loss
- Flaccidity

DX: Imaging studies (CT scan, MRI, angiography), EEG, ICP monitoring
TX: Medication (anticoagulants [if embolic], antihypertensives, osmotic diuretics, corticosteroids [if ICP is increased])
F/U: Referral to neurologist

HYPOXIC ENCEPHALOPATHY
Additional signs and symptoms
- Hypoactive DTRs
- Possible respiratory arrest

DX: History of hypoxic episode, imaging studies (CT scan, MRI), EEG
TX: Supportive measures, oxygen therapy
F/U: Referral to neurologist

PONTINE HEMORRHAGE
Additional signs and symptoms
- Sudden headache that's followed by coma in seconds to minutes
- Total paralysis
- Small reactive pupils
- Hyperpnea
- Severe hypertension
- Hyperhidrosis

DX: Imaging studies (CT scan, MRI)
TX: Supportive measures
F/U: Referral to neurologist

HEPATIC ENCEPHALOPATHY
Signs and symptoms
- Fetor hepaticus
- Positive Babinski's reflex
- Hyperactive DTRs

DX: Labs (electrolytes, serum ammonia level, coagulation studies), CT scan, EEG
TX: Lactulose, low- or no-protein diet
F/U: Referral to gastroenterologist

Additional differential diagnoses: brain stem tumor ▪ cerebral lesion ▪ hypoglycemic encephalopathy ▪ posterior fossa hemorrhage

Other cause: lumbar puncture

Decorticate posture

A sign of corticospinal damage, decorticate posture (decorticate rigidity, abnormal flexor response) is characterized by adduction of the arms and flexion of the elbows, with wrists and fingers flexed on the chest. The legs are extended and internally rotated, with plantar flexion of the feet. This posture may occur unilaterally or bilaterally. (See *Recognizing decorticate posture.*)

Decorticate posture usually results from stroke or head injury. It may be elicited by noxious stimuli or may occur spontaneously. The intensity of the required stimulus, the duration of the posture, and the frequency of spontaneous episodes vary with the severity and location of cerebral injury.

Although a serious sign, decorticate posture carries a more favorable prognosis than decerebrate posture. However, if the causative disorder extends lower in the brain stem, decorticate posture may progress to decerebrate posture.

 ALERT

If you observe decorticate posture:
* *obtain vital signs, and evaluate the patient's level of consciousness (LOC) (If LOC is impaired, insert an oropharyngeal airway, elevate his head 30 degrees, and turn his head to the side to prevent aspiration, unless spinal cord injury is suspected.)*
* *evaluate the patient's respiratory rate, rhythm, and depth (Prepare to institute emergency measures if necessary.)*
* *institute seizure precautions.*
  After the patient has stabilized, perform a focused assessment.

History
* Ask the patient about headache, dizziness, nausea, abnormal vision, and numbness or tingling.
* Ask the patient's family when decorticate posture was first noticed.
* Ask the patient's family about behavior changes.

* Review the patient's medical history for cerebrovascular disease, cancer, meningitis, encephalitis, upper respiratory tract infection, and recent trauma.

Physical assessment
* Take the patient's vital signs.
* Determine the patient's LOC, using the Glasgow Coma Scale as a reference. Be alert for signs of increased intracranial pressure (such as bradycardia, increasing systolic blood pressure, and widening pulse pressure) and neurologic deterioration (such as altered respiratory pattern and abnormal temperature).
* Test motor and sensory functions.
* Evaluate pupil size, equality, and response to light.
* Test cranial nerve and deep tendon reflexes.

Special considerations
Assess the patient frequently to detect subtle signs of neurologic deterioration.

Patient counseling
Instruct the patient and his family on what to expect from diagnostic testing and treatment. Provide emotional support.

Recognizing decorticate posture

Decorticate posture results from damage to one or both corticospinal tracts. With this posture, the arms are adducted and flexed, with the wrists and fingers flexed on the chest. The legs are usually extended and internally rotated, with plantar flexion of the feet.

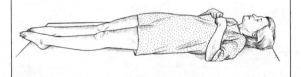

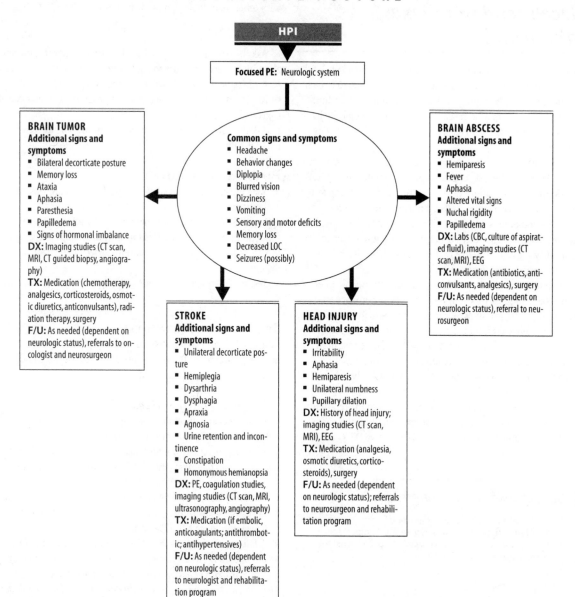

HPI

Focused PE: Neurologic system

Common signs and symptoms
- Headache
- Behavior changes
- Diplopia
- Blurred vision
- Dizziness
- Vomiting
- Sensory and motor deficits
- Memory loss
- Decreased LOC
- Seizures (possibly)

BRAIN TUMOR
Additional signs and symptoms
- Bilateral decorticate posture
- Memory loss
- Ataxia
- Aphasia
- Paresthesia
- Papilledema
- Signs of hormonal imbalance

DX: Imaging studies (CT scan, MRI, CT guided biopsy, angiography)
TX: Medication (chemotherapy, analgesics, corticosteroids, osmotic diuretics, anticonvulsants), radiation therapy, surgery
F/U: As needed (dependent on neurologic status), referrals to oncologist and neurosurgeon

BRAIN ABSCESS
Additional signs and symptoms
- Hemiparesis
- Fever
- Aphasia
- Altered vital signs
- Nuchal rigidity
- Papilledema

DX: Labs (CBC, culture of aspirated fluid), imaging studies (CT scan, MRI), EEG
TX: Medication (antibiotics, anticonvulsants, analgesics), surgery
F/U: As needed (dependent on neurologic status), referral to neurosurgeon

STROKE
Additional signs and symptoms
- Unilateral decorticate posture
- Hemiplegia
- Dysarthria
- Dysphagia
- Apraxia
- Agnosia
- Urine retention and incontinence
- Constipation
- Homonymous hemianopsia

DX: PE, coagulation studies, imaging studies (CT scan, MRI, ultrasonography, angiography)
TX: Medication (if embolic, anticoagulants; antithrombotic; antihypertensives)
F/U: As needed (dependent on neurologic status), referrals to neurologist and rehabilitation program

HEAD INJURY
Additional signs and symptoms
- Irritability
- Aphasia
- Hemiparesis
- Unilateral numbness
- Pupillary dilation

DX: History of head injury; imaging studies (CT scan, MRI), EEG
TX: Medication (analgesia, osmotic diuretics, corticosteroids), surgery
F/U: As needed (dependent on neurologic status); referrals to neurosurgeon and rehabilitation program

Deep tendon reflexes, abnormal

A hyperactive deep tendon reflex (DTR) is an abnormally brisk muscle contraction that occurs in response to a sudden stretch induced by sharply tapping the muscle's tendon of insertion. This elicited sign may be graded as brisk or pathologically hyperactive. Hyperactive DTRs are commonly accompanied by clonus.

The corticospinal tract and other descending tracts govern the reflex arc—the relay cycle that produces reflex response. A corticospinal lesion above the level of the reflex arc being tested may result in hyperactive DTRs. Abnormal neuromuscular transmission at the end of the reflex arc may also cause hyperactive DTRs. For example, a deficiency of calcium or magnesium may cause hyperactive DTRs because these electrolytes regulate neuromuscular excitability.

Although hyperactive DTRs commonly accompany other neurologic findings, they may be of specific diagnostic value. For example, they're an early, cardinal sign of hypocalcemia.

A hypoactive DTR is an abnormally diminished muscle contraction that occurs in response to a sudden stretch induced by sharply tapping the muscle's tendon of insertion. It may be graded as minimal (+) or absent (0). Symmetrically reduced (+) reflexes may be normal.

Hypoactive DTRs may result from damage to the reflex arc involving the specific muscle, the peripheral nerve, the nerve roots, or the spinal cord at that level. Hypoactive DTRs are an important sign of many disorders, especially when they appear with other neurologic signs and symptoms.

HISTORY

- Ask the patient about spinal cord injury or other trauma and about prolonged exposure to cold, wind, or water.
- If the patient is female, ask her if she's pregnant.
- Ask the patient about the onset and progression of associated signs and symptoms.
- Ask the patient about paresthesia, vomiting, and altered bladder habits.

PHYSICAL ASSESSMENT

- Take the patient's vital signs, and perform a neurologic examination.
- Evaluate level of consciousness, and test motor and sensory function in the limbs. (See *Documenting deep tendon reflexes.*)
- Check for ataxia or tremors and for speech and vision deficits.
- Test for Chvostek's and Trousseau's signs and for carpopedal spasm.

SPECIAL CONSIDERATIONS

Administer muscle relaxants and sedatives to relieve severe muscle contractions. Provide a quiet, calm atmosphere to decrease neuromuscular excitability.

Ⓐ PEDIATRIC POINTERS

- *Hyperreflexia may be a normal sign in neonates. After age 6, reflex responses are similar to those of adults.*
- *When testing DTRs in infants and small children, use distraction techniques to promote reliable results; assess motor function by watching the infant or child at play.*
- *Cerebral palsy commonly causes hyperactive DTRs in children.*
- *Reye's syndrome causes generalized hyperactive DTRs in stage II; however, in stage V, DTRs are absent.*
- *Adult causes of hyperactive DTRs may also appear in children.*
- *Hypoactive DTRs commonly occur in those with muscular dystrophy, Friedreich's ataxia, syringomyelia, and spinal cord injury. They also accompany progressive muscular atrophy, which affects preschoolers and adolescents.*

PATIENT COUNSELING

Provide emotional support to the patient and family. Teach them how to perform range-of-motion exercises to help the patient preserve muscle integrity.

DOCUMENTING DEEP TENDON REFLEXES

Record the patient's deep tendon reflex scores by drawing a stick figure and entering the grades on this scale at the proper location. The figure shown here indicates hypoactive deep tendon reflexes in the legs; other reflexes are normal.

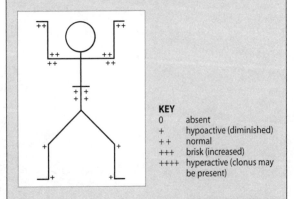

KEY
0	absent
+	hypoactive (diminished)
++	normal
+++	brisk (increased)
++++	hyperactive (clonus may be present)

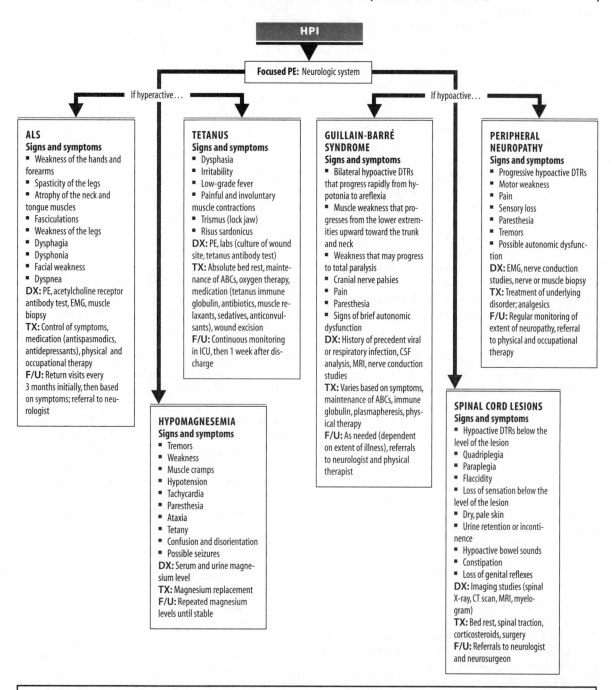

HPI

Focused PE: Neurologic system

If hyperactive...

If hypoactive...

ALS
Signs and symptoms
- Weakness of the hands and forearms
- Spasticity of the legs
- Atrophy of the neck and tongue muscles
- Fasciculations
- Weakness of the legs
- Dysphagia
- Dysphonia
- Facial weakness
- Dyspnea

DX: PE, acetylcholine receptor antibody test, EMG, muscle biopsy

TX: Control of symptoms, medication (antispasmodics, antidepressants), physical and occupational therapy

F/U: Return visits every 3 months initially, then based on symptoms; referral to neurologist

TETANUS
Signs and symptoms
- Dysphasia
- Irritability
- Low-grade fever
- Painful and involuntary muscle contractions
- Trismus (lock jaw)
- Risus sardonicus

DX: PE, labs (culture of wound site, tetanus antibody test)

TX: Absolute bed rest, maintenance of ABCs, oxygen therapy, medication (tetanus immune globulin, antibiotics, muscle relaxants, sedatives, anticonvulsants), wound excision

F/U: Continuous monitoring in ICU, then 1 week after discharge

HYPOMAGNESEMIA
Signs and symptoms
- Tremors
- Weakness
- Muscle cramps
- Hypotension
- Tachycardia
- Paresthesia
- Ataxia
- Tetany
- Confusion and disorientation
- Possible seizures

DX: Serum and urine magnesium level

TX: Magnesium replacement

F/U: Repeated magnesium levels until stable

GUILLAIN-BARRÉ SYNDROME
Signs and symptoms
- Bilateral hypoactive DTRs that progress rapidly from hypotonia to areflexia
- Muscle weakness that progresses from the lower extremities upward toward the trunk and neck
- Weakness that may progress to total paralysis
- Cranial nerve palsies
- Pain
- Paresthesia
- Signs of brief autonomic dysfunction

DX: History of precedent viral or respiratory infection, CSF analysis, MRI, nerve conduction studies

TX: Varies based on symptoms, maintenance of ABCs, immune globulin, plasmapheresis, physical therapy

F/U: As needed (dependent on extent of illness), referrals to neurologist and physical therapist

PERIPHERAL NEUROPATHY
Signs and symptoms
- Progressive hypoactive DTRs
- Motor weakness
- Pain
- Sensory loss
- Paresthesia
- Tremors
- Possible autonomic dysfunction

DX: EMG, nerve conduction studies, nerve or muscle biopsy

TX: Treatment of underlying disorder; analgesics

F/U: Regular monitoring of extent of neuropathy, referral to physical and occupational therapy

SPINAL CORD LESIONS
Signs and symptoms
- Hypoactive DTRs below the level of the lesion
- Quadriplegia
- Paraplegia
- Flaccidity
- Loss of sensation below the level of the lesion
- Dry, pale skin
- Urine retention or incontinence
- Hypoactive bowel sounds
- Constipation
- Loss of genital reflexes

DX: Imaging studies (spinal X-ray, CT scan, MRI, myelogram)

TX: Bed rest, spinal traction, corticosteroids, surgery

F/U: Referrals to neurologist and neurosurgeon

Additional differential diagnoses for hyperactive reflexes: brain tumor ▪ hepatic encephalopathy ▪ hyperthyroidism ▪ hypocalcemia ▪ hypothermia ▪ multiple sclerosis ▪ preeclampsia ▪ spinal cord lesion ▪ stroke

Additional differential diagnoses for hypoactive reflexes: botulism ▪ cerebellar dysfunction ▪ Eaton-Lambert syndrome ▪ hypothyroidism ▪ polymyositis ▪ syringomyelia ▪ tabes dorsalis

Other causes for hypoactive reflexes: barbiturates and paralyzants (such as pancuronium and curare)

Depression

Depression is a mental state of depressed mood, characterized by feelings of sadness, despair, and loss of interest or pleasure in activities. These feelings may be accompanied by somatic complaints, such as changes in appetite, sleep disturbances, restlessness or lethargy, and decreased concentration. Thoughts of death or suicide may also occur.

Clinical depression must be distinguished from "the blues," periodic bouts of dysphoria that are less persistent and severe than the clinical disorder. The criterion for major depression is one or more episodes of depressed mood, or decreased interest or the ability to take pleasure in all or most activities, lasting at least 2 weeks.

Major depression strikes 10% to 15% of adults and affects all racial, ethnic, age, and socioeconomic groups. It's twice as common in women as in men and is especially prevalent among adolescents. Depression has numerous causes, including genetic and family history, medical and psychiatric disorders, and the use of certain drugs. A complete psychiatric and physical assessment should be conducted to exclude possible medical causes.

HISTORY

- Ask the patient what's bothering him. Find out how his current mood differs from his usual mood.
- Review the patient's medical history for chronic illness.
- Ask the patient to describe the way he feels about himself. What are his plans and dreams? How realistic are they? Is he generally satisfied with what he has accomplished in his work, relationships, and other interests?
- Ask the patient about changes in his social interactions, sleep patterns, normal activities, or ability to make decisions and concentrate.
- Obtain a drug history, including prescription and over-the-counter drugs, herbal remedies, and recreational drugs. Also, ask the patient about alcohol intake.
- Listen for clues that the patient may be suicidal. Find out if he has an adequate support network to help him cope with his depression.
- Ask the patient about his family — its patterns of interaction and characteristic responses to success and failure. What part does he feel he plays in his family life? Ask if other family members have been depressed, and whether anyone important to the patient has been sick or has died in the past year.
- Ask the patient about his environment. Has his lifestyle changed in the past month? Six months? Year? When he's feeling blue, where does he go and what does he do to feel better? Find out how he feels about his role in the community and the resources that are available to him.

PHYSICAL ASSESSMENT

- Take the patient's vital signs.
- Evaluate physical complaints that the patient may have to help rule out a medical cause for depression.
- If the patient has a history of a chronic illness, focus your initial assessment on systems affected by that illness.

SPECIAL CONSIDERATIONS

Help the patient set realistic goals; encourage him to promote feelings of self-worth by asserting his opinions and making decisions. Try to determine his suicide potential, and take steps to help ensure his safety. The patient may require close surveillance to prevent a suicide attempt.

PEDIATRIC POINTERS

- *Because emotional lability is normal in adolescence, depression can be difficult to assess and diagnose in teenagers. Clues to underlying depression may include somatic complaints, sexual promiscuity, poor grades, and abuse of alcohol or drugs.*
- *Use of a family-systems model can help determine the cause of depression in adolescents. When family roles are determined, family therapy or group therapy with peers may help the patient overcome his depression.*

AGING ISSUES

Depressed older adults at highest risk for suicide are those who are age 85 or older, have high self-esteem, and need to be in control.

PATIENT COUNSELING

Because anger typically underlies depression, help the patient acknowledge this emotion and express it safely. Help foster feelings of competence by focusing on past and present experiences in which the patient was successful. Educate the patient about available treatment for depression. Arrange for follow-up counseling, or contact a mental health professional for a referral.

DEPRESSION

HPI

Focused PE: Mental health, HEENT, thyroid glands, abdomen, neurologic system

---

HYPOMAGNESEMIA
Signs and symptoms
- Weakness
- Muscle cramps
- Confusion
- Disorientation
- Delusions and hallucinations
- Emotional lability
- Tremors and muscle twitching
- Tetany

HYPONATREMIA
Signs and symptoms
- Lethargy
- Weakness
- Confusion
- Delirium
- Headache
- Short attention span
- Muscle twitching
- Tremors

HYPOPHOSPHATEMIA
Signs and symptoms
- Irritability
- Apprehension
- Anorexia
- Generalized muscle weakness
- Difficulty swallowing
- Confusion
- Dysarthria
- Seizures

HYPOTHYROIDISM
Signs and symptoms
- Fatigue
- Lethargy
- Weakness
- Arthralgia
- Dry skin
- Weight gain
- Cold intolerance

HYPOPARATHYROIDISM
Signs and symptoms
- Muscle spasms
- Paresthesia of the lips and extremities
- Chvostek's and Trousseau's signs

AFFECTIVE DISORDER
Signs and symptoms
- Hopelessness
- Sleep disturbances
- Suicidal tendencies
- Abrupt mood swings
- Prolonged symptoms that include agitation, preoccupation, memory loss, and poor concentration

CHRONIC ANXIETY DISORDER
Signs and symptoms
- Panic attacks
- Obsessive-compulsive behavior
- Free-floating anxiety

DX: Labs (electrolytes, thyroid studies)
TX: Fluid replacement as needed, medication (electrolyte replacement, thyroid hormone replacement)
F/U: Monitoring of electrolytes and thyroid levels until stable, then reevaluation every 3 to 6 months

DX: History of behavior, metabolic and endocrine imbalances ruled out, psychiatric evaluation
TX: Antidepressants, psychotherapy
F/U: Referral to a psychiatrist, advanced practice psychiatric nurse, or psychologist as needed (based on the extent of depression and response to treatment)

Other causes: alcohol abuse ▪ antiarrhythmics (such as disopyramide) ▪ anticonvulsants (such as diazepam) ▪ antiparkinsonian drugs ▪ barbiturates ▪ beta-adrenergic blockers (such as propranolol) ▪ centrally-acting antihypertensives (such as reserpine [common in high dosages], methyldopa, and clonidine) ▪ chemotherapeutics (such as asparaginase) ▪ corticosteroids ▪ cycloserine ▪ digoxin ▪ hormonal contraceptives ▪ indomethacin ▪ levodopa ▪ NSAIDs

Diaphoresis

Diaphoresis is profuse sweating—at times amounting to more than 1 qt (1 L) of sweat per hour. This sign represents an autonomic nervous system response to physical or psychogenic stress or to fever or high environmental temperature. When caused by stress, diaphoresis may be generalized or limited to the palms of the hands, soles of the feet, and forehead. When caused by fever or high environmental temperature, it's usually generalized.

Diaphoresis usually begins abruptly and may be accompanied by other autonomic system signs, such as tachycardia and increased blood pressure. Intermittent diaphoresis may accompany a chronic disorder characterized by recurrent fever; isolated diaphoresis may mark an episode of acute pain or fever. Night sweats may characterize intermittent fever because body temperature tends to return to normal between 2 a.m. and 4 a.m. before rising again. (Temperature is usually lowest around 6 a.m.)

Diaphoresis also commonly occurs during menopause, preceded by a sensation of intense heat (a hot flash). Other causes include exercise or exertion that accelerates metabolism and creates internal heat and mild to moderate anxiety that helps initiate the fight-or-flight response.

ALERT

If the patient is diaphoretic:
- *quickly take his vital signs*
- *assess him for chest pain or palpitations*
- *determine his blood glucose level if he complains of light-headedness or weakness or has a change in level of consciousness.*
  If the patient isn't diaphoretic, perform a focused assessment.

HISTORY

- Ask the patient to explain his chief complaint, then explore associated signs and symptoms. Ask whether diaphoresis occurs during the day or at night.
- Note general fatigue and weakness. Ask the patient if has insomnia, headache, or changes in vision or hearing. Is he often dizzy?
- Ask the patient if he experiences palpitations.
- Ask the patient about pleuritic pain, cough, sputum, difficulty breathing, nausea, vomiting, abdominal pain, and altered bowel or bladder habits.
- If the patient is a female, ask her about amenorrhea and changes in her menstrual cycle. Is she menopausal?
- Ask the patient about paresthesia, muscle cramps or stiffness, and joint pain.
- Ask the patient about recent weight loss or gain.

- Ask the patient if he has recently traveled to a tropical country, had recent exposure to high environmental temperatures or to pesticides, or experienced an insect bite.
- Review the patient's medical history for partial gastrectomy.
- Obtain a drug history, including prescription and over-the-counter drugs, herbal remedies, and recreational drugs. Also, ask the patient about alcohol intake.

PHYSICAL ASSESSMENT

- Determine the extent of diaphoresis by inspecting the trunk and extremities as well as the palms, soles, and forehead. Also, check the patient's clothing for dampness.
- Observe the patient for flushing, abnormal skin texture or lesions, and an increased amount of coarse body hair. Note poor skin turgor and dry mucous membranes.
- Evaluate the patient's mental status.
- Take the patient's vital signs.
- Observe the patient for fasciculations and flaccid paralysis. Be alert for seizures.
- Note the patient's facial expression and examine the eyes for pupillary dilation or constriction, exophthalmos, and excessive tearing. Test visual fields.
- Check for hearing loss.
- Check for tooth and gum disease.
- Percuss the lungs for dullness and auscultate for crackles, diminished or bronchial breath sounds, and increased vocal fremitus.
- Palpate for lymphadenopathy and hepatosplenomegaly.

SPECIAL CONSIDERATIONS

The patient experiencing profuse diaphoresis will require fluid and electrolyte replacement, especially children. Encourage oral fluids high in electrolytes or administer I.V. fluids.

PEDIATRIC POINTERS

Diaphoresis in children commonly results from environmental heat or overdressing the child; it's usually most apparent around the head. Other causes include drug withdrawal associated with maternal addiction, heart failure, thyrotoxicosis, and the effects of such drugs as antihistamines, ephedrine, haloperidol, and thyroid hormone.

AGING ISSUES

Keep in mind that older patients may not exhibit diaphoresis because of a decreased sweating mechanism. For this reason, they're at increased risk for developing heatstroke in high temperatures.

PATIENT COUNSELING

Explain to the patient and his family that diaphoresis signals a return to normal body temperature after it has risen for any reason. It can also occur spontaneously, after taking an antipyretic, or as a sympathetic response to pain or stress.

DIAPHORESIS

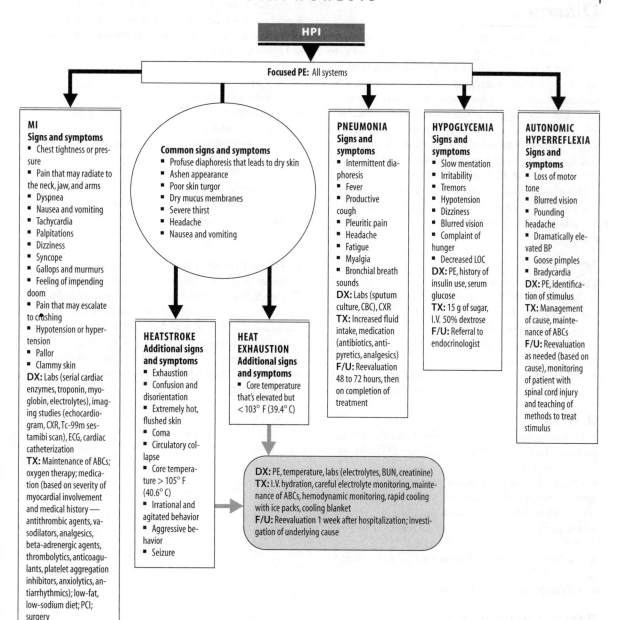

HPI

Focused PE: All systems

MI
Signs and symptoms
- Chest tightness or pressure
- Pain that may radiate to the neck, jaw, and arms
- Dyspnea
- Nausea and vomiting
- Tachycardia
- Palpitations
- Dizziness
- Syncope
- Gallops and murmurs
- Feeling of impending doom
- Pain that may escalate to crushing
- Hypotension or hypertension
- Pallor
- Clammy skin

DX: Labs (serial cardiac enzymes, troponin, myoglobin, electrolytes), imaging studies (echocardiogram, CXR, Tc-99m sestamibi scan), ECG, cardiac catheterization
TX: Maintenance of ABCs; oxygen therapy; medication (based on severity of myocardial involvement and medical history — antithrombic agents, vasodilators, analgesics, beta-adrenergic agents, thrombolytics, anticoagulants, platelet aggregation inhibitors, anxiolytics, antiarrhythmics); low-fat, low-sodium diet; PCI; surgery
F/U: Referral to cardiologist

Common signs and symptoms
- Profuse diaphoresis that leads to dry skin
- Ashen appearance
- Poor skin turgor
- Dry mucus membranes
- Severe thirst
- Headache
- Nausea and vomiting

HEATSTROKE
Additional signs and symptoms
- Exhaustion
- Confusion and disorientation
- Extremely hot, flushed skin
- Coma
- Circulatory collapse
- Core temperature > 105° F (40.6° C)
- Irrational and agitated behavior
- Aggressive behavior
- Seizure

HEAT EXHAUSTION
Additional signs and symptoms
- Core temperature that's elevated but < 103° F (39.4° C)

DX: PE, temperature, labs (electrolytes, BUN, creatinine)
TX: I.V. hydration, careful electrolyte monitoring, maintenance of ABCs, hemodynamic monitoring, rapid cooling with ice packs, cooling blanket
F/U: Reevaluation 1 week after hospitalization; investigation of underlying cause

PNEUMONIA
Signs and symptoms
- Intermittent diaphoresis
- Fever
- Productive cough
- Pleuritic pain
- Headache
- Fatigue
- Myalgia
- Bronchial breath sounds

DX: Labs (sputum culture, CBC), CXR
TX: Increased fluid intake, medication (antibiotics, antipyretics, analgesics)
F/U: Reevaluation 48 to 72 hours, then on completion of treatment

HYPOGLYCEMIA
Signs and symptoms
- Slow mentation
- Irritability
- Tremors
- Hypotension
- Dizziness
- Blurred vision
- Complaint of hunger
- Decreased LOC

DX: PE, history of insulin use, serum glucose
TX: 15 g of sugar, I.V. 50% dextrose
F/U: Referral to endocrinologist

AUTONOMIC HYPERREFLEXIA
Signs and symptoms
- Loss of motor tone
- Blurred vision
- Pounding headache
- Dramatically elevated BP
- Goose pimples
- Bradycardia

DX: PE, identification of stimulus
TX: Management of cause, maintenance of ABCs
F/U: Reevaluation as needed (based on cause), monitoring of patient with spinal cord injury and teaching of methods to treat stimulus

---

Additional differential diagnoses: acromegaly ▪ AIDS ▪ anxiety disorders ▪ drug and alcohol withdrawal syndromes ▪ empyema ▪ envenomation ▪ heart failure ▪ Hodgkin's disease ▪ immunoblastic lymphadenopathy ▪ infective endocarditis ▪ liver or lung abscess ▪ malaria ▪ Ménière's disease ▪ pheochromocytoma ▪ relapsing fever ▪ tetanus ▪ thyrotoxicosis ▪ tuberculosis

Other causes: acetaminophen and aspirin poisoning ▪ antipsychotics ▪ antipyretics ▪ dumping syndrome ▪ pesticide poisoning ▪ sympathomimetics ▪ thyroid hormone

Diarrhea

Usually a chief sign of an intestinal disorder, diarrhea is an increase in the volume of stools compared with the patient's normal bowel habits. It varies in severity and may be acute or chronic. Acute diarrhea may result from acute infection, food sensitivities, stress, fecal impaction, or the effects of certain drugs. Chronic diarrhea may result from food allergies, chronic infection, obstructive or inflammatory bowel disease, malabsorption syndrome, an endocrine disorder, or GI surgery. Periodic diarrhea may result from food intolerance or from ingestion of spicy or high-fiber foods or caffeine.

One or more pathophysiologic mechanisms may contribute to diarrhea. The fluid and electrolyte imbalances it produces may precipitate life-threatening arrhythmias or hypovolemic shock.

 ALERT

If the patient's diarrhea is profuse:
- *check for signs of shock, such as tachycardia, hypotension, and cool, pale, clammy skin*
- *check for electrolyte imbalances*
- *look for an irregular pulse, muscle weakness, anorexia, and nausea and vomiting*
- *keep emergency resuscitation equipment handy.*
If the patient isn't in shock, perform a focused assessment.

HISTORY

- Explore signs and symptoms associated with diarrhea. Does the patient have abdominal pain and cramps? Difficulty breathing? Is he weak or fatigued?
- Obtain a drug history, including prescription and over-the-counter drugs, herbal remedies, and recreational drugs. Also, ask the patient about alcohol intake.
- Ask the patient if he has had recent GI surgery or radiation therapy.
- Ask the patient to briefly describe his diet. Does he have any known food allergies?
- Ask the patient if he's under unusual stress.

PHYSICAL ASSESSMENT

- Take the patient's vital signs. Take his blood pressure with him lying, sitting, and standing. Take his temperature, and note any chills. Check his weight.
- Evaluate hydration, and check skin turgor. Also, look for rash.
- Inspect the abdomen for diffuse distention. Auscultate bowel sounds, and palpate for tenderness.

SPECIAL CONSIDERATIONS

Administer an analgesic for pain and an opiate to decrease intestinal motility. Ensure the patient's privacy during defecation. Maintain skin integrity by cleaning the perineum thoroughly and applying ointment.

 PEDIATRIC POINTERS

- *Diarrhea in children commonly results from infection, but chronic diarrhea may result from malabsorption syndrome, an anatomic defect, or allergies.*
- *Because dehydration and electrolyte imbalance occur rapidly in children, diarrhea can be life-threatening.*

 AGING ISSUES

In the elderly patient with new-onset segmental colitis, always consider ischemia before diagnosing his condition as Crohn's disease.

PATIENT COUNSELING

Advise the patient to avoid caffeine, milk, and spicy and high-fiber foods. Suggest smaller, more frequent meals if he has had GI surgery or disease. If appropriate, teach the patient stress-reducing exercises, such as guided imagery and deep-breathing techniques, or recommend counseling. If the patient has inflammatory bowel disease, stress the need for medical follow-up because his condition places him at increased risk for developing colon cancer.

DIARRHEA

HPI

Focused PE: Skin; GI, GU, pulmonary, and cardiovascular systems

Common signs and symptoms
- Watery diarrhea
- Abdominal cramping
- Nausea and vomiting

CROHN'S DISEASE
Signs and symptoms
- Nausea and vomiting
- Fever and chills
- Weakness
- Anorexia and weight loss

DX: Imaging studies (CT scan, barium enema), colonoscopy
TX: Medication (analgesics, electrolyte replacement, mesalamine, corticosteroids), surgery
F/U: Referral to gastroenterologist

Common signs and symptoms
- Increased intestinal motility
- Abdominal pain
- Abdominal tenderness and guarding
- Possible distention

GASTROENTERITIS
Additional signs and symptoms
- Sudden onset of diarrhea
- Fever

CLOSTRIDIUM DIFFICILE INFECTION
Additional signs and symptoms
- Foul-smelling or grossly bloody and watery diarrhea
- Leukocytosis

LACTOSE INTOLERANCE
Additional signs and symptoms
- Recent milk or milk product ingestion
- Bloating
- Borborygmi
- Flatus

LARGE-BOWEL CANCER
Additional signs and symptoms
- Bloody diarrhea
- Weakness and fatigue
- Anorexia
- Nausea and vomiting

DX: Labs (CBC, CEA, fecal occult blood), imaging studies (barium enema, CT scan, transrectal ultrasound), colonoscopy with biopsy if indicated
TX: Medication (analgesics, chemotherapy), surgery
F/U: Referrals to oncologist and surgeon; after surgery, CEA, LFT, and fecal occult blood test every 3 months for 2 years; annual colonoscopy

DX: History of recent antibiotic therapy (with *C. difficile*), labs (CBC, electrolytes, stool guaiac, stool culture)
TX: Rehydrate, medication (electrolyte replacement, antipyretics, antibiotics, if indicated)
F/U: If no resolution in 48 to 72 hours, reevaluation of lab work; referral to gastroenterologist

---

Additional differential diagnoses: acute appendicitis ▪ carcinoid syndrome ▪ irritable bowel syndrome ▪ ischemic bowel disease ▪ lead poisoning ▪ malabsorption syndrome ▪ pseudomembranous enterocolitis ▪ rotavirus gastroenteritis ▪ thyrotoxicosis

Other causes: antibiotics (ampicillin, cephalosporins, tetracyclines, clindamycin) ▪ colchicine ▪ dantrolene ▪ dehydration ▪ digoxin and quinidine (in high doses) ▪ ethacrynic acid ▪ gastrectomy ▪ gastroenterostomy ▪ guanethidine ▪ herbal medicines (ginkgo biloba, ginseng, licorice) ▪ high-dose radiation therapy ▪ lactulose ▪ laxative abuse ▪ magnesium-containing antacids ▪ mefenamic acid ▪ methotrexate ▪ metyrosine ▪ pyloroplasty

Diplopia

Diplopia is double vision—seeing one object as two. This symptom results when extraocular muscles fail to work together, causing images to fall on noncorresponding parts of the retinas. Orbital lesions, the effects of surgery, or impaired function of cranial nerves that supply extraocular muscles (oculomotor, CN III; trochlear, CN IV; abducens, CN VI) may be responsible for this muscular incoordination. (See *Testing extraocular muscles.*)

Diplopia usually begins intermittently and affects near or far vision exclusively. It can be classified as monocular or binocular. More common binocular diplopia may result from ocular deviation or displacement, extraocular muscle palsies, or psychoneurosis, or it may occur after retinal surgery. Monocular diplopia may result from an early cataract, retinal edema or scarring, iridodialysis, a subluxated lens, a poorly fitting contact lens, or an uncorrected refractive error such as astigmatism. Diplopia may also occur in those with hysteria or malingering.

HISTORY

- Ask the patient when he first noticed the diplopia.
- Ask the patient whether the images are side-by-side (horizontal), one above the other (vertical), or a combination. Ask him if it affects his near or far vision. Does it affect certain directions of gaze?

- Ask the patient whether the diplopia has worsened, remained the same, or subsided. Does its severity change throughout the day?
- Ask the patient about associated signs and symptoms, especially a severe headache. Also ask him about eye pain, hypertension, diabetes mellitus, allergies, and thyroid, neurologic, or muscular disorders.
- Review the patient's medical history for extraocular muscle disorders, trauma, or eye surgery.

PHYSICAL ASSESSMENT

- Take the patient's vital signs.
- Check the patient's neurologic status. Evaluate his level of consciousness, pupil size and response to light, and motor and sensory function.
- Find out if the patient can correct diplopia by tilting his head. If so, ask him to show you. (If the patient has a fourth nerve lesion, tilting of the head toward the opposite shoulder causes compensatory tilting of the unaffected eye. If he has incomplete sixth nerve palsy, tilting of the head toward the side of the paralyzed muscle may relax the affected lateral rectus muscle.)
- Observe the patient for ocular deviation, ptosis, proptosis, lid edema, and conjunctival injection.
- Determine whether the patient has monocular or binocular diplopia by asking him to occlude one eye. If he still sees double, he has monocular diplopia.
- Test visual acuity and extraocular muscles.

SPECIAL CONSIDERATIONS

Provide a safe environment. If the patient has severe diplopia, remove sharp obstacles and assist with ambulation. Also, institute seizure precautions, if indicated.

A PEDIATRIC POINTERS

- *Strabismus, which can be congenital or acquired at an early age, produces diplopia; however, in young children, the brain rapidly compensates for double vision by suppressing one image, so diplopia is a rare complaint.*
- *School-age children who complain of double vision require a careful examination to rule out serious disorders such as brain tumor.*

PATIENT COUNSELING

Instruct the patient on what to expect from diagnostic testing. If appropriate, refer him to an ophthalmologist for further evaluation and treatment.

TESTING EXTRAOCULAR MUSCLES

The coordinated action of six muscles controls eyeball movements. To test the function of each muscle and the cranial nerve (CN) that innervates it, ask the patient to look in the direction controlled by that muscle. The six directions you can test make up the *cardinal fields of gaze.* The patient's inability to turn the eye in the designated direction indicates muscle weakness or paralysis.

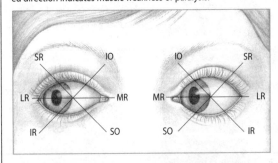

SR — superior rectus (CN III)
IR — inferior rectus (CN III)
MR — medial rectus (CN III)

LR — lateral rectus (CN VI)
IO — inferior oblique (CN III)
SO — superior oblique (CN IV)

DIPLOPIA

HPI

Focused PE: HEENT; neurologic, cardiovascular, and pulmonary systems; mental health

DISTURBANCE OF CN III, IV, OR VI
Signs and symptoms
- Misalignment of visual axes
- Phoria
- Nystagmus

DX: PE, direct ophthalmoscopy cover test
TX: Corrective lenses, muscle strengthening exercises, eye patch
F/U: Referral to ophthalmologist

HYPERTENSION
Signs and symptoms
- Systolic BP > 160 mm Hg
- Diastolic BP > 95 mm Hg
- Headache
- Nausea and vomiting

DX: Serial BP measurements, identification of underlying cause
TX: Reduction of risk factors, medication (diuretics, ACE inhibitors, calcium channel blockers, beta-adrenergic blockers), treatment of underlying cause (if any)
F/U: Once stable, reevaluation every 3 to 6 months

BRAIN TUMOR
Signs and symptoms
- Eye deviation
- Emotional lability
- Decreased LOC
- Headache
- Visual field deficits

DX: Imaging studies (CT scan, MRI)
TX: Medication (analgesics, chemotherapy), radiation therapy, surgery
F/U: Referrals to neurosurgeon and oncologist

OPHTHALMOLOGIC MIGRAINE
Signs and symptoms
- Diplopia that persists days after headache
- Unilateral pain
- Ptosis
- Extraocular muscle palsies
- Irritability and slight confusion

DX: History and PE, CT scan, ophthalmologic examination
TX: Medication (NSAIDs, beta-adrenergic blockers, anticonvulsants, antidepressants, steroids, calcium channel blockers, ergots), headache diary, low-fat, high-complex carbohydrate diet
F/U: Referrals to ophthalmologist and headache center, if necessary

INTRACRANIAL ANEURYSM
Signs and symptoms
- Eye deviation
- Ptosis and dilated pupil on the affected side
- Recurrent, severe, unilateral frontal headache
- Neck and spinal pain and rigidity
- Decreased LOC
- Tinnitus
- Dizziness
- Nausea and vomiting

DX: Imaging studies (CT scan, MRI, angiography)
TX: Varies according to the size of the aneurysm and patient history, reduction of risk factors for rupture, analgesics, surgery, or neuroradiologic nonsurgical procedure
F/U: As needed (based on neurologic symptoms), referral to neurosurgeon

STROKE
Signs and symptoms
- Unilateral motor weakness or paralysis
- Ataxia
- Decreased LOC
- Dizziness
- Aphasia
- Dysphagia
- Visual field deficits

DX: Labs (coagulation studies, lipid profile), imaging studies (duplex carotid ultrasonography, CT scan, cerebral angiography, MRI, MRA, echocardiogram)
TX: Maintenance of ABCs, medication (aspirin, platelet aggregation inhibitors, thrombolytics [if embolic]), symptom management
F/U: As needed (based on neurologic status); referral to neurologist; referral to rehabilitation center, if appropriate

Additional differential diagnoses: alcohol intoxication ▪ botulism ▪ cavernous sinus thrombosis ▪ diabetes mellitus ▪ encephalitis ▪ head injury ▪ multiple sclerosis ▪ myasthenia gravis ▪ orbital blowout fracture ▪ orbital cellulitis ▪ orbital tumors ▪ thyrotoxicosis

Other cause: eye surgery

Dizziness

A common symptom, dizziness is a sensation of imbalance or faintness, sometimes associated with giddiness, weakness, confusion, and blurred or double vision. Episodes of dizziness are usually brief; they may be mild or severe with abrupt or gradual onset. Dizziness may be aggravated by standing up quickly and alleviated by lying down and by rest.

Dizziness typically results from inadequate blood flow and oxygen supply to the cerebrum and spinal cord. It may occur with anxiety, a respiratory or cardiovascular disorder, and postconcussion syndrome. It's a key symptom of certain serious disorders, such as hypertension and vertebrobasilar artery insufficiency.

Dizziness is sometimes confused with vertigo — a sensation of revolving in space or of surroundings revolving about oneself. However, unlike dizziness, vertigo is commonly accompanied by nausea, vomiting, nystagmus, staggering gait, and tinnitus or hearing loss. Dizziness and vertigo may occur together, as in postconcussion syndrome.

 ALERT

If the patient complains of dizziness:
- *ask him to describe it (Is the dizziness associated with headache or blurred vision?)*
- *take his vital signs, and ask about a history of high blood pressure; then tell him to lie down, and recheck his vital signs*
- *ask about a history of diabetes and cardiovascular disease (Is he taking a drug prescribed for high blood pressure? If so, when did he take his last dose?)*

If the patient's blood pressure is normal, perform a focused assessment.

HISTORY

- Review the patient's medical history for hypertension, transient ischemic attack, anemia, chronic obstructive pulmonary disease, anxiety disorders, head injury, and anything that may predispose him to cardiac arrhythmias, such as myocardial infarction, heart failure, or atherosclerosis.
- Obtain a drug history, including prescription and over-the-counter drugs, herbal remedies, and recreational drugs. Also, ask the patient about alcohol intake.
- Ask the patient how often dizziness occurs and how long each episode lasts.
- Ask the patient if dizziness abates spontaneously or if it ever leads to loss of consciousness.
- Ask the patient if dizziness is triggered by sitting or standing up suddenly or stooping over.
- Ask the patient if being in a crowd makes him feel dizzy.

- Ask the patient about emotional stress. Has he been irritable or anxious lately? Does he have insomnia or difficulty concentrating?
- Ask the patient if he has experienced palpitations, chest pain, diaphoresis, shortness of breath, or chronic cough.

PHYSICAL ASSESSMENT

- Take the patient's vital signs, then take his blood pressure while he's lying, sitting, and standing to check for orthostatic hypotension.
- Assess the patient's level of consciousness, motor and sensory functions, and reflexes.
- Inspect for poor skin turgor and dry mucous membranes, which are signs of dehydration.
- Auscultate heart rate and rhythm.
- Inspect for barrel chest, clubbing, cyanosis, and use of accessory muscles. Also, auscultate breath sounds.
- Test capillary refill time in the extremities, and palpate for edema.

SPECIAL CONSIDERATIONS

Provide a safe environment, and assist with ambulation to ensure the patient's safety.

 PEDIATRIC POINTERS

- *Dizziness is less common in children than in adults.*
- *Children may have difficulty describing this symptom and instead complain of tiredness, stomachache, or feeling sick. If you suspect dizziness, assess the patient for vertigo as well.*
- *A more common symptom in children, vertigo may result from a vision disorder, an ear infection, or the effects of an antibiotic.*

PATIENT COUNSELING

Teach the patient ways to control dizziness. If he's hyperventilating, have him breathe and rebreathe into his cupped hands or a paper bag. If he experiences dizziness in an upright position, tell him to lie down and rest and then rise slowly. Advise the patient with carotid sinus hypersensitivity to avoid wearing garments that fit tightly at the neck. Instruct the patient who risks a transient ischemic attack from vertebrobasilar insufficiency to turn his body instead of sharply turning his head to one side.

Instruct the patient on what to expect from diagnostic testing, which may include blood studies, arteriography, computed tomography scan, EEG, and magnetic resonance imaging, as appropriate.

DIZZINESS

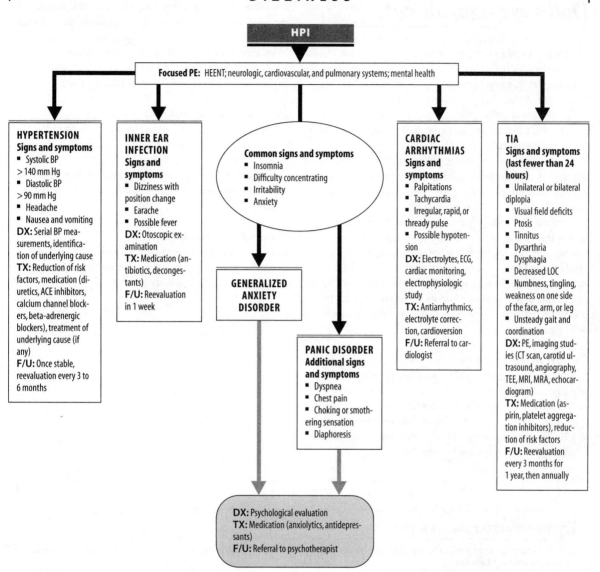

HPI

Focused PE: HEENT; neurologic, cardiovascular, and pulmonary systems; mental health

HYPERTENSION
Signs and symptoms
- Systolic BP >140 mm Hg
- Diastolic BP >90 mm Hg
- Headache
- Nausea and vomiting

DX: Serial BP measurements, identification of underlying cause

TX: Reduction of risk factors, medication (diuretics, ACE inhibitors, calcium channel blockers, beta-adrenergic blockers), treatment of underlying cause (if any)

F/U: Once stable, reevaluation every 3 to 6 months

INNER EAR INFECTION
Signs and symptoms
- Dizziness with position change
- Earache
- Possible fever

DX: Otoscopic examination

TX: Medication (antibiotics, decongestants)

F/U: Reevaluation in 1 week

Common signs and symptoms
- Insomnia
- Difficulty concentrating
- Irritability
- Anxiety

GENERALIZED ANXIETY DISORDER

PANIC DISORDER
Additional signs and symptoms
- Dyspnea
- Chest pain
- Choking or smothering sensation
- Diaphoresis

CARDIAC ARRHYTHMIAS
Signs and symptoms
- Palpitations
- Tachycardia
- Irregular, rapid, or thready pulse
- Possible hypotension

DX: Electrolytes, ECG, cardiac monitoring, electrophysiologic study

TX: Antiarrhythmics, electrolyte correction, cardioversion

F/U: Referral to cardiologist

TIA
Signs and symptoms (last fewer than 24 hours)
- Unilateral or bilateral diplopia
- Visual field deficits
- Ptosis
- Tinnitus
- Dysarthria
- Dysphagia
- Decreased LOC
- Numbness, tingling, weakness on one side of the face, arm, or leg
- Unsteady gait and coordination

DX: PE, imaging studies (CT scan, carotid ultrasound, angiography, TEE, MRI, MRA, echocardiogram)

TX: Medication (aspirin, platelet aggregation inhibitors), reduction of risk factors

F/U: Reevaluation every 3 months for 1 year, then annually

DX: Psychological evaluation
TX: Medication (anxiolytics, antidepressants)
F/U: Referral to psychotherapist

Additional differential diagnoses: carotid sinus hypersensitivity ▪ emphysema ▪ hyperventilation syndrome ▪ orthostatic hypotension ▪ postconcussion syndrome

Other causes: antianxiety drugs ▪ antihistamines ▪ antihypertensives ▪ CNS depressants ▪ decongestants ▪ narcotics ▪ St. John's wort ▪ vasodilators

Doll's eye sign, absent

An indicator of brain stem dysfunction, the absence of the doll's eye sign is detected by rapid, gentle turning of the patient's head from side to side. The eyes remain fixed in midposition, instead of moving laterally toward the side opposite the direction the head is turned. (See *Testing for absent doll's eye sign.*)

The absence of doll's eye sign, also known as negative oculocephalic reflex, indicates injury to the midbrain or pons, involving cranial nerves III, VI, and VIII. It typically accompanies coma caused by lesions of the cerebellum and brain stem. This sign usually can't be relied upon in a conscious patient because he can control eye movements voluntarily. Absent doll's eye sign is necessary for a diagnosis of brain death.

A variant of absent doll's eye sign that develops gradually is known as abnormal doll's eye sign: Because conjugate eye movement is lost, one eye may move laterally and the other remain fixed or move in the opposite direction. An abnormal doll's eye sign usually accompanies metabolic coma or increased intracranial pressure (ICP). Associated brain stem dysfunction may be reversible or may progress to deeper coma with absent doll's eye sign.

PHYSICAL ASSESSMENT

● Evaluate the patient's level of consciousness, using the Glasgow Coma Scale.
● Note decerebrate or decorticate posture.
● Examine the pupils for size, equality, and response to light.
● Check for signs of increased ICP — increased blood pressure, increasing pulse pressure, and bradycardia.

SPECIAL CONSIDERATIONS

Don't attempt to elicit doll's eye sign in a comatose patient with suspected cervical spine injury; doing so risks spinal cord damage. Instead, evaluate the oculovestibular reflex with the cold caloric test. Normally, instilling cold water in the ear causes the eyes to move slowly toward the irrigated ear. Cold caloric testing may also be done to confirm an absent doll's eye sign.

Ⓐ PEDIATRIC POINTERS

● Normally, the doll's eye sign isn't present for the first 10 days after birth, and it may be irregular until age 2. After that, this sign reliably indicates brain stem function.
● An absent doll's eye sign in a child may accompany coma associated with head injury, near drowning or suffocation, or brain stem astrocytoma.

PATIENT COUNSELING

An absent doll's eye sign is an ominous sign for the comatose patient. Support the family and provide information regarding the patient's outcome whenever possible.

TESTING FOR ABSENT DOLL'S EYE SIGN

To evaluate the patient's oculocephalic reflex, hold her upper eyelids open and quickly (but gently) turn her head from side to side, noting eye movements with each head turn.

With absent doll's eye sign, the eyes remain fixed in midposition.

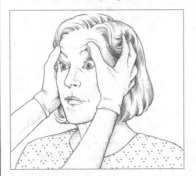 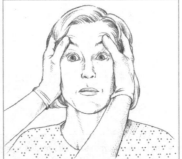 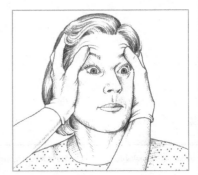

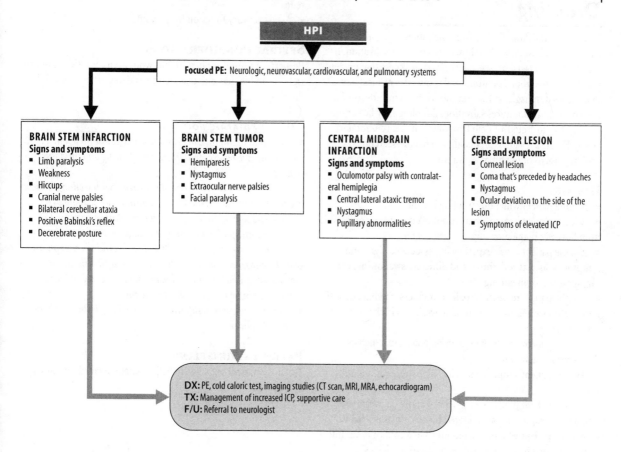

HPI

Focused PE: Neurologic, neurovascular, cardiovascular, and pulmonary systems

BRAIN STEM INFARCTION
Signs and symptoms
- Limb paralysis
- Weakness
- Hiccups
- Cranial nerve palsies
- Bilateral cerebellar ataxia
- Positive Babinski's reflex
- Decerebrate posture

BRAIN STEM TUMOR
Signs and symptoms
- Hemiparesis
- Nystagmus
- Extraocular nerve palsies
- Facial paralysis

CENTRAL MIDBRAIN INFARCTION
Signs and symptoms
- Oculomotor palsy with contralateral hemiplegia
- Central lateral ataxic tremor
- Nystagmus
- Pupillary abnormalities

CEREBELLAR LESION
Signs and symptoms
- Corneal lesion
- Coma that's preceded by headaches
- Nystagmus
- Ocular deviation to the side of the lesion
- Symptoms of elevated ICP

DX: PE, cold caloric test, imaging studies (CT scan, MRI, MRA, echocardiogram)
TX: Management of increased ICP, supportive care
F/U: Referral to neurologist

Other cause: barbiturates

Drooling

Drooling—the flow of saliva from the mouth—results from a failure to swallow or retain saliva, or from excess salivation. It may stem from facial muscle paralysis or weakness that prevents mouth closure, from a neuromuscular disorder or local pain that causes dysphagia or, less commonly, from the effects of a drug or toxin that induces salivation. Drooling may be scant or copious (up to 1 qt [1 L] daily) and may cause circumoral irritation. Because it signals an inability to handle secretions, drooling warns of potential aspiration.

HISTORY
- Ask the patient when the drooling began.
- Ask the patient how much he drools. Is it scant or copious? Is his pillow wet in the morning?
- Ask the patient if he's experiencing associated signs and symptoms, such as sore throat and difficulty swallowing, chewing, speaking, or breathing.
- Ask the patient to describe pain, numbness, tingling, or stiffness in the face and neck and muscle weakness in the face and extremities.
- Ask the patient about changes in mental status, such as drowsiness or agitation.
- Ask the patient about changes in vision, hearing, and sense of taste.
- Ask the patient if he has experienced anorexia, weight loss, fatigue, nausea, vomiting, or altered bowel or bladder habits.
- Ask the patient whether he recently had a cold or other infection, was bitten by an animal, or exposed to pesticides.
- Obtain a drug history, including prescription and over-the-counter drugs, herbal remedies, and recreational drugs. Also, ask the patient about alcohol intake.

PHYSICAL ASSESSMENT
- Take the patient's vital signs.
- Inspect for signs of facial paralysis or abnormal expression. Examine the mouth and neck for swelling, the throat for edema and redness, and the tonsils for exudate. Also inspect for circumoral irritation.
- Note foul breath odor. Examine the tongue for bilateral furrowing (trident tongue).
- Look for pallor and skin lesions and for frontal baldness. Carefully assess bite or puncture marks.
- Check pupillary size and response to light.
- Assess the patient's speech.
- Evaluate muscle strength, and palpate for tenderness or atrophy. Also palpate for lymphadenopathy, especially in the cervical area.

- Test for poor balance, hyperreflexia, and positive Babinski's reflex.
- Assess sensory function for paresthesia.

SPECIAL CONSIDERATIONS
Be alert for aspiration in a patient who drools. Position him upright or on his side, and use suction as necessary to control the drooling.

A PEDIATRIC POINTERS
- *Normally, an infant can't control saliva flow until about age 1, when muscular reflexes that initiate swallowing and lip closure mature.*
- *Salivation and drooling typically increase with teething, which begins at about the 5th month and continues until about age 2.*
- *Excessive salivation and drooling may occur in response to hunger or anticipation of feeding and in association with nausea.*
- *Common causes of drooling include epiglottiditis, retropharyngeal abscess, severe tonsillitis, stomatitis, herpetic lesions, esophageal atresia, cerebral palsy, mental deficiency, and drug withdrawal in neonates of addicted mothers.*
- *Drooling may also result from a foreign body in the esophagus, causing dysphagia.*

PATIENT COUNSELING
Teach the patient exercises to help strengthen facial muscles, if appropriate.

DROOLING

HPI

Focused PE: HEENT; skin; neurovascular and neurologic systems

BELL'S PALSY
Signs and symptoms
- Gradual onset of facial hemiplegia
- Pain in or behind the ear
- Mild transient tinnitus
- Slightly decreased hearing on the affected side
- Diminished or absent corneal reflex
- Decreased lacrimation

DX: PE
TX: Medication (corticosteroids, analgesic)
F/U: Monthly reevaluations for 6 to 12 months

STROKE
Signs and symptoms
- Unilateral motor weakness or paralysis
- Ataxia
- Decreased LOC
- Headache
- Dizziness
- Aphasia
- Dysphagia
- Visual field deficits
- Double, blurred vision

DX: Labs (coagulation studies, lipid profile, CBC) imaging studies (duplex carotid ultrasonography, CT scan, cerebral angiography, MRI, MRA, echocardiogram)
TX: Maintenance of ABCs, medication (aspirin, platelet aggregation inhibitors, thrombolytics [if embolic]), symptom management
F/U: As needed (based on neurologic status), referrals to neurologist and rehabilitation center (if appropriate)

ESOPHAGEAL TUMOR
Signs and symptoms
- Hematemesis
- Hoarseness
- Weight loss
- Progressively severe dysphagia
- Substernal back or neck pain

DX: PE, endoscopy
TX: Analgesics, mechanical modification of diet, surgery
F/U: Referrals to oncologist and surgeon

PARKINSON'S DISEASE
Signs and symptoms
- Resting tremor
- Rigidity
- Dysphagia
- Dysphonia
- Bradykinesia
- Shuffling gait
- Impaired postural reflexes

DX: Clinical examination
TX: Medication (anticholinergics, dopamine precursors, antivirals, dopamine agonists)
F/U: Referral to neurologist

Common signs and symptoms
- Moderate to copious drooling
- Severe sore throat
- Cervical lymphadenopathy
- Fever
- Pharyngeal edema and redness

PERITONSILLAR ABSCESS
Additional signs and symptoms
- Soft, gray exudate on the tonsils
- Rancid breath
- Uvula deviation

RETROPHARYNGEAL ABSCESS
Additional signs and symptoms
- Feeling of lump in the throat
- Dyspnea when sitting
- Coughing and choking
- Snoring
- Noisy breathing
- Stridor

DX: Labs (CBC, throat culture), lateral neck X-ray
TX: Medication (antipyretics, analgesics, antibiotics), surgical drainage
F/U: Reevaluation 1 week after treatment (sooner if symptoms worsen), ENT referrral if necessary

---

Additional differential diagnoses: achalasia ▪ acoustic neuroma ▪ ALS ▪ diphtheria ▪ envenomation ▪ glossopharyngeal neuralgia ▪ Guillain-Barré syndrome ▪ hypocalcemia ▪ Ludwig's angina ▪ paralytic poliomyelitis ▪ pesticide poisoning ▪ rabies

Other causes: clonazepam ▪ ethionamide ▪ haloperidol

Dysarthria

Dysarthria (poorly articulated speech) is characterized by slurring and labored, irregular rhythm. It may be accompanied by nasal voice tone caused by palate weakness. Whether it occurs abruptly or gradually, dysarthria is usually evident in ordinary conversation. It's confirmed by asking the patient to produce a few simple sounds and words, such as "ba," "sh," and "cat." However, dysarthria is occasionally confused with aphasia, loss of the ability to produce or comprehend speech.

Dysarthria results from damage to the brain stem that affects cranial nerve IX, X, or XI. Degenerative neurologic disorders commonly cause dysarthria. In fact, dysarthria is a chief sign of olivopontocerebellar degeneration. It may also result from ill-fitting dentures.

 ALERT

If the patient displays dysarthria:
- *ask him about associated difficulty swallowing*
- *determine respiratory rate and depth, measuring vital capacity with a Wright respirometer, if available*
- *assess blood pressure and heart rate (Tachycardia, slightly increased blood pressure, and shortness of breath are early indications of respiratory muscle weakness.)*
- *ensure a patent airway*
- *place the patient in Fowler's position*
- *keep emergency resuscitation equipment nearby.*

If dysarthria isn't accompanied by respiratory muscle weakness and dysphagia, perform a focused assessment.

HISTORY
- Ask the patient when the dysarthria began. Has it improved? Does it worsen during the day?
- Review the patient's medical history for seizures.
- Ask the patient if he has experienced numbness or tingling in his limbs.
- Obtain a drug history, including prescription and over-the-counter drugs, herbal remedies, and recreational drugs. Also, ask the patient about alcohol intake.

PHYSICAL ASSESSMENT
- Assess the patient for other neurologic deficits. Compare muscle strength and tone in the limbs.
- Evaluate tactile sensation. Test deep tendon reflexes, and note gait ataxia.
- Test visual fields, and ask the patient about double vision.
- Check for signs of facial weakness such as ptosis.
- Determine level of consciousness and mental status.

SPECIAL CONSIDERATIONS
Encourage the patient with dysarthria to speak slowly so that he can be understood. Give him time to express himself, and encourage him to use gestures.

 PEDIATRIC POINTERS
- *Dysarthria in children usually results from brain stem glioma, a slow-growing tumor that primarily affects children. It may also result from cerebral palsy.*
- *Dysarthria may be difficult to detect, especially in an infant or a young child who hasn't perfected speech. Be sure to look for other neurologic deficits.*

PATIENT COUNSELING
Dysarthria usually requires consultation with a speech therapist. Provide emotional support to the patient and his family. Teach the patient alternate ways to communicate.

DYSARTHRIA

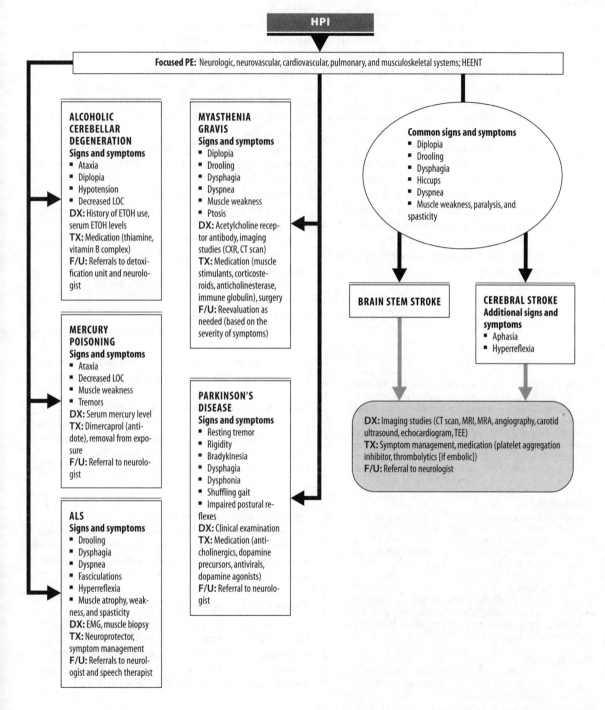

HPI

Focused PE: Neurologic, neurovascular, cardiovascular, pulmonary, and musculoskeletal systems; HEENT

ALCOHOLIC CEREBELLAR DEGENERATION
Signs and symptoms
- Ataxia
- Diplopia
- Hypotension
- Decreased LOC

DX: History of ETOH use, serum ETOH levels
TX: Medication (thiamine, vitamin B complex)
F/U: Referrals to detoxification unit and neurologist

MERCURY POISONING
Signs and symptoms
- Ataxia
- Decreased LOC
- Muscle weakness
- Tremors

DX: Serum mercury level
TX: Dimercaprol (antidote), removal from exposure
F/U: Referral to neurologist

ALS
Signs and symptoms
- Drooling
- Dysphagia
- Dyspnea
- Fasciculations
- Hyperreflexia
- Muscle atrophy, weakness, and spasticity

DX: EMG, muscle biopsy
TX: Neuroprotector, symptom management
F/U: Referrals to neurologist and speech therapist

MYASTHENIA GRAVIS
Signs and symptoms
- Diplopia
- Drooling
- Dysphagia
- Dyspnea
- Muscle weakness
- Ptosis

DX: Acetylcholine receptor antibody, imaging studies (CXR, CT scan)
TX: Medication (muscle stimulants, corticosteroids, anticholinesterase, immune globulin), surgery
F/U: Reevaluation as needed (based on the severity of symptoms)

PARKINSON'S DISEASE
Signs and symptoms
- Resting tremor
- Rigidity
- Bradykinesia
- Dysphagia
- Dysphonia
- Shuffling gait
- Impaired postural reflexes

DX: Clinical examination
TX: Medication (anticholinergics, dopamine precursors, antivirals, dopamine agonists)
F/U: Referral to neurologist

Common signs and symptoms
- Diplopia
- Drooling
- Dysphagia
- Hiccups
- Dyspnea
- Muscle weakness, paralysis, and spasticity

BRAIN STEM STROKE

CEREBRAL STROKE
Additional signs and symptoms
- Aphasia
- Hyperreflexia

DX: Imaging studies (CT scan, MRI, MRA, angiography, carotid ultrasound, echocardiogram, TEE)
TX: Symptom management, medication (platelet aggregation inhibitor, thrombolytics [if embolic])
F/U: Referral to neurologist

Other causes: anticonvulsants ▪ barbiturates

Dysmenorrhea

Dysmenorrhea—painful menstruation—affects more than 50% of menstruating women; in fact, it's the leading cause of lost time from school and work among women of childbearing age. Dysmenorrhea may involve sharp, intermittent pain or dull, aching pain. It's usually characterized by mild to severe cramping or colicky pain in the pelvis or lower abdomen that may radiate to the thighs and lower sacrum. This pain may precede menstruation by several days or may accompany it. The pain gradually subsides as bleeding tapers off.

Dysmenorrhea may be idiopathic, as in premenstrual syndrome and primary dysmenorrhea. It commonly results from endometriosis and other pelvic disorders. It may also result from structural abnormalities such as an imperforate hymen. Stress and poor health may aggravate dysmenorrhea; rest and mild exercise may relieve it. Other conditions that mimic dysmenorrhea include ovulation and normal uterine contractions that occur during pregnancy.

HISTORY

- Ask the patient how long she's been experiencing the pain.

- Ask the patient to describe her dysmenorrhea. Is it intermittent or continuous? Sharp, cramping, or aching? Ask her what relieves her cramps.
- Ask the patient where the pain is located and whether it's bilateral. Does it radiate to her back?
- Ask the patient when the pain begins and ends and when it's severe.
- Ask the patient about associated signs and symptoms, such as nausea and vomiting, altered bowel or urinary habits, bloating, pelvic or rectal pressure, and unusual fatigue, irritability, and depression.
- Obtain a menstrual and sexual history. Ask the patient if her menstrual flow is heavy or scant. Have her describe any vaginal discharge between menses. Find out if she experiences pain during sexual intercourse, and does it occur with menses? Note her method of contraception, and ask about a history of pelvic infection.
- Find out if the patient has any signs and symptoms of urinary system obstruction, such as pyuria, urine retention, and incontinence.
- Determine how the patient copes with stress.

PHYSICAL ASSESSMENT

- Take the patient's vital signs, noting fever and accompanying chills.
- Inspect the abdomen for distention, and palpate for tenderness and masses. Note costovertebral angle tenderness.

SPECIAL CONSIDERATIONS

In the past, women with dysmenorrhea were considered neurotic. Although current research suggests that prostaglandins contribute to this symptom, old attitudes persist. Encourage the patient to view dysmenorrhea as a medical problem, not as a sign of maladjustment.

Ⓐ PEDIATRIC POINTERS

Dysmenorrhea is rare during the first year of menstruation, before the menstrual cycle becomes ovulatory. However, the incidence of dysmenorrhea is generally higher among adolescents than older women.

PATIENT COUNSELING

If dysmenorrhea is idiopathic, advise the patient to place a heating pad on her abdomen to relieve pain. This therapy reduces abdominal muscle tension and increases blood flow. Giving a nonsteroidal anti-inflammatory 1 to 2 days before the onset of menses is usually helpful. (See *Relief for dysmenorrhea*.)

RELIEF FOR DYSMENORRHEA

To relieve cramping and other symptoms caused by primary dysmenorrhea or an intrauterine device, the patient may receive a prostaglandin inhibitor, such as aspirin, ibuprofen, indomethacin, or naproxen. These nonsteroidal anti-inflammatories block prostaglandin synthesis early in the inflammatory reaction, thereby inhibiting prostaglandin action at receptor sites. These drugs also have analgesic and antipyretic effects.

Make sure you and your patient are informed about the adverse effects and cautions associated with these drugs.

ADVERSE EFFECTS

Alert the patient to possible adverse effects of prostaglandin inhibitors. Central nervous system effects include dizziness, headache, and vision disturbances. GI effects include nausea, vomiting, heartburn, and diarrhea. Advise the patient to take the drug with milk or after meals to reduce gastric irritation.

CONTRAINDICATIONS

Because prostaglandin inhibitors are potentially teratogenic, be sure to rule out the possibility of pregnancy before starting therapy. Advise a patient who suspects she's pregnant to delay therapy until menstruation begins.

OTHER CAUTIONS

Use caution when administering a prostaglandin inhibitor to a patient with cardiac decompensation, hypertension, renal dysfunction, or a coagulation defect or to a patient receiving ongoing anticoagulant therapy. Because patients who are hypersensitive to aspirin may also be hypersensitive to other prostaglandin inhibitors, watch for signs of gastric ulceration and bleeding.

DYSMENORRHEA

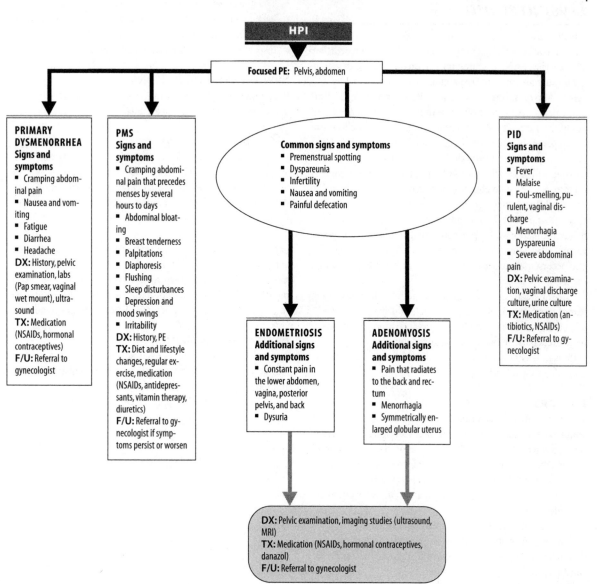

HPI

Focused PE: Pelvis, abdomen

PRIMARY DYSMENORRHEA
Signs and symptoms
- Cramping abdominal pain
- Nausea and vomiting
- Fatigue
- Diarrhea
- Headache

DX: History, pelvic examination, labs (Pap smear, vaginal wet mount), ultrasound
TX: Medication (NSAIDs, hormonal contraceptives)
F/U: Referral to gynecologist

PMS
Signs and symptoms
- Cramping abdominal pain that precedes menses by several hours to days
- Abdominal bloating
- Breast tenderness
- Palpitations
- Diaphoresis
- Flushing
- Sleep disturbances
- Depression and mood swings
- Irritability

DX: History, PE
TX: Diet and lifestyle changes, regular exercise, medication (NSAIDs, antidepressants, vitamin therapy, diuretics)
F/U: Referral to gynecologist if symptoms persist or worsen

Common signs and symptoms
- Premenstrual spotting
- Dyspareunia
- Infertility
- Nausea and vomiting
- Painful defecation

PID
Signs and symptoms
- Fever
- Malaise
- Foul-smelling, purulent, vaginal discharge
- Menorrhagia
- Dyspareunia
- Severe abdominal pain

DX: Pelvic examination, vaginal discharge culture, urine culture
TX: Medication (antibiotics, NSAIDs)
F/U: Referral to gynecologist

ENDOMETRIOSIS
Additional signs and symptoms
- Constant pain in the lower abdomen, vagina, posterior pelvis, and back
- Dysuria

ADENOMYOSIS
Additional signs and symptoms
- Pain that radiates to the back and rectum
- Menorrhagia
- Symmetrically enlarged globular uterus

DX: Pelvic examination, imaging studies (ultrasound, MRI)
TX: Medication (NSAIDs, hormonal contraceptives, danazol)
F/U: Referral to gynecologist

Other cause: intrauterine devices

Dyspareunia

A major obstacle to sexual enjoyment, dyspareunia is painful or difficult coitus. Although most sexually active women occasionally experience mild dyspareunia, persistent or severe dyspareunia is cause for concern. Dyspareunia may occur with attempted penetration or during or after coitus. It may stem from friction of the penis against perineal tissue or from jarring of deeper adnexal structures. The location of pain helps determine its cause.

Dyspareunia commonly accompanies pelvic disorders. However, it may also result from diminished vaginal lubrication associated with aging, the effects of certain drugs, or psychological factors—most notably, fear of pain or injury. A cycle of fear, pain, and tension may become established in which repeated episodes of painful coitus condition the patient to anticipate pain, causing fear, which prevents sexual arousal and adequate vaginal lubrication. Contraction of the pubococcygeus muscle also occurs, making penetration still more difficult and traumatic.

Other psychological factors include guilty feelings about sex, fear of pregnancy or of injury to the fetus during pregnancy, and anxiety caused by a disrupted sexual relationship or by a new sexual partner. Inadequate vaginal lubrication associated with insufficient foreplay and mental or physical fatigue may also cause dyspareunia.

History

- Ask the patient to describe the pain. Does it occur with attempted penetration or deep thrusting? How long does it last? Is the pain intermittent or does it always accompany intercourse? Ask whether changing coital position relieves the pain.
- Ask the patient about a history of pelvic, vaginal, or urinary infection. Does the patient have signs and symptoms of a current infection?
- Ask the patient to describe discharge, if present.
- Ask the patient about malaise, fever, headache, fatigue, abdominal or back pain, nausea and vomiting, and diarrhea or constipation.
- Obtain a sexual and menstrual history. Determine whether dyspareunia is related to the patient's menstrual cycle. Are her cycles regular? Ask about dysmenorrhea and metrorrhagia. Also, find out what contraceptive method the patient uses.
- Ask the patient if she recently had a baby. If so, did she have an episiotomy? Note whether she's breast-feeding. Ask about previous pregnancy, sexual abuse, or pelvic surgery.
- Try to determine the patient's attitude toward sexual intimacy. Does she feel tense during coitus? Is she satisfied with the length of foreplay? Does she usually achieve orgasm? Ask about a history of rape, incest, or sexual abuse as a child.

Physical assessment

- Take the patient's vital signs.
- Palpate the abdomen for tenderness, pain, or masses and for inguinal lymphadenopathy.
- Inspect the genitalia for lesions and vaginal discharge.

Special considerations

Radiation therapy for pelvic cancer may cause pelvic and vaginal scarring, resulting in dyspareunia.

 ### PEDIATRIC POINTERS

Dyspareunia can be an adolescent problem. Although about 40% of adolescents are sexually active by age 19, most are reluctant to initiate a frank sexual discussion. Obtain a thorough sexual history by asking the patient direct but nonjudgmental questions.

AGING ISSUES

In postmenopausal women, the absence of estrogen reduces vaginal diameter and elasticity, which causes tearing of the vaginal mucosa during intercourse. These tears as well as inflammatory reactions to bacterial invasion cause fibrous adhesions that occlude the vagina. Dyspareunia can result from any or all of these conditions.

Patient counseling

Encourage the patient to discuss dyspareunia openly. A women may hesitate to report dyspareunia because of embarrassment and modesty. If an antimicrobial or anti-inflammatory is prescribed, teach her how to apply the cream or insert a vaginal suppository.

DYSPAREUNIA

HPI

Focused PE: GU and GI systems, mental health

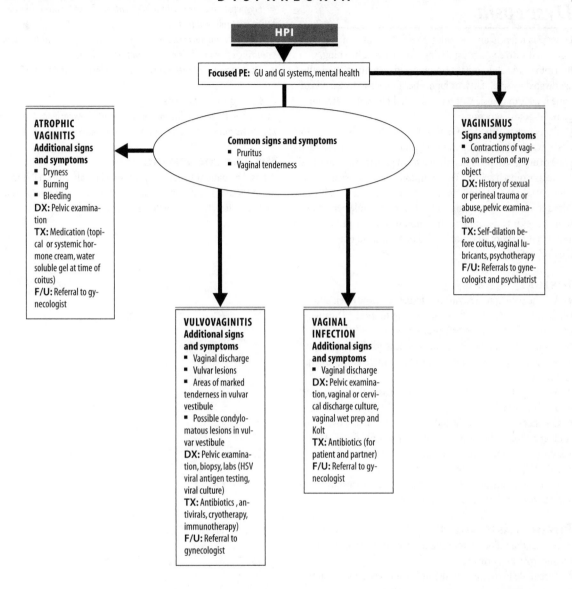

Common signs and symptoms
- Pruritus
- Vaginal tenderness

ATROPHIC VAGINITIS
Additional signs and symptoms
- Dryness
- Burning
- Bleeding

DX: Pelvic examination
TX: Medication (topical or systemic hormone cream, water soluble gel at time of coitus)
F/U: Referral to gynecologist

VAGINISMUS
Signs and symptoms
- Contractions of vagina on insertion of any object

DX: History of sexual or perineal trauma or abuse, pelvic examination
TX: Self-dilation before coitus, vaginal lubricants, psychotherapy
F/U: Referrals to gynecologist and psychiatrist

VULVOVAGINITIS
Additional signs and symptoms
- Vaginal discharge
- Vulvar lesions
- Areas of marked tenderness in vulvar vestibule
- Possible condylomatous lesions in vulvar vestibule

DX: Pelvic examination, biopsy, labs (HSV viral antigen testing, viral culture)
TX: Antibiotics, antivirals, cryotherapy, immunotherapy)
F/U: Referral to gynecologist

VAGINAL INFECTION
Additional signs and symptoms
- Vaginal discharge

DX: Pelvic examination, vaginal or cervical discharge culture, vaginal wet prep and Kolt
TX: Antibiotics (for patient and partner)
F/U: Referral to gynecologist

Other causes: diaphragms ▪ douches ▪ intrauterine devices ▪ spermicidal jellies ▪ vaginal creams and deodorants

Dyspepsia

Dyspepsia refers to an uncomfortable fullness after meals that's associated with epigastric gnawing pain, nausea, belching, heartburn, and abdominal cramping and distention. Typically aggravated by spicy, fatty, or high-fiber foods and by excess caffeine intake, dyspepsia without other pathology indicates impaired digestive function.

Dyspepsia is caused by GI disorders (such as ulcers) and, to a lesser extent, by cardiac, pulmonary, and renal disorders and adverse drug effects. It results when altered gastric secretions lead to excess stomach acidity. This symptom may also result from stress, overly rapid eating, or improper chewing. It usually occurs a few hours after eating and lasts for a variable period of time. Its severity depends on the amount and type of food eaten and on GI motility. Additional food or an antacid may relieve the discomfort.

HISTORY

- Ask the patient to describe his dyspepsia. How often and when does it occur, specifically in relation to meals? Do any drugs or activities relieve or aggravate it?
- Ask the patient if he experiences associated signs and symptoms, such as nausea, vomiting, melena, hematemesis, cough, and chest pain.
- Ask the patient if he has noticed a change in the amount or color of his urine?
- Obtain a drug history, including prescription and over-the-counter drugs, herbal remedies, and recreational drugs. Also, ask the patient about alcohol intake.
- Ask the patient about work-related problems.
- Review the patient's medical history for renal, cardiovascular, and pulmonary disease or recent surgery.

PHYSICAL ASSESSMENT

- Inspect the abdomen for distention, ascites, scars, jaundice, uremic frost, and bruising.
- Auscultate for bowel sounds, and characterize the motility.
- Palpate and percuss the abdomen, noting any tenderness, pain, guarding, rebound, organ enlargement, or tympany.
- Examine other body systems. Auscultate for gallops and crackles. Percuss the lungs to detect consolidation. Note peripheral edema and any swelling of lymph nodes.

SPECIAL CONSIDERATIONS

Changing the patient's position usually doesn't relieve dyspepsia but providing food or an antacid may. Because various drugs can cause dyspepsia, give these after meals, if possible.

PEDIATRIC POINTERS

- *Dyspepsia may occur in adolescents with peptic ulcer disease, but it isn't relieved by food.*
- *Congenital pyloric stenosis may cause dyspepsia, but projectile vomiting after meals is a more characteristic sign.*
- *Dyspepsia in infants may result from lactose intolerance.*

AGING ISSUES

Most older patients with chronic pancreatitis experience less-severe epigastric pain than younger adults; some have no pain at all.

PATIENT COUNSELING

Advise the patient to eat frequent, small meals. Also, tell him to avoid foods and substances that are known to cause dyspepsia, such as coffee, tea, chocolate, alcohol, and tobacco.

DYSPEPSIA

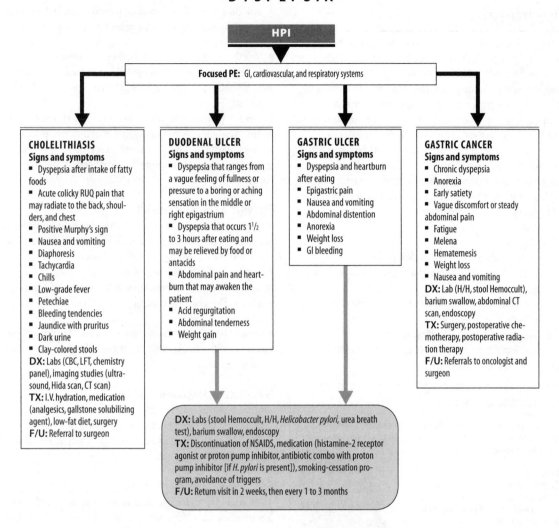

HPI

Focused PE: GI, cardiovascular, and respiratory systems

CHOLELITHIASIS
Signs and symptoms
- Dyspepsia after intake of fatty foods
- Acute colicky RUQ pain that may radiate to the back, shoulders, and chest
- Positive Murphy's sign
- Nausea and vomiting
- Diaphoresis
- Tachycardia
- Chills
- Low-grade fever
- Petechiae
- Bleeding tendencies
- Jaundice with pruritus
- Dark urine
- Clay-colored stools

DX: Labs (CBC, LFT, chemistry panel), imaging studies (ultrasound, Hida scan, CT scan)
TX: I.V. hydration, medication (analgesics, gallstone solubilizing agent), low-fat diet, surgery
F/U: Referral to surgeon

DUODENAL ULCER
Signs and symptoms
- Dyspepsia that ranges from a vague feeling of fullness or pressure to a boring or aching sensation in the middle or right epigastrium
- Dyspepsia that occurs $1^1/_2$ to 3 hours after eating and may be relieved by food or antacids
- Abdominal pain and heartburn that may awaken the patient
- Acid regurgitation
- Abdominal tenderness
- Weight gain

GASTRIC ULCER
Signs and symptoms
- Dyspepsia and heartburn after eating
- Epigastric pain
- Nausea and vomiting
- Abdominal distention
- Anorexia
- Weight loss
- GI bleeding

GASTRIC CANCER
Signs and symptoms
- Chronic dyspepsia
- Anorexia
- Early satiety
- Vague discomfort or steady abdominal pain
- Fatigue
- Melena
- Hematemesis
- Weight loss
- Nausea and vomiting

DX: Lab (H/H, stool Hemoccult), barium swallow, abdominal CT scan, endoscopy
TX: Surgery, postoperative chemotherapy, postoperative radiation therapy
F/U: Referrals to oncologist and surgeon

DX: Labs (stool Hemoccult, H/H, *Helicobacter pylori*, urea breath test), barium swallow, endoscopy
TX: Discontinuation of NSAIDS, medication (histamine-2 receptor agonist or proton pump inhibitor, antibiotic combo with proton pump inhibitor [if *H. pylori* is present]), smoking-cessation program, avoidance of triggers
F/U: Return visit in 2 weeks, then every 1 to 3 months

Additional differential diagnoses: gastric dilatation (acute) ▪ gastritis (chronic) ▪ heart failure ▪ hepatitis ▪ pancreatitis (chronic) ▪ pulmonary embolus ▪ pulmonary tuberculosis ▪ uremia

Other causes: ▪ antibiotics ▪ antihypertensives ▪ anti-inflammatory drugs ▪ aspirin ▪ diuretics ▪ surgery

Dysphagia

Dysphagia—difficulty swallowing—is a common symptom that's usually easy to localize. It may be constant or intermittent and is classified by the phase of swallowing it affects. (See *Classifying dysphagia*.) Among the factors that interfere with swallowing are severe pain, obstruction, abnormal peristalsis, impaired gag reflex, and excessive, scanty, or thick oral secretions.

Dysphagia is the most common—and sometimes the only—symptom of an esophageal disorder. However, it may also result from an oropharyngeal, respiratory, neurologic, or collagen disorder or from the effects of toxins or treatments. Dysphagia increases the risk of choking and aspiration and may lead to malnutrition and dehydration.

ALERT

If the patient suddenly complains of dysphagia:

- *assess him for signs of respiratory distress, such as dyspnea and stridor*
- *secure and maintain an open airway, performing the abdominal thrust maneuver if necessary*
- *initiate emergency measures, if necessary.*

If the patient's dysphagia doesn't suggest airway obstruction, perform a focused assessment.

CLASSIFYING DYSPHAGIA

Because swallowing occurs in three distinct phases, dysphagia can be classified by the phase that it affects. Each phase suggests a specific pathology for dysphagia.

PHASE 1
Swallowing begins in the *transfer phase* with chewing and moistening of food with saliva. The tongue presses against the hard palate to transfer the chewed food to the back of the throat; the fifth cranial nerve then stimulates the swallowing reflex. Phase 1 dysphagia typically results from a neuromuscular disorder.

PHASE 2
In the *transport phase*, the soft palate closes against the pharyngeal wall to prevent nasal regurgitation. At the same time, the larynx rises and the vocal cords close to keep food out of the lungs; breathing stops momentarily as the throat muscles constrict to move food into the esophagus. Phase 2 dysphagia usually indicates spasm or cancer.

PHASE 3
Peristalsis and gravity work together in the *entrance phase* to move food through the esophageal sphincter and into the stomach. Phase 3 dysphagia results from lower esophageal narrowing by diverticula, esophagitis, and other disorders.

HISTORY
- Ask the patient if swallowing is painful. If so, is the pain constant or intermittent? Have the patient point to where dysphagia feels most intense.
- Ask the patient if eating alleviates or aggravates the symptom. Are solids or liquids more difficult to swallow? If the answer is liquids, ask if hot, cold, and lukewarm fluids affect him differently.
- Ask the patient if the symptom disappears after several attempts to swallow. Is swallowing easier in different positions?
- Ask the patient if he has recently experienced vomiting, regurgitation, weight loss, anorexia, hoarseness, dyspnea, or a cough.

PHYSICAL ASSESSMENT
- Evaluate the swallowing reflex by placing your finger along the patient's thyroid notch and then instructing him to swallow. If you feel the larynx rise, the reflex is intact.
- Assess the cough and gag reflex.
- Listen closely to the patient's speech for signs of muscle weakness. Does he have aphasia or dysarthria? Is his voice nasal, hoarse, or breathy?
- Assess the patient's mouth carefully, check for dry mucous membranes and thick, sticky secretions. Check for tongue and facial weakness.

SPECIAL CONSIDERATIONS
Administer an anticholinergic or antiemetic to control excess salivation. If the patient has decreased saliva production, moisten his food with a little liquid. If he has a weak or absent cough reflex, begin tube feedings.

A *P*EDIATRIC POINTERS
- *In looking for dysphagia in an infant or a small child, be sure to pay close attention to his sucking and swallowing ability. Coughing, choking, or regurgitation during feeding suggests dysphagia.*
- *Corrosive esophagitis and esophageal obstruction by a foreign body are more common causes of dysphagia in children than in adults.*
- *Dysphagia may result from a congenital anomaly, such as annular stenosis, dysphagia lusoria, or esophageal atresia.*

AGING ISSUES
In patients older than age 50 with head or neck cancer, dysphagia is a common reason for seeking care. The incidence of such cancers increases markedly in this age-group.

PATIENT COUNSELING
Advise the patient to prepare foods that are easy to swallow. Consult with the dietitian to help the patient select foods with distinct temperatures and texture.

DYSPHAGIA

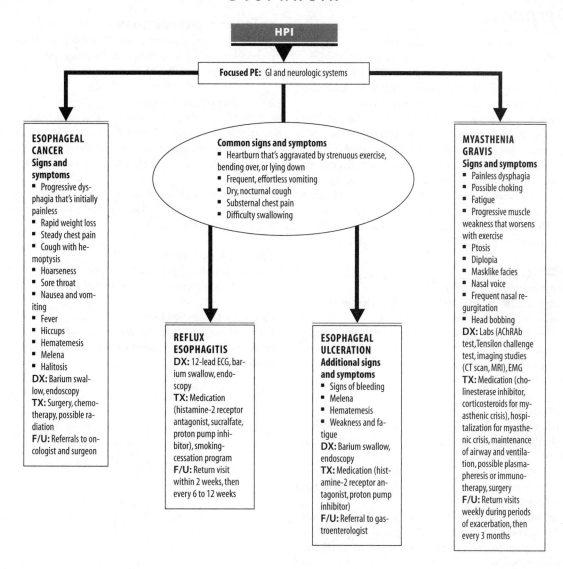

HPI

Focused PE: GI and neurologic systems

ESOPHAGEAL CANCER
Signs and symptoms
- Progressive dysphagia that's initially painless
- Rapid weight loss
- Steady chest pain
- Cough with hemoptysis
- Hoarseness
- Sore throat
- Nausea and vomiting
- Fever
- Hiccups
- Hematemesis
- Melena
- Halitosis

DX: Barium swallow, endoscopy
TX: Surgery, chemotherapy, possible radiation
F/U: Referrals to oncologist and surgeon

Common signs and symptoms
- Heartburn that's aggravated by strenuous exercise, bending over, or lying down
- Frequent, effortless vomiting
- Dry, nocturnal cough
- Substernal chest pain
- Difficulty swallowing

REFLUX ESOPHAGITIS
DX: 12-lead ECG, barium swallow, endoscopy
TX: Medication (histamine-2 receptor antagonist, sucralfate, proton pump inhibitor), smoking-cessation program
F/U: Return visit within 2 weeks, then every 6 to 12 weeks

ESOPHAGEAL ULCERATION
Additional signs and symptoms
- Signs of bleeding
- Melena
- Hematemesis
- Weakness and fatigue

DX: Barium swallow, endoscopy
TX: Medication (histamine-2 receptor antagonist, proton pump inhibitor)
F/U: Referral to gastroenterologist

MYASTHENIA GRAVIS
Signs and symptoms
- Painless dysphagia
- Possible choking
- Fatigue
- Progressive muscle weakness that worsens with exercise
- Ptosis
- Diplopia
- Masklike facies
- Nasal voice
- Frequent nasal regurgitation
- Head bobbing

DX: Labs (AChRAb test, Tensilon challenge test, imaging studies (CT scan, MRI), EMG
TX: Medication (cholinesterase inhibitor, corticosteroids for myasthenic crisis), hospitalization for myasthenic crisis, maintenance of airway and ventilation, possible plasmapheresis or immunotherapy, surgery
F/U: Return visits weekly during periods of exacerbation, then every 3 months

Additional differential diagnoses: achalasia ▪ airway obstruction ▪ ALS ▪ bulbar paralysis ▪ dysphagia lusoria ▪ esophageal compression (external) ▪ esophageal diverticulum ▪ esophageal leiomyoma ▪ esophageal obstruction by foreign body ▪ esophageal spasm ▪ esophagitis ▪ gastric carcinoma ▪ hypocalcemia ▪ laryngeal cancer (extrinsic) ▪ laryngeal nerve damage ▪ lead poisoning ▪ mediastinitis ▪ oral cavity tumor ▪ Parkinson's disease ▪ pharyngitis (chronic) ▪ Plummer-Vinson syndrome ▪ progressive systemic sclerosis ▪ SLE

Other causes: radiation therapy ▪ surgery (such as recent tracheostomy)

Dyspnea

Commonly a symptom of cardiopulmonary dysfunction, dyspnea is the sensation of difficult or uncomfortable breathing. It's usually reported as shortness of breath. The severity varies greatly and may be unrelated to the severity of the underlying cause. Dyspnea may be of sudden or gradual onset.

Most people experience dyspnea when they overexert themselves, but the severity depends on their overall physical condition. In a healthy person, dyspnea is quickly relieved by rest. Pathologic causes of dyspnea include pulmonary, cardiac, neuromuscular, and allergic disorders. Anxiety may also cause shortness of breath. (Because dyspnea is subjective and may be exacerbated by anxiety, patients from cultures that are highly emotional may complain of shortness of breath sooner than those who are more stoic about symptoms of illness.)

 ALERT

If a patient complains of dyspnea:
- *assess him for signs of respiratory distress, such as tachypnea, cyanosis, restlessness, and accessory muscle use*
- *administer oxygen, and initiate emergency measures, if necessary.*

  If the patient can answer questions without increasing his distress, perform a focused assessment.

HISTORY
- Ask the patient if the shortness of breath began suddenly or gradually. Is it constant or intermittent? Does it occur during activity or while at rest?
- Ask the patient if he has had dyspneic attacks before. If so, have the attacks increased in severity? What aggravates or alleviates the attacks?
- Review the patient's medical history for orthopnea, paroxysmal nocturnal dyspnea, progressive fatigue, upper respiratory tract infection, deep vein phlebitis, immobility, recent trauma and other disorders.
- Ask the patient if he has a productive or nonproductive cough or chest pain.
- Ask the patient about tobacco use and exposure to occupational irritants or toxic fumes.

PHYSICAL ASSESSMENT
- Look for signs of chronic dyspnea, such as accessory muscle hypertrophy (especially in the shoulders and neck). Also look for pursed-lip exhalation, finger clubbing, peripheral edema, barrel chest, diaphoresis, and jugular vein distention.
- Check blood pressure and auscultate for crackles, abnormal heart sounds or rhythms, egophony, bronchophony, and whispered pectoriloquy.

- Palpate the abdomen for hepatomegaly.

SPECIAL CONSIDERATIONS
Monitor the dyspneic patient closely. Be as calm and reassuring as possible to reduce his anxiety. Help the patient into a comfortable position, usually high Fowler's or forward leaning.

 PEDIATRIC POINTERS
- *Normally, an infant's respirations are abdominal, gradually changing to costal by age 7. Suspect dyspnea in an infant who breathes costally, in an older child who breathes abdominally, or in any child who uses his neck or shoulder muscles to help him breathe.*
- *Both acute epiglottiditis and laryngotracheobronchitis (croup) can cause severe dyspnea in a child and may even lead to respiratory or cardiovascular collapse.*

 AGING ISSUES
Older patients with dyspnea related to chronic illness may not be aware initially of a significant change in their breathing pattern.

PATIENT COUNSELING
Tell the patient that oxygen therapy isn't necessarily indicated for dyspnea. Encourage a patient with chronic dyspnea to pace his daily activities.

DYSPNEA

HPI

Focused PE: Abdomen; respiratory, cardiovascular, and neurologic systems

---

ASTHMA, ACUTE
Signs and symptoms
- Acute dyspneic attacks
- Audible or auscultated wheezing
- Dry cough
- Hyperpnea
- Chest tightness
- Accessory muscle use
- Nasal flaring
- Intercostal and supraclavicular retractions
- Tachypnea
- Tachycardia
- Diaphoresis
- Prolonged expiration
- Flushing or cyanosis
- Apprehension

DX: Labs (CBC, ABG, allergy skin testing), PFTs, CXR, peak flow meter

TX: Avoidance of allergens and tobacco, medication (beta-adrenergic blockers, inhaled beta$_2$-agonists, inhaled corticosteroid [nedocromil or cromolyn if age < 12], leukotriene receptor agonist, systemic corticosteroids during infections and exacerbations, mast cell stabilizer), peak expiratory flow monitoring

F/U: For acute exacerbation, return visit within 24 hours, then every 3 to 5 days, then every 1 to 3 months; referral to pulmonologist, if the treatment is ineffective

---

Common signs and symptoms
- Gradually developing dyspnea
- Chronic paroxysmal nocturnal dyspnea
- Orthopnea
- Tachypnea
- Tachycardia
- Palpitations
- S$_3$
- Fatigue
- Dependent peripheral edema
- Hepatomegaly
- Dry cough
- Anorexia
- Weight gain
- Loss of mental acuity
- Hemoptysis

HEART FAILURE

ACUTE ONSET HEART FAILURE
Additional signs and symptoms
- JVD
- Bibasilar crackles
- Oliguria
- Hypotension

DX: PE, labs (CBC, cardiac enzymes), imaging studies (CXR, echocardiogram), ECG

TX: Medication (ACE inhibitor, diuretics, carvedilol [possibly], digoxin [possibly]), inotropic agents

F/U: Return visit within 1 week after discharge, at 4 weeks, and then every 3 months; referral to cardiologist if chronic

---

Common signs and symptoms
- Acute dyspnea
- Sudden, stabbing chest pain that may radiate to the arms, face, back, or abdomen
- Anxiety
- Restlessness
- Dry cough
- Cyanosis
- Decreased vocal fremitus
- Tachypnea
- Tympany
- Decreased or absent breath sounds on the affected side
- Asymmetrical chest expansion
- Splinting
- Accessory muscle use

PNEUMOTHORAX

DX: ABG, CXR

TX: Chest tube insertion, oxygen therapy

F/U: Return visit in 1 to 2 weeks after hospitalization

TENSION PNEUMOTHORAX
Additional signs and symptoms
- Tracheal deviation
- Decreased BP
- Tachycardia
- JVD

DX: ABG, CXR

TX: Immediate needle decompression followed by chest tube insertion, oxygen therapy

F/U: Return visit in 1 to 2 weeks after hospitalization

PULMONARY EMBOLISM
Signs and symptoms
- Acute dyspnea
- Sudden pleuritic chest pain
- Tachycardia
- Low-grade fever
- Tachypnea
- Nonproductive or productive cough with blood-tinged sputum
- Pleural friction rub
- Crackles
- Possible hemoptysis
- Diffuse wheezing
- Dullness on percussion
- Decreased breath sounds
- Diaphoresis
- Restlessness
- Acute anxiety
- Signs of shock (possibly)

DX: Imaging studies (CXR, pulmonary $\dot{V}/\dot{Q}$ scan or pulmonary angiography, spiral chest CT scan), ECG

TX: Oxygen therapy, medication (anticoagulants, thrombolytic therapy)

F/U: Reevaluation within first week after hospitalization

Additional differential diagnoses: anemia ▪ ARDS ▪ aspiration of a foreign body ▪ cardiac arrhythmias ▪ COPD ▪ cor pulmonale ▪ emphysema ▪ flail chest ▪ inhalation injury ▪ interstitial fibrosis ▪ lung cancer ▪ MI ▪ pleural effusion ▪ pneumonia ▪ pulmonary edema

Dystonia

Dystonia is marked by slow, involuntary movements of large-muscle groups in the limbs, trunk, and neck. This extrapyramidal sign may involve flexion of the foot, hyperextension of the legs, extension and pronation of the arms, arching of the back, and extension and rotation of the neck (spasmodic torticollis). It's typically aggravated by walking and emotional stress and relieved by sleep.

Dystonia may be intermittent—lasting just a few minutes—or continuous and painful. Occasionally, it causes permanent contractures, resulting in a grotesque posture. Although dystonia may be hereditary or idiopathic, it usually results from an extrapyramidal disorder or from adverse drug effects.

HISTORY

If possible, include the patient's family when obtaining his history. The family may be more aware of behavior changes than the patient.
- Ask the patient when dystonia occurs. Is it aggravated by emotional upset? Does it disappear during sleep? Is there a family history of dystonia?
- Obtain a drug history, including prescription and over-the-counter drugs, herbal remedies, and recreational drugs. Note especially the use of phenothiazines or antipsychotics. Dystonia is a common adverse effect of these drugs, and dosage adjustments may be needed to minimize this effect. Also, ask the patient about alcohol intake.

PHYSICAL ASSESSMENT

- Check voluntary muscle movement by observing the patient's gait as he walks across the room. Have him squeeze your fingers to assess muscle strength. (See *Recognizing dystonia*.)
- Check coordination by having the patient touch your fingertip and then his nose repeatedly.
- Check gross-motor movement by placing the patient's heel on one knee, sliding it down his shin, and then returning it to his knee.
- Assess fine-motor movement by asking the patient to touch each finger to his thumb in succession.

SPECIAL CONSIDERATIONS

If dystonia is severe, protect the patient from injury by raising and padding his bed rails. Provide an uncluttered environment if he's ambulatory.

🅰 PEDIATRIC POINTERS

- *Children don't exhibit dystonia until after they can walk; it rarely occurs until after age 10.*
- *Common causes of dystonia in children include Fahr's syndrome, dystonia musculorum deformans, athetoid cerebral palsy, and the residual effects of anoxia at birth.*

PATIENT COUNSELING

Encourage the patient to obtain adequate sleep and avoid emotional upset. Avoid range of motion exercises, which can aggravate dystonia.

RECOGNIZING DYSTONIA

Dystonia, chorea, and athetosis may occur simultaneously. To differentiate between them, keep the following points in mind:
- *Dystonic movements* are slow and twisting and involve large muscle groups in the head, neck (as shown at right), trunk, and limbs. They may be intermittent or continuous.
- *Choreiform movements* are rapid, highly complex, and jerky.
- *Athetoid movements* are slow, sinuous, and writhing but always continuous; they typically affect the hands and extremities.

DYSTONIA OF THE NECK
(SPASMODIC TORTICOLLIS)

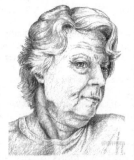

DYSTONIA

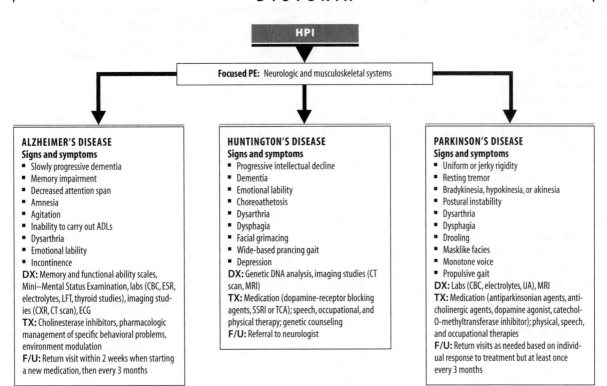

HPI

Focused PE: Neurologic and musculoskeletal systems

ALZHEIMER'S DISEASE
Signs and symptoms
- Slowly progressive dementia
- Memory impairment
- Decreased attention span
- Amnesia
- Agitation
- Inability to carry out ADLs
- Dysarthria
- Emotional lability
- Incontinence

DX: Memory and functional ability scales, Mini–Mental Status Examination, labs (CBC, ESR, electrolytes, LFT, thyroid studies), imaging studies (CXR, CT scan), ECG
TX: Cholinesterase inhibitors, pharmacologic management of specific behavioral problems, environment modulation
F/U: Return visit within 2 weeks when starting a new medication, then every 3 months

HUNTINGTON'S DISEASE
Signs and symptoms
- Progressive intellectual decline
- Dementia
- Emotional lability
- Choreoathetosis
- Dysarthria
- Dysphagia
- Facial grimacing
- Wide-based prancing gait
- Depression

DX: Genetic DNA analysis, imaging studies (CT scan, MRI)
TX: Medication (dopamine-receptor blocking agents, SSRI or TCA); speech, occupational, and physical therapy; genetic counseling
F/U: Referral to neurologist

PARKINSON'S DISEASE
Signs and symptoms
- Uniform or jerky rigidity
- Resting tremor
- Bradykinesia, hypokinesia, or akinesia
- Postural instability
- Dysarthria
- Dysphagia
- Drooling
- Masklike facies
- Monotone voice
- Propulsive gait

DX: Labs (CBC, electrolytes, UA), MRI
TX: Medication (antiparkinsonian agents, anti-cholinergic agents, dopamine agonist, catechol-O-methyltransferase inhibitor); physical, speech, and occupational therapies
F/U: Return visits as needed based on individual response to treatment but at least once every 3 months

---

Additional differential diagnoses: dystonia musculorum deformans ▪ Hallervorden-Spatz disease ▪ olivopontocerebellar atrophy ▪ Pick's disease ▪ supranuclear ophthalmoplegia (Steele-Richardson-Olszewski syndrome) ▪ Wilson's disease

Other causes: antiemetic doses of metoclopramide, risperidone, and metyrosine ▪ antipsychotics, such as haloperidol and loxapine ▪ excessive doses of levodopa ▪ phenothiazines

Dysuria

Dysuria — painful or difficult urination — is commonly accompanied by urinary frequency, urgency, or hesitancy. This symptom usually reflects lower urinary tract infection — a common disorder, especially in women.

Dysuria results from lower urinary tract irritation or inflammation, which stimulates nerve endings in the bladder and urethra. The pain's onset provides clues to its cause — for example, pain just *before* voiding usually indicates bladder irritation or distention, whereas pain at the *start* of urination typically results from bladder outlet irritation. Pain at the *end* of voiding may signal bladder spasms; in women, it may indicate vaginal candidiasis.

HISTORY

- Ask the patient when he first noticed the dysuria. Did anything precipitate it?
- Ask the patient to describe the dysuria's severity and location. Does anything aggravate or alleviate it?
- Review the patient's history for urinary or genital tract infections, intestinal disease, or a recent invasive procedure, such as cystoscopy or urethral dilatation.
- If the patient is female, ask her about menstrual disorders and use of products that irritate the urinary tract, such as bubble bath salts, feminine deodorants, contraceptive gels, or perineal lotions. Also ask her about vaginal discharge or pruritus.

PHYSICAL ASSESSMENT

- Take the patient's vital signs. Note increased temperature, if present.
- Inspect the abdomen. Palpate the abdomen for distention and tenderness. Note bladder distention, if present.
- Inspect the urethral meatus for discharge, irritation, or other abnormalities.

SPECIAL CONSIDERATIONS

Monitor vital signs, intake, and output. Administer prescribed drugs, and prepare the patient for such tests as urinalysis and cystoscopy.

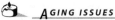

AGING ISSUES

Be aware that elderly patients tend to underreport their symptoms even though older men have an increased incidence of non–sexually related urinary tract infections and postmenopausal women have an increased incidence of noninfectious dysuria.

PATIENT COUNSELING

Teach a female patient (or her parents) that the perineum should be wiped from front to back after urination and defecation to prevent contamination with fecal material. Also, instruct the patient that feminine deodorants, douches, bubble baths, and similar irritants may cause dysuria.

DYSURIA

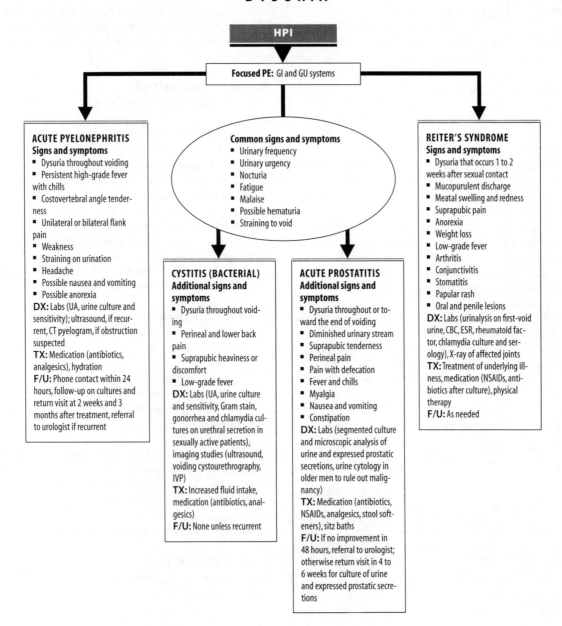

HPI

Focused PE: GI and GU systems

ACUTE PYELONEPHRITIS
Signs and symptoms
- Dysuria throughout voiding
- Persistent high-grade fever with chills
- Costovertebral angle tenderness
- Unilateral or bilateral flank pain
- Weakness
- Straining on urination
- Headache
- Possible nausea and vomiting
- Possible anorexia

DX: Labs (UA, urine culture and sensitivity); ultrasound, if recurrent, CT pyelogram, if obstruction suspected

TX: Medication (antibiotics, analgesics), hydration

F/U: Phone contact within 24 hours, follow-up on cultures and return visit at 2 weeks and 3 months after treatment, referral to urologist if recurrent

Common signs and symptoms
- Urinary frequency
- Urinary urgency
- Nocturia
- Fatigue
- Malaise
- Possible hematuria
- Straining to void

CYSTITIS (BACTERIAL)
Additional signs and symptoms
- Dysuria throughout voiding
- Perineal and lower back pain
- Suprapubic heaviness or discomfort
- Low-grade fever

DX: Labs (UA, urine culture and sensitivity, Gram stain, gonorrhea and chlamydia cultures on urethral secretion in sexually active patients), imaging studies (ultrasound, voiding cystourethrography, IVP)

TX: Increased fluid intake, medication (antibiotics, analgesics)

F/U: None unless recurrent

ACUTE PROSTATITIS
Additional signs and symptoms
- Dysuria throughout or toward the end of voiding
- Diminished urinary stream
- Suprapubic tenderness
- Perineal pain
- Pain with defecation
- Fever and chills
- Myalgia
- Nausea and vomiting
- Constipation

DX: Labs (segmented culture and microscopic analysis of urine and expressed prostatic secretions, urine cytology in older men to rule out malignancy)

TX: Medication (antibiotics, NSAIDs, analgesics, stool softeners), sitz baths

F/U: If no improvement in 48 hours, referral to urologist; otherwise return visit in 4 to 6 weeks for culture of urine and expressed prostatic secretions

REITER'S SYNDROME
Signs and symptoms
- Dysuria that occurs 1 to 2 weeks after sexual contact
- Mucopurulent discharge
- Meatal swelling and redness
- Suprapubic pain
- Anorexia
- Weight loss
- Low-grade fever
- Arthritis
- Conjunctivitis
- Stomatitis
- Papular rash
- Oral and penile lesions

DX: Labs (urinalysis on first-void urine, CBC, ESR, rheumatoid factor, chlamydia culture and serology), X-ray of affected joints

TX: Treatment of underlying illness, medication (NSAIDs, antibiotics after culture), physical therapy

F/U: As needed

Additional differential diagnoses: appendicitis • bladder cancer • chemical irritant • chronic prostatitis • cystitis • diverticulitis • paraurethral gland inflammation • urethral syndrome • urethritis • urinary system obstruction • vaginitis

Other causes: MAO inhibitors • metyrosine

E Earache

Earaches (otalgia) usually result from disorders of the external and middle ear associated with infection, obstruction, or trauma. Their severity ranges from a feeling of fullness or blockage to deep, boring pain; at times, they may be difficult to localize precisely. This common symptom may be intermittent or continuous and may develop suddenly or gradually.

HISTORY

● Ask the patient to characterize his earache. How long has he had it? Is it intermittent or continuous? Is it painful or slightly annoying? Can he localize the pain site? Does he have pain in another area such as the jaw?
● Ask the patient about recent ear injury or other trauma.
● Ask the patient if swimming or showering triggers ear discomfort? Has he been swimming lately in a lake or river?
● Ask the patient if there's discomfort associated with itching. If so, find out where the itching is most intense and when it began.
● Ask the patient about ear drainage and, if present, have him characterize it.
● Ask the patient if he recently had a head cold or problems with his eyes, mouth, teeth, jaws, sinuses, or throat. (Disorders in these areas may refer pain to the ear along the cranial nerves.)

● Ask the patient about associated signs and symptoms. Does he hear ringing or noise in his ears? Has he been dizzy? Does the earache worsen when he changes position? Does he have difficulty swallowing, hoarseness, neck pain, or pain when he opens his mouth?

PHYSICAL ASSESSMENT

● Inspect the external ear for redness, drainage, swelling, or deformity.
● Apply pressure to the mastoid process and tragus to elicit tenderness.
● Using an otoscope, examine the external auditory canal for lesions, bleeding or discharge, impacted cerumen, foreign bodies, tenderness, and swelling.
● Examine the tympanic membrane. Is it intact? Is it pearly gray (normal)? Look for tympanic membrane landmarks: the cone of light, umbo, pars tensa, and the handle and short process of the malleus. (See *Using an otoscope correctly*.)
● Perform the watch tick, whispered voice, Rinne, and Weber's tests to assess the patient for hearing loss.

SPECIAL CONSIDERATIONS

Administer an analgesic, and apply heat to relieve discomfort. Instill eardrops, if necessary.

A PEDIATRIC POINTERS

● *Common causes of earache in children are acute otitis media and insertion of foreign bodies that become lodged or infected.*
● *In a young child, be alert for nonverbal clues to earache, such as crying or ear tugging.*
● *To examine the child's ears, place him in a supine position with his arms extended and held securely by his parent. Then hold the otoscope with the handle pointing toward the top of the child's head, and brace it against him using one or two fingers.*
● *Because an ear examination may upset the child with an earache, save it for the end of your physical assessment.*

PATIENT COUNSELING

Teach the patient (or his parents) how to instill eardrops if they're prescribed for home use.

USING AN OTOSCOPE CORRECTLY

When the patient reports an earache, use an otoscope to inspect ear structures closely. Follow these techniques to obtain the best view and to ensure patient safety.

CHILD
To inspect an infant's or a young child's ear, grasp the *lower part* of the auricle and pull it *down and back* to straighten the upward S curve of the external canal. Then gently insert the speculum into the canal no more than ¹/₂″ (1.3 cm).

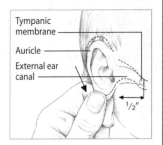

Tympanic membrane
Auricle
External ear canal
¹/₂″

ADULT
To inspect an adult's ear, grasp the *upper part* of the auricle and pull it *up and back* to straighten the external canal. Then insert the speculum about 1″ (2.5 cm). Also use this technique for children older than age 3.

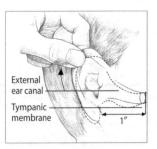

External ear canal
Tympanic membrane
1″

EARACHE

HPI

Focused PE: HEENT, neurologic and respiratory systems

ACUTE SUPPURATIVE OTITIS MEDIA
Signs and symptoms
- Severe, deep, throbbing ear pain
- Hearing loss or vertigo
- Otorrhea
- Fever that may reach 102° F (38.9° C)
- Nausea, vomiting, and diarrhea (in children)
- Reddened, bulging tympanic membrane
- Obscured, bony landmarks
- Distorted light reflex

DX: Ear examination, tympanometry, tympanocentesis for culture and sensitivity for recurrent infections

TX: Medication (antibiotics, analgesics)

F/U: Return visit in 2 to 3 days if condition isn't significantly improved, otherwise in 2 to 3 weeks

Common signs and symptoms
- Mild to moderate ear pain with tragus manipulation
- Low-grade fever initially (may reach 104° F [40° C] with progression)
- Sticky yellow or purulent ear discharge
- Conductive hearing loss
- Feeling of fullness in the ear
- Swelling of tragus, external meatus, and external canal
- Tympanic membrane erythema
- Lymphadenopathy
- Dizziness and malaise (possibly)

MÉNIÈRE'S DISEASE
Signs and symptoms
- Ear fullness
- Tinnitus
- Severe vertigo
- Sensorineural hearing loss

DX: Audiometry, electronystagmography

TX: Salt and fluid restriction, avoidance of nicotine, moderate caffeine and alcohol, medication (diuretics, antiemetic, antivertigo agents), hearing amplification, vestibular exercises

F/U: Reevaluation every 3 months, referral to otolaryngologist (if treatment is ineffective)

ACUTE OTITIS EXTERNA
DX: Ear examination

TX: Removal of exudate and epidermal debris, otic antibiotic, avoidance of swimming for 4 to 6 weeks, use of cotton covered with petroleum jelly to plug ear for bathing and showering for 4 to 6 weeks

F/U: Reevaluation in 3 to 7 days

MALIGNANT OTITIS EXTERNA
Additional signs and symptoms
- Intense itching
- Deep-seated nocturnal pain
- Parotid gland swelling
- Trismus
- Swollen external canal with exposed cartilage and temporal bone
- Cranial nerve palsy (possibly)

DX: Ear drainage culture

TX: I.V. antibiotics, surgical debridement

F/U: Referral to otolaryngologist

Additional differential diagnoses: abscess (extradural) ▪ barotrauma (acute) ▪ cerumen impaction ▪ chondrodermatitis nodularis chronica helicis ▪ ear canal obstruction by insect ▪ frostbite ▪ furunculosis ▪ herpes zoster oticus (Ramsay Hunt syndrome) ▪ keratosis obturans ▪ mastoiditis (acute) ▪ middle ear tumor ▪ myringitis bullosa ▪ otitis media ▪ perichondritis ▪ petrositis ▪ TMJ infection

Edema

A common sign in severely ill patients, *generalized edema* is the excessive accumulation of interstitial fluid throughout the body. Its severity varies widely; slight edema may be difficult to detect, especially if the patient is obese, whereas massive edema is immediately apparent.

Generalized edema may result from cardiac, renal, endocrine, or hepatic disorders as well as from severe burns, malnutrition, or the effects of certain drugs and treatments.

Facial edema refers to either localized swelling—for example, around the eyes—or more generalized facial swelling that may extend to the neck. Occasionally painful, this sign may develop gradually or abruptly. Sometimes it precedes onset of peripheral or generalized edema. Mild edema may be difficult to detect; the patient or someone familiar with his appearance may report it before it's noticed during assessment.

Leg edema results when excess interstitial fluid accumulates in one or both legs. It may affect just the foot and ankle, or it may extend to the thigh; it may be slight or dramatic, and pitting or nonpitting. It may result from a venous disorder, trauma, or a bone or cardiac disorder that disturbs normal fluid balance.

ALERT

If the patient has severe edema:
- *promptly take his vital signs, and check for jugular vein distention and cyanotic lips*
- *auscultate the lungs and heart; be alert for signs of heart failure*
- *place him in Fowler's position, if appropriate, and administer oxygen and a diuretic, as ordered*
- *initiate emergency measures (if facial edema is present and affecting the patient's airway).*

If the patient presents with generalized, facial, or leg edema, perform a focused assessment.

HISTORY

If the patient presents with generalized or leg edema, obtain a drug history, including prescription and over-the-counter drugs, herbal remedies, and recreational drugs as well as alcohol intake and recent I.V. therapy. Also ask these questions:
- When did the edema begin?
- Does the edema moves throughout the course of the day—for example, from the upper extremities to the lower extremities? Is it worse in the morning or at the end of the day or is it affected by position changes?
- Is the edema is accompanied by shortness of breath or pain in the arms or legs?
- Have you gained weight? How much? Describe your diet and fluid intake.
- Do you have previous cardiac, renal, hepatic, endocrine, or GI disorders?

If the patient has facial edema, also ask these questions:
- Did the edema developed suddenly or gradually?
- Do you have allergies? Have you been recently exposed to allergens?
- Have you had recent facial trauma?

PHYSICAL ASSESSMENT

If the patient presents with generalized edema:
- Compare the patient's arms and legs for symmetrical edema. Also, note ecchymoses and cyanosis. Assess the back, sacrum, and hips of the bedridden patient for dependent edema.
- Palpate peripheral pulses, noting whether hands and feet feel cold. Perform a complete cardiac and respiratory assessment.

If the patient presents with facial edema:
- Examine the oral cavity to evaluate dental hygiene, and look for signs of infection. Visualize the oropharynx, and look for soft-tissue swelling.

If the patient presents with leg edema:
- Examine each leg for pitting edema. Palpate peripheral pulses to detect possible insufficiency. Observe leg color and look for unusual vein patterns.
- Palpate each leg for warmth, tenderness, and cords, and gently squeeze the calf muscle against the tibia to check for deep pain. If leg edema is unilateral, dorsiflex the foot to look for Homans' sign, which is indicated by calf pain.
- Note skin thickening or ulceration in the edematous areas.

SPECIAL CONSIDERATIONS

If the patient has generalized edema, position him with his limbs above heart level to promote drainage. If he develops dyspnea, lower his limbs, elevate the head of the bed, and administer oxygen.

[A] PEDIATRIC POINTERS
- *Renal failure in children commonly causes generalized edema.*
- *Periorbital edema is more common than peripheral edema in children with such disorders as heart failure and acute glomerulonephritis. Pertussis may also cause periorbital edema.*
- *Uncommon in children, leg edema may result from osteomyelitis, leg trauma or, rarely, heart failure.*

AGING ISSUES
An older patient is more likely to develop edema for several reasons, including decreased cardiac and renal function and, in some cases, poor nutritional status.

PATIENT COUNSELING

Teach the patient with known heart failure or renal failure to recognize edema and to report it to his health care provider. Advise him to monitor his weight and report a gain of 2 lb (0.9 kg) in 1 day or 5 lb (2.3 kg) in 1 week.

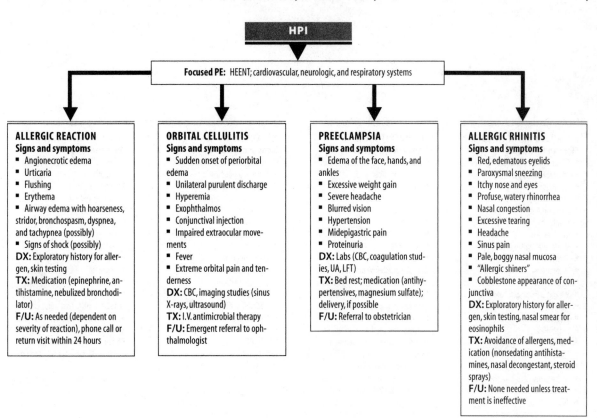

HPI

Focused PE: HEENT; cardiovascular, neurologic, and respiratory systems

ALLERGIC REACTION
Signs and symptoms
- Angionecrotic edema
- Urticaria
- Flushing
- Erythema
- Airway edema with hoarseness, stridor, bronchospasm, dyspnea, and tachypnea (possibly)
- Signs of shock (possibly)
DX: Exploratory history for allergen, skin testing
TX: Medication (epinephrine, antihistamine, nebulized bronchodilator)
F/U: As needed (dependent on severity of reaction), phone call or return visit within 24 hours

ORBITAL CELLULITIS
Signs and symptoms
- Sudden onset of periorbital edema
- Unilateral purulent discharge
- Hyperemia
- Exophthalmos
- Conjunctival injection
- Impaired extraocular movements
- Fever
- Extreme orbital pain and tenderness
DX: CBC, imaging studies (sinus X-rays, ultrasound)
TX: I.V. antimicrobial therapy
F/U: Emergent referral to ophthalmologist

PREECLAMPSIA
Signs and symptoms
- Edema of the face, hands, and ankles
- Excessive weight gain
- Severe headache
- Blurred vision
- Hypertension
- Midepigastric pain
- Proteinuria
DX: Labs (CBC, coagulation studies, UA, LFT)
TX: Bed rest; medication (antihypertensives, magnesium sulfate); delivery, if possible
F/U: Referral to obstetrician

ALLERGIC RHINITIS
Signs and symptoms
- Red, edematous eyelids
- Paroxysmal sneezing
- Itchy nose and eyes
- Profuse, watery rhinorrhea
- Nasal congestion
- Excessive tearing
- Headache
- Sinus pain
- Pale, boggy nasal mucosa
- "Allergic shiners"
- Cobblestone appearance of conjunctiva
DX: Exploratory history for allergen, skin testing, nasal smear for eosinophils
TX: Avoidance of allergens, medication (nonsedating antihistamines, nasal decongestant, steroid sprays)
F/U: None needed unless treatment is ineffective

Additional differential diagnoses: abscess (peritonsillar or periodontal) ▪ cavernous sinus thrombosis ▪ chalazion ▪ conjunctivitis ▪ corneal ulcers (fungal) ▪ dacryoadenitis ▪ dacryocystitis ▪ dermatomyositis ▪ facial burns ▪ facial trauma ▪ frontal sinus cancer ▪ generalized edema ▪ herpes zoster ophthalmicus (shingles) ▪ hordeolum (stye) ▪ malnutrition ▪ Melkersson's syndrome ▪ myxedema ▪ nephrotic syndrome ▪ osteomyelitis ▪ sinusitis ▪ superior vena cava syndrome ▪ trachoma ▪ richinosis

Other causes: allergic reaction to contrast medium ▪ drugs ▪ drugs that cause allergic reactions (aspirin, antipyretics, penicillin, sulfa preparations) ▪ long-term use of glucocorticoids ▪ surgery (cranial, nasal, or jaw)

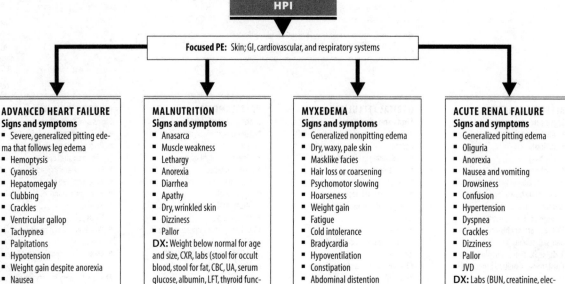

HPI

Focused PE: Skin; GI, cardiovascular, and respiratory systems

ADVANCED HEART FAILURE
Signs and symptoms
- Severe, generalized pitting edema that follows leg edema
- Hemoptysis
- Cyanosis
- Hepatomegaly
- Clubbing
- Crackles
- Ventricular gallop
- Tachypnea
- Palpitations
- Hypotension
- Weight gain despite anorexia
- Nausea
- Slowed mental response
- Diaphoresis
- Pallor
- Dyspnea
- Orthopnea
- Tachycardia
- Fatigue
- JVD

DX: Labs (cardiac enzymes, CBC, chemistry panel, ABG), imaging studies (CXR, echocardiogram), ECG
TX: Medication (ACE inhibitor, diuretics, I.V. inotropes)
F/U: Reevaluation within 1 week after hospitalization, then every 4 weeks if stabilized; referral to cardiologist

MALNUTRITION
Signs and symptoms
- Anasarca
- Muscle weakness
- Lethargy
- Anorexia
- Diarrhea
- Apathy
- Dry, wrinkled skin
- Dizziness
- Pallor

DX: Weight below normal for age and size, CXR, labs (stool for occult blood, stool for fat, CBC, UA, serum glucose, albumin, LFT, thyroid function studies, BUN, creatinine, electrolytes, amylase, lipase, serum iron, transferrin, TIBC, vitamin B_{12}, folate) anthropometric measurements, food intake diary
TX: Hospitalization if weight loss is more than 10%, treatment of underlying condition, vitamin supplementation, high-calorie diet with dietary supplementation, food diary
F/U: Reevaluation in 2 to 4 weeks, then every 6 to 12 weeks; referral to social worker for community resources

MYXEDEMA
Signs and symptoms
- Generalized nonpitting edema
- Dry, waxy, pale skin
- Masklike facies
- Hair loss or coarsening
- Psychomotor slowing
- Hoarseness
- Weight gain
- Fatigue
- Cold intolerance
- Bradycardia
- Hypoventilation
- Constipation
- Abdominal distention
- Menorrhagia
- Impotence
- Infertility

DX: Labs (electrolytes, thyroid studies), CXR, ECG
TX: Maintenance of ABCs, hemodynamic stabilization and monitoring, rewarming measures, thyroid hormone replacement
F/U: Referral to endocrinologist

ACUTE RENAL FAILURE
Signs and symptoms
- Generalized pitting edema
- Oliguria
- Anorexia
- Nausea and vomiting
- Drowsiness
- Confusion
- Hypertension
- Dyspnea
- Crackles
- Dizziness
- Pallor
- JVD

DX: Labs (BUN, creatinine, electrolytes, UA, ABG), imaging studies (ultrasound, IVP, KUB)
TX: Dialysis, medication (electrolyte replacement, antihypertensives)
F/U: Referral to nephrologist

Additional differential diagnoses: angioneurotic edema ▪ burns ▪ cirrhosis ▪ nephrotic syndrome ▪ pericardial effusion ▪ pericarditis (chronic constrictive) ▪ protein-losing enteropathy ▪ renal failure (chronic) ▪ septic shock

Other causes: drugs that cause sodium retention (antihypertensives, corticosteroids, androgenic and anabolic steroids, estrogens, NSAIDs) ▪ enteral feedings ▪ I.V. saline solution infusions

EDEMA (LEG)

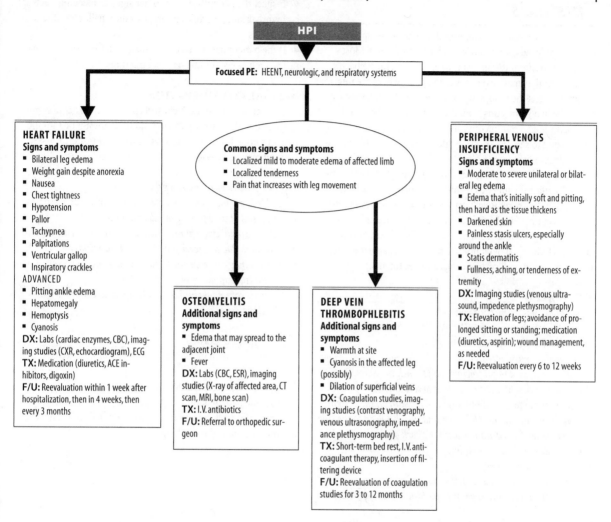

HPI

Focused PE: HEENT, neurologic, and respiratory systems

HEART FAILURE
Signs and symptoms
- Bilateral leg edema
- Weight gain despite anorexia
- Nausea
- Chest tightness
- Hypotension
- Pallor
- Tachypnea
- Palpitations
- Ventricular gallop
- Inspiratory crackles
ADVANCED
- Pitting ankle edema
- Hepatomegaly
- Hemoptysis
- Cyanosis
DX: Labs (cardiac enzymes, CBC), imaging studies (CXR, echocardiogram), ECG
TX: Medication (diuretics, ACE inhibitors, digoxin)
F/U: Reevaluation within 1 week after hospitalization, then in 4 weeks, then every 3 months

Common signs and symptoms
- Localized mild to moderate edema of affected limb
- Localized tenderness
- Pain that increases with leg movement

OSTEOMYELITIS
Additional signs and symptoms
- Edema that may spread to the adjacent joint
- Fever
DX: Labs (CBC, ESR), imaging studies (X-ray of affected area, CT scan, MRI, bone scan)
TX: I.V. antibiotics
F/U: Referral to orthopedic surgeon

DEEP VEIN THROMBOPHLEBITIS
Additional signs and symptoms
- Warmth at site
- Cyanosis in the affected leg (possibly)
- Dilation of superficial veins
DX: Coagulation studies, imaging studies (contrast venography, venous ultrasonography, impedance plethysmography)
TX: Short-term bed rest, I.V. anticoagulant therapy, insertion of filtering device
F/U: Reevaluation of coagulation studies for 3 to 12 months

PERIPHERAL VENOUS INSUFFICIENCY
Signs and symptoms
- Moderate to severe unilateral or bilateral leg edema
- Edema that's initially soft and pitting, then hard as the tissue thickens
- Darkened skin
- Painless stasis ulcers, especially around the ankle
- Statis dermatitis
- Fullness, aching, or tenderness of extremity
DX: Imaging studies (venous ultrasound, impedence plethysmography)
TX: Elevation of legs; avoidance of prolonged sitting or standing; medication (diuretics, aspirin); wound management, as needed
F/U: Reevaluation every 6 to 12 weeks

Additional differential diagnoses: burns ▪ envenomation ▪ leg trauma ▪ peripheral vascular disease ▪ phlegmasia cerulea dolens ▪ superficial vein thrombophlebitis

Epistaxis

Epistaxis (nosebleed) is a common sign that can be spontaneous or induced from the front or back of the nose. Most nosebleeds occur in the anterior nasal septum (Kiesselbach's plexus), but they may also occur at the point where the inferior turbinates meet the nasopharynx. Usually unilateral, they seem bilateral when blood runs from the bleeding side behind the nasal septum and out the opposite side. Epistaxis ranges from mild oozing to severe—possibly life-threatening—blood loss.

A rich supply of fragile blood vessels makes the nose particularly vulnerable to bleeding. Air moving through the nose can dry and irritate the mucous membranes, forming crusts that bleed when they're removed; dry mucous membranes are also more susceptible to infections, which can produce epistaxis as well. Trauma is another common cause of epistaxis. Additional causes include septal deviation; hematologic, coagulation, renal, and GI disorders; and certain drugs and treatments.

➤ **A**LERT

If the patient has severe epistaxis:
- *quickly take his vital signs (Be alert for tachypnea, hypotension, and other signs of hypovolemic shock.)*
- *attempt to control bleeding by pinching the nares closed (However, if you suspect a nasal fracture, don't pinch the nares. Instead, place gauze under the patient's nose to absorb the blood.)*
- *have him sit upright and tilt his head forward (If the patient has hypovolemia, have him lie down and turn his head to the side to prevent blood from draining down the back of his throat, which could cause aspiration or vomiting.)*
- *monitor airway patency*
- *initiate emergency measures, if necessary.*
  If the patient's condition permits, perform a focused assessment.

HISTORY
- Ask the patient about recent trauma. Also ask if he recently had surgery in the sinus area.
- Ask the patient about the frequency of his nosebleeds. Have they been long or unusually severe?
- Review the patient's medical history, noting especially hypertension, bleeding or liver disorders, and other recent illnesses. Also, ask the patient if he bruises easily.
- Obtain a drug history, including prescription and over-the-counter drugs (paying particular attention to his use of anti-inflammatories, such as aspirin, and anticoagulants such as warfarin), herbal remedies, and recreational drugs. Question the patient about cocaine or other illicit drug use nasally. Also, ask the patient about alcohol intake.

PHYSICAL ASSESSMENT
- Inspect the patient's skin for other signs of bleeding, such as ecchymoses and petechiae, noting jaundice, pallor, or other abnormalities.
- If the patient has suffered a trauma, look for associated injuries, such as eye trauma or facial fractures.

SPECIAL CONSIDERATIONS
If external pressure doesn't control epistaxis, insert cotton impregnated with a vasoconstrictor and local anesthetic into the patient's nose. If bleeding persists, anterior or posterior nasal packing may be inserted.

 PEDIATRIC **POINTERS**
- *Children are more likely to experience anterior nosebleeds, usually the result of nose picking or allergic rhinitis.*
- *Biliary atresia, cystic fibrosis, hereditary afibrinogenemia, and nasal trauma due to a foreign body can cause epistaxis.*
- *Rubeola may cause an oozing nosebleed along with the characteristic maculopapular rash.*
- *Epistaxis commonly begins at puberty in hereditary hemorrhagic telangiectasia.*

 AGING **ISSUES**
Older patients are more likely to have posterior nosebleeds.

PATIENT COUNSELING
Instruct the patient about proper pinching pressure techniques. For prevention, tell him to apply petroleum jelly to his nostrils to prevent drying and cracking.

EPISTAXIS

HPI

Focused PE: HEENT; integumentary, cardiovascular, and respiratory systems

ACUTE LEUKEMIA
Signs and symptoms
- Sudden epistaxis
- High fever
- Bleeding gums
- Ecchymoses
- Petechiae
- Easy bruising
- Prolonged menses
- Weakness
- Lassitude
- Pallor
- Chills
- Recurrent infections
- Lymphadenopathy
- Hepatosplenomegaly

CHRONIC LEUKEMIA
Signs and symptoms
- Extreme fatigue
- Weight loss
- Hepatosplenomegaly
- Bone tenderness
- Dyspnea
- Tachycardia
- Macular or nodular skin lesions

DX: CBC with differential, bone marrow biopsy
TX: Chemotherapy, radiation therapy, bone marrow transplant, if necessary
F/U: Referral to oncologist

COAGULATION DISORDERS
Signs and symptoms
- Ecchymoses
- Petechiae
- Bleeding from the gums, the mouth, and puncture sites
- Menorrhagia
- GI bleeding

DX: Labs (coagulation studies, CBC with differential)
TX: As needed (dependent on particular disorder)
F/U: Referral to hematologist

APLASTIC ANEMIA
Signs and symptoms
- Ecchymoses
- Retinal hemorrhages
- Menorrhagia
- Petechiae
- Bleeding from the mouth
- GI bleeding
- Fatigue
- Dyspnea
- Headache
- Tachycardia
- Pallor

DX: Labs (CBC, ferritin, serum iron, B_{12}, TIBC), bone marrow biopsy
TX: Treatment of underlying cause; blood transfusion; immunosuppressive therapy; bone marrow transplant, if necessary
F/U: Referral to hematologist

SEVERE HYPERTENSION
Signs and symptoms
- Extreme epistaxis with pulsation above middle turbinate
- BP > 180/110 mm Hg
- Dizziness
- Throbbing headache
- Vision changes
- Anxiety
- Peripheral edema
- Nocturia
- Nausea and vomiting
- Drowsiness
- Mental impairment

DX: Labs (CBC, BUN, creatinine, electrolytes, plasma renin, uric acid, cortisol, 24 hour urine for Bence Jones protein, VMA), renal X-ray, ECG
TX: Treatment of underlying condition, medication (beta-adrenergic blockers, ACE inhibitors, calcium channel blockers, I.V. diuretics, I.V. antihypertensives)
F/U: Reevaluation within 1 week after hospitalization, then every 4 weeks until BP is controlled

---

Additional differential diagnoses: angiofibroma (juvenile) ▪ barotrauma ▪ biliary obstruction ▪ cirrhosis ▪ glomerulonephritis (chronic) ▪ hepatitis ▪ hereditary hemorrhagic telangiectasia (Rendu-Osler-Weber syndrome) ▪ infectious mononucleosis ▪ influenza ▪ maxillofacial injury ▪ nasal fracture ▪ nasal tumor ▪ orbital floor fracture ▪ polycythemia vera ▪ renal failure ▪ sarcoidosis ▪ scleroma ▪ sinusitis (acute) ▪ skull fracture ▪ SLE ▪ syphilis ▪ typhoid fever

Other causes: anticoagulants (such as coumadin) ▪ anti-inflammatories (such as aspirin) ▪ chemical irritants ▪ facial and nasal surgery (rare), including septoplasty, rhinoplasty, antrostomy, endoscopic sinus procedures, orbital decompression, and dental extraction ▪ habitual illicit drug use, especially cocaine

Erythema

Dilated or congested blood vessels produce red skin, or erythema, the most common sign of skin inflammation or irritation. Erythema may be localized or generalized and may occur suddenly or gradually. Skin color can range from bright red (in someone with an acute condition) to pale violet or brown (in someone with a chronic condition). Erythema must be differentiated from purpura, which causes redness from bleeding into the skin. When pressure is applied directly to the skin, erythema blanches momentarily, but purpura doesn't.

Erythema usually results from changes in the arteries, veins, and small vessels that lead to increased small-vessel perfusion. Drugs and neurogenic mechanisms can also allow extra blood to enter the small vessels. In addition, erythema can result from trauma and tissue damage as well as from changes in supporting tissues, which increase vessel visibility. Many rare disorders can also cause this sign. (See *Rare causes of erythema.*)

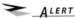

ALERT

If the patient has sudden progressive erythema:
- *quickly take his vital signs*
- *assess him for rapid pulse, dyspnea, hoarseness, and agitation, all of which may indicate anaphylactic shock*
- *initiate emergency measures, if necessary.*

If the patient's erythema isn't associated with anaphylaxis, perform a focused assessment.

HISTORY

- Ask the patient how long he has had the erythema and where it first began.
- Ask the patient if the erythema is associated with pain or itching.
- Ask the patient if he recently had a fever, upper respiratory tract infection, or joint pain.

RARE CAUSES OF ERYTHEMA

In exceptional cases, the patient's erythema may be caused by one of these rare disorders:
- *acute febrile neutrophilic dermatosis,* which produces erythematous lesions on the face, neck, and extremities after a high fever
- *erythema ab igne,* which produces lacy erythema and telangiectases after exposure to radiant heat
- *erythema chronicum migrans,* which produces erythematous macules and papules on the trunk, upper arms, or thighs after a tick bite
- *erythema gyratum repens,* which produces wavy bands of erythema and is commonly associated with internal malignancy
- *toxic epidermal necrolysis,* which causes severe, widespread erythema, tenderness, and skin loss as a result of staphylococci or, possibly, the use of certain drugs.

- Review the patient's medical history for skin disease and other illnesses. Also, ask the patient about a family history of allergies, asthma, or eczema.
- Ask the patient if he has been exposed to someone who has had a similar rash or is now ill.
- Obtain a drug history, including prescription and over-the-counter drugs, herbal remedies, and recreational drugs. Also, ask the patient about alcohol intake and recent immunizations.
- Ask the patient about food intake and exposure to chemicals.

PHYSICAL ASSESSMENT

- Assess the extent, distribution, and intensity of the erythema. Look for edema and other skin lesions, such as hives, scales, papules, and purpura.
- Examine the affected area for warmth, and gently palpate it to check for tenderness or crepitus.

SPECIAL CONSIDERATIONS

Because erythema can cause fluid loss, closely monitor and replace fluids and electrolytes, especially if the patient has burns or widespread erythema. Be sure to withhold all medication until the cause of erythema has been identified.

PEDIATRIC POINTERS

- *Erythema toxicum neonatorum (newborn rash), a pink papular rash, normally develops during the first 4 days after birth and spontaneously disappears by the 10th day.*
- *Neonates and infants can develop erythema from infections and other disorders. For instance, candidiasis can produce thick, white lesions over an erythematous base on the oral mucosa as well as diaper rash with beefy red erythema.*
- *Roseola, rubeola, scarlet fever, granuloma annulare, and cutis marmorata may all cause erythema in children.*

AGING ISSUES

Elderly patients commonly have well-demarcated purple macules or patches, usually on the back of the hands and on the forearms. Known as actinic purpura, this condition results from blood leaking through fragile capillaries. The lesions disappear spontaneously.

PATIENT COUNSELING

If the patient has a chronic disorder that causes erythema, teach him about the character of a typical rash so he can be alert to flare-ups. Also, advise him to avoid sun exposure and to use sunblock when appropriate.

HPI

Focused PE: Skin

BURNS
Signs and symptoms
FIRST DEGREE
- Pressure that causes blanching of skin
- Tenderness at site
- Involvement of superficial layers of the epidermis

SECOND DEGREE
- Deep or superficial blisters
- Increased tenderness at site
- Involvement of varying degrees of the epidermis and part of the dermis

THIRD DEGREE
- Tough and leathery affected area
- Nontender
- Destruction of all skin elements

DX: History of exposure to heat, chemicals, or electricity; PE; CXR for smoke inhalation
TX: Removal of cause of injury, rule of nines to estimate extent of injury and guide treatment, I.V. hydration, medication (analgesics, NSAIDs, topical antibacterial)
F/U: As needed (dependent on severity of burn), referral to burn center if injury is severe

ERYTHEMA MULTIFORME
Signs and symptoms
- Hivelike erythema with blisters
- Pathognomonic petechial or "iris" lesions
- Symmetrical lesions on the face, hands, and feet
- Lesions (less than 3 cm)
- Involvement of less than 20% of body surface area

DX: PE, skin biopsy
TX: Treatment of underlying cause, medication (analgesics, antipruritics)
F/U: None unless complications develop

SEBORRHEIC DERMATITIS
Signs and symptoms
- Dull red or yellow lesions
- Occurrence on the scalp, eyebrows, ears, and nasolabial folds
- Butterfly rash on the face, chest, or trunk

DX: PE, skin biopsy, allergic patch test
TX: Medication (antiseborrheic shampoo, selenium or zinc lotion, steroid creme)
F/U: Reevaluation every 2 to 12 weeks as necessary

ATOPIC DERMATITIS
Signs and symptoms
- Intense pruritus
- Small papules that redden, weep, scale, lichenify and commonly occur in skin folds of the extremities, neck, eyelids

DX: PE, skin biopsy, allergic patch test
TX: Topical corticosteroids
F/U: Reevaluation every 2 to 12 weeks as necessary

CONTACT DERMATITIS
Signs and symptoms
- History of exposure to irritant
- Vesicles, blisters, ulcerations that appear on exposed skin

DX: PE, skin biopsy, allergic patch test
TX: Cool compresses with astringent, soaks with oatmeal, medication (topical and systemic corticosteroids, antihistamines, antibiotics)
F/U: Reevaluation every 2 to 12 weeks as necessary

Additional differential diagnoses: allergic reaction ▪ candidiasis ▪ chronic liver disease ▪ dermatomyositis ▪ erysipelas ▪ erythema annulare centrifugum ▪ erythema marginatum rheumaticum ▪ erythema nodosum ▪ frostbite ▪ intertrigo ▪ necrotizing fasciitis ▪ polymorphous light eruption ▪ psoriasis ▪ Raynaud's disease ▪ rheumatoid arthritis ▪ rosacea ▪ rubella ▪ SLE ▪ thrombophlebitis ▪ toxic shock syndrome

Other causes: drugs ▪ ingestion of ginkgo biloba fruit pulp ▪ radiation therapy ▪ St. John's wort

Exophthalmos

Exophthalmos (proptosis)—the abnormal protrusion of one or both eyeballs—may result from hemorrhage, edema, or inflammation behind the eye; extraocular muscle relaxation; or space-occupying intraorbital lesions and metastatic tumors. This sign may occur suddenly or gradually, causing mild to dramatic protrusion. Occasionally, the affected eye also pulsates. The most common cause of exophthalmos in adults is dysthyroid eye disease.

Exophthalmos is usually easily observed. However, lid retraction may mimic exophthalmos even when protrusion is absent. Similarly, ptosis in one eye may make the other eye appear exophthalmic by comparison. An exophthalmometer can differentiate these signs by measuring ocular protrusion.

HISTORY
- Ask the patient when he first noticed exophthalmos.
- Ask the patient if the exophthalmos is associated with pain in or around the eye. If so, ask him how severe it is and how long he has had it.
- Find out if the patient has had a recent sinus infection or vision problems.

PHYSICAL ASSESSMENT
- Take the patient's vital signs, noting fever, which may accompany eye infection.

- Evaluate the severity of exophthalmos with an exophthalmometer. (See *Detecting unilateral exophthalmos.*) If the eyes bulge severely, look for cloudiness on the cornea, which may indicate ulcer formation. Describe eye discharge, and look for ptosis. Then check visual acuity, with and without correction, and evaluate extraocular movements.

SPECIAL CONSIDERATIONS
Protect the affected eye from trauma, especially drying of the cornea. Never place a gauze pad or other object over the affected eye; removal could damage the corneal epithelium.

A⃞   PEDIATRIC POINTERS
- *In children around age 5, a rare tumor—optic nerve glioma—may cause exophthalmos.*
- *Rhabdomyosarcoma, a more common tumor, usually affects children between ages 4 and 12 and produces rapid onset of exophthalmos.*

PATIENT COUNSELING
Exophthalmos usually makes the patient self-conscious. Provide privacy and emotional support. If necessary, refer him to an ophthalmologist for a complete examination.

DETECTING UNILATERAL EXOPHTHALMOS

If one of the patient's eyes seems more prominent than the other, examine both eyes from above the patient's head. Look down across his face, gently draw his lids up, and compare the relationship of the corneas to the lower lids. Abnormal protrusion of one eye suggests unilateral exophthalmos. *Remember:* Don't perform this test if you suspect eye trauma.

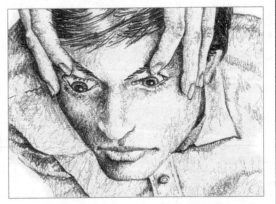

EXOPHTHALMOS

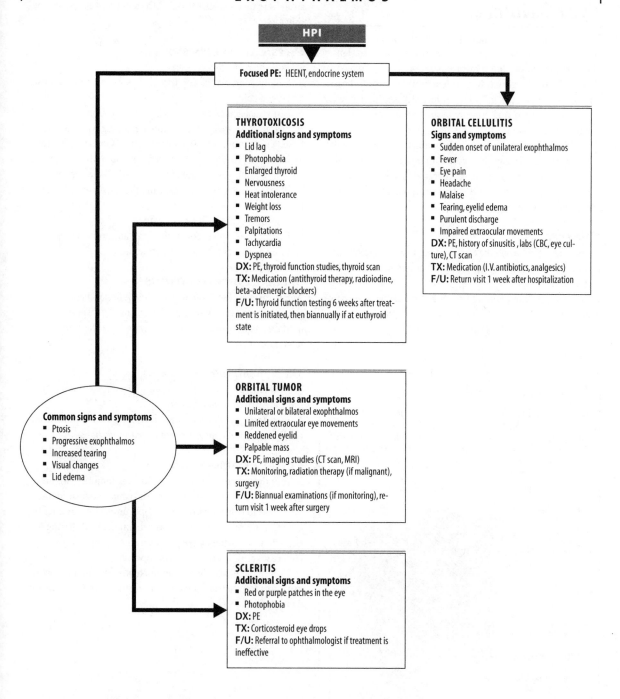

HPI

Focused PE: HEENT, endocrine system

THYROTOXICOSIS
Additional signs and symptoms
- Lid lag
- Photophobia
- Enlarged thyroid
- Nervousness
- Heat intolerance
- Weight loss
- Tremors
- Palpitations
- Tachycardia
- Dyspnea

DX: PE, thyroid function studies, thyroid scan
TX: Medication (antithyroid therapy, radioiodine, beta-adrenergic blockers)
F/U: Thyroid function testing 6 weeks after treatment is initiated, then biannually if at euthyroid state

ORBITAL CELLULITIS
Signs and symptoms
- Sudden onset of unilateral exophthalmos
- Fever
- Eye pain
- Headache
- Malaise
- Tearing, eyelid edema
- Purulent discharge
- Impaired extraocular movements

DX: PE, history of sinusitis , labs (CBC, eye culture), CT scan
TX: Medication (I.V. antibiotics, analgesics)
F/U: Return visit 1 week after hospitalization

ORBITAL TUMOR
Additional signs and symptoms
- Unilateral or bilateral exophthalmos
- Limited extraocular eye movements
- Reddened eyelid
- Palpable mass

DX: PE, imaging studies (CT scan, MRI)
TX: Monitoring, radiation therapy (if malignant), surgery
F/U: Biannual examinations (if monitoring), return visit 1 week after surgery

Common signs and symptoms
- Ptosis
- Progressive exophthalmos
- Increased tearing
- Visual changes
- Lid edema

SCLERITIS
Additional signs and symptoms
- Red or purple patches in the eye
- Photophobia

DX: PE
TX: Corticosteroid eye drops
F/U: Referral to ophthalmologist if treatment is ineffective

Additional differential diagnoses: cavernous sinus thrombosis ▪ dacryoadenitis ▪ foreign body ▪ Hodgkin's disease ▪ lacrimal gland tumor ▪ leiomyosarcoma ▪ leukemia ▪ lymphangioma ▪ ocular tuberculosis ▪ optic nerve meningioma ▪ orbital choristoma ▪ orbital emphysema ▪ orbital pseudotumor ▪ parasite infestation

Eye discharge

Usually associated with conjunctivitis, eye discharge is the excretion of any substance other than tears. This common sign may occur in one or both eyes, producing scant to copious discharge. The discharge may be purulent, frothy, mucoid, cheesy, serous, clear, or stringy and white. Sometimes, the discharge can be expressed by applying pressure to the tear sac, punctum, meibomian glands, or canaliculus.

Eye discharge is common with inflammatory and infectious eye disorders, but it may also occur with certain systemic disorders. (See *Sources of eye discharge*.) Because this sign may accompany a disorder that threatens vision, it must be assessed and treated immediately.

HISTORY

● Ask the patient when the discharge began and its frequency. Does it occur at certain times of the day or in connection with certain activities?

● If the patient complains of pain, ask him to show you its exact location and to describe its character. Is the pain dull, continuous, sharp, or stabbing?

● Ask the patient if his eyes itch or burn. Do they tear excessively? Are they sensitive to light? Does it feel like there's something in them?

PHYSICAL ASSESSMENT

● Take the patient's vital signs.

● Carefully inspect the eye discharge. Note its amount, consistency, and color.

● Test visual acuity, with and without correction.

● Examine external eye structures, beginning with the unaffected eye to prevent cross-contamination. Observe them for eyelid edema, entropion, crusts, lesions, and trichiasis. Ask the patient to blink as you watch for impaired lid movement.

● If the eyes seem to bulge, measure them with an exophthalmometer.

● Test the six cardinal fields of gaze.

● Examine the patient for conjunctival injection and follicles and for corneal cloudiness or white lesions.

SPECIAL CONSIDERATIONS

Apply warm soaks to soften crusts on eyelids and lashes, then gently wipe the eyes with soft gauze. Carefully dispose of all used dressings, tissues, and cotton swabs to prevent spread of infection.

A   PEDIATRIC POINTERS

● *In infants, prophylactic eye medication (silver nitrate) may cause eye irritation and discharge.*

● *In children, eye discharge usually results from eye trauma, an eye infection, or an upper respiratory tract infection.*

PATIENT COUNSELING

Inform the patient that bacterial and viral conjunctivitis are contagious. If the patient has bacterial conjunctivitis, advise him to avoid contact with other people until 24 hours after receiving antibiotic treatment. Also tell him to avoid sharing towels, pillows, or cosmetic eye products and to stop wearing contact lenses until the conjunctivitis resolves.

If the patient has allergic conjunctivitis, inform him that the inflammation that accompanies this form of conjunctivitis isn't contagious.

SOURCES OF EYE DISCHARGE

Eye discharge can come from the tear sac, punctum, meibomian glands, or canaliculi. If the patient reports discharge that isn't immediately apparent, you can express a sample by pressing your fingertip lightly over these structures. Then characterize the discharge, and note its source.

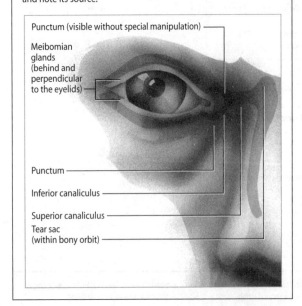

Punctum (visible without special manipulation)

Meibomian glands (behind and perpendicular to the eyelids)

Punctum

Inferior canaliculus

Superior canaliculus

Tear sac (within bony orbit)

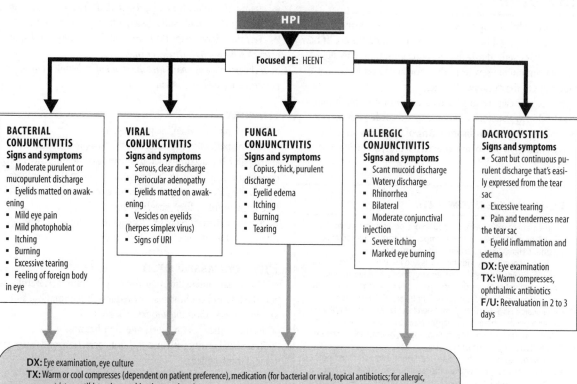

HPI

Focused PE: HEENT

BACTERIAL CONJUNCTIVITIS
Signs and symptoms
- Moderate purulent or mucopurulent discharge
- Eyelids matted on awakening
- Mild eye pain
- Mild photophobia
- Itching
- Burning
- Excessive tearing
- Feeling of foreign body in eye

VIRAL CONJUNCTIVITIS
Signs and symptoms
- Serous, clear discharge
- Periocular adenopathy
- Eyelids matted on awakening
- Vesicles on eyelids (herpes simplex virus)
- Signs of URI

FUNGAL CONJUNCTIVITIS
Signs and symptoms
- Copius, thick, purulent discharge
- Eyelid edema
- Itching
- Burning
- Tearing

ALLERGIC CONJUNCTIVITIS
Signs and symptoms
- Scant mucoid discharge
- Watery discharge
- Rhinorrhea
- Bilateral
- Moderate conjunctival injection
- Severe itching
- Marked eye burning

DACRYOCYSTITIS
Signs and symptoms
- Scant but continuous purulent discharge that's easily expressed from the tear sac
- Excessive tearing
- Pain and tenderness near the tear sac
- Eyelid inflammation and edema
DX: Eye examination
TX: Warm compresses, ophthalmic antibiotics
F/U: Reevaluation in 2 to 3 days

DX: Eye examination, eye culture
TX: Warm or cool compresses (dependent on patient preference), medication (for bacterial or viral, topical antibiotics; for allergic, vasoconstrictor-antihistamine combination eye drops)
F/U: As needed

Additional differential diagnoses: canaliculitis ▪ corneal ulcer ▪ dacryoadenitis ▪ erythema multiforme major ▪ herpes zoster ophthalmicus ▪ meibomianitis ▪ orbital cellulitis ▪ pemphigus ▪ psoriasis vulgaris ▪ trachoma

Eye pain

Eye pain (ophthalmalgia) may be described as a burning, throbbing, aching, or stabbing sensation in or around the eye. It may also be characterized as a foreign-body sensation. This sign varies from mild to severe; its duration and exact location provide clues to the causative disorder.

Eye pain usually results from corneal abrasion, but it may also be due to glaucoma or another eye disorder, trauma, or a neurologic or systemic disorder. Any of these may stimulate nerve endings in the cornea or external eye, producing pain.

EXAMINING THE EXTERNAL EYE

For the patient with eye pain or other ocular symptoms, examination of the external eye forms an important part of the ocular assessment. Here's how to examine the external eye.

First, inspect the eyelids for ptosis and incomplete closure. Also, observe the lids for edema, erythema, cyanosis, hematoma, and masses. Evaluate skin lesions, growths, swelling, and tenderness by gross palpation. Are the lids everted or inverted? Do the eyelashes turn inward? Have some of them been lost? Do the lashes adhere to one another or contain a discharge? Next, examine the lid margins, noting especially any debris, scaling, lesions, or unusual secretions. Also, watch for eyelid spasms.

Now gently retract the eyelid with your thumb and forefinger, and assess the conjunctiva for redness, cloudiness, follicles, and blisters or other lesions. Check for chemosis by pressing the lower lid against the eyeball and noting any bulging above this compression point. Observe the sclera, noting any change from its normal white color.

Next, shine a light across the cornea to detect scars, abrasions, or ulcers. Note any color changes, dots, or opaque or cloudy areas. Also, assess the anterior eye chamber, which should be clean, deep, shadow-free, and filled with clear aqueous humor.

Inspect the color, shape, texture, and pattern of the iris. Then assess the pupils' size, shape, and equality. Finally, evaluate their response to light. Are they sluggish, fixed, or unresponsive? Does pupil dilation or constriction occur only on one side?

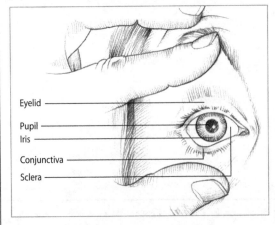

Eyelid

Pupil

Iris

Conjunctiva

Sclera

If the patient's eye pain is a result of a chemical burn:
- *remove his contact lenses, if present, and irrigate the eye with at least 1 qt (1 L) of normal saline solution over 10 minutes*
- *evert the lids and wipe the fornices with a cotton-tipped applicator to remove any particles or chemicals.*

If the patient's eye pain isn't the result of a chemical burn, perform a focused assessment.

HISTORY
- Ask the patient when the pain began.
- Ask the patient to fully describe the pain. Is it an ache or a sharp pain? Is it accompanied by burning or itching? How long does it last? Is it worse in the morning or late in the evening?
- Ask the patient about recent trauma or surgery, especially if he complains of sudden, severe pain.
- Ask the patient if he has headaches. If he does, find out how often and at what time of day they occur.

PHYSICAL ASSESSMENT
- Don't manipulate the eye if you suspect trauma. Carefully assess the lids and conjunctivae for redness, inflammation, and swelling. (See *Examining the external eye*.)
- Examine the eyes for ptosis or exophthalmos.
- Test visual acuity with and without correction, and assess extraocular movement.
- Characterize any discharge.

SPECIAL CONSIDERATIONS
Remember to ask a patient suffering from eye pain if he wears contact lenses; they may cause a foreign body sensation and be the source of the pain.

PEDIATRIC POINTERS
- *Trauma and infection are the most common causes of eye pain in children.*
- *Be alert for nonverbal clues to pain, such as tightly shutting or frequently rubbing the eyes.*

AGING ISSUES
Glaucoma, which can cause eye pain, is usually a disease of older patients, becoming clinically significant after age 40. It most commonly occurs bilaterally and leads to slowly progressive visual loss, especially in peripheral visual fields.

PATIENT COUNSELING
To help ease eye pain, tell the patient to lie down in a darkened, quiet room and close his eyes. Remind the patient not to rub his eyes, even if he feels a foreign body sensation.

EYE PAIN

HPI

Focused PE: HEENT

ACUTE ANGLE-CLOSURE GLAUCOMA
Signs and symptoms
- Sudden, excruciating eye pain
- Unilateral symptoms
- Photophobia
- Blurred vision
- Halo vision
- Rapidly decreasing visual acuity
- Fixed, nonreactive, moderately dilated pupil
- Nausea and vomiting

DX: Immediate eye examination, tonometric testing
TX: Medication (miotic eyedrops, carbonic anhydrase inhibitor, osmotic diuretics), immediate surgery
F/U: Immediate referral to ophthalmologist

HORDEOLUM
Signs and symptoms
- Localized eye pain that increases as the stye grows
- Eyelid erythema and edema
- Tender red nodule
- Slightly blurred vision

DX: Eye examination
TX: Warm compresses
F/U: None necessary unless stye persists

Common signs and symptoms
- Severe eye pain
- Purulent eye discharge
- Sticky eyelids
- Photophobia
- Impaired visual acuity
- Conjunctival injection
- Foreign body sensation

BACTERIAL CORNEAL ULCER
Additional signs and symptoms
- Grayish white, irregularly shaped ulcer on the cornea
- Unilateral pupil constriction

CORNEAL ULCER

FUNGAL CORNEAL ULCER
Additional signs and symptoms
- Eyelid edema and erythema
- Dense, cloudy, central ulcer surrounded by progressively clearer rings

DX: Eye examination, slit-lamp examination with fluorescein, eye culture
TX: Ophthalmic antibiotic
F/U: Referral to ophthalmologist

Additional differential diagnoses: astigmatism ■ blepharitis ■ burns ■ chalazion ■ conjunctivitis ■ corneal abrasion ■ corneal erosion ■ dacryoadenitis ■ dacryocystitis ■ episcleritis ■ foreign body ■ glaucoma ■ herpes zoster ophthalmicus ■ hyphema ■ interstitial keratitis ■ iritis (acute) ■ keratoconjunctivitis sicca ■ lacrimal gland tumor ■ migraine headache ■ optic neuritis ■ orbital cellulitis ■ pemphigus ■ scleritis ■ sclerokeratitis ■ trachoma ■ uveitis

Other causes: contact lenses ■ ocular surgery

F Fasciculations

Fasciculations are local muscle contractions representing the spontaneous discharge of a muscle fiber bundle innervated by a single motor nerve filament. These contractions cause visible dimpling or wavelike twitching of the skin, but they aren't strong enough to produce joint movement. They occur irregularly at frequencies ranging from once every several seconds to two or three times per second; infrequently, myokymia—continuous, rapid fasciculations that cause a rippling effect—may occur. Because fasciculations are brief and painless, they may go undetected or be ignored.

Benign, nonpathologic fasciculations are common and normal. They may occur in tense, anxious, or overtired people and commonly affect the eyelid, thumb, or calf. However, fasciculations may also indicate a severe neurologic disorder, most notably a diffuse motor neuron disorder that causes loss of control over muscle fiber discharge. They're also early signs of pesticide poisoning.

 ALERT

If onset of fasciculations is sudden:
- *ask the patient about the nature, onset, and duration of the fasciculations*
- *find out if the patient was exposed to pesticides*
- *institute emergency measures, if necessary.*

If the patient isn't in severe distress, perform a focused assessment.

HISTORY

- Ask the patient if he has experienced sensory changes, such as paresthesia, or difficulty speaking, swallowing, breathing, or controlling bowel or bladder function.
- Ask the patient if he's experiencing pain.
- Review the patient's medical history for neurologic disorders, cancer, and recent infections.
- Ask the patient about his lifestyle, especially stress at home, on the job, or at school.

PHYSICAL ASSESSMENT

- Observe the patient for fasciculations while the affected muscle is at rest.
- Test for motor and sensory abnormalities, particularly muscle atrophy and weakness, and decreased deep tendon reflexes.
- Perform a comprehensive neurologic examination.

SPECIAL CONSIDERATIONS

Fasciculations may progress, depending on the specific cause. Be sure to monitor the patient for progressive muscle weakness adjacent to where the fasciculations are occurring.

A *PEDIATRIC POINTERS*

Fasciculations, particularly of the tongue, are an important early sign of Werdnig-Hoffmann disease.

PATIENT COUNSELING

Help the patient with progressive neuromuscular degeneration to cope with activities of daily living, and provide appropriate assistive devices. Teach effective stress-management techniques to the patient with stress-induced fasciculations.

FASCICULATIONS

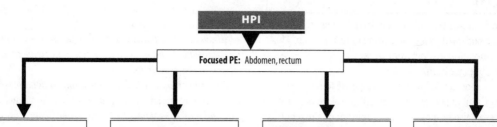

HPI

Focused PE: Abdomen, rectum

ALS
Signs and symptoms
- Coarse fasciculations of the hands and feet that spread to the forearms and legs
- Drooling
- Dysphagia
- Dyspnea
- Hyperreflexia
- Muscle atrophy, weakness, and spasticity

DX: EMG, muscle biopsy
TX: Neuroprotector, symptom management
F/U: Referral to neurologist

SPINAL CORD TUMOR
Signs and symptoms (depend on tumor site)
- Fasciculations that are initially asymmetrical, then bilateral
- Muscle atrophy and cramps
- Motor and sensory changes distal to tumor
- Back pain
- Loss of bowel and bladder control

DX: Spinal fluid analysis, imaging studies (CT scan, MRI, myelography, spinal X-rays, bone scan), biopsy
TX: Medication (chemotherapy, corticosteroids, analgesics), radiation therapy, surgery
F/U: Referral to neurosurgeon

HERNIATED DISK
Signs and symptoms
- Fasciculations of the muscles innervated by compressed nerve roots
- Severe lower back pain that may radiate unilaterally to the leg
- Pain that's exacerbated by coughing, sneezing, bending, and straining
- Muscle weakness, atrophy, and spasms
- Paresthesia
- Footdrop
- Steppage gait
- Hypoactive DTRs in the leg

DX: Imaging studies (spinal X-ray, MRI), nerve test
TX: Rest, medication (NSAIDs, epidural steroid injection, analgesics, muscle relaxants), physical therapy, surgery
F/U: As needed (dependent on symptoms), reevaluation 1 week after surgery

PESTICIDE POISONING
Signs and symptoms
- Acute onset of long, wavelike fasciculations
- Progressive muscle weakness to flaccid paralysis
- Nausea and vomiting
- Diarrhea
- Loss of bowel and bladder control
- Bradycardia
- Dyspnea or bradypnea
- Pallor
- Cyanosis
- Visual disturbances

DX: History of pesticide ingestion or exposure
TX: Maintenance of ABCs, antidote for specific pesticide
F/U: Referral to local poison control center, investigation of source of pesticide

---

Additional differential diagnoses: Guillain-Barré syndrome ▪ poliomyelitis ▪ syringomyelia

Fatigue

Fatigue is a feeling of excessive tiredness, lack of energy, or exhaustion accompanied by a strong desire to rest or sleep. This common symptom is distinct from weakness, which involves the muscles, but may occur with it.

Fatigue is a normal and important response to physical overexertion, prolonged emotional stress, and sleep deprivation. However, it can also be a nonspecific symptom of a psychological or physiologic disorder—especially viral infection and endocrine, cardiovascular, or neurologic disease.

Fatigue reflects hypermetabolic and hypometabolic states in which nutrients needed for cellular energy and growth are lacking because of overly rapid depletion, impaired replacement mechanisms, insufficient hormone production, or inadequate nutrient intake or metabolism.

HISTORY
- Ask the patient about related symptoms and recent viral illness or stressful changes in his lifestyle.
- Ask the patient about his nutritional habits and appetite or weight changes.
- Review the patient's medical and psychiatric history for chronic disorders that commonly produce fatigue. Ask the patient if there's a family history of such disorders.
- Obtain a drug history, including prescription and over-the-counter drugs, herbal remedies, and recreational drugs. Also, ask the patient about alcohol intake.

PHYSICAL ASSESSMENT
- Observe the patient's general appearance for overt signs of depression or organic illness.
- Evaluate the patient's mental status, noting especially mental clouding, attention deficits, agitation, psychomotor retardation, or depression.
- Conduct a full physical assessment to identify causation.

SPECIAL CONSIDERATIONS
Fatigue may result from various drugs, such as antihypertensives and sedatives. In cardiac glycoside therapy, fatigue may indicate toxicity.

A PEDIATRIC POINTERS
- *When evaluating a child for fatigue, ask his parents if they've noticed any change in his activity level.*
- *Fatigue without an organic cause occurs normally during accelerated growth phases in preschool-age and prepubescent children.*
- *Psychological causes of fatigue must be considered—for example, a depressed child may try to escape problems at home or school by taking refuge in sleep.*

- *In the pubescent child, consider the possibility of drug abuse, particularly of hypnotics and tranquilizers.*

AGING ISSUES
- *Always ask older patients about fatigue because this symptom may be insidious and mask more serious underlying conditions in patients of this age-group.*
- *Temporal arteritis, which is more common in people older than age 60, usually presents as fatigue, weight loss, jaw claudication, proximal muscle weakness, headache, vision disturbances, and associated anemia.*

PATIENT COUNSELING
Regardless of the cause of fatigue, help the patient alter his lifestyle to achieve a balanced diet, a program of regular exercise, and adequate rest. Teach stress-management techniques, as appropriate. Refer the patient to a community health nurse, housekeeping service, or psychological counseling, as necessary. If fatigue results from organic illness, help the patient determine which of his daily activities he may need help with and how to pace himself to ensure sufficient rest.

FATIGUE

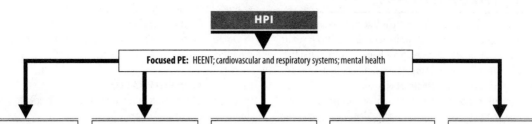

HPI

Focused PE: HEENT; cardiovascular and respiratory systems; mental health

ADRENOCORTICAL INSUFFICIENCY
Signs and symptoms
- Mild fatigue after exertion or stress that later becomes more severe and persistent
- Weakness
- Weight loss
- GI disturbances
- Hyperpigmentation
- Orthostatic hypotension
- Weak, irregular pulse

DX: Labs (electrolytes, ACTH level, CBC with differential, ferritin, TIBC, iron level), imaging studies (abdominal X-ray, CT scan)
TX: Medication (glucocorticoid and mineralocorticoid therapy), stress reduction
F/U: Regular monitoring of therapy

ANEMIA
Signs and symptoms
- Fatigue after mild activity
- Pallor
- Tachycardia
- Dyspnea
- Ecchymosis
- Petechiae
- Palpitations
- Weakness

DX: CBC
TX: Varies (dependent on cause and type of anemia)
F/U: Regular monitoring of CBC

DEPRESSION
Signs and symptoms
- Persistent fatigue that's unrelated to exertion
- Headache
- Change in appetite
- Sexual dysfunction
- Insomnia
- Agitation or bradykinesia
- Irritability
- Loss of concentration
- Feelings of worthlessness
- Poor appetite

DX: Psychological evaluation
TX: Antidepressants, psychotherapy
F/U: Referral to psychologist

CHRONIC FATIGUE SYNDROME
Signs and symptoms
- Incapacitating fatigue
- Unrefreshing sleep
- Sore throat
- Myalgia
- Cognitive dysfunction
- General muscle weakness
- Arthralgias
- Headache

DX: Exclude other illnesses, symptoms meet CDC criteria for diagnosis
TX: Treatment of symptoms, medication (analgesics, sedative-hypnotics), psychotherapy
F/U: As needed (dependent on symptoms and response to treatment)

HEART FAILURE
Signs and symptoms
- Persistent fatigue and lethargy
- Dyspnea
- JVD
- Nonproductive cough
- Tachycardia
- Tachypnea
- Dependent edema
- Crackles

DX: PE, ABG, CXR, echocardiogram
TX: Medication (diuretics, nitrates, analgesics, inotropic agents, ACE inhibitors)
F/U: As needed (dependent on recurrence of condition)

Additional differential diagnoses: AIDS ▪ anxiety ▪ cancer ▪ cirrhosis ▪ hypercortisolism ▪ hypopituitarism ▪ hypothyroidism ▪ infection ▪ Lyme disease ▪ malnutrition ▪ myasthenia gravis ▪ MI ▪ renal failure ▪ restrictive lung disease ▪ rheumatoid arthritis ▪ SLE ▪ sleep apnea ▪ thyrotoxicosis ▪ valvular heart disease

Other causes: antihypertensives ▪ cardiac glycosides ▪ sedatives ▪ surgery

Fecal incontinence

Fecal incontinence, the involuntary passage of feces, follows loss or impairment of external anal sphincter control. It can result from various GI, neurologic, and psychological disorders; the effects of certain drugs; and surgery. In some patients, it may even be a purposeful manipulative behavior.

Fecal incontinence may be temporary or permanent; its onset may be gradual, as in dementia, or sudden, as in spinal cord trauma. Although usually not a sign of severe illness, it can greatly affect the patient's physical and psychological well-being.

HISTORY

- Ask the patient (or the patient's family) with fecal incontinence about its onset, duration, and severity and about any discernible pattern — for example, at night or with diarrhea.
- Ask the patient (or the patient's family) to describe the frequency, consistency, and volume of stools passed within the last 24 hours.
- Review the patient's medical history for GI, neurologic, and psychological disorders.
- Obtain a drug history, including prescription and over-the-counter drugs, herbal remedies, and recreational drugs. Also, ask the patient about alcohol intake.

PHYSICAL ASSESSMENT

- If you suspect a brain or spinal cord lesion, perform a complete neurologic examination.
- If a GI disturbance seems likely, inspect the abdomen for distention, auscultate for bowel sounds, and percuss and palpate

for a mass. Inspect the anal area for signs of excoriation or infection.
- If not contraindicated, check for fecal impaction, which may be associated with incontinence.
- Obtain a stool sample. Note its consistency, color, and odor. Send the specimen for testing, as appropriate.

SPECIAL CONSIDERATIONS

While caring for the patient, maintain proper hygienic care, including control of foul odors.

⒜ PEDIATRIC POINTERS

Fecal incontinence is normal in infants and may occur temporarily in young children who experience stress-related psychological regression or a physical illness associated with diarrhea. It can also result from myelomeningocele.

AGING ISSUES

- *Age-related changes affecting smooth-muscle cells of the colon may change GI motility and lead to fecal incontinence. However, before age is determined to be the cause, pathology must be ruled out.*
- *Fecal incontinence is an important factor when long-term care is considered for an elderly patient.*
- *Leakage of liquid fecal material is especially common in males.*

PATIENT COUNSELING

Provide emotional support to decrease the feeling of embarrassment the patient may be experiencing. If the patient has intermittent or temporary incontinence, teach Kegel exercises to strengthen abdominal and perirectal muscles. If the patient has chronic incontinence but is neurologically capable of undergoing bowel retraining, institute a retraining program. (See *Bowel retraining tips*.)

BOWEL RETRAINING TIPS

You can help the patient control fecal incontinence by instituting a bowel retraining program. Here's how:
- Begin by establishing a specific time for defecation. A typical schedule is once per day or once every other day after a meal, usually breakfast. However, be flexible when establishing a schedule, and consider the patient's normal habits and preferences.
- If necessary, help ensure regularity by administering a suppository, either glycerin or bisacodyl, about 30 minutes before the scheduled defecation time. Avoid the routine use of enemas or laxatives because they can cause dependence.
- Provide privacy and a relaxed environment to encourage regularity. If "accidents" occur, assure the patient that they're normal and don't mean that he has failed in the program.
- Adjust the patient's diet to provide adequate bulk and fiber; encourage him to eat more raw fruits and vegetables and whole grains. Ensure a fluid intake of at least 1 qt (1 L)/day.
- If appropriate, encourage the patient to exercise regularly to help stimulate peristalsis.
- Be sure to keep accurate intake and elimination records.

FECAL INCONTINENCE

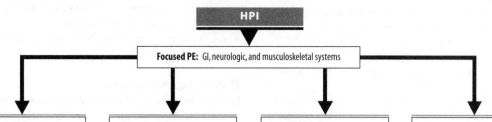

Focused PE: GI, neurologic, and musculoskeletal systems

INFLAMMATORY BOWEL SYNDROME
Signs and symptoms
- Nocturnal fecal incontinence
- Abdominal pain
- Anorexia
- Weight loss
- Blood in stools
- Hyperactive bowel sounds

DX: Characteristic history, barium studies, colonoscopy
TX: Treatment of symptoms (biofeedback, stress reduction, diet adjustment), anti-inflammatories
F/U: As needed (dependent on symptoms)

DEMENTIA
Signs and symptoms
- Urinary incontinence (possibly)
- Short- and long-term memory and intellectual impairment that cause significant social and occupational impairments

At least one of the following signs and symptoms
- Impairment in abstract thinking
- Impaired judgment
- Other disturbances of higher cortical function
- Personality change

One of the following signs and symptoms
- Evidence of an organic factor causing the impaired memory and intellect
- Impaired memory and intellect that can't be accounted for by a nonorganic mental disorder

DX: Characteristic history that meets the above criteria
TX: Environmental intervention, medication (benzodiazepines, antipsychotics)
F/U: As needed (dependent on level of dementia and social support)

GASTROENTERITIS
Signs and symptoms
- Temporary fecal incontinence (explosive diarrhea)
- Nausea and vomiting
- Colicky peristaltic abdominal pain
- Hyperactive bowel sounds
- Myalgia

DX: Characteristic history, stool culture
TX: Rehydration, clear liquid diet for 8 to 12 hours, gradual introduction of solid food
F/U: None necessary unless the illness persists for more than 48 to 72 hours

SPINAL CORD LESION
Signs and symptoms
- Permanent fecal incontinence (possibly)
- Motor and sensory disturbances below the level of the lesion

DX: Imaging studies (CT scan, MRI)
TX: Treatment of symptoms, medication (for spinal cord compression, corticosteroids; analgesics)
F/U: Referral to neurologist

Additional differential diagnoses: head trauma ▪ multiple sclerosis ▪ rectovaginal fistula ▪ stroke ▪ tabes dorsalis

Other causes: chronic laxative abuse ▪ colostomy ▪ ileostomy ▪ pelvic, prostate, or rectal surgery

Fever

Fever (pyrexia), a common sign, can arise from any one of several disorders affecting virtually any body system. As a result, fever in the absence of other signs usually has little diagnostic significance. A persistent high-grade fever, however, represents an emergency.

Fever can be classified as low-grade (oral reading of 99° to 100.4° F [37.2° to 38° C]), moderate (100.5° to 104° F [38.1° to 40° C]), or high-grade (above 104° F). Fever over 108° F (42.2° C) causes unconsciousness and, if sustained, leads to permanent brain damage and death.

Fever may also be classified as remittent, intermittent, sustained, relapsing, or undulant. Remittent fever, the most common type, is characterized by daily temperature fluctuations above the normal range. Intermittent fever is marked by a daily temperature drop into the normal range and then a rise back to above normal. An intermittent fever that fluctuates widely, typically producing chills and sweating, is called hectic or septic fever. Sustained fever involves persistent temperature elevation with little fluctuation. Relapsing fever consists of alternating feverish and afebrile periods. Undulant fever refers to a gradual increase in temperature that stays high for a few days and then decreases gradually.

Further classification involves duration—either brief (less than 3 weeks) or prolonged. Prolonged fevers include those of unknown origin, a classification used when careful examination fails to detect an underlying cause.

◣ ALERT

If you detect a fever higher than 106.7° F (41.5° C):
- *take the patient's other vital signs and determine his level of consciousness*
- *begin rapid cooling measures—for example, apply ice packs to the axillae and groin, give tepid sponge baths, or apply a hypothermia blanket*
- *continually monitor the patient's rectal temperature, using a rectal probe*
- *administer an antipyretic, as ordered.*

If the patient's fever is mild to moderate, perform a focused assessment.

History

- Ask the patient when the fever began and how high his temperature reached. Did the fever disappear, only to reappear later? Did he experience other symptoms, such as chills, fatigue, or pain?
- Review the patient's medical history, noting especially immunosuppressive disorders, infection, trauma, surgery, and diagnostic testing.

- Obtain a drug history, including prescription and over-the-counter drugs, herbal remedies, and recreational drugs. Note especially immunosuppressant therapy and use of anesthesia. Also, ask the patient about alcohol intake.
- Ask the patient about recent travel; certain diseases are endemic.

Physical assessment

Let the history findings direct your physical assessment. Because fever can accompany diverse disorders, the examination may range from a brief evaluation of one body system to a comprehensive review of all systems.

Special considerations

Regularly monitor the patient's temperature. Provide increased fluid and nutritional intake. When administering a prescribed antipyretic, minimize resultant chills and diaphoresis by following a regular dosing schedule.

A PEDIATRIC POINTERS

- *Infants and young children experience higher and more prolonged fevers, more rapid temperature increases, and greater temperature fluctuations than older children and adults.*
- *Keep in mind that seizures commonly accompany extremely high fever, so take appropriate precautions.*
- *Common pediatric causes of fever include varicella, croup syndrome, dehydration, meningitis, mumps, otitis media, pertussis, roseola infantum, rubella, rubeola, and tonsillitis.*
- *Instruct parents not to give aspirin to a child with varicella or flulike symptoms because of the risk of precipitating Reye's syndrome.*
- *Fever can occur as a reaction to immunizations and antibiotic therapy.*

❧ AGING ISSUES

- *An elderly patient may have an altered sweat mechanism that predisposes him to heatstroke when he's exposed to high temperatures.*
- *An elderly patient may have an impaired thermoregulatory mechanism, making temperature change a less reliable measure of disease severity.*

Patient counseling

If the patient isn't hospitalized, instruct him to measure and record his temperature at home. Explain that fever is a response to an underlying condition and that it plays an important role in fighting infection. Advise him not to take an antipyretic until his body temperature reaches 101° F (38.3° C).

FEVER

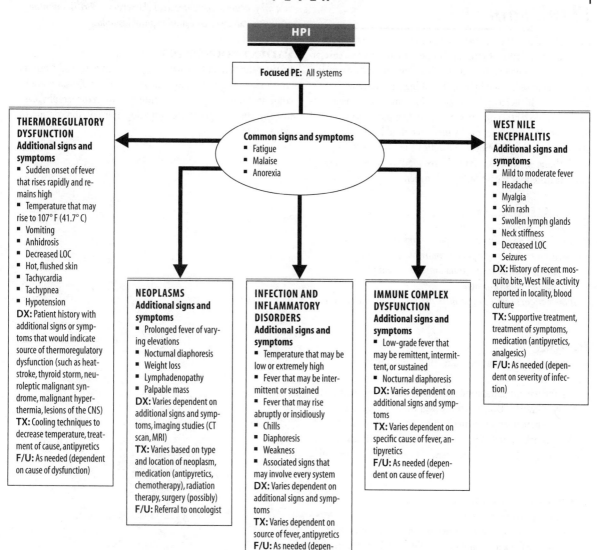

HPI

Focused PE: All systems

Common signs and symptoms
- Fatigue
- Malaise
- Anorexia

THERMOREGULATORY DYSFUNCTION
Additional signs and symptoms
- Sudden onset of fever that rises rapidly and remains high
- Temperature that may rise to 107° F (41.7° C)
- Vomiting
- Anhidrosis
- Decreased LOC
- Hot, flushed skin
- Tachycardia
- Tachypnea
- Hypotension

DX: Patient history with additional signs or symptoms that would indicate source of thermoregulatory dysfunction (such as heatstroke, thyroid storm, neuroleptic malignant syndrome, malignant hyperthermia, lesions of the CNS)
TX: Cooling techniques to decrease temperature, treatment of cause, antipyretics
F/U: As needed (dependent on cause of dysfunction)

NEOPLASMS
Additional signs and symptoms
- Prolonged fever of varying elevations
- Nocturnal diaphoresis
- Weight loss
- Lymphadenopathy
- Palpable mass

DX: Varies dependent on additional signs and symptoms, imaging studies (CT scan, MRI)
TX: Varies based on type and location of neoplasm, medication (antipyretics, chemotherapy), radiation therapy, surgery (possibly)
F/U: Referral to oncologist

INFECTION AND INFLAMMATORY DISORDERS
Additional signs and symptoms
- Temperature that may be low or extremely high
- Fever that may be intermittent or sustained
- Fever that may rise abruptly or insidiously
- Chills
- Diaphoresis
- Weakness
- Associated signs that may involve every system

DX: Varies dependent on additional signs and symptoms
TX: Varies dependent on source of fever, antipyretics
F/U: As needed (dependent on source of infection)

IMMUNE COMPLEX DYSFUNCTION
Additional signs and symptoms
- Low-grade fever that may be remittent, intermittent, or sustained
- Nocturnal diaphoresis

DX: Varies dependent on additional signs and symptoms
TX: Varies dependent on specific cause of fever, antipyretics
F/U: As needed (dependent on cause of fever)

WEST NILE ENCEPHALITIS
Additional signs and symptoms
- Mild to moderate fever
- Headache
- Myalgia
- Skin rash
- Swollen lymph glands
- Neck stiffness
- Decreased LOC
- Seizures

DX: History of recent mosquito bite, West Nile activity reported in locality, blood culture
TX: Supportive treatment, treatment of symptoms, medication (antipyretics, analgesics)
F/U: As needed (dependent on severity of infection)

Other causes: anticholinergics ▪ chemotherapy (especially with bleomycin, vincristine, and asparaginase) ▪ hypersensitivity to antifungals, sulfonamides, penicillins, cephalosporins, tetracyclines, barbiturates, phenytoin, quinidine, iodides, phenolphthalein, methyldopa, procainamide, and some antitoxins ▪ inhalant anesthetics ▪ MAO inhibitors ▪ muscle relaxants ▪ phenothiazines ▪ radiographic tests that use contrast medium ▪ surgery ▪ toxic doses of salicylates, amphetamines, and tricyclic antidepressants ▪ transfusion reactions

Flank pain

Pain in the flank, the area extending from the ribs to the ilium, is a leading indicator of renal and upper urinary tract disease or trauma. Depending on the cause, this symptom may vary from a dull ache to severe stabbing or throbbing pain and may be unilateral or bilateral and constant or intermittent. It's aggravated by costovertebral angle percussion and, in patients with renal or urinary tract obstruction, by increased fluid intake and ingestion of alcohol, caffeine, or diuretic drugs. Unaffected by position changes, flank pain typically responds only to an analgesic or to treatment of the underlying disorder.

ALERT

If the patient has suffered trauma:
- *quickly look for a visible or palpable flank mass, associated injuries, costovertebral angle pain, hematuria, Turner's sign, and signs of shock (such as tachycardia and cool, clammy skin)*
- *take the patient's vital signs.*
   If the patient's condition permits, perform a thorough assessment.

HISTORY

- Ask the patient about the pain's onset and apparent precipitating events.
- Ask the patient to describe the pain's location, intensity, pattern, and duration. Does anything aggravate or alleviate it?
- Ask the patient about changes in his normal pattern of fluid intake and urine output. Explore his history for urinary tract infection or obstruction, renal disease, or recent streptococcal infection.

PHYSICAL ASSESSMENT

- Take the patient's vital signs.
- Inspect the flank area for bruising or obvious injury.
- Palpate the flank area, and percuss the costovertebral angle to determine the extent of pain.
- Obtain a urine specimen, and inspect for color and odor. Send the specimen for testing, as appropriate.

SPECIAL CONSIDERATIONS

Administer pain medication. Continue to monitor the patient's vital signs, and maintain precise records of intake and output.

A PEDIATRIC POINTERS

- *Assessment of flank pain can be difficult if a child can't describe the pain. In such cases, transillumination of the abdomen and flanks may help in assessing bladder distention and identifying masses.*
- *Common causes of flank pain in a child include obstructive uropathy, acute poststreptococcal glomerulonephritis, infantile polycystic kidney disease, and nephroblastoma.*

PATIENT COUNSELING

Instruct the patient on what to expect from diagnostic testing, which may include excretory urography, flank ultrasonography, computed tomography scan, voiding cystourethrography, cystoscopy, and retrograde ureteropyelography, urethrography, or cystography.

FLANK PAIN

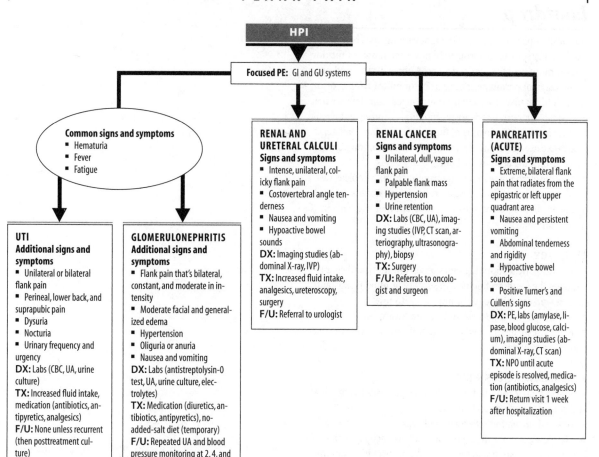

HPI

Focused PE: GI and GU systems

Common signs and symptoms
- Hematuria
- Fever
- Fatigue

UTI
Additional signs and symptoms
- Unilateral or bilateral flank pain
- Perineal, lower back, and suprapubic pain
- Dysuria
- Nocturia
- Urinary frequency and urgency

DX: Labs (CBC, UA, urine culture)
TX: Increased fluid intake, medication (antibiotics, antipyretics, analgesics)
F/U: None unless recurrent (then posttreatment culture)

GLOMERULONEPHRITIS
Additional signs and symptoms
- Flank pain that's bilateral, constant, and moderate in intensity
- Moderate facial and generalized edema
- Hypertension
- Oliguria or anuria
- Nausea and vomiting

DX: Labs (antistreptolysin-O test, UA, urine culture, electrolytes)
TX: Medication (diuretics, antibiotics, antipyretics), no-added-salt diet (temporary)
F/U: Repeated UA and blood pressure monitoring at 2, 4, and 8 weeks; then every 2 to 6 months as indicated

RENAL AND URETERAL CALCULI
Signs and symptoms
- Intense, unilateral, colicky flank pain
- Costovertebral angle tenderness
- Nausea and vomiting
- Hypoactive bowel sounds

DX: Imaging studies (abdominal X-ray, IVP)
TX: Increased fluid intake, analgesics, ureteroscopy, surgery
F/U: Referral to urologist

RENAL CANCER
Signs and symptoms
- Unilateral, dull, vague flank pain
- Palpable flank mass
- Hypertension
- Urine retention

DX: Labs (CBC, UA), imaging studies (IVP, CT scan, arteriography, ultrasonography), biopsy
TX: Surgery
F/U: Referrals to oncologist and surgeon

PANCREATITIS (ACUTE)
Signs and symptoms
- Extreme, bilateral flank pain that radiates from the epigastric or left upper quadrant area
- Nausea and persistent vomiting
- Abdominal tenderness and rigidity
- Hypoactive bowel sounds
- Positive Turner's and Cullen's signs

DX: PE, labs (amylase, lipase, blood glucose, calcium), imaging studies (abdominal X-ray, CT scan)
TX: NPO until acute episode is resolved, medication (antibiotics, analgesics)
F/U: Return visit 1 week after hospitalization

Additional differential diagnoses: bladder cancer ▪ cortical necrosis ▪ obstructive neuropathy ▪ papillary necrosis (acute) ▪ perirenal abscess ▪ polycystic kidney disease ▪ pyelonephritis (acute) ▪ renal infarction ▪ renal trauma ▪ renal vein thrombosis

Footdrop

Footdrop—plantar flexion of the foot with the toes bent toward the instep—results from weakness or paralysis of the dorsiflexor muscles of the foot and ankle. A characteristic and important sign of certain peripheral nerve or motor neuron disorders, footdrop may also stem from prolonged immobility when inadequate support, improper positioning, or infrequent passive exercise produces shortening of the Achilles tendon. Unilateral footdrop can result from compression of the common peroneal nerve against the head of the fibula.

Footdrop can range in severity from slight to complete, depending on the extent of muscle weakness or paralysis. It develops slowly in progressive muscle degeneration or suddenly in spinal cord injury.

HISTORY

- Ask the patient about the sign's onset, duration, and character. Does the footdrop fluctuate in severity or remain constant? Does it worsen with fatigue or improve with rest?
- Ask the patient if he feels weak or tires easily.
- Review the patient's medical history for neurologic disorders and spinal trauma.

PHYSICAL ASSESSMENT

- Assess muscle tone and strength in the patient's feet and legs, and compare findings on both sides.
- Assess deep tendon reflexes in both legs.
- Have the patient walk, if possible; look for steppage gait—a compensatory response to footdrop. Also inspect his shoes for wear.

SPECIAL CONSIDERATIONS

Prepare the patient for electromyography to evaluate nerve damage.

A PEDIATRIC POINTERS

Common causes of footdrop in children include spinal birth defects, such as spina bifida, and degenerative disorders such as muscular dystrophy.

PATIENT COUNSELING

Refer the patient for physical therapy for gait retraining and, possibly, for in-shoe splints or leg braces to maintain correct foot alignment for walking and standing.

FOOTDROP

HPI

Focused PE: Musculoskeletal and neurologic systems

Common signs and symptoms
- Steppage gait
- Muscle weakness
- Paresthesia
- Sensory loss

HERNIATED LUMBAR DISK
Additional signs and symptoms
- Fasciculations of the muscles innervated by compressed nerve roots
- Severe lower back pain that may radiate unilaterally to the leg
- Pain that's exacerbated by coughing, sneezing, bending, and straining
- Muscle atrophy and spasms
- Hypoactive DTRs in the leg

DX: Imaging studies (spinal X-ray, MRI), nerve test
TX: Rest, medication (NSAIDs, epidural steroid injection, analgesics, muscle relaxants), physical therapy, surgery
F/U: As needed (dependent on symptoms), return visit 1 week after surgery

MULTIPLE SCLEROSIS
Additional signs and symptoms
- Footdrop that may develop suddenly or slowly
- Facial pain
- Vision disturbances
- Incoordination
- Loss of position sensation and vibration in the ankles and toes

DX: CSF analysis, imaging studies (CT scan, MRI), evoked response testing
TX: Treatment of symptoms, medication (corticosteroids, antispasmodics, stool softeners, antidepressants)
F/U: As needed (dependent on symptoms and remissions)

PERONEAL NERVE DYSFUNCTION
Additional signs and symptoms
- Weakness or eversion of foot
- Footdrop
- Ankle instability
- Aching, cramping, coldness, and swelling in the feet and legs
- Cyanosis of the feet and legs

DX: Musculoskeletal examination, nerve conduction tests, muscle or nerve biopsy
TX: Treatment of underlying cause, medication (corticosteroids, analgesics), surgery, physical therapy
F/U: As needed (dependent on severity of dysfunction)

STROKE
Signs and symptoms
- Unilateral footdrop
- Unilateral arm and leg weakness or paralysis
- Sensorimotor disturbances
- Bowel and bladder dysfunction
- Personality changes
- Change in mental status
- Aphasia

DX: PE, imaging studies (CT scan, MRI, ultrasonography, angiography)
TX: Maintenance of ABCs, medication (aspirin; platelet aggregation inhibitors; if embolic, thrombolytics)
F/U: As needed (dependent on neurologic status), referral to neurologist

---

Additional differential diagnoses: Guillain-Barré syndrome ▪ myasthenia gravis ▪ poliomyelitis ▪ spinal cord trauma

G Gag reflex, abnormal

The gag reflex—a protective mechanism that prevents aspiration of food, fluid, and vomitus—can usually be elicited by touching the posterior wall of the oropharynx with a tongue depressor or by suctioning the throat. Prompt elevation of the palate, constriction of the pharyngeal musculature, and a sensation of gagging indicate a normal gag reflex. An abnormal gag reflex—either decreased or absent—interferes with the ability to swallow and, more important, increases susceptibility to life-threatening aspiration.

An impaired gag reflex can result from any lesion that affects its mediators—cranial nerves IX (glossopharyngeal) and X (vagus) or the pons or medulla. It can also occur during a coma; with muscle diseases, such as severe myasthenia gravis; or as a temporary result of anesthesia.

ALERT

If you detect an abnormal gag reflex:
- *quickly evaluate the patient's level of consciousness—if decreased, place him in a side-lying position to prevent aspiration; if not, place him in Fowler's position*
- *take steps to prevent aspiration by not allowing oral intake.*

After the patient has been stabilized, perform a focused assessment.

HISTORY
- Ask the patient (or a family member if the patient can't communicate) about the onset and duration of swallowing difficulties.
- Ask the patient if liquids are more difficult to swallow than solids.
- Ask the patient if swallowing is more difficult at certain times of the day.
- Ask the patient if he also has trouble chewing. If so, suspect more widespread neurologic involvement because chewing involves different cranial nerves.
- Review the patient's medical history for vascular and degenerative disorders.

PHYSICAL ASSESSMENT
- Assess the patient's respiratory status for evidence of aspiration.
- Perform a neurologic examination.

SPECIAL CONSIDERATIONS
Continually assess the patient's ability to swallow. If his gag reflex is absent, provide tube feedings; if it's diminished, the patient may attempt pureed foods, with supervision. Assess his nutritional status daily.

A PEDIATRIC POINTERS
Brain stem glioma is a major cause of abnormal gag reflex in children.

PATIENT COUNSELING
Advise the patient to eat small meals. Also tell him to chew slowly while sitting or in high Fowler's position.

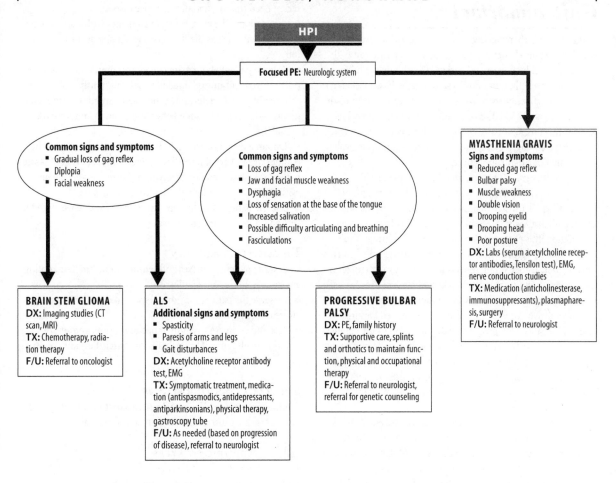

HPI

Focused PE: Neurologic system

Common signs and symptoms
- Gradual loss of gag reflex
- Diplopia
- Facial weakness

Common signs and symptoms
- Loss of gag reflex
- Jaw and facial muscle weakness
- Dysphagia
- Loss of sensation at the base of the tongue
- Increased salivation
- Possible difficulty articulating and breathing
- Fasciculations

MYASTHENIA GRAVIS
Signs and symptoms
- Reduced gag reflex
- Bulbar palsy
- Muscle weakness
- Double vision
- Drooping eyelid
- Drooping head
- Poor posture

DX: Labs (serum acetylcholine receptor antibodies, Tensilon test), EMG, nerve conduction studies
TX: Medication (anticholinesterase, immunosuppressants, plasmapharesis, surgery
F/U: Referral to neurologist

BRAIN STEM GLIOMA
DX: Imaging studies (CT scan, MRI)
TX: Chemotherapy, radiation therapy
F/U: Referral to oncologist

ALS
Additional signs and symptoms
- Spasticity
- Paresis of arms and legs
- Gait disturbances

DX: Acetylcholine receptor antibody test, EMG
TX: Symptomatic treatment, medication (antispasmodics, antidepressants, antiparkinsonians), physical therapy, gastroscopy tube
F/U: As needed (based on progression of disease), referral to neurologist

PROGRESSIVE BULBAR PALSY
DX: PE, family history
TX: Supportive care, splints and orthotics to maintain function, physical and occupational therapy
F/U: Referral to neurologist, referral for genetic counseling

Additional differential diagnoses: basilar artery occlusion ▪ cerebrovascular event ▪ compression tumor ▪ multiple sclerosis ▪ Parkinson's disease ▪ radiation injury ▪ Wallenberg's syndrome

Other causes: anesthesia (general and local [throat])

Gait, abnormal

A *bizarre gait* is characterized by a theatrical or bizarre quality with key organic elements missing, such as a spastic gait without hip circumduction or leg "paralysis" with normal reflexes and motor strength. It has no obvious organic basis; rather, it's produced unconsciously by a person with a somatoform disorder (hysterical neurosis) or consciously by a malingerer. The gait has no consistent pattern. Signs include wild gyrations, exaggerated stepping, leg dragging, or mimicking unusual walks such as that of a tightrope walker.

A *propulsive gait* is characterized by a stooped, rigid posture—the patient's head and neck are bent forward; his flexed, stiffened arms are held away from the body; his fingers are extended; and his knees and hips are stiffly bent. During ambulation, this posture results in a forward shifting of the body's center of gravity and consequent impairment of balance, causing increasingly rapid, short, shuffling steps with involuntary acceleration (festination) and lack of control over forward motion (propulsion) or backward motion (retropulsion).

A propulsive gait is a cardinal sign of advanced Parkinson's disease; it results from progressive degeneration of the ganglia, which are primarily responsible for smooth-muscle movement. Because this sign develops gradually and its accompanying effects can be wrongly attributed to aging, propulsive gait commonly goes unnoticed or unreported until severe disability results.

A *spastic gait*—sometimes referred to as a paretic or weak gait—is a stiff, foot-dragging walk caused by unilateral leg muscle hypertonicity. This gait indicates focal damage to the corticospinal tract. The affected leg becomes rigid, with a marked decrease in flexion at the hip and knee and, possibly, plantar flexion and equinovarus deformity of the foot. Because the patient's leg doesn't swing normally at the hip or knee, his foot tends to drag or shuffle, scraping his toes on the ground. To compensate, the pelvis of the affected side tilts upward in an attempt to lift the toes, causing the patient's leg to abduct and circumduct. Also, arm swing is hindered on the same side as the affected leg.

A spastic gait usually develops after a period of flaccidity (hypotonicity) in the affected leg. Whatever the cause, the gait is usually permanent after it develops.

HISTORY

- Ask the patient when he first noticed the gait impairment and whether it developed suddenly or gradually.
- Ask the patient if the impairment waxes and wanes or if it has progressively worsened.
- Ask the patient if fatigue, hot weather, or warm baths or showers worsen the gait.

- Review the patient's medical history for neurologic disorders, recent head trauma, and degenerative disease.
- Determine if the change in gait coincides with a stressful period or event, such as the death of a loved one or the loss of a job.
- Ask the patient about associated symptoms, and explore reports of frequent unexplained illnesses and multiple physician visits. Subtly try to determine if he'll gain anything from malingering—for example, added attention or an insurance settlement.
- Obtain a drug history, including prescription and over-the-counter drugs, herbal remedies, and recreational drugs. Ask the patient if he has been taking any tranquilizers, especially phenothiazines. Also ask him about alcohol intake.
- Ask the patient if he has been acutely or routinely exposed to carbon monoxide or manganese.

PHYSICAL ASSESSMENT

- Test the patient's reflexes and sensorimotor function, noting any abnormal response patterns.
- Observe the patient for normal movements when he's unaware of being watched.
- Test and compare strength, range of motion, and sensory function in all limbs. Also, palpate for muscle flaccidity or atrophy.

SPECIAL CONSIDERATIONS

A full neurologic workup may be necessary to completely rule out an organic cause of the patient's abnormal gait.

🅰 *PEDIATRIC POINTERS*

- *A bizarre gait is rare before age 8. More common in prepubescence, it usually results from conversion disorder.*
- *A propulsive gait, usually with severe tremors, typically occurs in juvenile parkinsonism, a rare form. Other possible but rare causes include Hallervorden-Spatz disease and kernicterus. Such effects are usually temporary, disappearing within a few weeks after therapy is discontinued.*
- *Causes of a spastic gait in children include sickle cell crisis, cerebral palsy, porencephalic cysts, and arteriovenous malformation that causes hemorrhage or ischemia.*

PATIENT COUNSELING

If the patient is learning to perform activities of daily living, assist him as appropriate. Encourage independence and self-reliance, and advise the family to allow plenty of time for these activities. Refer the patient to a physical therapist or for psychological counseling, as necessary.

GAIT (BIZARRE)

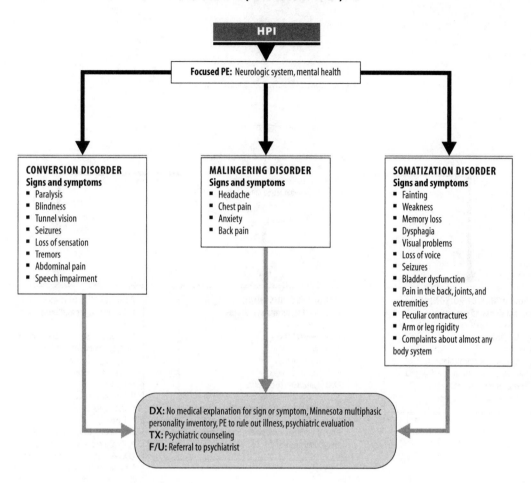

HPI

Focused PE: Neurologic system, mental health

CONVERSION DISORDER
Signs and symptoms
- Paralysis
- Blindness
- Tunnel vision
- Seizures
- Loss of sensation
- Tremors
- Abdominal pain
- Speech impairment

MALINGERING DISORDER
Signs and symptoms
- Headache
- Chest pain
- Anxiety
- Back pain

SOMATIZATION DISORDER
Signs and symptoms
- Fainting
- Weakness
- Memory loss
- Dysphagia
- Visual problems
- Loss of voice
- Seizures
- Bladder dysfunction
- Pain in the back, joints, and extremities
- Peculiar contractures
- Arm or leg rigidity
- Complaints about almost any body system

DX: No medical explanation for sign or symptom, Minnesota multiphasic personality inventory, PE to rule out illness, psychiatric evaluation
TX: Psychiatric counseling
F/U: Referral to psychiatrist

Additional differential diagnoses: orthopedic injury ▪ vestibular defects ▪ visual defects

GAIT (PROPULSIVE)

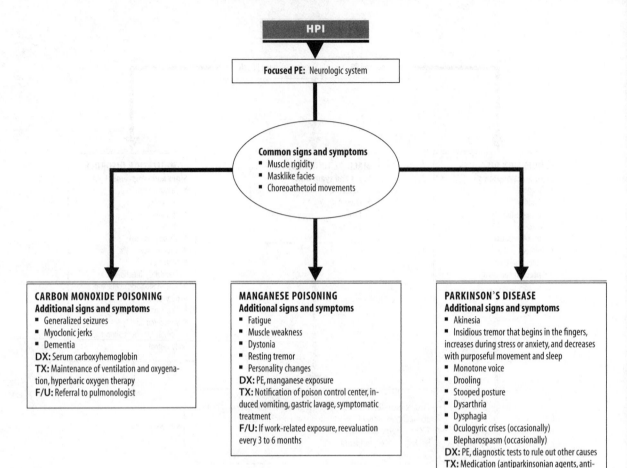

HPI

Focused PE: Neurologic system

Common signs and symptoms
- Muscle rigidity
- Masklike facies
- Choreoathetoid movements

CARBON MONOXIDE POISONING
Additional signs and symptoms
- Generalized seizures
- Myoclonic jerks
- Dementia

DX: Serum carboxyhemoglobin
TX: Maintenance of ventilation and oxygenation, hyperbaric oxygen therapy
F/U: Referral to pulmonologist

MANGANESE POISONING
Additional signs and symptoms
- Fatigue
- Muscle weakness
- Dystonia
- Resting tremor
- Personality changes

DX: PE, manganese exposure
TX: Notification of poison control center, induced vomiting, gastric lavage, symptomatic treatment
F/U: If work-related exposure, reevaluation every 3 to 6 months

PARKINSON'S DISEASE
Additional signs and symptoms
- Akinesia
- Insidious tremor that begins in the fingers, increases during stress or anxiety, and decreases with purposeful movement and sleep
- Monotone voice
- Drooling
- Stooped posture
- Dysarthria
- Dysphagia
- Oculogyric crises (occasionally)
- Blepharospasm (occasionally)

DX: PE, diagnostic tests to rule out other causes
TX: Medication (antiparkinsonian agents, anticholinergics, antivirals, antihistamines, antidepressants), physical and occupational therapy, speech therapy, surgery
F/U: As needed (based on the stage of the disease), referral to neurologist

Other causes: antipsychotics (haloperidol, thiothixene, loxapine) ▪ metoclopramide ▪ metyrosine ▪ phenothiazines

GAIT (SPASTIC)

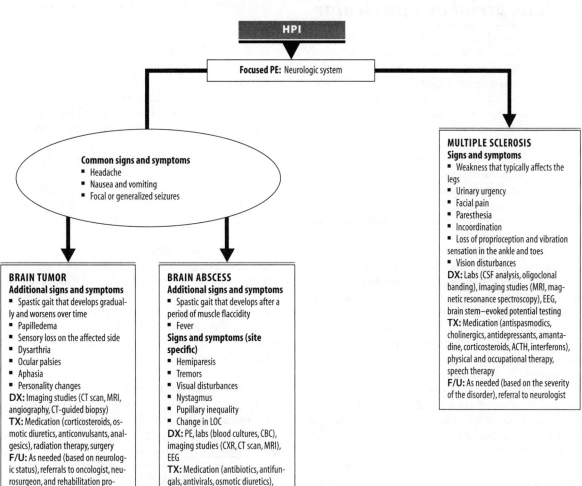

HPI

Focused PE: Neurologic system

Common signs and symptoms
- Headache
- Nausea and vomiting
- Focal or generalized seizures

BRAIN TUMOR
Additional signs and symptoms
- Spastic gait that develops gradually and worsens over time
- Papilledema
- Sensory loss on the affected side
- Dysarthria
- Ocular palsies
- Aphasia
- Personality changes

DX: Imaging studies (CT scan, MRI, angiography, CT-guided biopsy)
TX: Medication (corticosteroids, osmotic diuretics, anticonvulsants, analgesics), radiation therapy, surgery
F/U: As needed (based on neurologic status), referrals to oncologist, neurosurgeon, and rehabilitation program

BRAIN ABSCESS
Additional signs and symptoms
- Spastic gait that develops after a period of muscle flaccidity
- Fever

Signs and symptoms (site specific)
- Hemiparesis
- Tremors
- Visual disturbances
- Nystagmus
- Pupillary inequality
- Change in LOC

DX: PE, labs (blood cultures, CBC), imaging studies (CXR, CT scan, MRI), EEG
TX: Medication (antibiotics, antifungals, antivirals, osmotic diuretics), surgery
F/U: Referrals to neurologist or neurosurgeon and infectious disease specialist

MULTIPLE SCLEROSIS
Signs and symptoms
- Weakness that typically affects the legs
- Urinary urgency
- Facial pain
- Paresthesia
- Incoordination
- Loss of proprioception and vibration sensation in the ankle and toes
- Vision disturbances

DX: Labs (CSF analysis, oligoclonal banding), imaging studies (MRI, magnetic resonance spectroscopy), EEG, brain stem–evoked potential testing
TX: Medication (antispasmodics, cholinergics, antidepressants, amantadine, corticosteroids, ACTH, interferons), physical and occupational therapy, speech therapy
F/U: As needed (based on the severity of the disorder), referral to neurologist

---

Additional differential diagnoses: arthritis ▪ head trauma ▪ stroke

Other causes: antipsychotics (haloperidol, thiothixene, loxapine) ▪ metoclopramide ▪ metyrosine ▪ phenothiazines

Gallop, atrial or ventricular

An *atrial* or presystolic gallop is an extra heart sound (known as S_4) that's auscultated or palpated immediately before the first heart sound (S_1). This low-pitched sound is heard best with the bell of the stethoscope pressed lightly against the cardiac apex. Some clinicians say that an S_4 has the cadence of the "Ten" in Tennessee (Ten = S_4; nes = S_1; see = second heart sound [S_2]).

This gallop typically results from hypertension, conduction defects, valvular disorders, or other problems such as ischemia. It results from abnormal forceful atrial contraction caused by augmented ventricular filling or by decreased left ventricular compliance. An atrial gallop usually originates from left atrial contraction, is heard at the apex, and doesn't vary with inspiration. It may also originate from right atrial contraction. If so, it's heard best at the lower left sternal border and intensifies with inspiration.

A *ventricular* gallop is a heart sound (known as S_3) associated with rapid ventricular filling in early diastole. Usually palpable, this low-frequency sound occurs about 0.15 second after S_2. It may originate in either the right or left ventricle. A right-sided gallop usually sounds louder on inspiration and is heard best along the lower left sternal border or over the xiphoid region. A left-sided gallop usually sounds louder on expiration and is heard best at the apex.

Ventricular gallops are easily overlooked because they're usually faint. For better detection, auscultate in a quiet environment; examine the patient in the supine, left lateral, and semi-Fowler's positions; and have the patient cough or raise his legs to augment the sound.

Although the physiologic S_3 has the same timing as the pathologic S_3, its intensity waxes and wanes with respiration. It's also heard more faintly if the patient is sitting or standing.

A pathologic ventricular gallop may result from one of two mechanisms: rapid deceleration of blood entering a stiff, non-compliant ventricle, or rapid acceleration of blood associated with increased flow into the ventricle. A gallop that persists despite therapy indicates a poor prognosis.

Patients with cardiomyopathy or heart failure may develop a ventricular gallop and an atrial gallop—a condition known as a summation gallop.

➤ ALERT

If you auscultate an atrial gallop in a patient with chest pain:
- *take his vital signs and quickly look for signs of heart failure, such as dyspnea, crackles, and jugular vein distention*
- *connect him to a cardiac monitor, and obtain an electrocardiogram (ECG)*
- *elevate the head of the bed if he also has dyspnea, and then auscultate for abnormal breath sounds*

- *institute emergency measures, if necessary.*
  If the patient's condition permits, perform a focused assessment.

HISTORY

- Review the patient's medical history, noting especially hypertension, angina, valvular stenosis, cardiomyopathy, and other cardiac disorders.
- Ask the patient if he has had chest pain. If so, have him describe its character, location, frequency, duration, and any alleviating or aggravating factors. Also, ask about palpitations, dizziness, or syncope.
- Ask the patient if he has difficulty breathing after exertion, while lying down, or at rest.
- Obtain a drug history, including prescription and over-the-counter drugs, herbal remedies, and recreational drugs. Also, ask the patient about alcohol intake.

PHYSICAL ASSESSMENT

- Auscultate for murmurs or abnormalities in S_1 and S_2.
- Assess the patient for jugular vein distention and peripheral edema.
- Auscultate the lungs for pulmonary crackles.
- Assess peripheral pulses, noting an alternating strong and weak pulse.
- Palpate the liver to detect enlargement or tenderness.

SPECIAL CONSIDERATIONS

Monitor the patient with a gallop. Watch for and report tachycardia, dyspnea, crackles, and jugular vein distention.

Ⓐ PEDIATRIC POINTERS

- *An atrial gallop may result from a congenital heart disease, such as atrial septal defect, ventricular septal defect, patent ductus arteriosus, or severe pulmonary valvular stenosis.*
- *A ventricular gallop may accompany a congenital abnormality associated with heart failure, such as large ventricular septal defect or patent ductus arteriosus. It may also result from sickle cell anemia.*

🕐 AGING ISSUES

Because the absolute intensity of an atrial gallop doesn't decrease with age, as it does with an S_1, the relative intensity of an S_4 increases compared with an S_1. This explains the increased frequency of an audible S_4 in elderly patients and why this sound may be considered a normal finding.

PATIENT COUNSELING

Instruct the patient on what to expect from diagnostic testing, which may include an ECG, echocardiography, and cardiac catheterization.

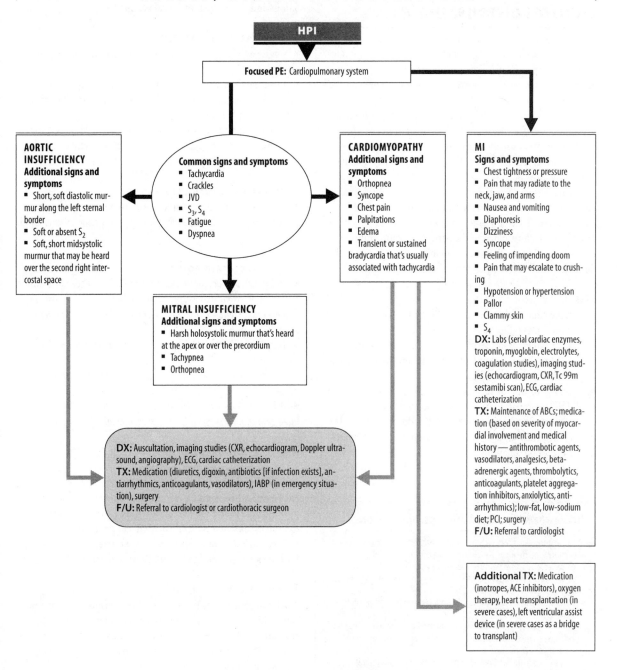

HPI

Focused PE: Cardiopulmonary system

Common signs and symptoms
- Tachycardia
- Crackles
- JVD
- S_3, S_4
- Fatigue
- Dyspnea

AORTIC INSUFFICIENCY
Additional signs and symptoms
- Short, soft diastolic murmur along the left sternal border
- Soft or absent S_2
- Soft, short midsystolic murmur that may be heard over the second right intercostal space

MITRAL INSUFFICIENCY
Additional signs and symptoms
- Harsh holosystolic murmur that's heard at the apex or over the precordium
- Tachypnea
- Orthopnea

CARDIOMYOPATHY
Additional signs and symptoms
- Orthopnea
- Syncope
- Chest pain
- Palpitations
- Edema
- Transient or sustained bradycardia that's usually associated with tachycardia

MI
Signs and symptoms
- Chest tightness or pressure
- Pain that may radiate to the neck, jaw, and arms
- Nausea and vomiting
- Diaphoresis
- Dizziness
- Syncope
- Feeling of impending doom
- Pain that may escalate to crushing
- Hypotension or hypertension
- Pallor
- Clammy skin
- S_4

DX: Labs (serial cardiac enzymes, troponin, myoglobin, electrolytes, coagulation studies), imaging studies (echocardiogram, CXR, Tc 99m sestamibi scan), ECG, cardiac catheterization
TX: Maintenance of ABCs; medication (based on severity of myocardial involvement and medical history — antithrombotic agents, vasodilators, analgesics, beta-adrenergic agents, thrombolytics, anticoagulants, platelet aggregation inhibitors, anxiolytics, antiarrhythmics); low-fat, low-sodium diet; PCI; surgery
F/U: Referral to cardiologist

DX: Auscultation, imaging studies (CXR, echocardiogram, Doppler ultrasound, angiography), ECG, cardiac catheterization
TX: Medication (diuretics, digoxin, antibiotics [if infection exists], antiarrhythmics, anticoagulants, vasodilators), IABP (in emergency situation), surgery
F/U: Referral to cardiologist or cardiothoracic surgeon

Additional TX: Medication (inotropes, ACE inhibitors), oxygen therapy, heart transplantation (in severe cases), left ventricular assist device (in severe cases as a bridge to transplant)

Additional differential diagnoses for atrial gallop: anemia ▪ angina ▪ aortic stenosis ▪ AV block ▪ hypertension ▪ pulmonary embolism

Additional differential diagnoses for ventricular gallop: heart failure ▪ thyrotoxicosis

Genital lesions, male

Among the diverse lesions that may affect the male genitalia are warts, papules, ulcers, scales, and pustules. These common lesions may be painful or painless, singular or multiple. They may be limited to the genitalia or may also occur elsewhere on the body.

Genital lesions may result from infection, neoplasms, parasites, allergy, or the effects of drugs. These lesions can profoundly affect the patient's self-image. In fact, the patient may hesitate to seek medical attention because he fears cancer or a sexually transmitted disease (STD).

Genital lesions that arise from an STD could mean that the patient is at risk for human immunodeficiency virus (HIV). Genital ulcers make HIV transmission between sexual partners more likely. Unfortunately, if the patient is treating himself, he may alter the lesions, making differential diagnosis especially difficult. (See *Recognizing common male genital lesions*.)

HISTORY

- Ask the patient when he noticed the first lesion.
- Ask the patient if he has recently traveled.
- Ask the patient if has recently started on a new medication.
- Ask the patient if he has had similar lesions before. If so, did he get medical treatment for them?
- Ask the patient if he has been treating the lesion himself. If so, did the treatment make the lesion better or worse?
- Ask the patient if the lesion itches. If it does, ask him if the itching is constant or if it bothers him only at night. Also, ask him if the lesion is painful.

RECOGNIZING COMMON MALE GENITAL LESIONS

Many lesions can affect the male genitalia. Some of the more common ones and their causes are discussed here.

- *Chancroid* causes a painful ulcer that's usually less than 2 cm in diameter and bleeds easily. The lesion may be deep and covered by gray or yellow exudate at its base.
- *Fixed drug eruptions* cause bright-red to purplish lesions on the glans penis.
- *Genital herpes* begins as a swollen, slightly pruritic wheal and later becomes a group of small vesicles or blisters on the foreskin, glans penis, or penile shaft.
- *Genital warts* are marked by clusters of flesh-colored papillary growths that range in size from barely visible to several inches in diameter.
- *Penile cancer* causes a painless ulcerative lesion on the glans penis or foreskin, possibly accompanied by a foul-smelling discharge.
- *Tinea cruris* (commonly known as jock itch) produces itchy patches of well-defined, slightly raised, scaly lesions that usually affect the inner thighs and groin.

- Obtain a complete sexual history, noting the frequency of relations and the number of sexual partners.

PHYSICAL ASSESSMENT

- Observe the fit of the patient's clothing, noting if his pants fit properly.
- Examine the skin surface in the genital area, noting the location, size, color, and pattern of the lesions. Note any lesions on other parts of the body.
- Palpate for nodules, masses, and tenderness. Also, look for bleeding, edema, or signs of infection such as erythema.
- Take the patient's vital signs.

SPECIAL CONSIDERATIONS

Many disorders produce penile lesions that resemble those of syphilis. Expect to screen every patient with penile lesions for an STD.

A PEDIATRIC POINTERS

- *In infants, contact dermatitis (diaper rash) may produce minor irritation or bright red, weepy, excoriated lesions. Use of disposable diapers and careful cleaning of the penis and scrotum can help reduce diaper rash.*
- *In children, impetigo may cause pustules with thick, yellow, weepy crusts.*
- *Children with an STD must be evaluated for signs of sexual abuse.*
- *Adolescents ages 15 to 19 have a high incidence of STDs and related genital lesions. Syphilis, however, may also be congenital.*

AGING ISSUES

- *All patients — including the elderly — who are sexually active with multiple partners are at high risk for developing an STD. However, because many elderly patients have decreased immunity, poor hygiene, poor symptom reporting, and several concurrent conditions, they may present with different symptoms.*
- *Seborrheic dermatitis lasts longer and is more extensive in bedridden patients and those with Parkinson's disease.*

PATIENT COUNSELING

Teach the patient how to use prescribed ointments or creams. Advise him to use a heat lamp to dry moist lesions or to take a sitz bath to relieve crusting or itching. Instruct him to report changes in the lesions. If appropriate, counsel the patient on safer sex practices.

GENITAL LESIONS (MALE)

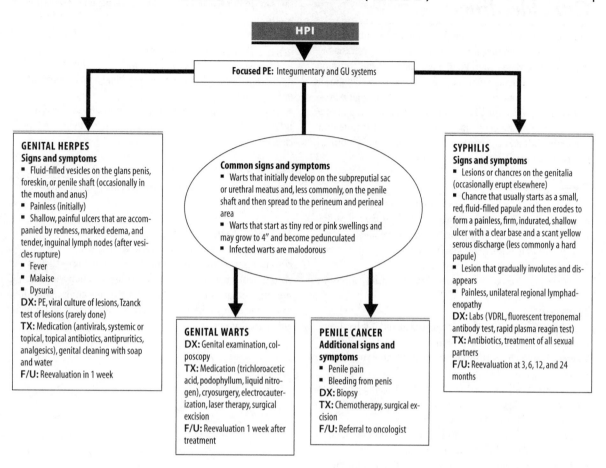

HPI

Focused PE: Integumentary and GU systems

GENITAL HERPES
Signs and symptoms
- Fluid-filled vesicles on the glans penis, foreskin, or penile shaft (occasionally in the mouth and anus)
- Painless (initially)
- Shallow, painful ulcers that are accompanied by redness, marked edema, and tender, inguinal lymph nodes (after vesicles rupture)
- Fever
- Malaise
- Dysuria

DX: PE, viral culture of lesions, Tzanck test of lesions (rarely done)
TX: Medication (antivirals, systemic or topical, topical antibiotics, antipruritics, analgesics), genital cleaning with soap and water
F/U: Reevaluation in 1 week

Common signs and symptoms
- Warts that initially develop on the subpreputial sac or urethral meatus and, less commonly, on the penile shaft and then spread to the perineum and perineal area
- Warts that start as tiny red or pink swellings and may grow to 4" and become pedunculated
- Infected warts are malodorous

GENITAL WARTS
DX: Genital examination, colposcopy
TX: Medication (trichloroacetic acid, podophyllum, liquid nitrogen), cryosurgery, electrocauterization, laser therapy, surgical excision
F/U: Reevaluation 1 week after treatment

PENILE CANCER
Additional signs and symptoms
- Penile pain
- Bleeding from penis

DX: Biopsy
TX: Chemotherapy, surgical excision
F/U: Referral to oncologist

SYPHILIS
Signs and symptoms
- Lesions or chancres on the genitalia (occasionally erupt elsewhere)
- Chancre that usually starts as a small, red, fluid-filled papule and then erodes to form a painless, firm, indurated, shallow ulcer with a clear base and a scant yellow serous discharge (less commonly a hard papule)
- Lesion that gradually involutes and disappears
- Painless, unilateral regional lymphadenopathy

DX: Labs (VDRL, fluorescent treponemal antibody test, rapid plasma reagin test)
TX: Antibiotics, treatment of all sexual partners
F/U: Reevaluation at 3, 6, 12, and 24 months

Additional differential diagnoses: balanitis ▪ balanoposthitis ▪ Bowen's disease ▪ candidiasis ▪ chancroid ▪ erythroplasia of Queyrat ▪ folliculitis ▪ Fournier's gangrene ▪ furunculosis ▪ granuloma inguinale ▪ leukoplakia ▪ lichen planus ▪ lymphogranuloma venereum ▪ pediculosis pubis ▪ psoriasis ▪ scabies ▪ seborrheic dermatitis ▪ tinea cruris ▪ urticaria

Other causes: barbiturates ▪ broad-spectrum antibiotics (tetracycline, sulfonamides) ▪ phenolphthalein

Gum bleeding

Gum bleeding (gingival bleeding) usually results from a dental disorder; less commonly, it may stem from blood dyscrasia or the effects of certain drugs. Physiologic causes of this common sign include pregnancy, which can produce gum swelling in the first or second trimester (pregnancy epulis); atmospheric pressure changes, which usually affect divers and aviators; and oral trauma. Bleeding ranges from slight oozing to life-threatening hemorrhage. It may be spontaneous, or it may follow trauma. Occasionally, direct pressure can control it.

▶ ALERT
If you detect profuse, spontaneous bleeding in the oral cavity:
- *quickly check the patient's airway and look for signs of cardiovascular collapse, such as tachycardia and hypotension*
- *apply direct pressure to the bleeding site, if able*
- *institute emergency measures, if necessary.*
  If the patient's condition permits, perform a focused assessment.

HISTORY
- Ask the patient when the bleeding began and if it has been continuous or intermittent. Does it occur spontaneously or when he brushes his teeth? Have the patient show you the site of the bleeding, if possible.
- Review the patient's medical history for bleeding tendencies and a history of liver or spleen disease. Also, ask him if there's a family history of such disorders.
- Check the patient's dental history. Ask him how often he brushes his teeth and visits the dentist.
- Ask the patient about his normal diet to evaluate his nutritional status.
- Obtain a drug history, including prescription and over-the-counter drugs, herbal remedies, and recreational drugs. Also, ask the patient about alcohol intake.

PHYSICAL ASSESSMENT
- Perform a complete oral examination. Examine the gums to determine the site and amount of bleeding.
- Check for inflammation, pockets around the teeth, swelling, retraction, hypertrophy, discoloration, and gum hyperplasia.
- Note obvious decay; discoloration; foreign material, such as food; and absence of teeth.

SPECIAL CONSIDERATIONS
Warfarin and heparin interfere with blood clotting and may cause profuse gum bleeding. Abuse of aspirin and nonsteroidal anti-inflammatory drugs may alter platelet function, producing bleeding gums. Localized gum bleeding may occur with mucosal "aspirin burn," caused by dissolving aspirin near an aching tooth.

ⓐ PEDIATRIC POINTERS
- *In neonates, bleeding gums may result from vitamin K deficiency associated with a lack of normal intestinal flora or poor maternal nutrition.*
- *In infants who primarily drink cow's milk and don't receive vitamin supplements, bleeding gums can result from vitamin C deficiency.*

⬡ AGING ISSUES
In patients who have no teeth, constant gum trauma and bleeding may result from using a dental prosthesis.

PATIENT COUNSELING
Teach the patient proper mouth and gum care. If he has a chronic disorder that predisposes him to bleeding — such as chronic leukemia, cirrhosis, or idiopathic thrombocytopenic purpura — make sure he's aware that bleeding gums may indicate a worsening of his condition, which would require immediate medical attention.

GUM BLEEDING

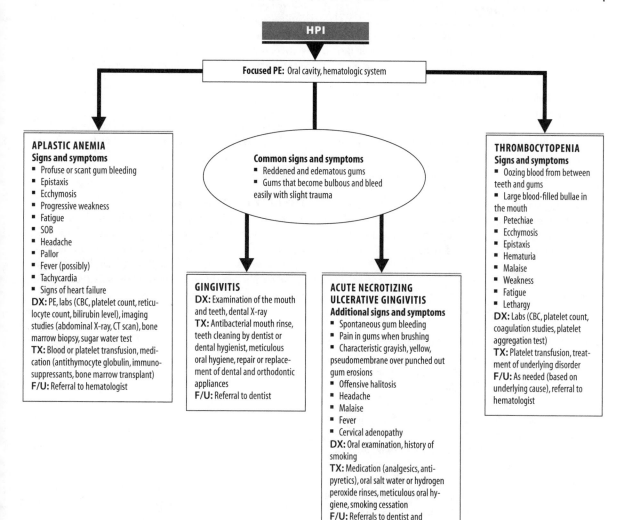

HPI

Focused PE: Oral cavity, hematologic system

APLASTIC ANEMIA
Signs and symptoms
- Profuse or scant gum bleeding
- Epistaxis
- Ecchymosis
- Progressive weakness
- Fatigue
- SOB
- Headache
- Pallor
- Fever (possibly)
- Tachycardia
- Signs of heart failure

DX: PE, labs (CBC, platelet count, reticulocyte count, bilirubin level), imaging studies (abdominal X-ray, CT scan), bone marrow biopsy, sugar water test
TX: Blood or platelet transfusion, medication (antithymocyte globulin, immunosuppressants, bone marrow transplant)
F/U: Referral to hematologist

Common signs and symptoms
- Reddened and edematous gums
- Gums that become bulbous and bleed easily with slight trauma

GINGIVITIS
DX: Examination of the mouth and teeth, dental X-ray
TX: Antibacterial mouth rinse, teeth cleaning by dentist or dental hygienist, meticulous oral hygiene, repair or replacement of dental and orthodontic appliances
F/U: Referral to dentist

ACUTE NECROTIZING ULCERATIVE GINGIVITIS
Additional signs and symptoms
- Spontaneous gum bleeding
- Pain in gums when brushing
- Characteristic grayish, yellow, pseudomembrane over punched out gum erosions
- Offensive halitosis
- Headache
- Malaise
- Fever
- Cervical adenopathy

DX: Oral examination, history of smoking
TX: Medication (analgesics, antipyretics), oral salt water or hydrogen peroxide rinses, meticulous oral hygiene, smoking cessation
F/U: Referrals to dentist and smoking-cessation program

THROMBOCYTOPENIA
Signs and symptoms
- Oozing blood from between teeth and gums
- Large blood-filled bullae in the mouth
- Petechiae
- Ecchymosis
- Epistaxis
- Hematuria
- Malaise
- Weakness
- Fatigue
- Lethargy

DX: Labs (CBC, platelet count, coagulation studies, platelet aggregation test)
TX: Platelet transfusion, treatment of underlying disorder
F/U: As needed (based on underlying cause), referral to hematologist

---

Additional differential diagnoses: agranulocytosis ▪ chemical irritants ▪ cirrhosis ▪ Ehlers-Danlos syndrome ▪ giant cell epulis ▪ hemophilia ▪ hereditary hemorrhagic telangiectasia hypofibrinogenemia ▪ leukemia ▪ malnutrition ▪ pemphigoid (benign mucosal) ▪ periodontal disease ▪ pernicious anemia ▪ polycythemia vera ▪ pyogenic granuloma ▪ thrombasthenia (familial) ▪ thrombocytopenic purpura (idiopathic) ▪ vitamin C deficiency

Other causes: abuse of aspirin and NSAIDs ▪ coumadin ▪ heparin ▪ mucosal "aspirin burn"

Gum swelling

Gum swelling may result from one of two mechanisms: enlarged existing gum cells (hypertrophy) or an increase in their number (hyperplasia). This common sign may involve one or many papillae—the triangular bits of gum between adjacent teeth. Occasionally, the gums swell markedly, obscuring the teeth altogether. Usually, the swelling is most prominent on the labia and bucca.

Gum swelling usually results from the effects of phenytoin; less commonly, from nutritional deficiency and certain systemic disorders. Physiologic gum swelling and bleeding may occur during the first and second trimesters of pregnancy when hormonal changes make the gums highly vascular; even slight irritation causes swelling and gives the papillae a characteristic raspberry hue (pregnancy epulis). Irritating dentures may also cause swelling associated with red, soft, movable masses on the gums.

HISTORY

- Ask the patient to fully describe the swelling. Has he had it before? Is it painful?
- Ask the patient when the swelling began and about aggravating or alleviating factors.
- Review the patient's medical history, focusing on major illnesses, bleeding disorders and, if the patient is female, pregnancies.
- Check the patient's dental history. Ask him if he wears dentures. If he does, ask if they're new.
- Obtain a drug history, including prescription and over-the-counter drugs, herbal remedies, and recreational drugs. Also, ask the patient about alcohol intake and tobacco use.
- Ask the patient about his normal diet to evaluate nutritional status. Ask about his intake of citrus fruits and vegetables.

PHYSICAL ASSESSMENT

- Inspect the patient's mouth and note the color and texture of the gums. Note ulcers, lesions, masses, lumps, or debris-filled pockets around the teeth.
- Inspect the patient's teeth for discoloration, obvious decay, and looseness.

SPECIAL CONSIDERATIONS

When performing mouth care, avoid using lemon-glycerin swabs, which can irritate the gums.

A PEDIATRIC POINTERS

- *Gum swelling in children commonly results from nutritional deficiency.*

- *Gum swelling may accompany phenytoin therapy; drug-induced gum swelling is more common in children than in adults. Fortunately, this dramatic swelling is usually painless and limited to one or two papillae.*
- *Gum swelling may result from idiopathic fibrous hyperplasia and from inflammatory gum hyperplasia, which is especially common in pubertal girls.*

AGING ISSUES

- *Always ask an elderly patient if he wears dentures. If he does and they are the cause of the gum inflammation, he may require a new set.*
- *Ask the patient when he last visited the dentist.*

PATIENT COUNSELING

To prevent further swelling, teach the patient the basics of good nutrition. Advise him to eat foods high in vitamin C, such as fresh fruits and vegetables, daily. Encourage him to avoid gum irritants, such as commercial mouthwashes, alcohol, and tobacco. Advise him to see a periodontist at least once every 6 months.

GUM SWELLING

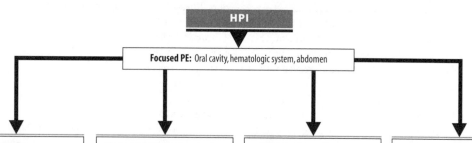

HPI

Focused PE: Oral cavity, hematologic system, abdomen

CROHN'S DISEASE
Signs and symptoms
- Granular or cobblestone gum swelling
- Cramping abdominal pain and diarrhea
- Nausea
- Fever
- Tachycardia
- Abdominal distention and pain
- Diarrhea
- Foul-smelling stools
- Weight loss

DX: Fecal occult blood, imaging studies (barium enema, upper GI series, enteroclysis), endoscopy, colonoscopy, sigmoidoscopy with small bowel biopsy
TX: Antibiotics, dietary changes, surgery (if obstruction occurs)
F/U: Referral to gastroenterologist

FIBROUS HYPERPLASIA (IDIOPATHIC)
Signs and symptoms
- Gums that are diffusely enlarged (may cover the teeth)
- Large, firm, painless masses of fibrous tissue that form on the gums
- Lip protrusion
- Difficulty chewing
- Bone pain
- Fractures

DX: PE, X-ray of involved bones
TX: No specific treatment, treatment of bone fractures, monitoring for development of endocrine disorders
F/U: Lab testing every 6 to 12 months, referral to endocrinologist if appropriate

VITAMIN C DEFICIENCY (SCURVY)
Signs and symptoms
- Spongy, tender, edematous gums
- Papillae that appear red or purple
- Gums that bleed easily
- Pockets filled with clotted blood around loose teeth
- Pallor
- Anorexia
- Weakness and lethargy
- Muscle and joint pain
- Insomnia
- Scaly dermatitis
- Skin hemorrhages

DX: Dietary history, labs (serum ascorbic acid levels, WBC ascorbic acid concentration)
TX: Vitamin C (P.O. or I.V.), diet modification
F/U: Monitoring as needed until the condition is improved, referral to dietitian

LEUKEMIA
Signs and symptoms
- Localized, necrotic gum swelling (early sign)
- Tender gums that appear blue and glossy and bleed easily
- High fever
- Severe prostration
- Signs of abnormal bleeding
- Dyspnea
- Tachycardia
- Palpitations
- Abdominal or bone pain

DX: PE, CBC, bone marrow aspiration
TX: Blood or platelet transfusion, chemotherapy, bone marrow transplant
F/U: Referrals to oncologist and hematologist

Additional differential diagnoses: infection ■ malnutrition ■ vitamin K deficiency

Other causes: cyclosporine ■ dentures ■ phenytoin

Gynecomastia

Occurring only in males, gynecomastia refers to increased breast size due to excessive mammary gland development. This change in breast size may be barely palpable or immediately obvious. Usually bilateral, gynecomastia may be associated with breast tenderness and milk secretion.

Normally, several hormones regulate breast development. Estrogens, growth hormone, and corticosteroids stimulate ductal growth, and progesterone and prolactin stimulate growth of the alveolar lobules. Although the pathophysiology of gynecomastia isn't fully understood, a hormonal imbalance — particularly a change in the estrogen-androgen ratio and an increase in prolactin — is a likely contributing factor. This explains why gynecomastia commonly results from the effects of estrogens and other drugs. It may also result from a hormone-secreting tumor or from an endocrine, genetic, hepatic, or adrenal disorder. Physiologic gynecomastia may occur in neonatal, pubertal, and elderly males because of normal fluctuations in hormone levels.

HISTORY

- Ask the patient when he first noticed his breast enlargement. How old was he at the time?
- Ask the patient whether his breasts have become progressively larger or smaller or whether they've stayed the same.
- Ask the patient if he has breast tenderness or discharge.
- Obtain a drug history, including prescription and over-the-counter drugs, herbal remedies, and recreational drugs. Also, ask the patient about alcohol intake.
- Ask the patient about associated signs and symptoms, such as a testicular mass or pain, loss of libido, decreased potency, and loss of chest, axillary, or facial hair.

PHYSICAL ASSESSMENT

- Examine the breasts, noting asymmetry, dimpling, abnormal pigmentation, or ulceration.
- Inspect the testicles for size and symmetry. Then palpate them to detect nodules, tenderness, or unusual consistency.
- Look for normal penile development after puberty, and note hypospadias if present.

SPECIAL CONSIDERATIONS

To make the patient as comfortable as possible, apply cold compresses to his breasts, and administer an analgesic. Prepare him for diagnostic tests, including chest and skull X-rays and blood hormone levels.

 PEDIATRIC POINTERS

- In neonates, gynecomastia may be associated with galactorrhea. This sign usually disappears within a few weeks, but may persist until age 2.
- Most males have physiologic gynecomastia at some time during adolescence, usually around age 14. This gynecomastia is usually asymmetrical and tender; it commonly resolves within 2 years and rarely persists beyond age 20.

PATIENT COUNSELING

Because gynecomastia may alter the patient's body image, provide emotional support. Reassure the patient that treatment can reduce gynecomastia.

GYNECOMASTIA

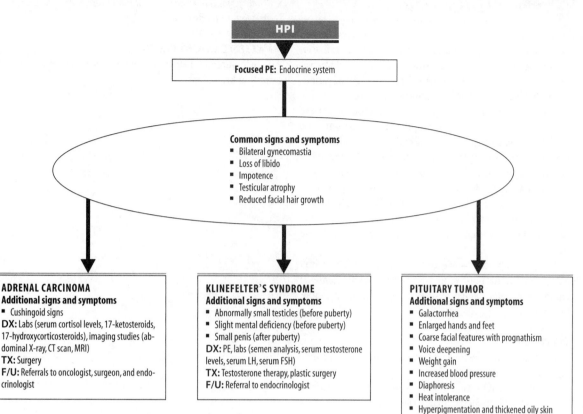

HPI

Focused PE: Endocrine system

Common signs and symptoms
- Bilateral gynecomastia
- Loss of libido
- Impotence
- Testicular atrophy
- Reduced facial hair growth

ADRENAL CARCINOMA
Additional signs and symptoms
- Cushingoid signs

DX: Labs (serum cortisol levels, 17-ketosteroids, 17-hydroxycorticosteroids), imaging studies (abdominal X-ray, CT scan, MRI)
TX: Surgery
F/U: Referrals to oncologist, surgeon, and endocrinologist

KLINEFELTER'S SYNDROME
Additional signs and symptoms
- Abnormally small testicles (before puberty)
- Slight mental deficiency (before puberty)
- Small penis (after puberty)

DX: PE, labs (semen analysis, serum testosterone levels, serum LH, serum FSH)
TX: Testosterone therapy, plastic surgery
F/U: Referral to endocrinologist

PITUITARY TUMOR
Additional signs and symptoms
- Galactorrhea
- Enlarged hands and feet
- Coarse facial features with prognathism
- Voice deepening
- Weight gain
- Increased blood pressure
- Diaphoresis
- Heat intolerance
- Hyperpigmentation and thickened oily skin
- Paresthesia or sensory loss
- Muscle weakness

DX: PE, labs (CSF analysis, endocrine function tests, growth hormone, urine cortisol, 17-hydroxycorticosteroids), imaging studies (skull X-ray, CT scan, MRI, angiogram)
TX: Radiation therapy, surgery
F/U: Referrals to oncologist, surgeon, and endocrinologist

Additional differential diagnoses: breast cancer ▪ cirrhosis ▪ hermaphroditism ▪ hypogonadism ▪ hypothyroidism ▪ liver cancer ▪ lung cancer ▪ malnutrition ▪ obesity ▪ puberty ▪ Reifenstein's syndrome ▪ renal failure (chronic) ▪ testicular failure (secondary) ▪ testicular tumor ▪ thyrotoxicosis

Other causes: alcohol ▪ antihypertensives ▪ cardiac glycosides ▪ chlorotrianisene ▪ cimetidine ▪ cyproterone ▪ diethylstilbestrol ▪ estramustine ▪ flutamide ▪ hemodialysis ▪ heroin ▪ human chorionic gonadotropin ▪ ketoconazole ▪ major surgery ▪ marijuana ▪ phenothiazines ▪ spironolactone ▪ testicular irradiation ▪ tricyclic antidepressants

Halo vision

Halo vision refers to seeing rainbowlike, colored rings around lights or bright objects. The rainbowlike effect can be explained by this physical principle: As light passes through water (in the eye, through tears or the cells of various antiretinal media), it breaks up into spectral colors.

Halo vision usually develops suddenly; its duration depends on the causative disorder. This symptom may occur with those disorders in which excessive tearing and corneal epithelial edema are present. Among these causes, the most common and significant is acute angle-closure glaucoma, which can lead to blindness. With this disorder, increased intraocular pressure forces fluid into corneal tissues anterior to Bowman's membrane, causing edema. Halo vision is also an early symptom of cataracts, resulting from dispersion of light by abnormal opacities on the lens.

Nonpathologic causes of excessive tearing associated with halo vision include poorly fitted or overworn contact lenses, emotional extremes, and exposure to intense light, as in snow blindness.

HISTORY

- Ask the patient how long he has been seeing halos around lights and when he usually sees them.
- Ask the patient if light bothers his eyes or if he's experiencing eye pain. If he is, have him describe it.
- Ask the patient if he wears contact lenses.
- Review the patient's medical history for glaucoma and cataracts.

PHYSICAL ASSESSMENT

- Examine the patient's eyes, noting conjunctival injection, excessive tearing, and lens changes.
- Examine pupil size, shape, and response to light.

SPECIAL CONSIDERATIONS

Halos associated with excruciating eye pain or a severe headache may point to acute angle-closure glaucoma, which constitutes an emergency.

A PEDIATRIC POINTERS

- *Halo vision in a child usually results from a congenital cataract or glaucoma.*
- *In a young child, limited verbal ability may make halo vision difficult to assess.*

AGING ISSUES

Primary glaucoma, the most common cause of halo vision, is more common in elderly patients.

PATIENT COUNSELING

To help minimize halo vision, remind the patient not to look directly at bright light.

HALO VISION

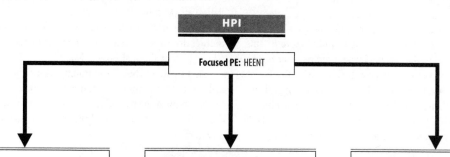

HPI

Focused PE: HEENT

CATARACT
Signs and symptoms
- Blurred vision
- Double vision
- Impaired visual acuity
- Changes in color vision
- Lens opacity

DX: Ophthalmic examination, slit-lamp examination, ultrasonography of the eye
TX: Glasses, magnifying glass, surgery
F/U: Referral to ophthalmologist

CORNEAL ENDOTHELIAL DYSTROPHY
Signs and symptoms
- Impaired visual acuity
- Foreign body sensation
- Eye pain upon wakening

DX: Slit-lamp examination, keratometry, CT scan
TX: Medication (hypertonic drops or ointments, nonhypertonic lubricating drops or ointments), patching (acute episodes of associated corneal erosion), hard or gas permeable contact lenses, surgery
F/U: Referral to ophthalmologist

GLAUCOMA
Signs and symptoms
ACUTE ANGLE-CLOSURE
- Blurred vision
- Severe headache
- Excruciating pain in and around the affected eye
- Mild dilated fixed pupil
- Conjunctival injection
- Cloudy cornea
- Impaired visual acuity
- Nausea and vomiting

CHRONIC ANGLE-CLOSURE
- Pain and blindness in advanced disease

CHRONIC OPEN-ANGLE
- Mild eye ache
- Peripheral vision loss
- Impaired visual acuity

DX: Ophthalmic examination, slit-lamp examination, tonometry examination, visual field measurement refraction, pupillary reflex response
TX: Medication (beta-adrenergic blocker, ophthalmic drops, epinephrine ophthalmic drops, pilocarpine), surgery for acute angle-closure
F/U: Referral to ophthalmologist

Headache

Headaches, which are the most common neurologic symptom, may be localized or generalized, producing mild to severe pain. About 90% of all headaches are benign and can be described as muscle-contraction, vascular, or a combination of both. Occasionally, however, headaches indicate a severe neurologic disorder associated with intracranial inflammation, increased intracranial pressure (ICP), or meningeal irritation. They may also result from ocular or sinus disorders or the effects of drugs, tests, or treatments.

Other causes of headache include fever, eyestrain, dehydration, and systemic febrile illnesses. Headaches may occur with certain metabolic disturbances—such as hypoxemia, hypercapnia, hyperglycemia, or hypoglycemia—but they aren't a diagnostic or prominent symptom. Some individuals get headaches after seizures or from coughing, sneezing, heavy lifting, or stooping. (See *Comparing benign headaches.*)

HISTORY

- Ask the patient to describe the characteristics of the headache, including its location, recurrence, and duration. Does it waken him from sleep or recur at certain times of the day? Does anything alleviate or aggravate it?
- Ask the patient if the headache is associated with neck pain.

- Ask the patient about precipitating factors, such as certain foods, exposure to bright lights, stress, trouble sleeping, hunger, elation, or yawning.
- Obtain a drug history, including prescription and over-the-counter drugs, herbal remedies, and recreational drugs. Also, ask the patient about alcohol intake.
- Ask the patient about head trauma within the last 4 weeks and about nausea, vomiting, photophobia, or vision changes.
- Determine if the patient feels drowsy, confused, or dizzy.
- Ask the patient if he recently developed seizures or has a history of seizures.

PHYSICAL ASSESSMENT

- Evaluate the patient's level of consciousness. Note signs of increased ICP—widened pulse pressure, bradycardia, altered respiratory pattern, and increased blood pressure.
- Check pupil size and response to light, and note neck stiffness.

Ⓐ PEDIATRIC POINTERS

- *In an infant, a shrill cry or bulging fontanels may indicate increased ICP and headache.*
- *In children older than age 3, headache is the most common symptom of a brain tumor.*

PATIENT COUNSELING

Advise the patient to take an analgesic, darken the room, and minimize other stimuli when a headache occurs.

COMPARING BENIGN HEADACHES

Benign headaches, which comprise 90% of all headaches, may be classified as muscle-contraction (tension), vascular (migraine and cluster), or a combination of both. When caring for a patient with headaches, it's important to know the particular signs and symptoms of each type.

CHARACTERISTICS	MUSCLE-CONTRACTION HEADACHES	VASCULAR HEADACHES
Incidence	• Most common type, accounting for 80% of all headaches	• More common in women and those with a family history of migraines • Onset after puberty
Precipitating factors	• Stress, anxiety, tension, improper posture, and body alignment • Prolonged muscle contraction without structural damage • Eye, ear, and paranasal sinus disorders that produce reflex muscle contractions	• Hormone fluctuations • Alcohol • Emotional upset • Too little or too much sleep • Foods, such as chocolate, cheese, monosodium glutamate, and cured meats; caffeine withdrawal
Intensity and duration	• Produce an aching tightness or a band of pain around the head, especially in the neck and in occipital and temporal areas • Occur frequently and usually last for several hours	• Weather changes such as shifts in barometric pressure • May begin with an awareness of an impending migraine or a 5- to 15-minute prodrome of neurologic deficits, such as vision disturbances, dizziness, unsteady gait, or tingling of the face, lips, or hands • Produce severe, constant, throbbing pain that's typically unilateral and may be incapacitating • Last for 4 to 6 hours
Associated signs and symptoms	• Tense neck and facial muscles	• Anorexia, nausea, and vomiting • Occasionally, photophobia, sensitivity to loud noises, weakness, and fatigue • Depending on the type (cluster headache or classic, common, or hemiplegic migraine), possibly chills, depression, eye pain, ptosis, tearing, rhinorrhea, diaphoresis, and facial flushing

HEADACHE

HPI

Focused PE: Neurologic and musculoskeletal systems, HEENT, neck, mental health, lymph nodes

SINUSITIS
Signs and symptoms
- Dull periorbital headache
- Unilateral or bilateral frontal or maxillary sinus pain that's increased by palpation or bending over
- Fever
- Malaise
- Nasal turbinate edema
- Sore throat
- Nasal discharge

DX: PE, transillumination, sinus X-ray
TX: Medication (decongestants, analgesics, antibiotics)
F/U: None unless signs and symptoms worsen or reoccur

BRAIN ABSCESS
Signs and symptoms
- Localized headache that increases over a few days
- Possible nausea and vomiting
- Focal or generalized seizures
- Drowsiness

EPIDURAL HEMORRHAGE
Signs and symptoms
- Progressively severe headache
- Unilateral seizures
- Decrease in LOC
- Hemiparesis or hemiplegia
- High-grade fever

CEREBRAL ANEURYSM (RUPTURED)
Signs and symptoms
- Sudden, severe headache
- Possible unilateral headache
- Possible nausea and vomiting
- Change in LOC
- Vision changes

SUBDURAL HEMATOMA
Signs and symptoms
- Decreased LOC
- Acute drowsiness, confusion, or agitation
- Pounding headache
- Giddiness
- Personality changes
- Dizziness
- Confusion

ENCEPHALITIS
Signs and symptoms
- Severe, generalized headache
- Deteriorating LOC within 48 hours of initial headache
- Fever
- Nuchal rigidity
- Irritability
- Seizures
- Nausea and vomiting
- Photophobia

INTRACRANIAL HEMORRHAGE
Signs and symptoms
- Severe general headache
- Rapid, steady decrease in LOC
- Hemiparesis or hemiplegia
- Aphasia
- Dizziness
- Nausea and vomiting
- Irregular respirations
- Positive Babinski's reflex

BRAIN TUMOR
Signs and symptoms
- Localized or general headache
- Intermittent deep pain
- More intense pain in the morning
- Associated personality changes
- Changes in LOC
- Increased pain with Valsalva's maneuver

DX: Possible history of head trauma, lumbar puncture, imaging studies (CT scan, MRI, arteriography)
TX: Medication (antibiotics, if indicated; analgesics, anticonvulsants, osmotic diuretics); surgery if appropriate; if malignancy is present, chemotherapy, radiation therapy
F/U: Referral to neurologist or neurosurgeon

Additional differential diagnoses: acute angle glaucoma ▪ cervical spine disorder ▪ dental cause ▪ Ebola virus ▪ hantavirus pulmonary syndrome ▪ hypertension ▪ influenza ▪ meningitis ▪ migraine headache ▪ postconcussional syndrome ▪ subarachnoid hemorrhage ▪ temporal arteritis ▪ tension headache ▪ trigeminal neuralgia ▪ West Nile encephalitis

Other causes: cervical traction ▪ herbal medicines, such as St. John's wort, ginseng, and ephedra ▪ indomethacin ▪ lumbar puncture ▪ myelogram ▪ nitrates ▪ vasodilators ▪ withdrawal from vasopressors, such as caffeine, ergotamine, and sympathomimetic drugs

Hearing loss

Hearing loss, which affects nearly 16 million Americans, may be temporary or permanent and partial or complete. This common symptom may involve reception of low-, middle-, or high-frequency tones. If the hearing loss doesn't affect speech frequencies, the patient may be unaware of it.

Hearing loss can be classified as conductive, sensorineural, mixed, or functional. Conductive hearing loss results from external or middle ear disorders that block sound transmission. This type of hearing loss usually responds to medical or surgical intervention (or in some cases, both). Sensorineural hearing loss results from disorders of the inner ear or of the eighth cranial nerve. Mixed hearing loss combines aspects of conductive and sensorineural hearing loss. Functional hearing loss results from psychological factors rather than identifiable organic damage.

Hearing loss may also result from trauma, infection, allergy, tumors, certain systemic and hereditary disorders, and the effects of ototoxic drugs and treatments. In most cases, however, it results from presbycusis, a type of sensorineural hearing loss that typically affects people older than age 50. Other physiologic causes of hearing loss include cerumen impaction; barotitis media associated with descent in an airplane or elevator, diving, or close proximity to an explosion; and chronic exposure to noise over 90 dB.

HISTORY

- Ask the patient to fully describe the hearing loss. Is it unilateral or bilateral? Is it continuous or intermittent?
- Review the patient's medical history, noting especially chronic ear infections, ear surgery, and ear or head trauma. Ask him if he has recently had an upper respiratory tract infection. Also, ask him about a family history of hearing loss.
- Obtain a drug history, including prescription and over-the-counter drugs, herbal remedies, and recreational drugs. Also, ask the patient about alcohol intake.
- Ask the patient to describe his occupation and work environment.
- Ask the patient about associated signs and symptoms. Does he have ear pain? If so, ask him whether it's unilateral or bilateral, continuous or intermittent.
- Ask the patient if he has noticed discharge from one or both ears. If he has, ask him when it began. Also, ask him to describe the discharge's color and consistency.
- Ask the patient if he hears ringing, buzzing, hissing, or other noises in one or both ears. If he does, ask him whether the noises are constant or intermittent.
- Ask the patient if he gets dizzy. If he does, ask him when he first noticed it.

PHYSICAL ASSESSMENT

- Inspect the external ear for inflammation, boils, foreign bodies, and discharge.
- Apply pressure to the tragus and mastoid to elicit tenderness.
- Using an otoscope, note color change, perforation, bulging, or retraction of the tympanic membrane, which normally looks like a shiny, pearl gray cone.
- Evaluate the patient's hearing acuity, using the ticking watch and whispered voice tests. Perform the Weber's and Rinne tests to obtain a preliminary evaluation of the type and degree of hearing loss.

SPECIAL CONSIDERATIONS

When talking with the patient, remember to face him and speak slowly. Don't shout, smoke, eat, or chew gum when talking.

⒜ PEDIATRIC POINTERS

- *Hereditary disorders (such as Paget's disease and Alport's, Hurler's, and Klippel-Feil syndromes) cause sensorineural hearing loss at birth.*
- *Nonhereditary disorders associated with congenital sensorineural hearing loss include Usher's syndrome, albinism, onychodystrophy syndrome, cochlear dysplasias, and Pendred's, Waardenburg's, and Jervell and Lange-Nielsen syndromes. This type of hearing loss may also result from maternal use of ototoxic drugs, birth trauma, and anoxia during or after birth.*
- *Mumps is the most common pediatric cause of unilateral sensorineural hearing loss. Other causes are meningitis, measles, influenza, and acute febrile illness.*
- *Disorders that may produce congenital conductive hearing loss include atresia, ossicle malformation, and other abnormalities. Serous otitis media commonly causes bilateral conductive hearing loss in children.*
- *Conductive hearing loss may occur in children who put foreign objects in their ears.*
- *When assessing an infant or a young child for hearing loss, remember that you can't use a tuning fork. Instead, test the startle reflex in infants younger than age 6 months, or have an audiologist test brain stem evoked response in neonates, infants, and young children. Also, obtain a gestational, perinatal, and family history from the parents.*

🔔 AGING ISSUES

In older patients, presbycusis may be aggravated by exposure to noise as well as other factors.

PATIENT COUNSELING

Instruct the patient to avoid exposure to loud noise and to use ear protection to arrest loss.

HEARING LOSS

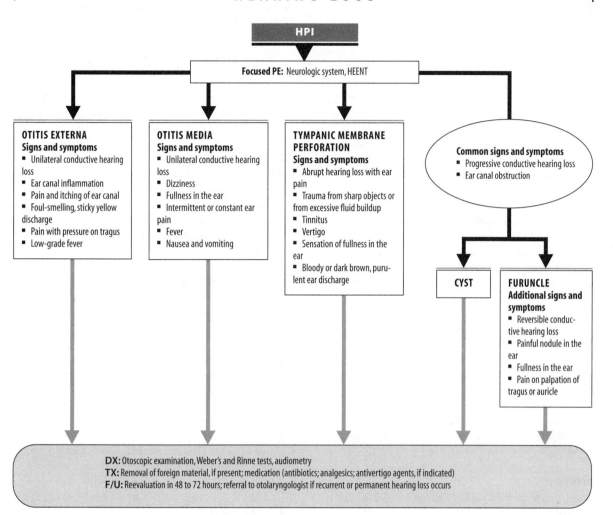

HPI

Focused PE: Neurologic system, HEENT

OTITIS EXTERNA
Signs and symptoms
- Unilateral conductive hearing loss
- Ear canal inflammation
- Pain and itching of ear canal
- Foul-smelling, sticky yellow discharge
- Pain with pressure on tragus
- Low-grade fever

OTITIS MEDIA
Signs and symptoms
- Unilateral conductive hearing loss
- Dizziness
- Fullness in the ear
- Intermittent or constant ear pain
- Fever
- Nausea and vomiting

TYMPANIC MEMBRANE PERFORATION
Signs and symptoms
- Abrupt hearing loss with ear pain
- Trauma from sharp objects or from excessive fluid buildup
- Tinnitus
- Vertigo
- Sensation of fullness in the ear
- Bloody or dark brown, purulent ear discharge

Common signs and symptoms
- Progressive conductive hearing loss
- Ear canal obstruction

CYST

FURUNCLE
Additional signs and symptoms
- Reversible conductive hearing loss
- Painful nodule in the ear
- Fullness in the ear
- Pain on palpation of tragus or auricle

DX: Otoscopic examination, Weber's and Rinne tests, audiometry
TX: Removal of foreign material, if present; medication (antibiotics; analgesics; antivertigo agents, if indicated)
F/U: Reevaluation in 48 to 72 hours; referral to otolaryngologist if recurrent or permanent hearing loss occurs

Additional differential diagnoses: acoustic neuroma ▪ adenoid hypertrophy ▪ allergies ▪ aural polyps ▪ cerebellopontine tumor ▪ cholesteatoma ▪ external ear canal tumor ▪ glomus jugulare tumor or glomus tympanicum tumor ▪ granuloma ▪ hypothyroidism ▪ Ménière's disease ▪ multiple sclerosis ▪ myringitis nasopharyngeal cancer ▪ osteoma ▪ otosclerosis ▪ Ramsay Hunt syndrome ▪ skull fracture ▪ temporal arteritis ▪ temporal bone fracture ▪ Wegener's granulomatosis

Other causes: aminoglycosides (especially neomycin, kanamycin, and amikacin) ▪ chloroquine ▪ cisplatin ▪ fenestrations ▪ head trauma ▪ high doses of erythromycin or salicylates (such as aspirin) ▪ loop diuretics, such as furosemide, ethacrynic acid, and bumetanide ▪ myringoplasty ▪ myringotomy ▪ ototoxic drugs ▪ quinidine ▪ quinine ▪ radiation therapy ▪ simple or radical mastoidectomy ▪ vancomycin

Hematemesis

Hematemesis, the vomiting of blood, usually indicates GI bleeding above the ligament of Treitz, which suspends the duodenum at its junction with the jejunum. Bright red or blood-streaked vomitus indicates fresh or recent bleeding. Dark red, brown, or black vomitus (the color and consistency of coffee grounds) indicates that blood has been retained in the stomach and partially digested.

Although hematemesis usually results from a GI disorder, it may stem from a coagulation disorder or from a treatment that irritates the GI tract. Swallowed blood from epistaxis or oropharyngeal erosion may also cause bloody vomitus.

Hematemesis is always an important sign, but its severity depends on the amount, source, and rapidity of the bleeding. Massive hematemesis (vomiting of 500 to 1,000 ml of blood) may rapidly be life-threatening. Hematemesis may be precipitated by straining, emotional stress, anti-inflammatory therapy, or alcohol consumption. (See *Rare causes of hematemesis*.)

➤ ALERT

If the patient has massive hematemesis:
- *quickly check his vital signs*
- *look for signs of shock, such as tachypnea, hypotension, and tachycardia*
- *place him in a supine position and elevate his feet 20 to 30 degrees*
- *prepare for emergency endoscopy, if necessary.*

If the patient's hematemesis isn't immediately life-threatening, perform a focused assessment.

HISTORY

- Ask the patient when the hematemesis began. Has he ever had it before?
- Ask the patient to describe the amount, color, and consistency of the vomitus.

RARE CAUSES OF HEMATEMESIS

Two rare disorders commonly cause hematemesis. *Malaria* produces this and other GI signs, but its most characteristic effects are chills, fever, headache, muscle pain, and splenomegaly. *Yellow fever* causes hematemesis as well as sudden fever, bradycardia, jaundice, and severe prostration.

Two relatively common disorders may cause hematemesis in rare cases. When *acute diverticulitis* affects the duodenum, GI bleeding and resultant hematemesis occur with abdominal pain and fever. With GI involvement, *secondary syphilis* can cause hematemesis; more characteristic signs and symptoms include a primary chancre, rash, fever, weight loss, malaise, anorexia, and headache.

- Ask the patient if he has bloody or black tarry stools and whether hematemesis is usually preceded by nausea, flatulence, diarrhea, or weakness.
- Ask the patient if he recently had bouts of retching with or without vomiting.
- Ask the patient about a history of ulcers and liver and coagulation disorders.
- Ask the patient about his alcohol intake and if he regularly takes aspirin or another nonsteroidal anti-inflammatory drug (NSAID), such as phenylbutazone or indomethacin.

PHYSICAL ASSESSMENT

- Take the patient's vital signs. Take his blood pressure and pulse while he's in a supine, sitting, and standing position.
- Inspect the mucous membranes, nasopharynx, and skin for signs of bleeding or other abnormalities.
- Palpate the abdomen for tenderness, pain, or masses. Note lymphadenopathy.

SPECIAL CONSIDERATIONS

Closely monitor the patient's vital signs, and watch for signs of shock. Check the patient's stools for occult blood, and keep accurate intake and output records.

A PEDIATRIC POINTERS

- *Hematemesis is less common in children than in adults and may be related to foreign-body ingestion.*
- *Occasionally, neonates develop hematemesis after swallowing maternal blood during delivery or breast-feeding from a cracked nipple.*
- *Hemorrhagic disease of the neonate and esophageal erosion may cause hematemesis in infants; such cases require immediate fluid replacement.*

AGING ISSUES

- *In elderly patients, hematemesis may result from a vascular anomaly, an aortoenteric fistula, or upper GI cancer.*
- *Chronic obstructive pulmonary disease, chronic liver or renal failure, and chronic NSAID use all predispose elderly patients to hemorrhage secondary to a coexisting ulcerative disorder.*

PATIENT COUNSELING

Instruct the patient on what to expect from diagnostic testing, which may include complete blood count, endoscopy, and barium swallow.

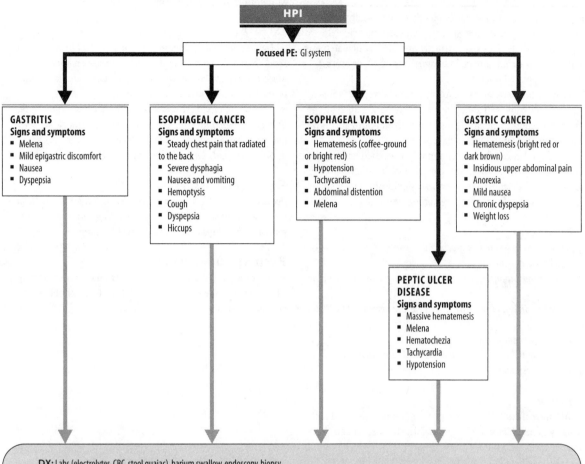

HPI

Focused PE: GI system

GASTRITIS
Signs and symptoms
- Melena
- Mild epigastric discomfort
- Nausea
- Dyspepsia

ESOPHAGEAL CANCER
Signs and symptoms
- Steady chest pain that radiated to the back
- Severe dysphagia
- Nausea and vomiting
- Hemoptysis
- Cough
- Dyspepsia
- Hiccups

ESOPHAGEAL VARICES
Signs and symptoms
- Hematemesis (coffee-ground or bright red)
- Hypotension
- Tachycardia
- Abdominal distention
- Melena

GASTRIC CANCER
Signs and symptoms
- Hematemesis (bright red or dark brown)
- Insidious upper abdominal pain
- Anorexia
- Mild nausea
- Chronic dyspepsia
- Weight loss

PEPTIC ULCER DISEASE
Signs and symptoms
- Massive hematemesis
- Melena
- Hematochezia
- Tachycardia
- Hypotension

DX: Labs (electrolytes, CBC, stool guaiac), barium swallow, endoscopy, biopsy
TX: Fluid replacement, medication (histamine-2 blockers, antacids, proton pump inhibitors, antibiotics [if indicated]), chemotherapy if appropriate, NG irrigation, blood transfusion, surgery if indicated
F/U: As needed (dependent on diagnosis), referral to gastroenterologist or oncologist if appropriate

Additional differential diagnoses: achalasia ▪ arteriovenous malformation ▪ coagulation disorders ▪ duodenal ulcer ▪ esophageal fistula ▪ esophageal injury ▪ esophageal rupture ▪ GI leiomyoma ▪ Mallory-Weiss syndrome

Other causes: nose or throat surgery ▪ traumatic nasogastric or endotracheal intubation

Hematochezia

Hematochezia, or the passage of bloody stools, usually indicates—and may be the first sign of—GI bleeding below the ligament of Treitz. This sign is usually preceded by hematemesis and may also accompany rapid hemorrhage of 1 L or more from the upper GI tract.

Hematochezia ranges from formed, blood-streaked stools to liquid, bloody stools that may be bright red, dark mahogany, or maroon in color (melena). This sign usually develops abruptly and is heralded by abdominal pain.

Although hematochezia is commonly associated with GI disorders, it may also result from a coagulation disorder, exposure to toxins, or a diagnostic test. Always a significant sign, hematochezia may precipitate life-threatening hypovolemia.

◢ ALERT

If the patient has severe hematochezia:
- *quickly check his vital signs*
- *look for indications of shock, such as hypotension and tachycardia*
- *place him in a supine position, and elevate his feet 20 to 30 degrees*
- *prepare for endoscopy, if necessary.*

If the hematochezia isn't immediately life-threatening, perform a focused assessment.

HISTORY

- Ask the patient to fully describe the amount, color, and consistency of his bloody stools. (If possible, also inspect and characterize the stools yourself.)
- Ask the patient how long the stools have been bloody. Do they always look the same or does the amount of blood vary?
- Ask the patient about associated signs and symptoms, such as abdominal pain, dizziness, or signs of bleeding elsewhere in the body, such as bruising or bleeding gums.
- Review the patient's medical history, noting especially GI and coagulation disorders.
- Ask the patient about the use of GI irritants, such as alcohol, aspirin, and other nonsteroidal anti-inflammatory drugs.

PHYSICAL ASSESSMENT

- Take the patient's vital signs. Take his blood pressure and pulse while he's in a supine, sitting, and standing position.
- Examine the skin for petechiae and spider angiomas.
- Palpate the abdomen for tenderness, pain, or masses. Also, note lymphadenopathy.
- Perform a digital rectal examination, and obtain a stool sample.

SPECIAL CONSIDERATIONS

Monitor the patient's vital signs, and watch for signs of shock. Monitor his intake and output.

Ⓐ PEDIATRIC POINTERS

- *Hematochezia is less common in children than in adults. It may result from a structural disorder, such as intussusception and Meckel's diverticulum, or from an inflammatory disorder, such as peptic ulcer disease and ulcerative colitis.*
- *In children, ulcerative colitis typically produces chronic, rather than acute, signs and symptoms and may also cause slow growth and maturation related to malnutrition.*
- *Suspect sexual abuse in all cases of rectal bleeding in children.*

◒ AGING ISSUES

Because older people have an increased risk of colon cancer, hematochezia should be evaluated with colonoscopy after perirectal lesions have been ruled out as the cause of bleeding.

PATIENT COUNSELING

Instruct the patient on what to expect from diagnostic testing, which may include endoscopy and GI X-ray. Teach the patient how to test his stools for occult blood.

HPI

Focused PE: Abdomen, rectum, GI system

Common signs and symptoms
- Painful defecation that leads to constipation
- Anemia
- Fatigue (weakness, if prolonged)

COLITIS
Signs and symptoms
- Bloody diarrhea
- Severe cramping
- Lower abdominal pain
- Hypotension
- Abdominal distention
- Absent bowel sounds

DIVERTICULITIS
Signs and symptoms
- Sudden mild to moderate rectal bleeding after the urge to defecate
- Blood loss (may be life-threatening)
- Left lower quadrant abdominal pain that's relieved by defecation
- Alternating diarrhea and constipation

Additional common signs and symptoms
- Slight hematochezia
- Severe rectal pain

HEMORRHOIDS
DX: Rectal examination, CBC
TX: Medication (stool softener, topical corticosteroid cream), diet modification, surgery
F/U: Based on severity of disorder

ANORECTAL FISTULA
Additional signs and symptoms
- Blood, pus, and mucus draining from fistula
- Rectal pain
- Pruritus
DX: History of recurrent abscesses, rectal examination, anoscopy, sigmoidoscopy
TX: Antibiotics, if indicated; surgery
F/U: Return visit 1 week after surgery

ANAL FISSURE
DX: Rectal examination
TX: Gentle cleansing, sitz bath, medication (stool softener, anesthetic ointment)
F/U: As needed, referral to general surgeon if appropriate

DX: Lab (CBC, stool guaiac), imaging studies (abdominal X-ray, CT scan), sigmoidoscopy, colonoscopy
TX: Antibiotics, cauterization of bleeding source, surgery, diet modification
F/U: Referrals to gastroenterologist and surgeon if disorder is severe or recurrent

---

Additional differential diagnoses: amyloidosis ▪ angiodysplasia lesions ▪ arteriovenous malformation ▪ coagulation disorders ▪ colon cancer ▪ colorectal polyps ▪ Crohn's disease ▪ dysentery ▪ esophageal varices ▪ food poisoning ▪ heavy metal poisoning ▪ rectal melanoma ▪ small intestine cancer ▪ typhoid fever ▪ ulcerative proctitis

Other causes: bowel perforation (rare) ▪ colonoscopy ▪ polypectomy ▪ proctosigmoidoscopy

Hematuria

A cardinal sign of renal and urinary tract disorders, hematuria is the abnormal presence of blood in the urine. Strictly defined, it means three or more red blood cells (RBCs) per high-power microscopic field in the urine. Microscopic hematuria is confirmed by an occult blood test, whereas macroscopic hematuria is immediately visible. However, macroscopic hematuria must be distinguished from pseudohematuria. Macroscopic hematuria may be continuous or intermittent, is commonly accompanied by pain, and may be aggravated by prolonged standing or walking.

Hematuria may be classified by the stage of urination it predominantly affects. Bleeding at the start of urination (initial hematuria) usually indicates urethral pathology; bleeding at the end of urination (terminal hematuria) usually indicates pathology of the bladder neck, posterior urethra, or prostate; bleeding throughout urination (total hematuria) usually indicates pathology above the bladder neck.

Hematuria may result from one of two mechanisms: rupture or perforation of vessels in the renal system or urinary tract or impaired glomerular filtration, which allows RBCs to seep into the urine. The color of the bloody urine provides a clue to the source of the bleeding. Generally, dark or brownish blood indicates renal or upper urinary tract bleeding, whereas bright red blood indicates lower urinary tract bleeding.

Although hematuria usually results from a renal or urinary tract disorder, it may also result from a GI, prostate, vaginal, or coagulation disorder or therapy with certain drugs. Invasive therapy and diagnostic tests that involve manipulative instrumentation of the renal and urologic systems may also cause hematuria. Nonpathologic hematuria may result from fever and hypercatabolic states. Transient hematuria may follow strenuous exercise.

HISTORY

- Ask the patient when he first noticed blood in his urine and if he has ever experienced this problem before.
- Ask the patient if the bleeding varies in severity between voidings. Also, ask him if it's worse at the beginning, middle, or end of urination.
- Ask the patient if he has noticed any clots. To rule out artifactitious hematuria, ask him about bleeding hemorrhoids. If the patient is female, ask her about the onset of menses.
- Ask the patient if he has had recent abdominal or flank trauma.
- Ask the patient if he has been exercising strenuously.
- Review the patient's medical history for renal, urinary, prostatic, or coagulation disorders.

- Obtain a drug history, including prescription and over-the-counter drugs, herbal remedies, and recreational drugs. Also, ask the patient about alcohol intake.

PHYSICAL ASSESSMENT

- Palpate and percuss the abdomen and flanks. Next, percuss the costovertebral angle to elicit tenderness.
- Check the urinary meatus for bleeding or other abnormalities.
- Using a chemical reagent strip, test a urine specimen for protein.
- A vaginal or digital rectal examination may be necessary.
- Obtain a urine specimen, and note its color.

SPECIAL CONSIDERATIONS

Monitor the patient's vital signs and intake and output.

PEDIATRIC POINTERS

- *Cyclophosphamide is more likely to cause hematuria in children than in adults.*
- *Common causes of hematuria that chiefly affect children include congenital anomalies, such as obstructive uropathy and renal dysplasia; birth trauma; hematologic disorders, such as vitamin K deficiency, hemophilia, and hemolytic uremic syndrome; certain neoplasms, such as Wilms' tumor, bladder cancer, and rhabdomyosarcoma; allergies; foreign bodies in the urinary tract; and venous thrombosis. Artifactitious hematuria may result from recent circumcision.*

AGING ISSUES

Evaluation of hematuria in elderly patients should include a urine culture, excretory urography or sonography, and consultation with an urologist.

PATIENT COUNSELING

Because hematuria may frighten and upset the patient, be sure to provide emotional support. Teach the patient to collect serial urine specimens using the three-glass technique to help determine whether hematuria marks the beginning, end, or entire course of urination.

HEMATURIA

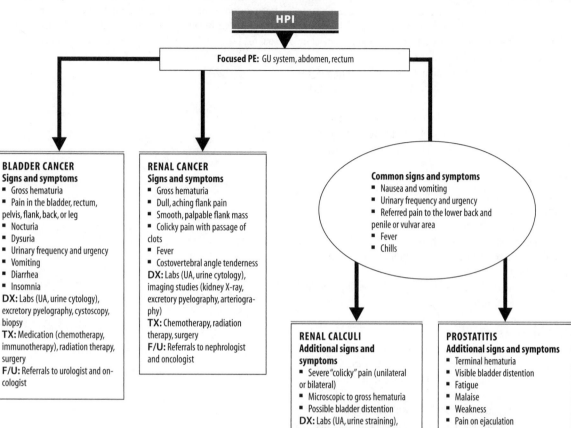

HPI

Focused PE: GU system, abdomen, rectum

BLADDER CANCER
Signs and symptoms
- Gross hematuria
- Pain in the bladder, rectum, pelvis, flank, back, or leg
- Nocturia
- Dysuria
- Urinary frequency and urgency
- Vomiting
- Diarrhea
- Insomnia

DX: Labs (UA, urine cytology), excretory pyelography, cystoscopy, biopsy

TX: Medication (chemotherapy, immunotherapy), radiation therapy, surgery

F/U: Referrals to urologist and oncologist

RENAL CANCER
Signs and symptoms
- Gross hematuria
- Dull, aching flank pain
- Smooth, palpable flank mass
- Colicky pain with passage of clots
- Fever
- Costovertebral angle tenderness

DX: Labs (UA, urine cytology), imaging studies (kidney X-ray, excretory pyelography, arteriography)

TX: Chemotherapy, radiation therapy, surgery

F/U: Referrals to nephrologist and oncologist

Common signs and symptoms
- Nausea and vomiting
- Urinary frequency and urgency
- Referred pain to the lower back and penile or vulvar area
- Fever
- Chills

RENAL CALCULI
Additional signs and symptoms
- Severe "colicky" pain (unilateral or bilateral)
- Microscopic to gross hematuria
- Possible bladder distention

DX: Labs (UA, urine straining), imaging studies (ultrasound, retrograde pyelography, CT scan, MRI)

TX: Increased fluid intake, medications (analgesics, diuretics, antibiotics, alkalinizing agents), diet modification, lithotripsy, surgery

F/U: None if calculi passes spontaneously, referral to urologist if recurrent

PROSTATITIS
Additional signs and symptoms
- Terminal hematuria
- Visible bladder distention
- Fatigue
- Malaise
- Weakness
- Pain on ejaculation
- Scrotal swelling
- Swollen prostate gland that's warm and tender on palpation

DX: Rectal examination, labs (UA, urine culture)

TX: Increased fluid intake, antibiotics

F/U: Return visit 1 week after treatment, referral to urologist if recurrent

---

Additional differential diagnoses: coagulation disorder ▪ cortical necrosis ▪ cystitis ▪ diverticulitis ▪ endocarditis ▪ glomerulonephritis ▪ infection ▪ nephritis ▪ obstructive nephropathy ▪ polycystic kidney disease ▪ prostatic hypertrophy ▪ pyelonephritis ▪ renal infarction ▪ renal papillary necrosis ▪ renal tuberculosis ▪ renal vein thrombosis ▪ schistosomiasis ▪ sickle cell anemia ▪ SLE ▪ vaginitis ▪ vasculitis

Other causes: analgesics ▪ anticoagulation therapy ▪ biopsy or manipulative instrumentation of the urinary tract ▪ bladder, kidney, or urethral trauma ▪ cyclophosphamide (Cytoxan) ▪ herbal medicines, such as garlic and ginkgo biloba, when taken with anticoagulants ▪ metyrosine ▪ penicillin ▪ phenylbutazone ▪ renal biopsy ▪ rifampin ▪ thiabendazole

Hemianopsia

Hemianopsia is the loss of vision in half the visual field of one or both eyes. However, if the visual field defects are identical in both eyes but affect less than half the field of vision in each eye (incomplete homonymous hemianopsia), the lesion may be in the occipital lobe; otherwise, it probably involves the parietal or temporal lobe.

Hemianopsia is caused by a lesion affecting the optic chiasm, tract, or radiation. Defects in visual perception due to cerebral lesions are usually associated with impaired color vision.

HISTORY

● Ask the patient when the vision problems began. Has he ever experienced hemianopsia before?
● Ask the patient if he has recently experienced headache, dysarthria, or seizures. Does he have ptosis or facial or extremity weakness? Is he experiencing hallucinations or loss of color vision?
● Obtain a medical history, noting especially eye disorders, hypertension, and diabetes mellitus.

PHYSICAL ASSESSMENT

Suspect a visual field defect if the patient seems startled when you approach him from one side or if he fails to see objects placed directly in front of him. To help determine the type of defect, perform the following:
● Compare the patient's visual fields with your own — assuming that yours are normal. First, ask the patient to cover his right eye while you cover your left eye. Then move a pen or similarly shaped object from the periphery of his (and your) uncovered eye into his field of vision. Ask the patient to indicate when he first sees the object. Does he see it at the same time as you? After you? Repeat this test in each quadrant of both eyes.
● For each eye, plot the defect by shading the area of a circle that corresponds to the area of vision loss.
● Evaluate the patient's level of consciousness, take his vital signs, and check his pupillary reaction and motor response.

SPECIAL CONSIDERATIONS

If the patient's visual field defect is significant, further visual field testing, such as perimetry or a tangent screen examination, may be indicated.

Ⓐ   PEDIATRIC POINTERS

In children, a brain tumor is the most common cause of hemianopsia. To help detect this sign, look for nonverbal clues such as the child reaching for a toy but missing it.

PATIENT COUNSELING

Explain to the patient the extent of his defect so that he can learn to compensate for it. Advise him to scan his surroundings frequently, turning his head in the direction of the defective visual field so that he can directly view objects he'd normally notice only peripherally.

HEMIANOPSIA

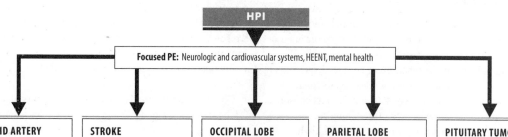

HPI

Focused PE: Neurologic and cardiovascular systems, HEENT, mental health

CAROTID ARTERY ANEURYSM
Signs and symptoms
- Contralateral or bilateral defects in the visual fields
- Hemiplegia
- Decreased LOC
- Headache
- Aphasia
- Behavior disturbances
- Unilateral hypoesthesia
- Carotid bruit

DX: PE, imaging studies (carotid Doppler ultrasound, CT scan, angiography)
TX: Surgery
F/U: Referral to vascular surgeon

STROKE
Signs and symptoms
- Vision changes
- Ataxia
- Dysarthria
- Dysphagia
- Hearing loss
- Decreased LOC
- Motor and sensory deficits
- Emotional lability
- Headache

DX: PE, imaging studies (CT scan, MRI, MRA, angiography, carotid Doppler ultrasound, echocardiogram)
TX: Symptomatic, medication (anticonvulsants; anticoagulants; if embolic, thrombolytics; antiplatelet); surgery, if carotid stenosis or hematoma is present
F/U: As needed (dependent on neurologic status), referrals to rehabilitation program and neurologist

OCCIPITAL LOBE LESION
Signs and symptoms
- Incomplete homonymous hemianopsia
- Scotomata
- Impaired color vision
- Diplopia
- Visual hallucinations
- Flashes of light or color

PARIETAL LOBE LESION
Signs and symptoms
- Homonymous hemianopsia
- Inability to perceive body position or passive movement or to localize tactile, thermal, or vibratory stimuli
- Apraxia

DX: PE, CT scan, visual field testing, perimetry, tangent screen examination
TX: Anticonvulsants, surgery
F/U: Referral to neurosurgeon

PITUITARY TUMOR
Signs and symptoms
- Complete or partial bitemporal hemianopsia that occurs in the upper visual fields and can progress to blindness
- Blurred vision
- Diplopia
- Headache
- Somnolence
- Hypothermia
- Seizures

DX: PE, eye examination, labs (endocrine function studies, growth hormone, urine cortisol levels, 17-hydroxycorticosteroids), imaging studies (skull X-ray, CT scan, MRI, angiogram)
TX: Radiation therapy, surgery
F/U: Referrals to neurosurgeon, endocrinologist, and oncologist

Hemoptysis

Frightening to the patient and usually ominous, hemoptysis is the expectoration of blood or bloody sputum from the lungs or tracheobronchial tree. It's sometimes confused with bleeding from the mouth, throat, nasopharynx, or GI tract. Expectoration of 200 ml of blood in a single episode suggests severe bleeding, whereas expectoration of 400 ml in 3 hours or more than 600 ml in 16 hours signals a life-threatening crisis.

Hemoptysis usually results from chronic bronchitis, lung cancer, or bronchiectasis. However, it may also result from an inflammatory, infectious, cardiovascular, or coagulation disorder or, rarely, from a ruptured aortic aneurysm. In up to 15% of patients, the cause is unknown. The most common causes of massive hemoptysis are lung cancer, bronchiectasis, active tuberculosis, and cavitary pulmonary disease from necrotic infection or tuberculosis.

A number of pathophysiologic processes can cause hemoptysis.

ALERT

If the patient coughs up copious amounts of blood:
- *maintain his airway*
- *prepare for endotracheal intubation, if appropriate*
- *prepare for an emergency bronchoscopy, if necessary*
- *take his vital signs, and look for signs of shock.*

If the hemoptysis is mild, perform a focused assessment.

HISTORY
- Ask the patient when the hemoptysis began. Has he ever coughed up blood before?
- Ask the patient how much blood he's coughing up and how often.
- Review the patient's medical history for cardiac, pulmonary, and bleeding disorders.
- Obtain a drug history, including prescription and over-the-counter (OTC) drugs, herbal remedies, and recreational drugs. If the patient is receiving anticoagulant therapy, find out the name of the drug, its dosage and schedule, and the duration of therapy. Also, ask him about alcohol intake.
- Ask the patient if he smokes. If so, establish how many packs per year he smokes.

PHYSICAL ASSESSMENT
- Take the patient's vital signs, and examine his nose, mouth, and pharynx for sources of bleeding.
- Inspect the configuration of the patient's chest, and look for abnormal movement during breathing, use of accessory muscles, and retractions. Observe his respiratory rate, depth, and rhythm.

- Examine the skin for lesions.
- Palpate the chest for diaphragm level and for tenderness, respiratory excursion, fremitus, and abnormal pulsations; then percuss for flatness, dullness, resonance, hyperresonance, and tympany. Auscultate the lungs, paying attention to the quality and intensity of breath sounds.
- Auscultate for heart murmurs, bruits, and pleural friction rubs.
- Obtain a sputum sample and examine it for overall quantity, for the amount of blood it contains, and for color, odor, and consistency.

SPECIAL CONSIDERATIONS
Place the patient in a slight Trendelenburg position to promote drainage of blood from the lung.

PEDIATRIC POINTERS
Hemoptysis in children may stem from Goodpasture's syndrome, cystic fibrosis, or (rarely) idiopathic primary pulmonary hemosiderosis.

AGING ISSUES
If the patient is receiving an anticoagulant, determine changes that need to be made in his diet or drug therapy (including OTC drugs and herbal remedies) because these factors may affect clotting.

PATIENT COUNSELING
Many chronic disorders cause recurrent hemoptysis. Instruct the patient to report recurring episodes and to bring a sputum specimen containing blood when he returns for reevaluation. Comfort and reassure the patient, who may react to this alarming sign with anxiety and apprehension.

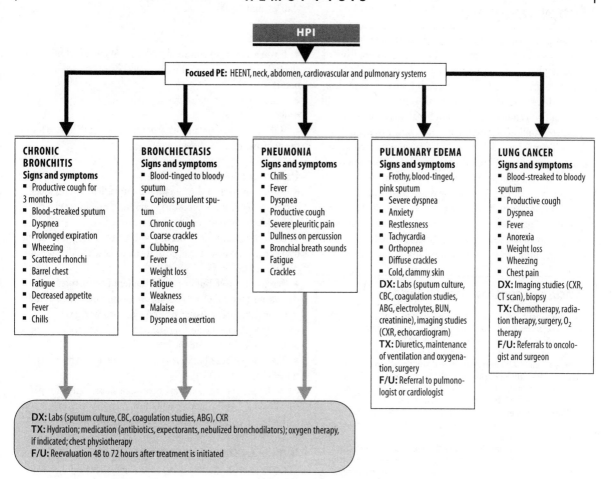

HPI

Focused PE: HEENT, neck, abdomen, cardiovascular and pulmonary systems

CHRONIC BRONCHITIS
Signs and symptoms
- Productive cough for 3 months
- Blood-streaked sputum
- Dyspnea
- Prolonged expiration
- Wheezing
- Scattered rhonchi
- Barrel chest
- Fatigue
- Decreased appetite
- Fever
- Chills

BRONCHIECTASIS
Signs and symptoms
- Blood-tinged to bloody sputum
- Copious purulent sputum
- Chronic cough
- Coarse crackles
- Clubbing
- Fever
- Weight loss
- Fatigue
- Weakness
- Malaise
- Dyspnea on exertion

PNEUMONIA
Signs and symptoms
- Chills
- Fever
- Dyspnea
- Productive cough
- Severe pleuritic pain
- Dullness on percussion
- Bronchial breath sounds
- Fatigue
- Crackles

PULMONARY EDEMA
Signs and symptoms
- Frothy, blood-tinged, pink sputum
- Severe dyspnea
- Anxiety
- Restlessness
- Tachycardia
- Orthopnea
- Diffuse crackles
- Cold, clammy skin

DX: Labs (sputum culture, CBC, coagulation studies, ABG, electrolytes, BUN, creatinine), imaging studies (CXR, echocardiogram)
TX: Diuretics, maintenance of ventilation and oxygenation, surgery
F/U: Referral to pulmonologist or cardiologist

LUNG CANCER
Signs and symptoms
- Blood-streaked to bloody sputum
- Productive cough
- Dyspnea
- Fever
- Anorexia
- Weight loss
- Wheezing
- Chest pain

DX: Imaging studies (CXR, CT scan), biopsy
TX: Chemotherapy, radiation therapy, surgery, O_2 therapy
F/U: Referrals to oncologist and surgeon

DX: Labs (sputum culture, CBC, coagulation studies, ABG), CXR
TX: Hydration; medication (antibiotics, expectorants, nebulized bronchodilators); oxygen therapy, if indicated; chest physiotherapy
F/U: Reevaluation 48 to 72 hours after treatment is initiated

---

Additional differential diagnoses: aortic aneurysm (ruptured) ▪ bronchial adenoma ▪ coagulation disorder ▪ laryngeal cancer ▪ lung abscess ▪ pulmonary contusion ▪ pulmonary embolism with infarction ▪ pulmonary hypertension ▪ pulmonary tuberculosis ▪ silicosis ▪ SLE ▪ tracheal trauma ▪ Wegener's granulomatosis

Other causes: lung or airway injury from bronchoscopy, laryngoscopy, mediastinoscopy, or lung biopsy

Hepatomegaly

Hepatomegaly, an enlarged liver, indicates potentially reversible primary or secondary liver disease. This sign may stem from diverse pathophysiologic mechanisms, including dilated hepatic sinusoids (with heart failure), persistently high venous pressure leading to liver congestion (with chronic constrictive pericarditis), dysfunction and engorgement of hepatocytes (with hepatitis), fatty infiltration of parenchymatous cells causing fibrous tissue (with cirrhosis), distention of liver cells with glycogen (with diabetes), and infiltration of amyloid (with amyloidosis).

Hepatomegaly is seldom a patient's chief complaint. It usually comes to light during palpation and percussion of the abdomen and may be confirmed by imaging studies and further palpation and percussion. Also, hepatomegaly may be mistaken for displacement of the liver by the diaphragm in a patient with a respiratory disorder; by an abdominal tumor; by a spinal deformity, such as kyphosis; by the gallbladder; or by fecal material or a tumor in the colon.

HISTORY

- If you suspect hepatomegaly, ask the patient about his use of alcohol and possible ways he could have been exposed to hepatitis.
- Ask the patient if he's currently ill or taking any prescribed drugs.
- If the patient complains of abdominal pain, ask him to locate the pain and describe how it feels.

PHYSICAL ASSESSMENT

- Inspect the skin and sclera for jaundice, dilated veins (suggesting generalized congestion), scars from previous surgery, and spider angiomas (common with cirrhosis).
- Inspect the contour of the abdomen. Note if it's protuberant over the liver or distended (possibly from ascites). Measure abdominal girth.
- Percuss the liver, but be careful to identify structures and conditions that can obscure dull percussion notes, such as the sternum, ribs, breast tissue, pleural effusions, and gas in the colon. (See *Percussing for liver size and position.*) Next, during deep inspiration, palpate the liver's edge.
- Take the patient's baseline vital signs, and assess his nutritional status.
- Evaluate the patient's level of consciousness. Watch for personality changes, irritability, agitation, memory loss, inability to concentrate, and—in a severely ill patient—coma.

SPECIAL CONSIDERATIONS

The patient with hepatomegaly may experience dyspnea, so position him in semi-Fowler's position.

A PEDIATRIC POINTERS

Childhood hepatomegaly may stem from Reye's syndrome; biliary atresia; a rare disorder, such as Wilson's, Gaucher's, or Niemann-Pick disease; or poorly controlled type 1 diabetes mellitus.

PATIENT COUNSELING

Advise the patient to remain on bed rest, avoid stress, and get adequate nutrition by going on a low-protein diet. Tell him to avoid alcohol to help protect the liver cells from further damage and to promote the regeneration of functioning cells. Also, instruct him on what to expect from diagnostic testing, which may include blood studies, X-rays, liver scan, celiac arteriography, computed tomography scan, and ultrasonography.

PERCUSSING FOR LIVER SIZE AND POSITION

With the patient in a supine position, begin at the right iliac crest to percuss up the right midclavicular line (MCL), as shown below. The percussion note becomes dull when you reach the liver's inferior border — usually at the costal margin, but sometimes at a lower point in a patient with liver disease. Mark this point and then percuss down from the right clavicle, again along the right MCL. The liver's superior border usually lies between the fifth and seventh intercostal spaces. Mark the superior border.

The distance between the two marked points represents the approximate span of the liver's right lobe, which normally ranges from 2³/₈″ to 4³/₄″ (6 to 12 cm).

Next, assess the liver's left lobe similarly, percussing along the sternal midline. Again, mark the points where you hear dull percussion notes. Also, measure the span of the left lobe, which normally ranges from 1¹/₂″ to 3¹/₈″ (4 to 8 cm). Record your findings for use as a baseline.

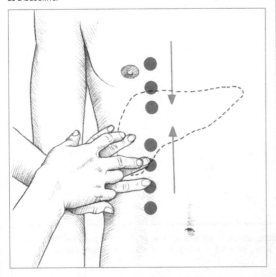

HEPATOMEGALY

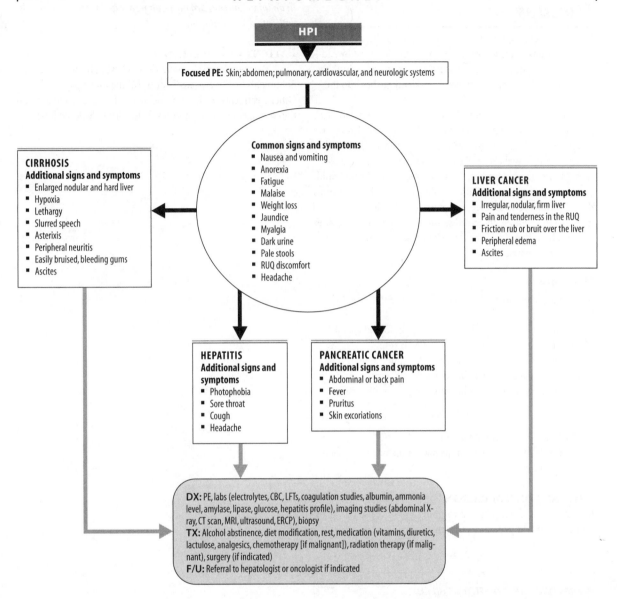

HPI

Focused PE: Skin; abdomen; pulmonary, cardiovascular, and neurologic systems

Common signs and symptoms
- Nausea and vomiting
- Anorexia
- Fatigue
- Malaise
- Weight loss
- Jaundice
- Myalgia
- Dark urine
- Pale stools
- RUQ discomfort
- Headache

CIRRHOSIS
Additional signs and symptoms
- Enlarged nodular and hard liver
- Hypoxia
- Lethargy
- Slurred speech
- Asterixis
- Peripheral neuritis
- Easily bruised, bleeding gums
- Ascites

LIVER CANCER
Additional signs and symptoms
- Irregular, nodular, firm liver
- Pain and tenderness in the RUQ
- Friction rub or bruit over the liver
- Peripheral edema
- Ascites

HEPATITIS
Additional signs and symptoms
- Photophobia
- Sore throat
- Cough
- Headache

PANCREATIC CANCER
Additional signs and symptoms
- Abdominal or back pain
- Fever
- Pruritus
- Skin excoriations

DX: PE, labs (electrolytes, CBC, LFTs, coagulation studies, albumin, ammonia level, amylase, lipase, glucose, hepatitis profile), imaging studies (abdominal X-ray, CT scan, MRI, ultrasound, ERCP), biopsy
TX: Alcohol abstinence, diet modification, rest, medication (vitamins, diuretics, lactulose, analgesics, chemotherapy [if malignant]), radiation therapy (if malignant), surgery (if indicated)
F/U: Referral to hepatologist or oncologist if indicated

Additional differential diagnoses: amyloidosis ▪ diabetes mellitus ▪ granulomatous disorders ▪ hepatic abscess ▪ leukemia ▪ lymphoma ▪ obesity ▪ pericarditis

Hiccups

Hiccups (singultus) occur as a two-stage process: an involuntary, spasmodic contraction of the diaphragm followed by sudden closure of the glottis. Their characteristic sound reflects the vibration of closed vocal cords as air suddenly rushes into the lungs.

Usually benign and transient, hiccups are common and usually subside spontaneously or with simple treatment. However, in a patient with a neurologic disorder, they may indicate increasing intracranial pressure or extension of a brain stem lesion. They may also occur after ingestion of a hot or cold liquid or other irritant, after exposure to cold, or with irritation from a drainage tube. Persistent hiccups cause considerable distress and may lead to vomiting. Increased serum levels of carbon dioxide may inhibit hiccups; decreased levels may accentuate them. (See *Treating and preventing hiccups.*)

History
- Ask the patient when the hiccups began and if they're tiring him.
- Ask the patient if he has had the hiccups before. If so, ask him what caused them and what made them stop.
- Review the patient's medical history for abdominal or thoracic disorders and recent abdominal surgery. (Occasionally, mild and transient attacks of hiccups may follow abdominal surgery.)

Physical assessment
Base the physical assessment on the patient history and associated symptoms.

Special considerations
If a patient with hiccups is also vomiting and unconscious, turn him on his side to prevent aspiration.

In an infant, hiccups usually result from rapid ingestion of liquids without adequate burping.

Patient counseling
Teach the patient simple methods of relieving hiccups, such as holding his breath repeatedly or breathing into a paper bag. Other treatments for hiccups include gastric lavage and application of finger pressure on the eyeballs (through closed lids).

Treating and preventing hiccups

Hiccups commonly occur without an underlying medical cause. Some home remedies to treat hiccups include:
- holding one's breath as long as possible
- breathing into a paper bag
- ingesting a spoonful of sugar
- drinking cold water from the wrong side of the glass while bending forward.
    The following actions may help to prevent hiccups:
- avoiding extremely hot or cold foods
- avoiding spicy foods
- avoiding the use of straws
- burping frequently (for infants).

HICCUPS

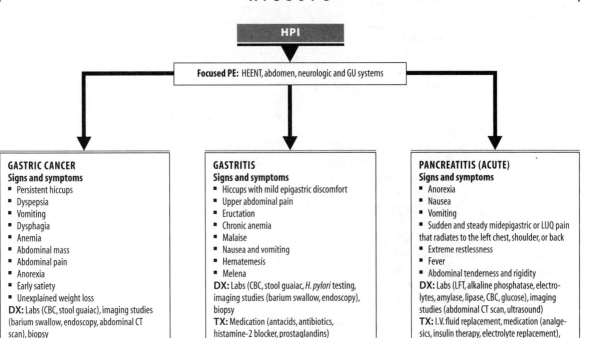

HPI

Focused PE: HEENT, abdomen, neurologic and GU systems

GASTRIC CANCER
Signs and symptoms
- Persistent hiccups
- Dyspepsia
- Vomiting
- Dysphagia
- Anemia
- Abdominal mass
- Abdominal pain
- Anorexia
- Early satiety
- Unexplained weight loss

DX: Labs (CBC, stool guaiac), imaging studies (barium swallow, endoscopy, abdominal CT scan), biopsy
TX: Chemotherapy, radiation therapy, surgery
F/U: Referrals to gastroenterologist and oncologist

GASTRITIS
Signs and symptoms
- Hiccups with mild epigastric discomfort
- Upper abdominal pain
- Eructation
- Chronic anemia
- Malaise
- Nausea and vomiting
- Hematemesis
- Melena

DX: Labs (CBC, stool guaiac, *H. pylori* testing, imaging studies (barium swallow, endoscopy), biopsy
TX: Medication (antacids, antibiotics, histamine-2 blocker, prostaglandins)
F/U: As needed (dependent on symptoms), referral to gastroenterologist if recurrent

---

PANCREATITIS (ACUTE)
Signs and symptoms
- Anorexia
- Nausea
- Vomiting
- Sudden and steady midepigastric or LUQ pain that radiates to the left chest, shoulder, or back
- Extreme restlessness
- Fever
- Abdominal tenderness and rigidity

DX: Labs (LFT, alkaline phosphatase, electrolytes, amylase, lipase, CBC, glucose), imaging studies (abdominal CT scan, ultrasound)
TX: I.V. fluid replacement, medication (analgesics, insulin therapy, electrolyte replacement), alcohol abstinence, diet modification, rest
F/U: Return visit 1 week after hospitalization

Additional differential diagnoses: brain stem lesion ▪ increased ICP ▪ multiple sclerosis ▪ pleurisy ▪ pneumonia ▪ renal failure

Other causes: abdominal surgery ▪ alcohol ingestion ▪ bloating ▪ hot and spicy foods or liquids ▪ hyponatremia ▪ noxious fumes ▪ pscyhogenic

Hirsutism

Hirsutism is the excessive growth of dark, coarse body hair in females. Excessive androgen production stimulates hair growth on the pubic region, axilla, chin, upper lip, cheeks, anterior neck, sternum, linea alba, forearms, abdomen, back, and upper arms. Altered androgen metabolism is the most common cause of hirsutism.

With mild hirsutism, fine and pigmented hair appears on the sides of the face and the chin (but doesn't form a complete beard) and on the extremities, chest, abdomen, and perineum. With moderate hirsutism, coarse and pigmented hair appears on the same areas. With severe hirsutism, coarse hair also covers the whole beard area, the proximal interphalangeal joints, and the ears and nose.

Depending on the degree of excess androgen production, hirsutism may be associated with acne and increased skin oiliness, increased libido, and menstrual irregularities (including anovulation and amenorrhea). Extremely high androgen levels cause further virilization, including such signs as breast atrophy, loss of female body contour, frontal balding, and deepening of the voice.

Hirsutism may result from endocrine abnormalities and idiopathic causes. It may also occur during pregnancy from transient androgen production by the placenta or corpus luteum, and during menopause from increased androgen and decreased estrogen production. Some patients have a strong familial predisposition to hirsutism, which may be considered normal in the context of their genetic background.

HISTORY

- Ask the patient where on her body she first noticed excessive hair growth. Ask her how old she was and where and how quickly other hirsute areas developed.
- Ask the patient if she uses hair removal techniques. If so, how often does she use it, and when did she use it last?
- Obtain a menstrual history: the patient's age at menarche, the duration of her menses, the usual amount of blood flow, and the number of days between menses.
- Obtain a drug history, including prescription and over-the-counter drugs, herbal remedies, and recreational drugs. Also, ask the patient about alcohol intake.

PHYSICAL ASSESSMENT

- Examine the hirsute areas. Note whether excessive hair appears on other body parts as well.
- Determine if the hair is fine, pigmented, dense, or coarse.
- Assess whether the patient is obese. Observe her for signs of virilization. (See *Recognizing signs of virilization.*)

SPECIAL CONSIDERATIONS

Prepare the patient for hormone studies.

 PEDIATRIC POINTERS

- *Childhood hirsutism can stem from congenital adrenal hyperplasia. This disorder is almost always detected at birth because affected infants have ambiguous genitalia. Rarely, a mild form becomes apparent after puberty when hirsutism, irregular bleeding or amenorrhea, and signs of virilization appear.*
- *Hirsutism that occurs at or after puberty commonly results from polycystic ovary disease.*

AGING ISSUES

Hirsutism can occur after menopause if peripheral conversion of estrogen is poor.

PATIENT COUNSELING

At the patient's request, provide information on hair removal methods, such as bleaching, tweezing, hot wax treatments, chemical depilatories, shaving, and electrolysis.

RECOGNIZING SIGNS OF VIRILIZATION

Excessive androgen levels produce severe hirsutism and other marked signs of virilization, as shown in the figure below.

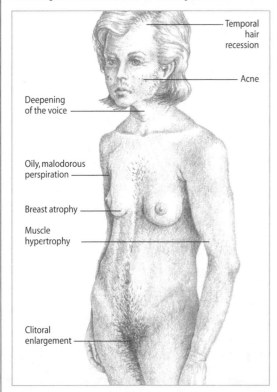

- Temporal hair recession
- Acne
- Deepening of the voice
- Oily, malodorous perspiration
- Breast atrophy
- Muscle hypertrophy
- Clitoral enlargement

HIRSUTISM

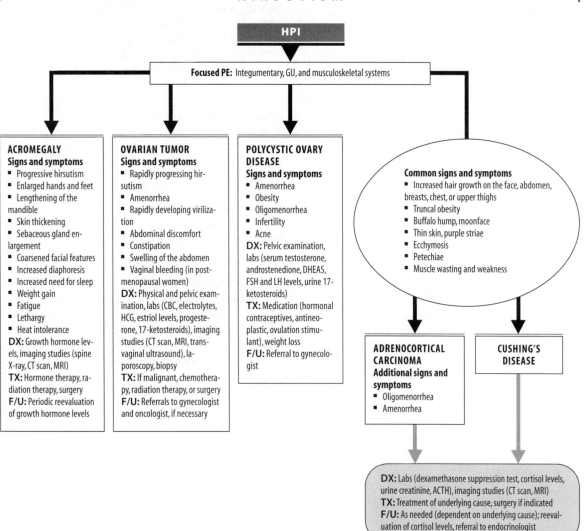

HPI

Focused PE: Integumentary, GU, and musculoskeletal systems

ACROMEGALY
Signs and symptoms
- Progressive hirsutism
- Enlarged hands and feet
- Lengthening of the mandible
- Skin thickening
- Sebaceous gland enlargement
- Coarsened facial features
- Increased diaphoresis
- Increased need for sleep
- Weight gain
- Fatigue
- Lethargy
- Heat intolerance

DX: Growth hormone levels, imaging studies (spine X-ray, CT scan, MRI)
TX: Hormone therapy, radiation therapy, surgery
F/U: Periodic reevaluation of growth hormone levels

OVARIAN TUMOR
Signs and symptoms
- Rapidly progressing hirsutism
- Amenorrhea
- Rapidly developing virilization
- Abdominal discomfort
- Constipation
- Swelling of the abdomen
- Vaginal bleeding (in postmenopausal women)

DX: Physical and pelvic examination, labs (CBC, electrolytes, HCG, estriol levels, progesterone, 17-ketosteroids), imaging studies (CT scan, MRI, transvaginal ultrasound), laporoscopy, biopsy
TX: If malignant, chemotherapy, radiation therapy, or surgery
F/U: Referrals to gynecologist and oncologist, if necessary

POLYCYSTIC OVARY DISEASE
Signs and symptoms
- Amenorrhea
- Obesity
- Oligomenorrhea
- Infertility
- Acne

DX: Pelvic examination, labs (serum testosterone, androstenedione, DHEAS, FSH and LH levels, urine 17-ketosteroids)
TX: Medication (hormonal contraceptives, antineoplastic, ovulation stimulant), weight loss
F/U: Referral to gynecologist

Common signs and symptoms
- Increased hair growth on the face, abdomen, breasts, chest, or upper thighs
- Truncal obesity
- Buffalo hump, moonface
- Thin skin, purple striae
- Ecchymosis
- Petechiae
- Muscle wasting and weakness

ADRENOCORTICAL CARCINOMA
Additional signs and symptoms
- Oligomenorrhea
- Amenorrhea

CUSHING'S DISEASE

DX: Labs (dexamethasone suppression test, cortisol levels, urine creatinine, ACTH), imaging studies (CT scan, MRI)
TX: Treatment of underlying cause, surgery if indicated
F/U: As needed (dependent on underlying cause); reevaluation of cortisol levels, referral to endocrinologist

---

Additional differential diagnoses: hyperprolactemia ▪ idiopathic hirsutism

Other causes: aminoglutethimide ▪ cyclosporine ▪ drugs containing androgens or progestins ▪ glucocorticoids ▪ metoclopramide ▪ minoxidil

Hoarseness

Hoarseness—a rough or harsh sound to the voice—can result from an infection or inflammatory lesion or exudate of the larynx, from laryngeal edema, or from compression or disruption of the vocal cords or recurrent laryngeal nerve. This common sign can also result from a thoracic aortic aneurysm, vocal cord paralysis, or a systemic disorder, such as Sjögren's syndrome or rheumatoid arthritis. It's characteristically worsened by excessive alcohol intake, smoking, inhalation of noxious fumes, excessive talking, and shouting.

Hoarseness can be acute or chronic. For example, chronic hoarseness and laryngitis result when irritating polyps or nodules develop on the vocal cords. Gastroesophageal reflux into the larynx should also be considered as a possible cause of chronic hoarseness. Hoarseness may also result from progressive atrophy of the laryngeal muscles and mucosa due to aging, which leads to diminished control of the vocal cords.

HISTORY

- Ask the patient about the onset of hoarseness.
- Ask the patient if he has been overusing his voice; has experienced shortness of breath, a sore throat, dry mouth, or a cough; or has had difficulty swallowing dry food. In addition, ask if he has been in or near a fire within the past 48 hours.
- Explore associated symptoms, and review the patient's medical history for cancer, rheumatoid arthritis, and an aortic aneurysm.
- Ask the patient if he regularly smokes or drinks alcohol.

PHYSICAL ASSESSMENT

- Inspect the oral cavity and pharynx for redness or exudate, possibly indicating an upper respiratory tract infection.
- Palpate the neck for masses and the cervical lymph nodes and the thyroid for enlargement.
- Palpate the trachea. (Is it midline?)
- Ask the patient to stick out his tongue; if he can't, he may have paralysis from cranial nerve involvement.
- Examine the eyes for corneal ulcers and enlarged lacrimal ducts (signs of Sjögren's syndrome).
- Assess the patient for dilated neck and chest veins.
- Take the patient's vital signs, noting especially fever and bradycardia.
- Assess the patient for asymmetrical chest expansion or signs of respiratory distress, such as nasal flaring, stridor, and intercostal retractions.
- Auscultate for crackles, rhonchi, wheezing, and tubular sounds, and percuss for dullness.

SPECIAL CONSIDERATIONS

Carefully observe the patient for stridor, which may indicate bilateral vocal cord paralysis. Be aware that inhalation injury can cause sudden airway obstruction.

When hoarseness lasts longer than two weeks, indirect or fiber-optic laryngoscopy is indicated to observe the larynx at rest and during phonation.

A. PEDIATRIC POINTERS

- *In children, hoarseness may result from congenital anomalies, such as laryngocele and dysphonia plicae ventricularis.*
- *In prepubescent boys, hoarseness can stem from juvenile papillomatosis of the upper respiratory tract.*
- *In infants and young children, hoarseness commonly stems from acute laryngotracheobronchitis (croup).*
- *Temporary hoarseness frequently results from laryngeal irritation due to aspiration of liquids, foreign bodies, or stomach contents.*

PATIENT COUNSELING

Stress to the patient the importance of resting his voice. Talking—even whispering—further traumatizes the vocal cords. Suggest other ways to communicate, such as writing or using body language. Urge the patient to avoid alcohol, smoking, and exposure to secondhand smoke.

HOARSENESS

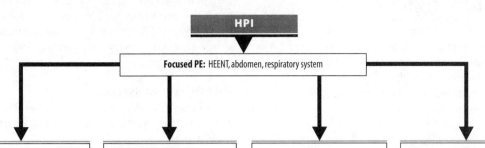

GERD
Signs and symptoms
- Throat pain
- Dyspepsia
- Heartburn
- Regurgitation
- Dysphagia
- Cough
- Throat clearing
- Sensation of a lump in the throat
- Red and swollen vocal cords

DX: History, barium swallow, manometry, endoscopy
TX: Smoking-cessation program, weight management, elevation of HOB while sleeping, diet modification, medication (histamine-2 receptor antagonists, antacids, proton pump inhibitors)
F/U: Reevaluation in 1 to 2 weeks, then every 8 weeks

LARYNGEAL CANCER
Signs and symptoms
- Mild, dry cough
- Minor throat discomfort
- Dysphagia
- Otalgia
- Possible hemoptysis

DX: CT scan, laryngoscopy
TX: Chemotherapy, radiation therapy, surgery
F/U: Referrals to otolaryngologist and oncologist

ACUTE LARYNGITIS
Signs and symptoms
- Sudden hoarseness or loss of voice
- Throat pain
- Dysphagia
- Odynophagia
- Cough
- Rhinorrhea
- Diaphoresis
- Fever

DX: Throat culture, laryngoscopy
TX: Rest, increased fluid intake, medication (analgesics; if bacterial, antibiotics)
F/U: Reevaluation 48 to 72 hours after treatment is initiated

THORACIC AORTIC ANEURYSM
Signs and symptoms
- Asymptomatic (possibly)
- Hoarseness
- Severe penetrating pain while supine
- Brassy cough
- Dyspnea
- Wheezing

DX: Radiologic studies (CT scan, MRI, angiography)
TX: Antihypertensives, surgery, aggressive fluid management
F/U: Referral to thoracic surgeon

Additional differential diagnoses: hypothyroidism ▪ laryngeal leukoplakia ▪ rheumatoid arthritis ▪ Sjögren's syndrome ▪ vocal cord polyps or nodules

Other causes: inhalation injury ▪ prolonged endotracheal intubation ▪ surgical trauma ▪ tracheal trauma ▪ vocal cord paralysis

Homans' sign

Homans' sign is the elicitation of deep calf pain from strong and abrupt dorsiflexion of the ankle. This pain results from venous thrombosis or inflammation of the calf muscles. However, because a positive Homans' sign appears in only 35% of patients with these conditions, it's an unreliable indicator. (See *Eliciting Homans' sign.*) Even when accurate, a positive Homans' sign doesn't indicate the extent of the venous disorder.

This elicited sign may be confused with continuous calf pain, which can result from strains, contusions, cellulitis, or arterial occlusion or with pain in the posterior ankle or Achilles tendon (for example, in a woman with Achilles' tendons shortened from wearing high heels).

 ALERT

If you strongly suspect deep vein thrombosis (DVT), elicit Homans' sign carefully to avoid detaching the clot, which could cause pulmonary embolism, a life-threatening condition.

HISTORY

● Ask the patient about associated signs and symptoms, such as throbbing, aching, heavy, or tight sensations in the calf. Also, ask about leg pain during or after exercise or routine activity.

● Ask the patient if he has experienced shortness of breath or chest pain, which may indicate pulmonary embolism.
● Ask the patient about predisposing events, such as leg injury, recent surgery, childbirth, use of hormonal contraceptives, associated diseases (cancer, nephrosis, hypercoagulable states), and prolonged inactivity.

PHYSICAL ASSESSMENT

● Inspect and palpate the patient's calf for warmth, tenderness, redness, swelling, and the presence of a palpable pulse in the lower extremity.
● Measure the circumferences of the patient's calves. The calf with a positive Homans' sign may be larger because of edema and swelling.

SPECIAL CONSIDERATIONS

Be sure to place the patient on bed rest, with the affected leg elevated above heart level. Apply warm, moist compresses to the affected area, and administer a mild oral analgesic.

 PEDIATRIC POINTERS

Homans' sign is seldom assessed in children, who rarely have DVT or thrombophlebitis.

PATIENT COUNSELING

If the patient is put on long-term anticoagulant therapy, instruct him to report signs of prolonged clotting time. These include black tarry stools, brown or red urine, bleeding gums, and bruises. Also, stress the importance of keeping follow-up visits so that coagulation studies can be done to monitor treatment.

ELICITING HOMANS' SIGN

To elicit Homans' sign, first support the patient's thigh with one hand and his foot with the other. Bend his leg slightly at the knee; then firmly and abruptly dorsiflex the ankle. Resulting deep calf pain indicates a positive Homans' sign. (The patient may also resist ankle dorsiflexion or flex the knee involuntarily if Homans' sign is positive.)

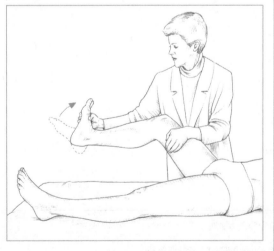

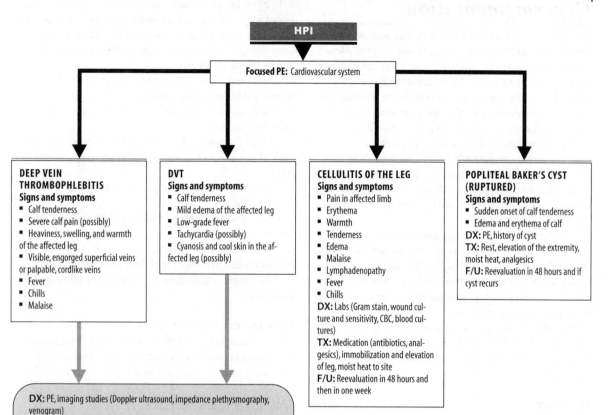

HPI

Focused PE: Cardiovascular system

DEEP VEIN THROMBOPHLEBITIS
Signs and symptoms
- Calf tenderness
- Severe calf pain (possibly)
- Heaviness, swelling, and warmth of the affected leg
- Visible, engorged superficial veins or palpable, cordlike veins
- Fever
- Chills
- Malaise

DVT
Signs and symptoms
- Calf tenderness
- Mild edema of the affected leg
- Low-grade fever
- Tachycardia (possibly)
- Cyanosis and cool skin in the affected leg (possibly)

CELLULITIS OF THE LEG
Signs and symptoms
- Pain in affected limb
- Erythema
- Warmth
- Tenderness
- Edema
- Malaise
- Lymphadenopathy
- Fever
- Chills

DX: Labs (Gram stain, wound culture and sensitivity, CBC, blood cultures)
TX: Medication (antibiotics, analgesics), immobilization and elevation of leg, moist heat to site
F/U: Reevaluation in 48 hours and then in one week

POPLITEAL BAKER'S CYST (RUPTURED)
Signs and symptoms
- Sudden onset of calf tenderness
- Edema and erythema of calf

DX: PE, history of cyst
TX: Rest, elevation of the extremity, moist heat, analgesics
F/U: Reevaluation in 48 hours and if cyst recurs

DX: PE, imaging studies (Doppler ultrasound, impedance plethysmography, venogram)
TX: Bed rest, medication (anticoagulants, analgesic, antipyretics)
F/U: Referral to vascular specialist

Hyperpigmentation

Hyperpigmentation, also known as hypermelanosis or excessive skin coloring, usually reflects overproduction, abnormal location, or mal distribution of melanin — the dominant brown or black pigment found in skin, hair, mucous membranes, nails, brain tissue, cardiac muscle, and parts of the eye. This sign can also reflect abnormalities of other skin pigments: carotenoids (yellow), oxyhemoglobin (red), and hemoglobin (blue).

Hyperpigmentation usually results from exposure to sunlight. However, it can also result from a metabolic, endocrine, neoplastic, or inflammatory disorder; chemical poisoning; use of certain drugs; a genetic defect; thermal burns; ionizing radiation; or localized activation by sunlight of certain photosensitizing chemicals on the skin.

Many types of benign hyperpigmented lesions occur normally. Some, such as acanthosis nigricans and carotenemia, may also accompany certain disorders, but their significance is unproven. Chronic nutritional insufficiency may lead to dyspigmentation — increased pigmentation in some areas and decreased pigmentation in others.

Typically asymptomatic and chronic, hyperpigmentation is a common problem that can have distressing psychological and social implications. It varies in location and intensity and may fade over time.

HISTORY

- Ask the patient when he first noticed the hyperpigmentation.
- Ask the patient if other signs or symptoms, such as rash, accompany or precede the hyperpigmentation. Is it related to exposure to sunlight or seasonal changes?
- Review the patient's medical history, especially noting endocrine disorders. Also, ask the patient if there is a family history of hyperpigmentation.
- If the patient is female, ask if she's pregnant.
- Ask the patient if he's been in contact with or ingested chemicals, metals, plants, vegetables, citrus fruits, or perfumes.
- Obtain a drug history, including prescription and over-the-counter drugs, herbal remedies, and recreational drugs. Also, ask the patient about alcohol intake.
- Ask the patient about other signs and symptoms, such as fatigue; weakness; muscle aches; chills; irritability; fainting; itching; cough; shortness of breath; swelling of the ankles, hands, or other areas; anorexia; nausea; vomiting; weight loss; abdominal pain; diarrhea; constipation; epigastric fullness; dark or pink urine; increased or decreased urination; menstrual irregularities; and loss of libido.

PHYSICAL ASSESSMENT

- Examine the skin. Note the color of hyperpigmented areas: Brown suggests excess melanin in the epidermis; slate gray or a bluish tone suggests excess pigment in the dermis. Inspect for other changes, such as thickened and leathered skin texture and changes in hair distribution.
- Check the skin and sclera for jaundice, and note spider angiomas, palmar erythema, or purpura.
- Take the patient's vital signs, noting fever, hypotension, or pulse irregularities.
- Evaluate the patient's general appearance. Does he have exophthalmos, an enlarged jaw, an enlarged nose, or enlarged hands?
- Palpate for an enlarged thyroid, and auscultate for a bruit over the gland.
- Palpate muscles for atrophy and joints for swelling and tenderness.
- Assess the abdomen for ascites and edema, and palpate and percuss the liver and spleen to evaluate their size and position.
- If the patient is male, check for testicular atrophy and gynecomastia.

SPECIAL CONSIDERATIONS

A Wood's lamp is a special ultraviolet light that helps enhance the contrast between normal and hyperpigmented epidermis. A skin biopsy can help confirm the cause of hyperpigmentation.

[A]   *PEDIATRIC POINTERS*

- *Bizarre arrangements of linear or streaky hyperpigmented lesions on a child's sun-exposed lower legs suggest phytophotodermatitis.*
- *Congenital hyperpigmented lesions include mongolian spots (which are benign) and sharply defined or diffuse lesions occurring in such disorders as neurofibromatosis xeroderma pigmentosum; Gaucher's, Niemann-Pick, and Wilson's diseases; Albright's, Fanconi's, and Peutz-Jeghers syndromes; and phenylketonuria.*

PATIENT COUNSELING

Advise patients to use corrective cosmetics, to avoid excessive sun exposure, and to apply sunscreen or sunblock when outdoors. Advise patients who stop using bleaching agents to continue using sunscreen because rebound hyperpigmentation can occur. Warn every patient with a benign hyperpigmented area to consult his health care provider if the lesion's size, shape, or color changes; this may signal developing skin cancer.

HYPERPIGMENTATION

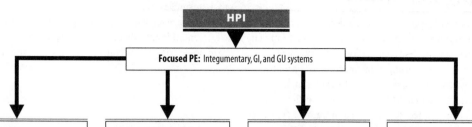

HPI

Focused PE: Integumentary, GI, and GU systems

ADRENOCORTICAL INSUFFICIENCY
Signs and symptoms
- Diffuse tan, brown, or bronze-to-black hyperpigmentation of the face, knees, knuckles, elbows, beltline, palmar creases, lips, gums, tongue, and buccal mucosa
- Hyperpigmentation of scars and moles
- Loss of axillary and pubic hair
- Possible vitiligo
- Slowly progressive fatigue
- Mental sluggishness
- Postural hypotension
- Weakness
- Anorexia
- Nausea and vomiting
- Weight loss
- Abdominal pain
- Orthostatic hypotension
- Irritability
- Diarrhea or constipation
- Decreased libido
- Amenorrhea
- Syncope
- Weak, irregular pulse
- Enhanced sense of taste, smell, and hearing (possibly)

DX: Labs (CBC, BUN, creatinine, electrolytes, cortisol levels, serum calcium, thyroid studies, ACTH stimulation test), imaging studies (CXR, CT scan), ECG
TX: Ventilatory and circulatory support, medication (glucocorticoid and mineral corticoid hormone replacement therapy), fluid and electrolyte replacement, treatment of underlying condition
F/U: Referral to endocrinologist

HEMOCHROMATOSIS, HEREDITARY
Signs and symptoms
- Early and progressive hyperpigmentation
- Generalized bronzing and metallic gray areas over sun-exposed areas, genitalia, and scars
- Weakness
- Lassitude
- Weight loss
- Abdominal pain
- Peripheral neuritis
- Arthritis
- Testicular atrophy
- Loss of libido
- Liver and cardiac involvement (late sign)

SIGNS OF DIABETES
- Polydipsia
- Polyuria

DX: Labs (iron level, ferritin level, CBC with differential), liver biopsy
TX: Weekly phlebotomy
F/U: Reevaluation every 3 months, referrals to hepatologist and hematologist

MALIGNANT MELANOMA
Signs and symptoms
- Hyperpigmented lesions of the skin (commonly moles) that are usually asymmetrical with border irregularity, color variegation, and a diameter > 6 mm
- Inflamed, itchy, ulcerated, and bleeding lesions

DX: Skin examination, biopsy
TX: Surgery, sun exposure protection
F/U: Referrals to dermatologist and oncologist

CUSHING'S DISEASE
Signs and symptoms
- Increased hair growth on the face, abdomen, breasts, chest, or upper thighs
- Truncal obesity
- Buffalo hump
- Moonface
- Thin skin, purple striae
- Ecchymosis
- Petechiae
- Muscle wasting and weakness

DX: Labs (dexamethasone suppression test, cortisol levels, urine creatinine, ACTH), imaging studies (CT scan, MRI)
TX: Treatment of underlying cause, surgery if indicated
F/U: As needed (dependent on underlying cause), reevaluation of cortisol levels, referral to endocrinologist

---

Additional differential diagnoses: acromegaly ▪ biliary cirrhosis ▪ Laënnec's cirrhosis ▪ porphyria cutanea tarda ▪ scleroderma ▪ thyrotoxicosis ▪ venous insufficiency

Other causes: antimalarial drugs such as hydroxychloroquine ▪ arsenic poisoning ▪ barbiturates ▪ chemotherapeutic drugs, such as busulfan, cyclophosphamide, procarbazine, and nitrogen mustard ▪ chlorpromazine ▪ corticotropin ▪ hydantoin ▪ metals, such as silver and gold ▪ minocycline ▪ phenolphthalein ▪ phenothiazines ▪ salicylates

Hypopigmentation

Hypopigmentation (hypomelanosis) is a decrease in normal skin, hair, mucous membrane, or nail color resulting from deficiency, absence, or abnormal degradation of the pigment melanin. This sign may be congenital or acquired, asymptomatic, or associated with other findings. Its causes include genetic disorders, nutritional deficiency, exposure to chemicals or drugs, inflammation, infection, and physical trauma. Typically chronic, hypopigmentation can be difficult to identify if the patient is light-skinned or has only slightly decreased coloring.

HISTORY

● Ask the patient if the hypopigmentation was present from birth or developed after skin lesions or a rash. Have other family members experienced hypopigmentation?
● Ask the patient if the lesions are painful.
● Ask the patient if he has medical problems or a history of burns, physical injury, or physical contact with chemicals.
● Obtain a drug history, including prescription and over-the-counter drugs, herbal remedies, and recreational drugs. Also, ask the patient about alcohol intake.
● Find out if the patient has noticed other skin changes, such as erythema, scaling, ulceration, or hyperpigmentation or if sun exposure causes unusually severe burning.

PHYSICAL ASSESSMENT

● Examine the patient's skin, noting erythema, scaling, ulceration, areas of hyperpigmentation, and other findings.

SPECIAL CONSIDERATIONS

In fair-skinned patients, a Wood's lamp, which is a special ultraviolet (UV) light, can help differentiate hypopigmented lesions, which appear pale, from depigmented lesions, which appear white.

A PEDIATRIC POINTERS

● *In children, hypopigmentation results from genetic or acquired disorders, including albinism, phenylketonuria, and tuberous sclerosis.*
● *In neonates, hypopigmentation may indicate a metabolic or nervous system disorder.*

AGING ISSUES

In elderly people, hypopigmentation is usually the result of cumulative exposure to UV light.

PATIENT COUNSELING

Advise patients to use corrective cosmetics to help hide skin lesions and to use a sunblock when outdoors because hypopigmented areas may sunburn easily. Advise patients with associated eye problems, such as albinism, to avoid the midday sun and to wear sunglasses.

Encourage regular examinations for early detection and treatment of lesions that may become premalignant or malignant. Refer patients for counseling if lesions cause stress.

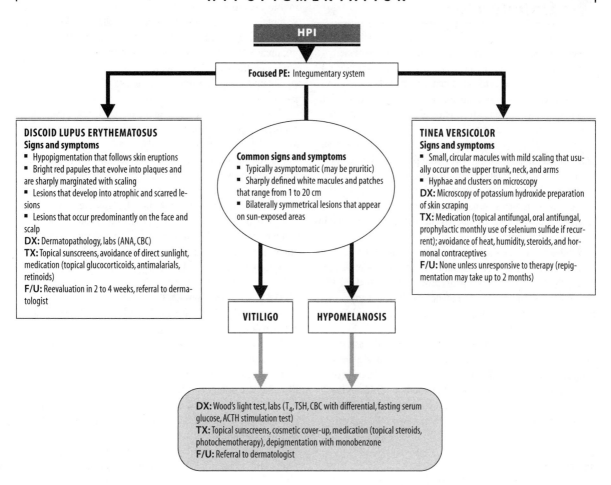

HPI

Focused PE: Integumentary system

DISCOID LUPUS ERYTHEMATOSUS
Signs and symptoms
- Hypopigmentation that follows skin eruptions
- Bright red papules that evolve into plaques and are sharply marginated with scaling
- Lesions that develop into atrophic and scarred lesions
- Lesions that occur predominantly on the face and scalp

DX: Dermatopathology, labs (ANA, CBC)
TX: Topical sunscreens, avoidance of direct sunlight, medication (topical glucocorticoids, antimalarials, retinoids)
F/U: Reevaluation in 2 to 4 weeks, referral to dermatologist

Common signs and symptoms
- Typically asymptomatic (may be pruritic)
- Sharply defined white macules and patches that range from 1 to 20 cm
- Bilaterally symmetrical lesions that appear on sun-exposed areas

TINEA VERSICOLOR
Signs and symptoms
- Small, circular macules with mild scaling that usually occur on the upper trunk, neck, and arms
- Hyphae and clusters on microscopy

DX: Microscopy of potassium hydroxide preparation of skin scraping
TX: Medication (topical antifungal, oral antifungal, prophylactic monthly use of selenium sulfide if recurrent); avoidance of heat, humidity, steroids, and hormonal contraceptives
F/U: None unless unresponsive to therapy (repigmentation may take up to 2 months)

VITILIGO

HYPOMELANOSIS

DX: Wood's light test, labs (T_4, TSH, CBC with differential, fasting serum glucose, ACTH stimulation test)
TX: Topical sunscreens, cosmetic cover-up, medication (topical steroids, photochemotherapy), depigmentation with monobenzone
F/U: Referral to dermatologist

Additional differential diagnoses: burns ▪ inflammatory and infectious disorders ▪ tuberculoid leprosy

Other causes: chloroquine ▪ germicides ▪ phenolic compounds (paratertiary butylphenol) ▪ topical or intralesional administration of corticosteroids

I

Impotence

Impotence is the inability to achieve and maintain penile erection sufficient to complete satisfactory intercourse; ejaculation may or may not be affected. Impotence varies from occasional and minimal to permanent and complete. Occasional impotence occurs in about one-half of adult men in the United States, whereas chronic impotence affects about 1 in 8 million men in the United States.

Impotence can be classified as primary or secondary. A man with primary impotence has never been potent with a partner, but may achieve normal erections in other situations. This uncommon condition is difficult to treat. Secondary impotence carries a more favorable prognosis because, despite present erectile dysfunction, the patient has succeeded in completing intercourse in the past.

Penile erection involves increased arterial blood flow secondary to psychological, tactile, and other sensory stimulation. Trapping of blood within the penis produces increased length, circumference, and rigidity. Impotence results when any component of this process—psychological, vascular, neurologic, or hormonal—malfunctions.

Organic causes of impotence include vascular disease, diabetes mellitus, hypogonadism, a spinal cord lesion, alcohol and drug abuse, and surgical complications. (The incidence of organic impotence associated with other medical problems increases after age 50.) Psychogenic causes range from performance anxiety and marital discord to moral or religious conflicts.

HISTORY

- If the patient complains of impotence or of a condition that may be causing it, let him describe his problem without interruption.
- Ask the patient when his impotence began. How did it progress? What's its current status? Make your questions specific, but remember that the patient may have difficulty discussing sexual problems or may not understand the physiology involved.
- Ask the patient if he's married, single, or widowed. How long has he been married or had a sexual relationship? What's the age and health status of his sexual partner?
- If you can do so discreetly, ask the patient about sexual activity outside marriage or his primary sexual relationship.
- Ask the patient about his job history, his typical daily activities, and his living situation. How well does he get along with others in his household?
- Review the patient's medical history for type 2 diabetes mellitus, hypertension, or heart disease, noting information on on-set and treatment. Also, ask about neurologic diseases such as multiple sclerosis.
- Obtain a surgical history, noting especially neurologic, vascular, and urologic surgery. If trauma may be causing the patient's impotence, find out the date of the injury as well as its severity, associated effects, and treatment.
- Obtain a urologic history, including voiding problems and past injury.
- Obtain a drug history, including prescription and over-the-counter drugs, herbal remedies, and recreational drugs. Also, ask the patient about alcohol intake.
- Ask the patient if he smokes. If so, ask him how many packs he smokes in a year.
- Ask the patient about his diet and exercise regimen.
- Ask the patient to rate the quality of a typical erection on a scale of 0 to 10, with 0 being completely flaccid and 10 being completely erect. Using the same scale, also ask him to rate his ability to ejaculate during sexual activity, with 0 being never and 10 being always.

PHYSICAL ASSESSMENT

- Inspect and palpate the genitalia and prostate for structural abnormalities.
- Assess the patient's sensory function, concentrating on the perineal area.
- Test motor strength and deep tendon reflexes in all extremities, and note other neurologic deficits.
- Take the patient's vital signs and palpate his pulses for quality. Note signs of peripheral vascular disease, such as cyanosis and cool extremities.
- Auscultate for abdominal aortic, femoral, carotid, or iliac bruits, and palpate for thyroid gland enlargement.

SPECIAL CONSIDERATIONS

Sildenafil can be used for the treatment of erectile dysfunction and is an alternative to surgery.

AGING ISSUES

In elderly people who suffer from sexual dysfunction, organic disease must be ruled out first.

PATIENT COUNSELING

Keep in mind that impotence is potentially frustrating, humiliating, and devastating to self-esteem and significant relationships. Encourage the patient to talk openly about his needs and desires, fears, and anxieties or misconceptions. Urge him to discuss these issues with his partner as well as the role they want sexual activity to play in their lives.

IMPOTENCE

HPI

Focused PE: Cardiovascular, respiratory, neurologic, and GU systems

PERIPHERAL NEUROPATHY
Signs and symptoms
- Progressive impotence
- Bladder distention with overflow incontinence
- Orthostatic hypotension
- Syncope
- Paresthesia
- Muscle weakness
- Leg atrophy

DX: Labs (lipid profile, TSH, blood glucose, UA, CBC, BUN, creatinine), noninvasive portable monitoring of nocturnal erectile activity, penile nerve conduction studies

TX: Management of the underlying cause of neuropathy, intracavernosal or penile injection therapy, vacuum and constrictive devices, surgery

F/U: Reevaluation every 3 months, referral to urologist, APN, psychologist, or psychiatrist

PSYCHOLOGICAL DISTRESS
Signs and symptoms
- Stress
- Anxiety
- Depression (possibly)
- Fatigue

DX: Noninvasive portable monitoring of nocturnal erectile activity, psychological evaluation

TX: Treatment of underlying depression and anxiety, antidepressants

F/U: Reevaluation every 3 months, referral to sexual therapist

VASCULAR DISORDERS
Signs and symptoms
- Progressive impotence
- Decreased peripheral pulses
- Cool, pale extremities

DX: Labs (testing of intracorporeal prostaglandin E1, phentolamine, and papaverine, lipid profile BUN, creatinine, UA), noninvasive portable monitoring of nocturnal erectile activity, imaging studies (duplex ultrasound, angiography)

TX: Sildenafil citrate, intracavernosal or penile injection therapy, vacuum and constrictive devices, treatment of underlying vascular disorder, surgery

F/U: Reevaluation every 3 months; referral to APN, psychologist, or psychiatrist

TRAUMA
Signs and symptoms
- Structural alteration
- Nerve damage
- Interrupted blood flow

DX: History of injury to the penis, prostate, or pelvis

TX: Treatment of causative injury

F/U: As needed (based on type and severity of injury)

Additional differential diagnoses: CNS disorders such as stroke ▪ endocrine disorders such as diabetes mellitus ▪ liver disease

Other causes: alcohol abuse ▪ antihypertensives ▪ drug abuse ▪ radiation therapy ▪ surgery ▪ urologic procedures such as prostatectomy ▪ various drugs

Insomnia

Insomnia is the inability to fall asleep, remain asleep, or feel refreshed by sleep. Acute and transient during periods of stress, insomnia may become chronic, causing constant fatigue, extreme anxiety as bedtime approaches, and even psychiatric disorders. This common complaint is experienced occasionally by about 25% of Americans, chronically by another 10%.

Physiologic causes of insomnia include jet lag, stress, and lack of exercise. Pathophysiologic causes range from medical and psychiatric disorders to pain, adverse drug effects, and idiopathic factors. Complaints of insomnia are subjective and require close investigation; the patient may mistakenly attribute his insomnia to fatigue from an organic cause such as anemia.

TIPS FOR RELIEVING INSOMNIA

COMMON PROBLEMS	INTERVENTIONS
Acroparesthesia	Teach the patient to assume a comfortable position in bed, with his limbs unrestricted. If he tends to awaken with a numb leg or arm, tell him to massage and move it until sensation returns completely and then to assume an unrestricted position.
Anxiety	Encourage the patient to discuss his fears and concerns, and teach him relaxation techniques, such as guided imagery and deep breathing. If ordered, administer a mild sedative, such as diazepam, before bedtime.
Dyspnea	Elevate the head of the bed, or provide at least two pillows or a reclining chair to help the patient sleep. Suction him when he awakens, and encourage deep breathing every 2 to 4 hours. Also, provide supplementary oxygen by nasal cannula.
Pain	Administer pain medication, as ordered, 20 minutes before bedtime, and teach deep, even, slow breathing to promote relaxation. Help the patient with back pain lie on his side with his legs flexed. Encourage the patient with epigastric pain to take an antacid before bedtime and to sleep with the head of the bed elevated.
Pruritus	Wash the patient's skin with mild soap and water, and dry the skin thoroughly. Apply moisturizing lotion on dry, unbroken skin and an antipruritic, such as calamine lotion, on pruritic areas.
Restless leg	Help the patient exercise his legs gently by slowly walking with him around the room and down the hall. If ordered, administer a muscle relaxant such as diazepam.

HISTORY

● Ask the patient when his insomnia began and the attending circumstances. Is he trying to stop using sedatives? Does he use central nervous system stimulants, such as amphetamines, pseudoephedrine, theophylline derivatives, phenylpropanolamine, cocaine, and caffeine-containing drugs or beverages? Does he use herbal remedies?

● Review the patient's medical history for a chronic or acute condition that may be disturbing his sleep, particularly a cardiac or respiratory disease or a painful or pruritic condition. Also, check for a history of endocrine or neurologic disorders and drug or alcohol abuse.

● Ask the patient if he's a frequent traveler who suffers from jet lag.

● Ask the patient if he uses his legs a lot during the day only to feel restless at night.

● Ask the patient about daytime fatigue and regular exercise. Also, ask if he experiences periods of gasping for air or apnea and frequent body repositioning. If possible, consult the patient's spouse or sleep partner because the patient may not be aware of his own behavior.

● Assess the patient's emotional status, and try to estimate his level of self-esteem. Ask about personal and professional problems and psychological stress.

● Ask the patient if he has had hallucinations, and note behavior that may indicate alcohol withdrawal.

PHYSICAL ASSESSMENT

● Take the patient's vital signs.

● Perform a complete physical assessment. Note skin abnormalities, and observe for areas of pain or tenderness.

● Closely assess the patient's heart and thyroid gland for abnormalities.

SPECIAL CONSIDERATIONS

Herbal remedies, such as ginseng and green tea, can cause adverse effects, including insomnia.

Ⓐ PEDIATRIC POINTERS

● *Insomnia in early childhood may develop along with separation anxiety between ages 2 and 3, after a stressful or tiring day, or during illness or teething.*

● *In children ages 6 to 11, insomnia usually reflects residual excitement from the day's activities; a few children continue to have bedtime fears.*

PATIENT COUNSELING

Teach the patient comfort and relaxation techniques to promote natural sleep. (See *Tips for relieving insomnia*.)

INSOMNIA

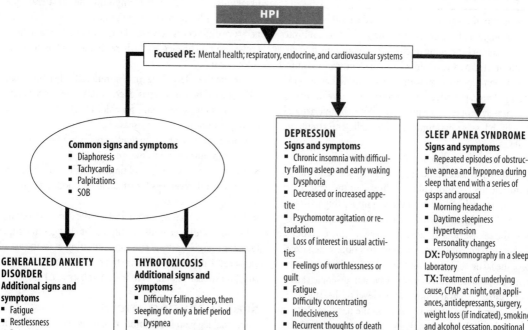

HPI

Focused PE: Mental health; respiratory, endocrine, and cardiovascular systems

Common signs and symptoms
- Diaphoresis
- Tachycardia
- Palpitations
- SOB

GENERALIZED ANXIETY DISORDER
Additional signs and symptoms
- Fatigue
- Restlessness
- Dyspepsia
- Dry mouth
- Lightheadedness
- Nausea
- Diarrhea
- Flushes or chills
- Excessive worry
- Irritability
- Difficulty concentrating

DX: Psychological evaluation
TX: Medication (SSRIs, antidepressants, beta-adrenergic blockers [for physical symptoms], short-term benzodiazepines), cognitive and behavioral therapies
F/U: Reevaluation every 2 to 3 weeks until stabilized on medication

THYROTOXICOSIS
Additional signs and symptoms
- Difficulty falling asleep, then sleeping for only a brief period
- Dyspnea
- Atrial or ventricular gallop
- Inability to concentrate
- Emotional lability
- Weight loss despite increased appetite
- Tremors
- Nervousness
- Diaphoresis
- Hypersensitivity to heat
- Enlarged thyroid
- Exophthalmos

DX: PE, labs (TSH, T_3, T_4, thyroid resin uptake)
TX: Medication (antithyroid agents, therapeutic radioiodine, beta-adrenergic blockers)
F/U: Reevaluation of thyroid function every 6 months; reevaluation at 6 weeks and 12 weeks, and then every 6 months, if undergoing radionuclide therapy

DEPRESSION
Signs and symptoms
- Chronic insomnia with difficulty falling asleep and early waking
- Dysphoria
- Decreased or increased appetite
- Psychomotor agitation or retardation
- Loss of interest in usual activities
- Feelings of worthlessness or guilt
- Fatigue
- Difficulty concentrating
- Indecisiveness
- Recurrent thoughts of death
- Possible suicidal ideation

DX: Beck Depression Inventory, Zung Self-Rating Depression Scale, Geriatric Depression Scale, labs (CBC, ESR, VDRL, electrolytes, thyroid profile, drug screening)
TX: Medication (SSRIs, tricyclic antidepressants), cognitive therapy, support groups, exercise program
F/U: Initial reevaluation at 2 weeks, then every 4 to 8 weeks, then every 3 months; referral to psychologist

SLEEP APNEA SYNDROME
Signs and symptoms
- Repeated episodes of obstructive apnea and hypopnea during sleep that end with a series of gasps and arousal
- Morning headache
- Daytime sleepiness
- Hypertension
- Personality changes

DX: Polysomnography in a sleep laboratory
TX: Treatment of underlying cause, CPAP at night, oral appliances, antidepressants, surgery, weight loss (if indicated), smoking and alcohol cessation, positional therapy
F/U: Referrals to sleep specialist and pulmonologist

Additional differential diagnoses: alcohol withdrawal syndrome ▪ mood (affective) disorders ▪ nocturnal myoclonus ▪ pain ▪ pheochromocytoma ▪ pruritus

Other causes: amphetamines ▪ caffeine-containing beverages ▪ cocaine ▪ ginseng ▪ green tea ▪ phenylpropanolamine ▪ pseudoephedrine ▪ theophylline derivatives ▪ withdrawal from sedatives or hypnotics

Intermittent claudication

Most common in the legs, intermittent claudication is cramping limb pain brought on by exercise and relieved by 1 to 2 minutes of rest. This pain may be acute or chronic; when acute, it may signal acute arterial occlusion. Intermittent claudication is most common in men ages 50 to 60 with a history of diabetes mellitus, hyperlipidemia, hypertension, or tobacco use. Without treatment, it may progress to pain at rest. With chronic arterial occlusion, limb loss is uncommon because collateral circulation usually develops.

With occlusive artery disease, intermittent claudication results from an inadequate blood supply. Pain in the calf (the most common area) or foot indicates disease of the femoral or popliteal arteries; pain in the buttocks and upper thigh, disease of the aortoiliac arteries. During exercise, the pain typically results from the release of lactic acid due to anaerobic metabolism in the ischemic segment secondary to obstruction. When exercise stops, the lactic acid clears and the pain subsides.

Intermittent claudication may also have a neurologic cause: narrowing of the vertebral column at the level of the cauda equina. This condition creates pressure on the nerve roots to the lower extremities. Walking stimulates circulation to the cauda equina, causing increased pressure on those nerves and resultant pain.

◤ ALERT
If the patient has sudden intermittent claudication with severe or aching leg pain at rest:
- *check the leg's temperature and color and palpate pulses*
- *ask about numbness and tingling*
- *don't elevate the leg; protect it and let nothing press on it*
- *arrange for an immediate surgical consult.*

If the patient has chronic intermittent claudication, perform a focused assessment.

HISTORY
- Ask the patient how far he can walk before pain occurs and how long he must rest before it subsides. Can he walk less far now than before, or does he need to rest longer? Does the pain-rest pattern vary? Has this symptom affected his lifestyle?
- Review the patient's medical history for risk factors of atherosclerosis, such as smoking, diabetes, hypertension, and hyperlipidemia.
- Ask the patient about associated signs and symptoms, such as paresthesia in the affected limb and visible changes in the color of the fingers (white to blue to pink) when he's smoking, exposed to cold, or under stress. If the patient is male, ask him if he experiences impotence.

PHYSICAL ASSESSMENT
- Palpate for femoral, popliteal, dorsalis pedis, and posterior tibial pulses. Note character, amplitude, and bilateral equality.
- Listen for bruits over the major arteries. Note color and temperature differences between the legs or compared with the arms; also note the leg level where changes in temperature and color occur.
- Elevate the affected leg for 2 minutes; if it becomes pale or white, blood flow is severely decreased. When the leg hangs down, how long does it take for color to return? (Thirty seconds or longer indicates severe disease.)
- Check the patient's deep tendon reflexes after exercise; note if they're diminished in his lower extremities.
- Examine the feet, toes, and fingers for ulceration, and inspect the hands and lower legs for small, tender nodules and erythema along blood vessels.
- If the patient has arm pain, inspect the arms for a change in color (to white) on elevation. Palpate for changes in temperature, for muscle wasting, and for a pulsating mass in the subclavian area. Palpate and compare the radial, ulnar, brachial, axillary, and subclavian pulses to identify obstructed areas.

SPECIAL CONSIDERATIONS
Nocturnal leg pain is common in older adults. It may indicate ischemic rest pain or restless leg syndrome.

Ⓐ PEDIATRIC POINTERS
- *Intermittent claudication rarely occurs in children. Although it sometimes develops in patients with coarctation of the aorta, extensive compensatory collateral circulation typically prevents manifestation of this sign.*
- *Muscle cramps from exercise and growing pains may be mistaken for intermittent claudication in children.*

PATIENT COUNSELING
Encourage the patient to exercise to improve collateral circulation and increase venous return. Advise him to avoid prolonged sitting or standing as well as crossing his legs at the knees.

Counsel the patient with intermittent claudication about risk factors. Encourage him to stop smoking, and refer him to a support group, if appropriate. Teach him to inspect his legs and feet for ulcers; to keep his extremities warm, clean, and dry; and to avoid injury.

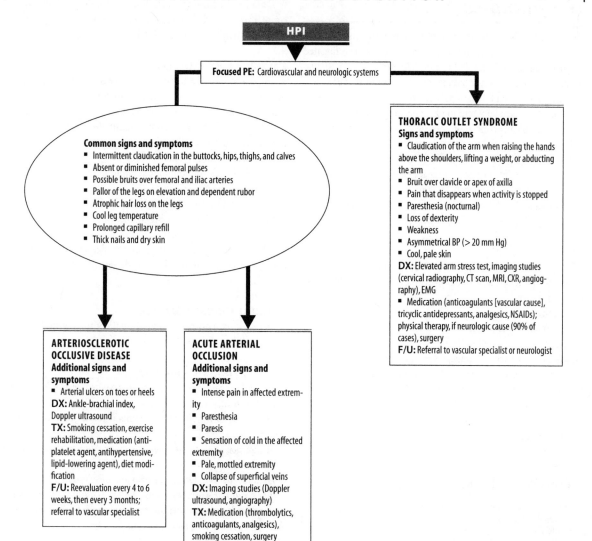

HPI

Focused PE: Cardiovascular and neurologic systems

Common signs and symptoms
- Intermittent claudication in the buttocks, hips, thighs, and calves
- Absent or diminished femoral pulses
- Possible bruits over femoral and iliac arteries
- Pallor of the legs on elevation and dependent rubor
- Atrophic hair loss on the legs
- Cool leg temperature
- Prolonged capillary refill
- Thick nails and dry skin

ARTERIOSCLEROTIC OCCLUSIVE DISEASE
Additional signs and symptoms
- Arterial ulcers on toes or heels
DX: Ankle-brachial index, Doppler ultrasound
TX: Smoking cessation, exercise rehabilitation, medication (anti-platelet agent, antihypertensive, lipid-lowering agent), diet modification
F/U: Reevaluation every 4 to 6 weeks, then every 3 months; referral to vascular specialist

ACUTE ARTERIAL OCCLUSION
Additional signs and symptoms
- Intense pain in affected extremity
- Paresthesia
- Paresis
- Sensation of cold in the affected extremity
- Pale, mottled extremity
- Collapse of superficial veins
DX: Imaging studies (Doppler ultrasound, angiography)
TX: Medication (thrombolytics, anticoagulants, analgesics), smoking cessation, surgery
F/U: Referral to vascular surgeon

THORACIC OUTLET SYNDROME
Signs and symptoms
- Claudication of the arm when raising the hands above the shoulders, lifting a weight, or abducting the arm
- Bruit over clavicle or apex of axilla
- Pain that disappears when activity is stopped
- Paresthesia (nocturnal)
- Loss of dexterity
- Weakness
- Asymmetrical BP (> 20 mm Hg)
- Cool, pale skin
DX: Elevated arm stress test, imaging studies (cervical radiography, CT scan, MRI, CXR, angiography), EMG
- Medication (anticoagulants [vascular cause], tricyclic antidepressants, analgesics, NSAIDs); physical therapy, if neurologic cause (90% of cases), surgery
F/U: Referral to vascular specialist or neurologist

Additional differential diagnoses: arteriosclerosis obliterans ▪ Buerger's disease ▪ Leriche's syndrome ▪ neurogenic claudication

J

Jaundice

The yellow discoloration of the skin or mucous membranes, jaundice indicates excessive levels of conjugated or unconjugated bilirubin in the blood. In fair-skinned patients, it's most noticeable on the face, trunk, and sclerae; in dark-skinned patients, on the hard palate, sclerae, and conjunctivae.

Jaundice is most apparent in natural sunlight. In fact, it may be undetectable in artificial or poor light. It's commonly accompanied by pruritus (because bile pigment damages sensory nerves), dark urine, and clay-colored stools.

Jaundice presents in one of three forms: prehepatic jaundice, hepatic jaundice, and posthepatic jaundice. It may be the only warning sign of certain disorders such as pancreatic cancer. (See *Classifying jaundice.*)

HISTORY

- Ask the patient when he first noticed the jaundice.
- Ask the patient if he also has pruritus, clay-colored stools, or dark urine.
- Ask the patient if he has ever had past episodes of jaundice. Is there a family history of the disease?
- Ask the patient whether he has experienced associated signs and symptoms, such as fatigue, fever, or chills; GI signs or symptoms, such as anorexia, abdominal pain, nausea, or vomiting; or cardiopulmonary symptoms, such as shortness of breath or palpitations.
- Review the patient's medical history for liver or gallbladder disease and cancer.

- Ask the patient if he recently lost weight.
- Obtain a drug history, including prescription and over-the-counter drugs, herbal remedies, and recreational drugs. Also, ask the patient about alcohol intake.

PHYSICAL EXAMINATION

- Inspect the skin for texture and dryness and for hyperpigmentation and xanthomas. Look for spider angiomas or petechiae, clubbed fingers, and gynecomastia.
- If the patient has heart failure, auscultate for arrhythmias, murmurs, and gallops. For all patients, auscultate for crackles and abnormal bowel sounds.
- Palpate the lymph nodes for swelling and the abdomen for tenderness, pain, and swelling.
- Palpate and percuss the liver and spleen for enlargement, and test for ascites with the shifting dullness and fluid wave techniques.
- Obtain baseline data on the patient's mental status: Slight changes in sensorium may be an early sign of deteriorating hepatic function.

SPECIAL CONSIDERATIONS

To help decrease pruritus, bathe the patient frequently, and apply an antipruritic lotion such as calamine.

🅰 *PEDIATRIC POINTERS*

- *Physiologic jaundice is common in neonates, developing 3 to 5 days after birth.*
- *In infants, obstructive jaundice usually results from congenital biliary atresia.*
- *A choledochal cyst—a congenital cystic dilation of the common bile duct—may also cause jaundice in children, particularly those of Japanese descent. Other causes of jaundice include Crigler-Najjar syndrome, Gilbert's disease, Rotor's syndrome, thalassemia major, hereditary spherocytosis, erythroblastosis fetalis, Hodgkin's disease, and infectious mononucleosis.*

🖐 *AGING ISSUES*

In patients older than age 60, jaundice is usually caused by cholestasis resulting from extrahepatic obstruction.

PATIENT COUNSELING

Encourage the patient with a hepatic disorder to decrease protein intake and increase carbohydrate intake. If he has obstructive jaundice, encourage a balanced, nutritious diet (avoiding high-fat foods) and frequent small meals.

CLASSIFYING JAUNDICE

Jaundice occurs in three forms: prehepatic, hepatic, and posthepatic. In all three, bilirubin levels in the blood increase due to impaired metabolism.

With *prehepatic jaundice,* certain conditions and disorders, such as transfusion reactions and sickle cell anemia, cause massive hemolysis. Red blood cells rupture faster than the liver can conjugate bilirubin, so large amounts of unconjugated bilirubin pass into the blood, causing increased intestinal conversion of this bilirubin to water-soluble urobilinogen for excretion in urine and stools. (Unconjugated bilirubin is insoluble in water, so it can't be directly excreted in urine.)

Hepatic jaundice results from the liver's inability to conjugate or excrete bilirubin, leading to increased blood levels of conjugated and unconjugated bilirubin. This occurs in such disorders as hepatitis, cirrhosis, and metastatic cancer and during prolonged use of drugs metabolized by the liver.

With *posthepatic jaundice,* which occurs in patients with biliary or pancreatic disorders, bilirubin forms at its normal rate, but inflammation, scar tissue, a tumor, or gallstones block the flow of bile into the intestine. This causes an accumulation of conjugated bilirubin in the blood. Water-soluble, conjugated bilirubin is excreted in the urine.

JAUNDICE

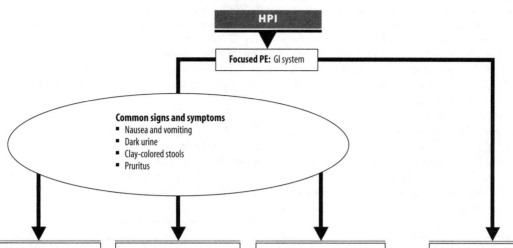

HPI

Focused PE: GI system

Common signs and symptoms
- Nausea and vomiting
- Dark urine
- Clay-colored stools
- Pruritus

CHOLELITHIASIS
Additional signs and symptoms
- Biliary colic
- Severe, steady pain in RUQ or epigastrium that radiates to the right scapula
- Positive Murphy's sign
- Tachycardia
- Restlessness
- Dyspepsia after a fatty meal

DX: Lab (CBC, LFT, electrolytes), imaging studies (ultrasound, CT scan, ERCP, cholecystogram, hida scan)
TX: Gallstone solubilizing agent, diet modification, surgery
F/U: Reevaluation every 3 months; referral to surgeon, if acute

ACUTE HEPATITIS
Additional signs and symptoms
- Fatigue
- Malaise
- Arthralgia
- Myalgia
- Headache
- Anorexia
- Photophobia
- Cough
- Sore throat
- Liver and lymph node enlargement

DX: Hepatitis surface antigen or antibody based testing (A, B, C, D)
TX: Based on symptoms, rest, avoidance of alcohol and hepatotoxic substances, safer sex practices
F/U: For hepatitis A and E, reevaluation every 2 to 4 weeks; for hepatitis B, C, D, referral to hepatologist or gastroenterologist

CHOLESTASIS
Additional signs and symptoms
- Prolonged attacks of jaundice
- Fatigue
- Weight loss
- Anorexia
- RUQ pain

DX: History, LFT, imaging studies (CT scan, MRI, cholangiography, ultrasound, ERCP)
TX: Treatment of causative factor (such as certain drugs), diet modification, medication (antibacterial, phenobarbital), surgery
F/U: Referral to gastroenterologist

ACUTE PANCREATITIS
Signs and symptoms
- Severe relentless epigastric pain that radiates to the back
- Nausea
- Persistent vomiting
- Abdominal distention
- Turner's or Cullen's sign (possibly)
- Fever
- Tachycardia
- Hypoactive bowel sounds
- Abdominal rigidity and tenderness
- Shock (if severe)

DX: Labs (amylase, lipase, CBC, electrolytes, calcium, albumin, LFT), imaging studies (CT scan, ultrasound)
TX: Based on symptoms, I.V. hydration, medication (analgesics, electrolyte replacement, insulin therapy)
F/U: Referral to gastroenterologist

Additional differential diagnoses: agnogenic ▪ cholangitis ▪ cholecystitis ▪ cirrhosis ▪ Dubin-Johnson syndrome ▪ glucose-6-phosphate dehydrogenase deficiency ▪ hemolytic anemia (acquired) ▪ hepatic abscess ▪ hepatic cancer ▪ leptospirosis ▪ myeloid metaplasia ▪ pancreatic cancer ▪ sickle cell anemia ▪ Zieve syndrome

Other causes: androgenic steroids ▪ erythromycin estolate ▪ HMG-CoA reductase inhibitors ▪ hormonal contraceptives ▪ isoniazid ▪ I.V. tetracycline ▪ mercaptopurine ▪ niacin ▪ phenothiazines ▪ phenylbutazone ▪ portocaval shunt ▪ sulfonamides ▪ troleandomycin ▪ upper abdominal surgery

Jaw pain

Jaw pain may arise from either or both of the bones that hold the teeth in the jaw—the maxilla (upper jaw) and the mandible (lower jaw). Jaw pain also includes pain in the temporomandibular joint (TMJ), where the mandible meets the temporal bone. Life-threatening disorders, such as myocardial infarction and tetany, also produce jaw pain, as do drugs (especially phenothiazine) and dental or surgical procedures.

Jaw pain may develop gradually or abruptly and may range from barely noticeable to excruciating, depending on its cause. It usually results from a disorder of the teeth, soft tissue, or glands of the mouth or throat or from local trauma or infection. Systemic causes include musculoskeletal, neurologic, cardiovascular, endocrine, immunologic, metabolic, and infectious disorders.

Jaw pain is seldom a primary indicator of any one disorder; however, some of its causes are medical emergencies.

 ALERT

If the patient complains of sudden severe jaw pain:
- *take his vital signs*
- *find out if the pain radiates to other areas*
- *place him on a cardiac monitor and administer oxygen*
- *assess him for associated symptoms of a life-threatening disorder, such as chest pain or shortness of breath*
- *initiate emergency measures, if necessary.*
  If the patient's condition permits, perform a focused assessment.

HISTORY
- Ask the patient to describe the character, intensity, and frequency of the pain. When did he first notice the jaw pain? Did it arise suddenly or gradually? Has it become more severe or frequent? Also, ask about recent trauma.
- Ask the patient where on the jaw he feels pain. Does the pain radiate to other areas? Ask the patient about aggravating or alleviating factors.
- Ask the patient about associated signs and symptoms, such as joint or chest pain, fatigue, headache, malaise, anorexia, weight loss, intermittent claudication, diplopia, and hearing loss.

PHYSICAL EXAMINATION
- Inspect the painful area for redness, and palpate for edema or warmth. Facing the patient directly, look for facial asymmetry indicating swelling.
- Check the TMJ. Place your fingertips just anterior to the external auditory meatus. Ask the patient to open and close his mouth, and then ask him to thrust out and retract his jaw. Note the presence of crepitus, an abnormal scraping or grinding sensation in the joint. (Clicks heard when the jaw is widely spread apart are normal.)
- Observe how wide the patient can open his mouth. Less than 1¼″ (3 cm) or more than 2¼″ (6 cm) between the upper and lower teeth is abnormal.
- Palpate the parotid area for pain and swelling, and inspect and palpate the oral cavity for lesions, elevation of the tongue, or masses.

SPECIAL CONSIDERATIONS
If the patient is in severe pain, withhold food, liquids, and medications he normally takes until the diagnosis is confirmed. Apply an ice pack if the jaw is swollen, and discourage the patient from talking or moving his jaw.

 PEDIATRIC POINTERS
- *Be alert for nonverbal signs of jaw pain, such as rubbing the affected area or wincing while talking or swallowing.*
- *Mumps cause unilateral or bilateral swelling from the lower mandible to the zygomatic arch.*
- *Parotiditis due to cystic fibrosis may cause jaw pain.*
- *When trauma causes jaw pain in children, always consider the possibility of abuse.*

PATIENT COUNSELING
If jaw pain is the result of abuse, encourage the patient to seek counseling and protection. If the patient is a child and abuse is suspected, consult social services.

JAW PAIN

HPI

Focused PE: Cardiovascular and neurologic systems, HEENT

Common signs and symptoms
- Chest pain that may radiate to the neck, jaw, and arms
- Chest tightness or pressure
- Dyspnea
- Nausea and vomiting
- Tachycardia
- Palpitations
- Diaphoresis
- Dizziness
- Syncope
- Gallops and murmurs

MI
Additional signs and symptoms
- Feeling of impending doom
- Pain that may escalate to crushing
- Hypotension or hypertension
- Pallor
- Clammy skin

ACUTE SINUSITIS
Signs and symptoms
- Maxillary, cheek, and tooth pain
- Yellow or green nasal discharge
- Fever
- Pain that gets worse with lying down or bending over
- Malaise
- Early morning periorbital swelling
- Halitosis
- Sore throat
- Headache
- Increased pain on percussion over sinuses
- Negative transillumination

DX: PE, imaging studies (sinus X-ray, CT scan)
TX: Medication (antibiotics, decongestants), air humidification, increased fluid intake
F/U: Reevaluation after 48 hours, then in 10 days

TEMPORAL ARTERITIS
Signs and symptoms
- Headache, focal pain that's unvarying in location
- Jaw claudication
- Tenderness over temporal artery
- Diplopia
- Hemianopsia
- Malaise
- Fever
- Weight loss

DX: ESR, biopsy
TX: Corticosteroids
F/U: Reevaluation in 48 to 72 hours

ANGINA
Additional signs and symptoms
- Pain that typically lasts 2 to 10 minutes and may be provoked by exertion, heavy stress, or a heavy meal

DX: Labs (serial cardiac enzymes, troponin, myoglobin, electrolytes), imaging studies (echocardiogram, CXR, Tc 99m sestamibi scan), ECG, cardiac catheterization
TX: Maintenance of ABCs; medication (based on severity of myocardial involvement and medical history — antithrombic agents, vasodilators, analgesics, beta-adrenergic agents, thrombolytics, anticoagulants, platelet aggregation inhibitors, anxiolytics, antiarrhythmics); low-fat, low-sodium diet; PCI; surgery
F/U: Referral to cardiologist

Additional differential diagnoses: arthritis ▪ head and neck cancer ▪ hypocalcemic tetany ▪ Ludwig's angina ▪ osteomyelitis ▪ sialolithiasis ▪ suppurative parotitis ▪ tetanus ▪ TMJ syndrome ▪ trauma ▪ trigeminal neuralgia

Other causes: drugs that reduce calcium ▪ phenothiazines

Jugular vein distention

Jugular vein distention (JVD) is the abnormal fullness and height of the pulse waves in the internal or external jugular veins. When a patient in a supine position has his head elevated 45 degrees, a pulse wave height greater than 1½" (4 cm) above the angle of Louis indicates distention. Engorged, distended veins reflect increased venous pressure in the right side of the heart. This sign characteristically occurs in heart failure and other cardiovascular disorders. (See *Evaluating jugular vein distention.*)

 ALERT

If you detect JVD and the patient is in respiratory distress:
- *take his vital signs*
- *assess his skin for paleness, coolness, and clamminess*
- *auscultate lung sounds*
- *provide supplemental oxygen and monitor cardiac status.*

If the patient isn't in respiratory distress, perform a focused assessment.

HISTORY
- Ask the patient if he has gained weight recently. Does he have difficulty putting on shoes? Are his ankles swollen?
- Ask the patient if he has experienced chest pain, shortness of breath, paroxysmal nocturnal dyspnea, anorexia, nausea, and vomiting.
- Review the patient's medical history for cancer and heart, pulmonary, or renal disease.

- Ask the patient if he has experienced a decrease in urine output.

PHYSICAL EXAMINATION
- Take the patient's vital signs, and then weigh him, if possible.
- Inspect and palpate the extremities and face for edema.
- Auscultate the lungs for crackles and the heart for gallops and a pericardial friction rub.
- Inspect the abdomen for distention, and palpate and percuss for an enlarged liver.

SPECIAL CONSIDERATIONS
If the patient has cardiac tamponade, prepare him for pericardiocentesis. If he doesn't have cardiac tamponade, restrict fluids and monitor his intake and output.

 PEDIATRIC POINTERS
Jugular vein distention is difficult (sometimes impossible) to evaluate in most infants and toddlers because of their short, thick necks. Even in school-age children, measurement of jugular vein distention can be unreliable because the sternal angle may not be the same distance (5 to 7 cm) above the right atrium, as it is in adults.

PATIENT COUNSELING
Teach the patient with chronic heart failure about appropriate treatments, including dietary restrictions such as a low-sodium diet. Also, instruct him to report edema of the lower extremities and weight gain of 2 lb (0.9 kg) in one day or 5 lb (2.3 kg) in one week.

EVALUATING JUGULAR VEIN DISTENTION

To evaluate jugular vein distention (JVD), first place the patient in the supine position so that you can visualize pulsations reflected from the right atrium. Then elevate the head of the bed 45 to 90 degrees. (Normally, veins distend only when a patient lies flat.) Next, locate the angle of Louis (sternal notch) — the reference point for measuring venous pressure. To do so, palpate the clavicles where they join the sternum (the suprasternal notch). Place your first two fingers on the suprasternal notch. Then, without lifting them from the skin, slide them down the sternum until you feel a bony protuberance — this is the angle of Louis.

Find the internal jugular vein (which indicates venous pressure more reliably than the external jugular vein). Shine a flashlight across the patient's neck to create shadows that highlight his venous pulse. Be sure to distinguish jugular venous pulsations from carotid arterial pulsations. One way to do this is to palpate the vessel: Arterial pulsations continue, whereas venous pulsations disappear with light finger pressure. Also, venous pulsations increase or decrease with changes in body position, but arterial pulsations remain constant.

Next, locate the highest point along the vein

where you can see pulsations. Using a centimeter ruler, measure the distance between that high point and the sternal notch. Record this finding as well as the angle at which the patient was lying. A finding greater than 4 cm above the sternal notch, with the head of the bed at a 45-degree angle, indicates JVD.

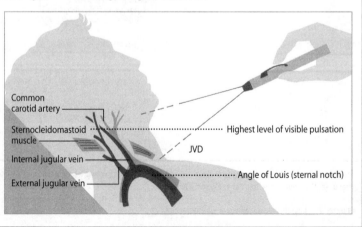

Common carotid artery

Sternocleidomastoid muscle

Internal jugular vein

External jugular vein

Highest level of visible pulsation

JVD

Angle of Louis (sternal notch)

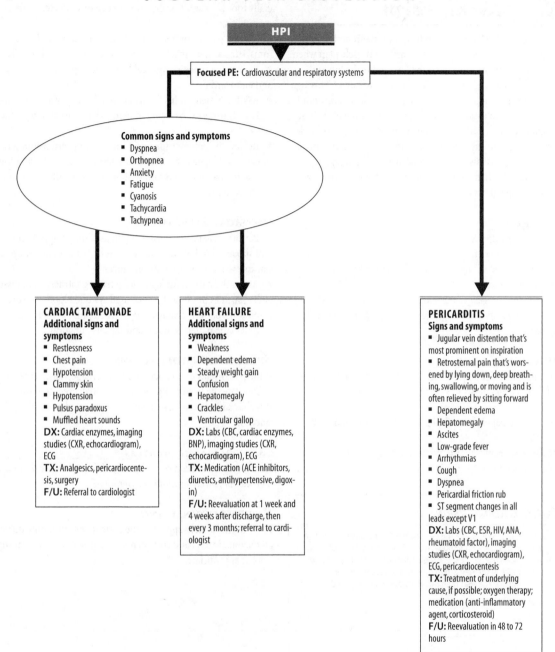

HPI

Focused PE: Cardiovascular and respiratory systems

Common signs and symptoms
- Dyspnea
- Orthopnea
- Anxiety
- Fatigue
- Cyanosis
- Tachycardia
- Tachypnea

CARDIAC TAMPONADE
Additional signs and symptoms
- Restlessness
- Chest pain
- Hypotension
- Clammy skin
- Hypotension
- Pulsus paradoxus
- Muffled heart sounds

DX: Cardiac enzymes, imaging studies (CXR, echocardiogram), ECG
TX: Analgesics, pericardiocentesis, surgery
F/U: Referral to cardiologist

HEART FAILURE
Additional signs and symptoms
- Weakness
- Dependent edema
- Steady weight gain
- Confusion
- Hepatomegaly
- Crackles
- Ventricular gallop

DX: Labs (CBC, cardiac enzymes, BNP), imaging studies (CXR, echocardiogram), ECG
TX: Medication (ACE inhibitors, diuretics, antihypertensive, digoxin)
F/U: Reevaluation at 1 week and 4 weeks after discharge, then every 3 months; referral to cardiologist

PERICARDITIS
Signs and symptoms
- Jugular vein distention that's most prominent on inspiration
- Retrosternal pain that's worsened by lying down, deep breathing, swallowing, or moving and is often relieved by sitting forward
- Dependent edema
- Hepatomegaly
- Ascites
- Low-grade fever
- Arrhythmias
- Cough
- Dyspnea
- Pericardial friction rub
- ST segment changes in all leads except V1

DX: Labs (CBC, ESR, HIV, ANA, rheumatoid factor), imaging studies (CXR, echocardiogram), ECG, pericardiocentesis
TX: Treatment of underlying cause, if possible; oxygen therapy; medication (anti-inflammatory agent, corticosteroid)
F/U: Reevaluation in 48 to 72 hours

Additional differential diagnoses: hypervolemia ▪ leiomyosarcoma ▪ superior vena cava obstruction

Kernig's sign

A reliable early indicator of meningeal irritation, Kernig's sign elicits resistance and hamstring muscle pain when the examiner attempts to extend the knee while the hip and knee are flexed 90 degrees. (See *Eliciting Kernig's sign.*) This sign is usually positive in patients with meningitis or subarachnoid hemorrhage. With these potentially life-threatening disorders, hamstring muscle resistance results from stretching the blood- or exudate-irritated meninges surrounding spinal nerve roots.

Kernig's sign can also indicate a herniated disk or spinal tumor. In these disorders, sciatic pain results from disk or tumor pressure on spinal nerve roots.

➤ **ALERT**

If you elicit a positive Kernig's sign:
- *take the patient's vital signs*
- *test for Brudzinski's sign to obtain further evidence of meningeal irritation*
- *prepare for emergency intervention.*

If you don't suspect meningeal irritation, perform a focused assessment.

HISTORY

- Ask the patient if he feels back pain that radiates down one or both legs. Does he also feel leg numbness, tingling, or weakness?
- Review the patient's medical history for cancer and back injury.

If you suspect meningitis, proceed with these steps:
- Ask the patient or his family to describe the onset of illness.

- Ask the patient or his family about recent infections, especially tooth abscesses or exposure to persons infected with meningitis.
- Ask the patient or his family about other signs and symptoms, such as headache, confusion, fever, and nuchal rigidity.
- Review the patient's medical history for open-head injury and endocarditis.
- Ask the patient or his family about a history of I.V. drug use.

If you suspect subarachnoid hemorrhage, proceed with these steps:
- Review the patient's medical history for hypertension, cerebral aneurysm, head trauma, and arteriovenous malformation.
- Ask the patient or his family about sudden withdrawal of an antihypertensive.

PHYSICAL ASSESSMENT

- Perform a neurologic assessment, including pupil reaction and size and level of consciousness. Test for hemiparesis, aphasia, and sensory or visual disturbances.
- Assess the patient for signs of increasing intracranial pressure (ICP), such as bradycardia, increased systolic blood pressure, respiratory pattern change, and widened pulse pressure.
- Assess the patient's motor and sensory function.

SPECIAL CONSIDERATIONS

If the patient has a subarachnoid hemorrhage, darken the room and elevate the head of the bed at least 30 degrees to reduce ICP. If he has a herniated disk or spinal tumor, he may require pelvic traction.

 PEDIATRIC POINTERS

Kernig's sign is considered ominous in children because they have a greater potential for rapid deterioration.

PATIENT COUNSELING

Provide emotional support to the patient and his family during all diagnostic tests and treatments. Refer them for spiritual support, if appropriate.

ELICITING KERNIG'S SIGN

To elicit Kernig's sign, place the patient in a supine position. Flex her leg at the hip and knee, as shown here. Then try to extend the leg while you keep the hip flexed. If the patient experiences pain and possibly spasm in the hamstring muscle and resists further extension, you can assume that meningeal irritation has occurred.

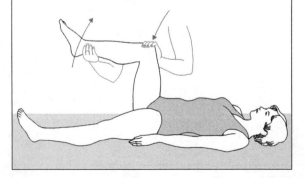

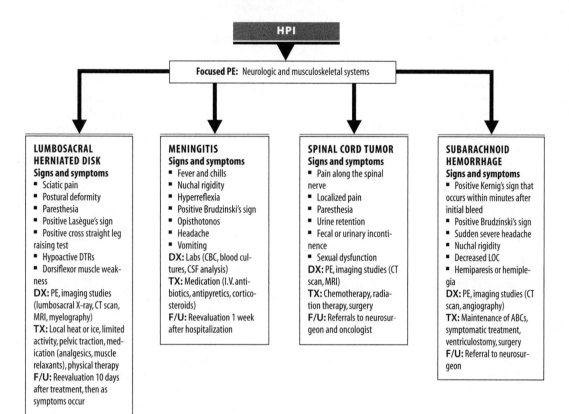

HPI

Focused PE: Neurologic and musculoskeletal systems

LUMBOSACRAL HERNIATED DISK
Signs and symptoms
- Sciatic pain
- Postural deformity
- Paresthesia
- Positive Lasègue's sign
- Positive cross straight leg raising test
- Hypoactive DTRs
- Dorsiflexor muscle weakness

DX: PE, imaging studies (lumbosacral X-ray, CT scan, MRI, myelography)
TX: Local heat or ice, limited activity, pelvic traction, medication (analgesics, muscle relaxants), physical therapy
F/U: Reevaluation 10 days after treatment, then as symptoms occur

MENINGITIS
Signs and symptoms
- Fever and chills
- Nuchal rigidity
- Hyperreflexia
- Positive Brudzinski's sign
- Opisthotonos
- Headache
- Vomiting

DX: Labs (CBC, blood cultures, CSF analysis)
TX: Medication (I.V. antibiotics, antipyretics, corticosteroids)
F/U: Reevaluation 1 week after hospitalization

SPINAL CORD TUMOR
Signs and symptoms
- Pain along the spinal nerve
- Localized pain
- Paresthesia
- Urine retention
- Fecal or urinary incontinence
- Sexual dysfunction

DX: PE, imaging studies (CT scan, MRI)
TX: Chemotherapy, radiation therapy, surgery
F/U: Referrals to neurosurgeon and oncologist

SUBARACHNOID HEMORRHAGE
Signs and symptoms
- Positive Kernig's sign that occurs within minutes after initial bleed
- Positive Brudzinski's sign
- Sudden severe headache
- Nuchal rigidity
- Decreased LOC
- Hemiparesis or hemiplegia

DX: PE, imaging studies (CT scan, angiography)
TX: Maintenance of ABCs, symptomatic treatment, ventriculostomy, surgery
F/U: Referral to neurosurgeon

L Leg pain

Although leg pain commonly signifies a musculoskeletal disorder, it can also result from a more serious vascular or neurologic disorder. The pain may arise suddenly or gradually and may be localized or affect the entire leg. Constant or intermittent, it may feel dull, burning, sharp, shooting, or tingling. Leg pain commonly affects locomotion, limiting weight bearing. Severe leg pain that follows cast application for a fracture may signal limb-threatening compartment syndrome. Sudden onset of severe leg pain in a patient with underlying vascular insufficiency may signal acute deterioration, possibly requiring an arterial graft or amputation. (See *Highlighting causes of local leg pain.*)

➤ ALERT

If the patient has acute leg pain and a history of trauma:
- *quickly take his vital signs and determine the leg's neurovascular status by assessing distal pulses, skin color, and temperature*
- *observe his leg position, and check for swelling, gross deformities, or abnormal rotation*
- *prepare for emergency surgery, if appropriate.*
  If the patient's condition permits, perform a focused assessment.

HISTORY

- Ask the patient when the pain began and have him describe its intensity, character, and pattern. Is the pain worse in the morning, at night, or with movement? If the pain doesn't prevent him from walking, ask him if he uses a crutch or other assistive device.
- Ask the patient if he's experiencing other associated signs and symptoms.
- Review the patient's medical history for leg injury or surgery and joint, vascular, or back problems. Also, ask the patient if there's a family history of these disorders.
- Obtain a drug history, including prescription and over-the-counter drugs, herbal remedies, and recreational drugs. Also, ask the patient about alcohol intake.

PHYSICAL ASSESSMENT

- Observe the patient walk, if his condition permits.
- Observe how he holds his leg while standing and sitting.
- Palpate the legs, buttocks, and lower back to determine the extent of pain and tenderness. If fracture has been ruled out, test range of motion (ROM) in the hip and knee.
- Test reflexes with the patient's leg straightened and raised, noting any action that causes pain.
- Compare both legs for symmetry, movement, and active ROM. Also, assess pulses, color, sensation, and strength.
- If the patient wears a leg cast, splint, or restrictive dressing, carefully check distal circulation, sensation, and mobility, and stretch his toes to elicit associated pain.

SPECIAL CONSIDERATIONS

If the patient has acute leg pain, closely monitor his neurovascular status by frequently assessing distal pulses, temperature, and color of both legs.

🅰 PEDIATRIC POINTERS

- *Common pediatric causes of leg pain include fracture, osteomyelitis, and bone cancer.*
- *If parents fail to give an adequate explanation for a leg fracture, consider the possibility of child abuse.*

PATIENT COUNSELING

If the patient has chronic leg pain, advise him on the appropriate anti-inflammatory regimen and teach him to perform ROM exercises. If necessary, teach him how to use a cane, walker, or other assistive device.

HIGHLIGHTING CAUSES OF LOCAL LEG PAIN

Various disorders cause hip, knee, ankle, or foot pain, which may radiate to surrounding tissues and be reported as leg pain. Local pain is commonly accompanied by tenderness, swelling, and deformity in the affected area.

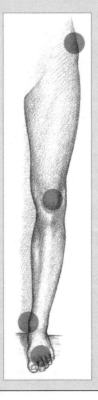

ANKLE PAIN
Achilles tendon
   contracture
Arthritis
Dislocation
Fracture
Sprain
Tenosynovitis

KNEE PAIN
Arthritis
Bursitis
Chondromalacia
Contusion
Cruciate ligament
   injury
Dislocation
Fracture
Meniscal injury
Osteochondritis
   dissecans
Phlebitis
Popliteal cyst
Radiculopathy
Ruptured extensor
   mechanism
Sprain

HIP PAIN
Arthritis
Avascular necrosis
Bursitis
Dislocation
Fracture
Sepsis
Tumor

FOOT PAIN
Arthritis
Bunion
Callus or corn
Dislocation
Flatfoot
Fracture
Gout
Hallux rigidus
Hammer toe
Ingrown toenail
Köhler's disease
Morton's neuroma
Occlusive vascular
   disease
Plantar fasciitis
Plantar wart
Radiculopathy
Tabes dorsalis
Tarsal tunnel syn-
   drome

HPI

Focused PE: Neurovascular and musculoskeletal systems

Common signs and symptoms
- Ecchymosis of the affected leg
- Edema
- Loss of mobility

FRACTURE
Additional signs and symptoms
- Severe pain in affected leg that increases with movement
- Impaired neurovascular status
- Deformity
- Muscle spasm
- Bony crepitation

Common signs and symptoms
- Calf tenderness or severe pain, swelling, and warmth
- Engorged, palpable superficial veins

COMPARTMENT SYNDROME
Signs and symptoms
- Progressive, intense lower leg pain that increases with passive muscle stretching
- Pain that increases with restrictive dressing or treatment
- Muscle weakness and paresthesia
- Normal distal circulation

DX: History of injury or compression of limb, PE
TX: Analgesics, surgery
F/U: Immediate referral to orthopedic or vascular surgeon

STRAIN OR SPRAIN
Additional signs and symptoms
- Sharp transient pain (acute)
- Stiffness, soreness, and generalized leg tenderness (chronic)
- Pain with active or passive motion

DX: PE, X-ray of affected leg
TX: RICE therapy, orthosis, crutches, analgesics
F/U: For fracture, referral to orthopedic surgeon; for strain or sprain, reevaluation after 6 to 8 weeks (unless symptoms worsen, then referral to orthopedic surgeon)

DEEP VEIN THROMBOPHLEBITIS
Additional signs and symptoms
- Positive Homans' sign
DX: PE, imaging studies (contrast venography, impedence plethysmography, Doppler ultrasound)
TX: Bed rest for 1 to 2 days, medication (anticoagulants, thrombolytics [investigational])
F/U: For initial episodes, monitoring of PT weekly for 3 weeks, then monthly for up to 6 months; for recurrent episodes, treatment and monitoring once per year

THROMBOPHLEBITIS (SUPERFICIAL)
DX: PE, labs (WBC, blood culture [septic], coagulation studies, platelet function test [aseptic]), ultrasound
TX: Medication (antibiotics [septic], anticoagulants, NSAIDs [aseptic]), bed rest, local heat, surgery
F/U: Reevaluation in 1 week

Additional differential diagnoses: bone cancer ▪ infection ▪ occlusive vascular disease ▪ sciatica ▪ varicose veins ▪ venous stasis ulcers

Level of consciousness decrease

A decrease in level of consciousness (LOC), from lethargy to stupor to coma, usually results from a neurologic disorder and commonly signals life-threatening complications of hemorrhage, trauma, or cerebral edema. However, this sign can also result from a metabolic, GI, musculoskeletal, urologic, or cardiopulmonary disorder; severe nutritional deficiency; exposure to a toxin; or drug use. LOC can deteriorate suddenly or gradually and can remain altered temporarily or permanently.

Consciousness is affected by the reticular activating system (RAS), an intricate network of neurons whose axons extend from the brain stem, thalamus, and hypothalamus to the cerebral cortex. A disturbance in any part of this integrated system prevents the intercommunication that makes consciousness possible. Loss of consciousness can result from a bilateral cerebral disturbance, an RAS disturbance, or both. Cerebral dysfunction characteristically produces the least dramatic decrease in a patient's LOC. In contrast, dysfunction of the RAS produces the most dramatic decrease in LOC—coma.

The most sensitive indicator of a decreased LOC is a change in the patient's mental status. The Glasgow Coma Scale, which measures the ability to respond to verbal, sensory, and motor stimulation, can be used to quickly evaluate a patient's LOC. (See *Glasgow Coma Scale*.)

⚠ ALERT

If the patient has a decreased LOC:
- *evaluate his airway, breathing, and circulation*
- *use the Glasgow Coma Scale to quickly determine LOC and obtain baseline data. If the patient's score is 13 or less, he should be immediately evaluated for a life-threatening occurrence.*

If the patient's condition permits, perform a focused assessment.

HISTORY

- Obtain history information from the patient (if he's lucid) or his family. Ask if the patient complained of headache, dizziness, nausea, visual or hearing disturbances, weakness, fatigue, or other problems before his LOC decreased.
- Ask the patient's family if they noticed changes in the patient's behavior, personality, memory, or temperament.
- Review the patient's medical history for neurologic disease, cancer, and recent trauma.
- Obtain a drug history, including prescription and over-the-counter drugs, herbal remedies, and recreational drugs. Also, ask the patient about alcohol intake.

PHYSICAL ASSESSMENT

Perform a complete neurologic assessment. Because a decreased LOC can result from any one of several disorders that can affect any body system, tailor the physical assessment according to the patient's associated symptoms.

SPECIAL CONSIDERATIONS

Reassess the patient's LOC and neurologic status at least hourly. Ensure airway patency. Take precautions to help ensure the patient's safety.

🅰 PEDIATRIC POINTERS

The primary cause of decreased LOC in children is head trauma, which commonly results from physical abuse or a motor vehicle accident. Other causes include accidental poisoning, hydrocephalus, and meningitis or brain abscess following an ear or respiratory tract infection.

PATIENT COUNSELING

Advise the family to talk to the patient even if he appears comatose; their voices may help reorient the patient to reality.

GLASGOW COMA SCALE

You've probably heard such terms as *lethargic, obtunded,* and *stuporous* used to describe a progressive decrease in a patient's level of consciousness (LOC). However, the Glasgow Coma Scale provides a more accurate, less subjective method of recording such changes, grading consciousness in relation to eye opening and motor and verbal responses.

To use the Glasgow Coma Scale, test the patient's ability to respond to verbal, motor, and sensory stimulation. The scoring system doesn't determine an exact LOC, but it does provide an easy way to describe the patient's basic status and helps to detect and interpret changes from baseline findings. A decreased reaction score in one or more categories may signal an impending neurologic crisis. A score of 7 or less indicates severe neurologic damage.

TEST	REACTION	SCORE
Eyes	Open spontaneously	4
	Open to verbal command	3
	Open to pain	2
	No response	1
Best motor response	Obeys verbal command	6
	Localizes painful stimulus	5
	Flexion — withdrawal	4
	Flexion — abnormal (decorticate rigidity)	3
	Extension (decerebrate rigidity)	2
	No response	1
Best verbal response	Oriented and converses	5
	Disoriented and converses	4
	Inappropriate words	3
	Incomprehensible sounds	2
	No response	1
Total		3 to 15

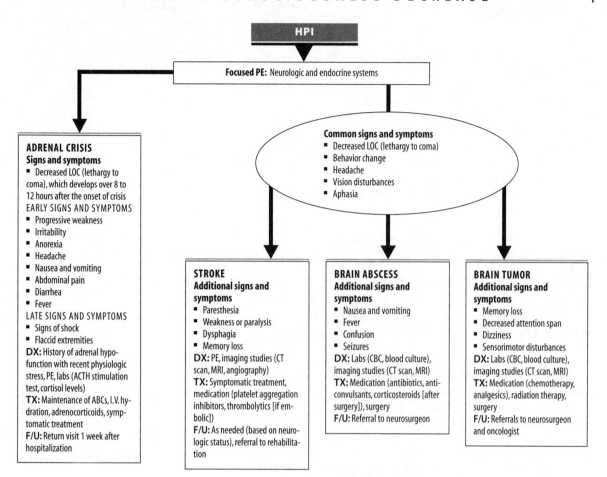

HPI

Focused PE: Neurologic and endocrine systems

Common signs and symptoms
- Decreased LOC (lethargy to coma)
- Behavior change
- Headache
- Vision disturbances
- Aphasia

ADRENAL CRISIS
Signs and symptoms
- Decreased LOC (lethargy to coma), which develops over 8 to 12 hours after the onset of crisis

EARLY SIGNS AND SYMPTOMS
- Progressive weakness
- Irritability
- Anorexia
- Headache
- Nausea and vomiting
- Abdominal pain
- Diarrhea
- Fever

LATE SIGNS AND SYMPTOMS
- Signs of shock
- Flaccid extremities

DX: History of adrenal hypofunction with recent physiologic stress, PE, labs (ACTH stimulation test, cortisol levels)
TX: Maintenance of ABCs, I.V. hydration, adrenocorticoids, symptomatic treatment
F/U: Return visit 1 week after hospitalization

STROKE
Additional signs and symptoms
- Paresthesia
- Weakness or paralysis
- Dysphagia
- Memory loss

DX: PE, imaging studies (CT scan, MRI, angiography)
TX: Symptomatic treatment, medication (platelet aggregation inhibitors, thrombolytics [if embolic])
F/U: As needed (based on neurologic status), referral to rehabilitation

BRAIN ABSCESS
Additional signs and symptoms
- Nausea and vomiting
- Fever
- Confusion
- Seizures

DX: Labs (CBC, blood culture), imaging studies (CT scan, MRI)
TX: Medication (antibiotics, anticonvulsants, corticosteroids [after surgery]), surgery
F/U: Referral to neurosurgeon

BRAIN TUMOR
Additional signs and symptoms
- Memory loss
- Decreased attention span
- Dizziness
- Sensorimotor disturbances

DX: Labs (CBC, blood culture), imaging studies (CT scan, MRI)
TX: Medication (chemotherapy, analgesics), radiation therapy, surgery
F/U: Referrals to neurosurgeon and oncologist

Additional differential diagnoses: cerebral aneurysm (ruptured) ▪ cerebral contusion ▪ diabetic ketoacidosis ▪ encephalitis ▪ encephalomyelitis (postvaccinal) ▪ encephalopathy ▪ epidural hemorrhage (acute) ▪ heatstroke ▪ hypercapnia with pulmonary disease ▪ hyperglycemic hyperosmolar nonketotic coma ▪ hypernatremia ▪ hyperventilation syndrome ▪ hypokalemia ▪ hyponatremia ▪ hypothermia ▪ intracerebral hemorrhage ▪ meningitis ▪ myxedema crisis ▪ poisoning ▪ pontine hemorrhage ▪ seizure disorders ▪ shock ▪ subdural hematoma (chronic) ▪ subdural hemorrhage (acute) ▪ thyroid storm ▪ TIA ▪ West Nile encephalitis

Other causes: alcohol ▪ aspirin ▪ barbiturate overdose ▪ CNS

Light flashes

A cardinal symptom of vision-threatening retinal detachment, light flashes (photopsias) can occur locally or throughout the visual field. The patient usually reports seeing spots, stars, or lightning-type streaks. Flashes can occur suddenly or gradually and can indicate temporary or permanent vision impairment.

In most cases, light flashes signal the splitting of the posterior vitreous membrane into two layers; the inner layer detaches from the retina and the outer layer remains fixed. The sensation of light flashes may result from vitreous traction on the retina, hemorrhage caused by a tear in the retinal capillary, or strands of solid vitreous floating in a local pool of liquid vitreous.

HISTORY

● Ask the patient when the light flashes began. Can he pinpoint their location, or do they occur throughout the visual field?

● If the patient is experiencing eye pain or headache, have him describe it.

● Ask the patient if he wears or has ever worn corrective lenses and if he or a family member has a history of eye or vision problems.

● Review the patient's medical history for other problems, noting especially hypertension or diabetes mellitus, which can cause retinopathy and retinal detachment.

● Obtain an occupational history because light flashes may be related to job stress or eye strain.

PHYSICAL ASSESSMENT

● Inspect the external eye, lids, lashes, and tear puncta for abnormalities and the iris and sclera for signs of bleeding.

● Observe pupil size and shape. Check for reaction to light, accommodation, and consensual light response.

● Test visual acuity in each eye. Also test visual fields; document light flashes the patient reports during this test.

SPECIAL CONSIDERATIONS

Provide emotional support because the patient may be upset about the potential loss of vision.

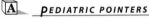 **PEDIATRIC POINTERS**

Children may experience light flashes after minor head trauma.

PATIENT COUNSELING

If the patient has retinal detachment, prepare him for reattachment surgery. If he doesn't have retinal detachment, reassure him that his light flashes are temporary and don't indicate eye damage. Advise him to take an analgesic, darken the room, minimize other stimuli, and obtain adequate sleep when a headache occurs.

LIGHT FLASHES

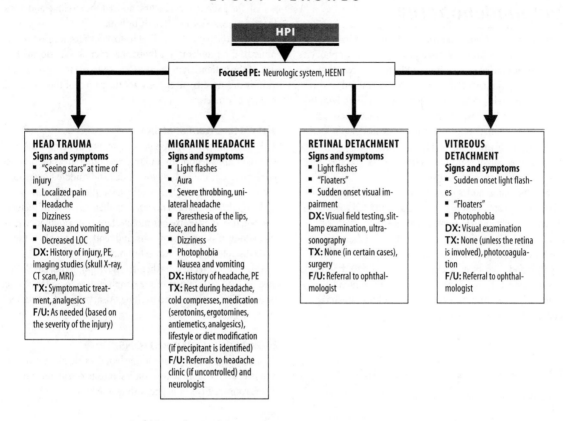

HPI

Focused PE: Neurologic system, HEENT

HEAD TRAUMA
Signs and symptoms
- "Seeing stars" at time of injury
- Localized pain
- Headache
- Dizziness
- Nausea and vomiting
- Decreased LOC

DX: History of injury, PE, imaging studies (skull X-ray, CT scan, MRI)
TX: Symptomatic treatment, analgesics
F/U: As needed (based on the severity of the injury)

MIGRAINE HEADACHE
Signs and symptoms
- Light flashes
- Aura
- Severe throbbing, unilateral headache
- Paresthesia of the lips, face, and hands
- Dizziness
- Photophobia
- Nausea and vomiting

DX: History of headache, PE
TX: Rest during headache, cold compresses, medication (serotonins, ergotomines, antiemetics, analgesics), lifestyle or diet modification (if precipitant is identified)
F/U: Referrals to headache clinic (if uncontrolled) and neurologist

RETINAL DETACHMENT
Signs and symptoms
- Light flashes
- "Floaters"
- Sudden onset visual impairment

DX: Visual field testing, slit-lamp examination, ultrasonography
TX: None (in certain cases), surgery
F/U: Referral to ophthalmologist

VITREOUS DETACHMENT
Signs and symptoms
- Sudden onset light flashes
- "Floaters"
- Photophobia

DX: Visual examination
TX: None (unless the retina is involved), photocoagulation
F/U: Referral to ophthalmologist

Additional differential diagnoses: CNS disorders such as stroke ▪ endocrine disorders such as diabetes mellitus ▪ liver disease

Other causes: alcohol abuse ▪ antihypertensives ▪ drug abuse ▪ radiation therapy ▪ surgery ▪ urologic procedures such as prostatectomy

Lymphadenopathy

Lymphadenopathy—enlargement of one or more lymph nodes—may result from increased production of lymphocytes or reticuloendothelial cells or from infiltration of cells that aren't normally present. This sign may be generalized (involving three or more node groups) or localized. Generalized lymphadenopathy may be caused by an inflammatory process, such as bacterial or viral infection; connective tissue disease; endocrine disorder; or neoplasm. Localized lymphadenopathy usually results from infection or trauma affecting the drained area. (See *Causes of localized lymphadenopathy*.)

Normally, lymph nodes range from ¼″ to 1″ (0.5 to 2.5 cm) in diameter and are discrete, mobile, nontender and, except in children, nonpalpable. (However, palpable nodes may be normal in adults.) Nodes that exceed 1⅛″ (3 cm) in diameter are cause for concern. They may be tender, and the skin overlying the lymph node may be erythematous, suggesting a draining lesion. Or they may be hard and fixed, tender or nontender, suggesting a malignant tumor. Assess the patient for unilateral versus bilateral areas of lymphadenopathy.

HISTORY

- Ask the patient when he first noticed the swelling and if it's located on one side of his body or both.
- Review the patient's medical history for recent infection and other health problems. If a biopsy has ever been performed on one of the patient's lymph nodes, check to see if it revealed previously diagnosed cancer. Also, ask the patient if there's a family history of cancer.

PHYSICAL ASSESSMENT

- Palpate the entire lymph node system to determine the extent of lymphadenopathy and to detect other areas of local enlargement. Use the pads of your index and middle fingers to move the skin over underlying tissues at the nodal area.
- If you detect enlarged nodes, note their size in centimeters and whether they're fixed or mobile, tender or nontender, erythematous or nonerythematous, and tender or rough. Is the node discrete or does the area feel matted?
- If you detect tender, erythematous lymph nodes, check the area drained by that part of the lymph system for signs of infection, such as erythema and swelling. Also, palpate for and percuss the spleen.

SPECIAL CONSIDERATIONS

Expect to obtain blood for routine blood work, platelet count, and liver and renal function studies. If tests reveal infection, check your facility's policy regarding infection control.

Ⓐ PEDIATRIC POINTERS

Infection is the most common cause of lymphadenopathy in children. The condition is commonly associated with otitis media and pharyngitis.

PATIENT COUNSELING

Tell the patient that a fever under 101° F (38.3° C) may assist recovery and shouldn't be treated with an antipyretic, unless he's very uncomfortable. Advise him to try and soothe the fever with tepid baths.

CAUSES OF LOCALIZED LYMPHADENOPATHY

Various disorders can cause localized lymphadenopathy, but this sign usually results from infection or trauma affecting the drained area. Here you'll find some common causes of lymphadenopathy listed according to the areas affected.

AURICULAR
- Erysipelas
- Herpes zoster ophthalmicus
- Infection
- Rubella
- Squamous cell carcinoma
- Styes or chalazion
- Tularemia

AXILLARY
- Breast cancer
- Lymphoma
- Mastitis

CERVICAL
- Cat-scratch fever
- Facial or oral cancer
- Infection
- Mononucleosis
- Mucocutaneous lymph node syndrome
- Rubella
- Rubeola
- Thyrotoxicosis
- Tonsillitis
- Tuberculosis
- Varicella

INGUINAL AND FEMORAL
- Carcinoma
- Chancroid
- Lymphogranuloma venereum
- Syphilis

OCCIPITAL
- Roseola
- Scalp infection
- Seborrheic dermatitis
- Tick bite
- Tinea capitis

POPLITEAL
- Infection

SUBMAXILLARY AND SUBMENTAL
- Cystic fibrosis
- Dental infection
- Gingivitis
- Glossitis

SUPRACLAVICULAR
- Neoplastic disease

LYMPHADENOPATHY

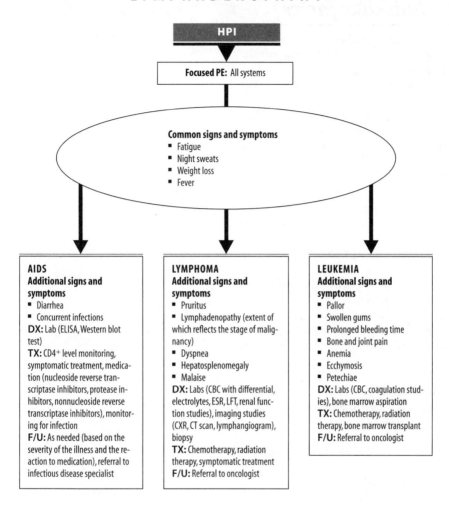

HPI

Focused PE: All systems

Common signs and symptoms
- Fatigue
- Night sweats
- Weight loss
- Fever

AIDS
Additional signs and symptoms
- Diarrhea
- Concurrent infections

DX: Lab (ELISA, Western blot test)
TX: CD4+ level monitoring, symptomatic treatment, medication (nucleoside reverse transcriptase inhibitors, protease inhibitors, nonnucleoside reverse transcriptase inhibitors), monitoring for infection
F/U: As needed (based on the severity of the illness and the reaction to medication), referral to infectious disease specialist

LYMPHOMA
Additional signs and symptoms
- Pruritus
- Lymphadenopathy (extent of which reflects the stage of malignancy)
- Dyspnea
- Hepatosplenomegaly
- Malaise

DX: Labs (CBC with differential, electrolytes, ESR, LFT, renal function studies), imaging studies (CXR, CT scan, lymphangiogram), biopsy
TX: Chemotherapy, radiation therapy, symptomatic treatment
F/U: Referral to oncologist

LEUKEMIA
Additional signs and symptoms
- Pallor
- Swollen gums
- Prolonged bleeding time
- Bone and joint pain
- Anemia
- Ecchymosis
- Petechiae

DX: Labs (CBC, coagulation studies), bone marrow aspiration
TX: Chemotherapy, radiation therapy, bone marrow transplant
F/U: Referral to oncologist

Additional differential diagnoses: brucellosis ▪ chronic fatigue syndrome ▪ cytomegalovirus infection ▪ leptospirosis ▪ Lyme disease ▪ mononucleosis (infectious) ▪ mycosis fungoides ▪ rheumatoid arthritis ▪ sarcoidosis ▪ Sjögren's syndrome ▪ syphilis (secondary) ▪ SLE ▪ tuberculous lymphadenitis ▪ Waldenström's macroglobulinemia

Other causes: immunizations such as typhoid vaccination ▪ phenytoin

M Masklike facies

A total loss of facial expression, masklike facies results from bradykinesia, usually due to extrapyramidal damage. Even the rate of eye blinking is reduced to 1 to 4 blinks/minute, producing a characteristic "reptilian" stare. Although a neurologic disorder is the most common cause, masklike facies can also result from certain systemic diseases and the effects of drugs and toxins. The sign typically develops insidiously, at first mistaken by the observer for depression or apathy.

HISTORY

- Ask the patient and his family or friends when they first noticed the masklike facial expression.
- Ask the patient if he's experiencing facial pain. If so, ask him to describe it.
- Ask the patient if he's experiencing limb weakness, paresthesia, or vision disturbances.
- Review the patient's medical history, noting especially neurological disorders and viral infections.
- Obtain a drug history, including prescription and over-the-counter drugs, herbal remedies, and recreational drugs. Ask about changes in dosage or schedule. Also, ask the patient about alcohol intake.

PHYSICAL ASSESSMENT

- Determine the degree of facial muscle weakness by asking the patient to smile and to wrinkle his forehead. Typically, the patient's responses are slowed.
- Inspect the patient's face, and note edema, rash, or facial weakness.
- Perform a neurological assessment.
- Test motor reflexes, noting weakness.

SPECIAL CONSIDERATIONS

If the patient's facial weakness results from Guillain-Barré syndrome or myasthenia gravis, be prepared to initiate emergency respiratory support.

A PEDIATRIC POINTERS

Masklike facies occurs in the juvenile form of Parkinson's disease.

PATIENT COUNSELING

If the patient's masklike facies results from Parkinson's disease, explain to his family that the sign may hide facial clues to depression — a common occurrence with Parkinson's disease.

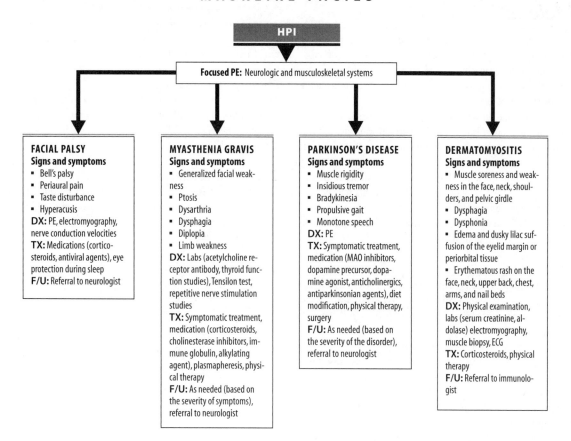

HPI

Focused PE: Neurologic and musculoskeletal systems

FACIAL PALSY
Signs and symptoms
- Bell's palsy
- Periaural pain
- Taste disturbance
- Hyperacusis

DX: PE, electromyography, nerve conduction velocities
TX: Medications (corticosteroids, antiviral agents), eye protection during sleep
F/U: Referral to neurologist

MYASTHENIA GRAVIS
Signs and symptoms
- Generalized facial weakness
- Ptosis
- Dysarthria
- Dysphagia
- Diplopia
- Limb weakness

DX: Labs (acetylcholine receptor antibody, thyroid function studies), Tensilon test, repetitive nerve stimulation studies
TX: Symptomatic treatment, medication (corticosteroids, cholinesterase inhibitors, immune globulin, alkylating agent), plasmapheresis, physical therapy
F/U: As needed (based on the severity of symptoms), referral to neurologist

PARKINSON'S DISEASE
Signs and symptoms
- Muscle rigidity
- Insidious tremor
- Bradykinesia
- Propulsive gait
- Monotone speech

DX: PE
TX: Symptomatic treatment, medication (MAO inhibitors, dopamine precursor, dopamine agonist, anticholinergics, antiparkinsonian agents), diet modification, physical therapy, surgery
F/U: As needed (based on the severity of the disorder), referral to neurologist

DERMATOMYOSITIS
Signs and symptoms
- Muscle soreness and weakness in the face, neck, shoulders, and pelvic girdle
- Dysphagia
- Dysphonia
- Edema and dusky lilac suffusion of the eyelid margin or periorbital tissue
- Erythematous rash on the face, neck, upper back, chest, arms, and nail beds

DX: Physical examination, labs (serum creatinine, aldolase) electromyography, muscle biopsy, ECG
TX: Corticosteroids, physical therapy
F/U: Referral to immunologist

Additional differential diagnoses: Guillain-Barré syndrome ▪ scleroderma

---

Other causes: antipsychotics ▪ carbon monoxide poisoning ▪ manganese poisoning (chronic) ▪ metoclopramide ▪ metyrosine ▪ phenothiazines (particularly piperazine derivatives)

Melena

A common sign of upper GI bleeding, melena is the passage of black, tarry stools. Characteristic color results from bacterial degradation and hydrochloric acid acting on the blood as it travels through the GI tract. At least 60 ml of blood is needed to produce this sign.

Severe melena can signal acute bleeding and life-threatening hypovolemic shock. Although melena usually indicates bleeding from the esophagus, stomach, or duodenum, it can also indicate bleeding from the jejunum, ileum, or ascending colon. This sign can also result from swallowing blood as in epistaxis, from certain drugs, and from alcohol. Because false melena may be caused by ingestion of lead, iron, bismuth, or licorice (which produces black stools without the presence of blood), all black stools should be tested for occult blood.

 ALERT

If the patient is experiencing severe melena:
- *quickly take orthostatic vital signs to detect hypovolemic shock*
- *look for other signs of shock, such as tachycardia, tachypnea, and cool, clammy skin*
- *institute emergency measures, if necessary.*
  If the patient's condition permits, perform a focused assessment.

HISTORY
- Ask the patient when he first noticed that his stools were black and tarry.
- Ask the patient about the frequency and quantity of his bowel movements.
- Ask the patient if he has had melena before.
- Ask the patient about other signs and symptoms, notably hematemesis or hematochezia.
- Obtain a drug history, including prescription and over-the-counter drugs, herbal remedies, and recreational drugs, especially anti-inflammatory drugs and other GI irritants. Also, ask the patient about alcohol intake.
- Review the patient's medical history for GI lesions.

PHYSICAL ASSESSMENT
- Inspect the patient's mouth and nasopharynx for evidence of bleeding.
- Perform an abdominal examination that includes inspection, auscultation, palpation, and percussion.

SPECIAL CONSIDERATIONS
For general comfort, encourage bed rest and keep the patient's perineal area clean and dry to prevent skin irritation and breakdown.

 PEDIATRIC POINTERS
- *Neonates may experience melena neonatorum due to extravasation of blood into the alimentary canal.*
- *In older children, melena usually results from peptic ulcer, gastritis, and Meckel's diverticulum.*

 AGING ISSUES

In elderly patients with recurrent intermittent GI bleeding without a clear cause, angiography or exploratory laparotomy should be considered when the risk from continued anemia is deemed to outweigh the risk associated with the procedures.

PATIENT COUNSELING
Instruct the patient on what to expect from diagnostic testing, which may include blood tests, gastroscopy or other endoscopic studies, barium swallow, and upper GI series.

MELENA

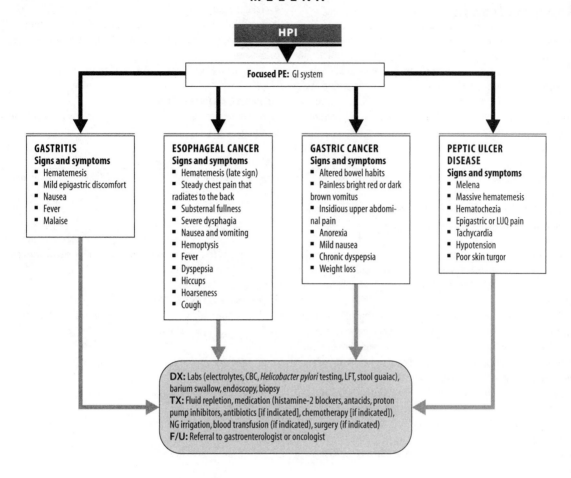

HPI

Focused PE: GI system

GASTRITIS
Signs and symptoms
- Hematemesis
- Mild epigastric discomfort
- Nausea
- Fever
- Malaise

ESOPHAGEAL CANCER
Signs and symptoms
- Hematemesis (late sign)
- Steady chest pain that radiates to the back
- Substernal fullness
- Severe dysphagia
- Nausea and vomiting
- Hemoptysis
- Fever
- Dyspepsia
- Hiccups
- Hoarseness
- Cough

GASTRIC CANCER
Signs and symptoms
- Altered bowel habits
- Painless bright red or dark brown vomitus
- Insidious upper abdominal pain
- Anorexia
- Mild nausea
- Chronic dyspepsia
- Weight loss

PEPTIC ULCER DISEASE
Signs and symptoms
- Melena
- Massive hematemesis
- Hematochezia
- Epigastric or LUQ pain
- Tachycardia
- Hypotension
- Poor skin turgor

DX: Labs (electrolytes, CBC, *Helicobacter pylori* testing, LFT, stool guaiac), barium swallow, endoscopy, biopsy
TX: Fluid repletion, medication (histamine-2 blockers, antacids, proton pump inhibitors, antibiotics [if indicated], chemotherapy [if indicated]), NG irrigation, blood transfusion (if indicated), surgery (if indicated)
F/U: Referral to gastroenterologist or oncologist

Additional differential diagnoses: colon cancer ▪ Ebola virus ▪ esophageal varices (ruptured) ▪ Mallory-Weiss syndrome ▪ pancreatic cancer ▪ small bowel tumors ▪ thrombocytopenia ▪ typhoid fever ▪ yellow fever

Other causes: alcohol ▪ aspirin ▪ NSAIDs

Menorrhagia

Heavy, or significantly heavier menstrual bleeding, menorrhagia may occur as a single episode or a chronic sign. In menorrhagia, bleeding is heavier than the patient's normal menstrual flow; menstrual blood loss is 80 ml or more per monthly period. A form of dysfunctional uterine bleeding, menorrhagia can result from endocrine and hematologic disorders, stress, and certain drugs and procedures.

 ALERT

If the patient is experiencing severe menorrhagia:
- *take her vital signs*
- *assess her for signs of hypovolemic shock, such as pallor, tachycardia, tachypnea, and cool, clammy skin*
- *administer I.V. fluids*
- *prepare her for a pelvic examination.*
  If the patient's condition permits, perform a focused assessment.

HISTORY

- Ask the patient her age at menarche, the normal duration of her menstrual periods, and the normal interval between them.
- Ask the patient the date of her last menses and about recent changes in her normal menstrual pattern. Ask her to describe the character and amount of bleeding.
- Ask the patient about the development of other signs and symptoms before and during the menstrual period.
- Ask the patient if she's sexually active and which type of birth control she uses, if any.
- Obtain a pregnancy history, noting the outcome of each as well as pregnancy-related complications.
- Find out the dates of the patient's most recent pelvic examination and Papanicolaou test and the details of previous gynecologic infections or neoplasms.
- Ask the patient about previous episodes of abnormal bleeding and the outcome of treatment.
- If possible, obtain a pregnancy history of the patient's mother and determine if the patient was exposed to diethylstilbestrol in utero.
- Review the patient's medical history, noting especially surgical procedures; thyroid, adrenal, or hepatic disease; blood dyscrasias; and tuberculosis. Also, ask the patient about a family history of these disorders.
- Ask the patient about her general health and if she's under emotional stress.
- Obtain a drug history, including prescription and over-the-counter drugs, herbal remedies, and recreational drugs. Also, ask the patient about alcohol intake.

PHYSICAL ASSESSMENT

- Take the patient's vital signs.
- Inspect the skin, hair, and nails. Note color and texture.
- Palpate and percuss the abdomen. Note areas of tenderness or masses.
- Assist with a pelvic examination, as appropriate.

SPECIAL CONSIDERATIONS

Herbal remedies, such as ginseng, can cause postmenopausal bleeding.

 PEDIATRIC POINTERS

Irregular menstrual function in young girls may be accompanied by hemorrhage and resulting anemia.

 AGING ISSUES

In postmenopausal women, menorrhagia can't occur. In such patients, vaginal bleeding is usually caused by endometrial atrophy. Malignancy should be ruled out.

PATIENT COUNSELING

Explain to the patient the need for a pelvic examination as well as the need for blood studies and a pregnancy test.

MENORRHAGIA

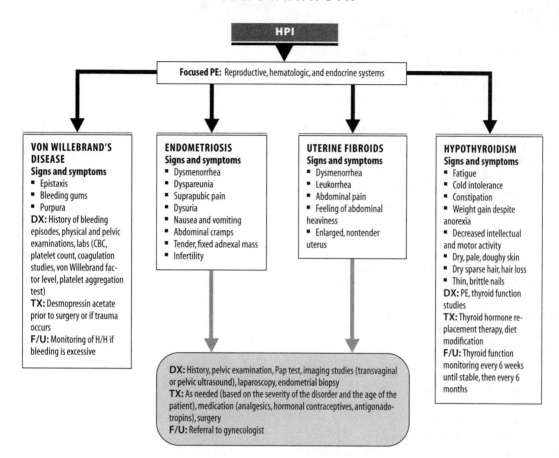

HPI

Focused PE: Reproductive, hematologic, and endocrine systems

VON WILLEBRAND'S DISEASE
Signs and symptoms
- Epistaxis
- Bleeding gums
- Purpura

DX: History of bleeding episodes, physical and pelvic examinations, labs (CBC, platelet count, coagulation studies, von Willebrand factor level, platelet aggregation test)

TX: Desmopressin acetate prior to surgery or if trauma occurs

F/U: Monitoring of H/H if bleeding is excessive

ENDOMETRIOSIS
Signs and symptoms
- Dysmenorrhea
- Dyspareunia
- Suprapubic pain
- Dysuria
- Nausea and vomiting
- Abdominal cramps
- Tender, fixed adnexal mass
- Infertility

UTERINE FIBROIDS
Signs and symptoms
- Dysmenorrhea
- Leukorrhea
- Abdominal pain
- Feeling of abdominal heaviness
- Enlarged, nontender uterus

HYPOTHYROIDISM
Signs and symptoms
- Fatigue
- Cold intolerance
- Constipation
- Weight gain despite anorexia
- Decreased intellectual and motor activity
- Dry, pale, doughy skin
- Dry sparse hair, hair loss
- Thin, brittle nails

DX: PE, thyroid function studies

TX: Thyroid hormone replacement therapy, diet modification

F/U: Thyroid function monitoring every 6 weeks until stable, then every 6 months

DX: History, pelvic examination, Pap test, imaging studies (transvaginal or pelvic ultrasound), laparoscopy, endometrial biopsy
TX: As needed (based on the severity of the disorder and the age of the patient), medication (analgesics, hormonal contraceptives, antigonadotropins), surgery
F/U: Referral to gynecologist

Other causes: anticoagulants ▪ ginseng ▪ hormonal contraceptives ▪ injectable or implanted contraceptives ▪ intrauterine contraceptive devices

Miosis

Miosis—pupillary constriction caused by contraction of the sphincter muscle in the iris—occurs normally as a response to fatigue, increased light, and miotic drugs; as part of the eye's accommodation reflex; and as part of the aging process (pupil size steadily decreases from adolescence to about age 60). However, it can also stem from an ocular or neurologic disorder, trauma, systemic drug therapy, or contact lens overuse. A rare form of miosis—Argyll Robertson pupils—can stem from tabes dorsalis or any one of several neurologic disorders. Occurring bilaterally, these miotic (often pinpoint), unequal, and irregularly shaped pupils don't dilate properly with mydriatic drug use and fail to react to light, although they do constrict on accommodation.

HISTORY

- Ask the patient if he has experienced other ocular signs and symptoms. If so, have him describe their onset, duration, and intensity.
- Ask the patient if he wears contact lenses.
- Review the patient's medical history, noting especially trauma and serious systemic disease.
- Obtain a drug history, including prescription and over-the-counter drugs, herbal remedies, and recreational drugs. Also, ask the patient about alcohol intake.

PHYSICAL ASSESSMENT

- Examine and compare both pupils for size (many persons have a normal discrepancy), color, shape, reaction to light, accommodation, and consensual light response.
- Examine both eyes for additional signs, and then evaluate extraocular muscle function by assessing the six cardinal fields of gaze.
- Test visual acuity in each eye, with and without correction, paying particular attention to blurred or decreased vision in the miotic eye.

SPECIAL CONSIDERATIONS

Certain topical drugs, such as acetylcholine, carbachol, demecarium bromide, echothiophate iodide, and pilocarpine, are used to treat eye disorders specifically for their miotic effect.

A _PEDIATRIC POINTERS_

- _Miosis occurs frequently in the neonate because he's asleep or sleepy most of the time._
- _Bilateral miosis occurs in congenital microcoria._

PATIENT COUNSELING

Instruct the patient on what to expect from diagnostic testing, which may include a complete ophthalmologic examination and a neurologic workup.

MIOSIS

HPI

Focused PE: Neurologic system, HEENT

CLUSTER HEADACHE
Signs and symptoms
- Ipsilateral miosis
- Severe headache
- Tearing
- Conjunctival injection
- Ptosis
- Facial flushing
- Diaphoresis
- Rhinorrhea
- Nasal stuffiness

DX: History, PE
TX: Rest during headache, cold compresses, medication (serotonins, ergotamines, antiemetics, analgesics), lifestyle or diet modification (if precipitant is identified)
F/U: Referral to headache clinic (if uncontrolled)

Common signs and symptoms
- Eye pain
- Photophobia
- Conjunctival injection

CORNEAL FOREIGN BODY
Additional signs and symptoms
- Foreign body sensation or irritation
- Slight vision loss
- Profuse tearing

DX: History, eye examination
TX: Flushing of eye with sterile solution; antibiotic eyedrops; if able, removal of object — if unable, covering of eye until patient can be seen by ophthalmologist
F/U: None if the foreign object is removed; otherwise, referral to ophthalmologist

IRITIS (ACUTE)
Additional signs and symptoms
- Decreased pupillary response
- Pus accumulation in the anterior chamber

POSTERIOR UVEITIS
Additional signs and symptoms
- "Floaters"
- Visual blurring
- Distorted pupil size

HORNER'S SYNDROME
Signs and symptoms
- Moderate miosis ipsilateral to the lesion
- Sluggish pupillary response
- Slight enophthalmos
- Moderate ptosis
- Facial anhidrosis
- Transient conjunctival injection
- Vascular headache

DX: Eye examination, cocaine and hydroxyamphetamine testing
TX: Treatment of underlying cause
F/U: Referral to ophthalmologist

DX: Slit-lamp examination
TX: Medication (topical corticosteroids, mydriatics), treatment of the underlying cause (for posterior uveitis)
F/U: Referral to ophthalmologist

Additional differential diagnoses: cerebrovascular arteriosclerosis ▪ corneal ulcer ▪ hyphema ▪ neuropathy ▪ Parry-Romberg syndrome ▪ pontine hemorrhage ▪ sun stroke ▪ tabes dorsalis

Other causes: chemical burns ▪ contact lens overuse ▪ deep anesthesia ▪ systemic drugs (barbiturates, cholinergics, cholinesterase inhibitors, clonidine [overdose], guanethidine, opiates, reserpine) ▪ topical drugs (acetylcholine, carbachol, demecarium bromide, echothiophate iodide, pilocarpine) ▪ trauma

Mouth lesions

Mouth lesions include ulcers (the most common type), cysts, firm nodules, hemorrhagic lesions, papules, vesicles, bullae, and erythematous lesions. They may occur anywhere on the lips, cheeks, hard and soft palate, salivary glands, tongue, gingivae, or mucous membranes. Many are painful and can be readily detected. Some, however, are asymptomatic; when these occur deep in the mouth, they may be discovered only through a complete oral examination. (See *Common mouth lesions*.)

Mouth lesions can result from trauma, infection, systemic disease, drugs, and radiation therapy.

HISTORY

- Ask the patient when the lesions appeared and whether he has noticed pain, odor, or drainage.
- Ask the patient about associated symptoms, particularly skin lesions.
- Obtain a drug history, including prescription and over-the-counter drugs, herbal remedies, and recreational drugs. Ask the patient about drug allergies. Also, ask him about alcohol intake.
- Review the patient's medical history, noting especially malignancies, sexually transmitted disease, recent infection, and trauma.
- Ask the patient about his dental history, including oral hygiene habits, frequency of dental examinations, and the date of his most recent dental visit.

PHYSICAL ASSESSMENT

- Examine the lips for color and texture.
- Inspect and palpate the buccal mucosa and tongue for color, texture, and contour; note especially any painless ulcers on the sides or base of the tongue. Hold the tongue with a piece of gauze, lift it, and examine its underside and the floor of the mouth. Depress the tongue with a tongue blade, and examine the oropharynx.
- Inspect the teeth and gums, noting missing, broken, or discolored teeth; dental caries; excessive debris; and bleeding, inflamed, swollen, or discolored gums.
- Palpate the neck for adenopathy, especially in a patient older than age 45 who smokes tobacco or uses alcohol excessively.

SPECIAL CONSIDERATIONS

If the patient's mouth lesions are painful, a topical anesthetic may be given.

A | PEDIATRIC POINTERS

- *In neonates, mouth ulcers can result from candidiasis or congenital syphilis.*
- *Causes of mouth ulcers in children include chickenpox, measles, scarlet fever, diphtheria, and hand-foot-and-mouth disease.*

PATIENT COUNSELING

Instruct the patient to avoid irritants, such as highly seasoned foods, citrus fruits, alcohol, and tobacco. As appropriate, teach the patient proper oral hygiene. Tell him to report mouth lesions that don't heal within 2 weeks.

COMMON MOUTH LESIONS

SQUAMOUS CELL CARCINOMA

LICHEN PLANUS

ULCERATION FROM TONGUE BITING

GINGIVAL HYPERPLASIA

RECURRENT APHTHOUS STOMATITIS

SYPHILITIC CHANCRE (RARE)

MOUTH LESIONS

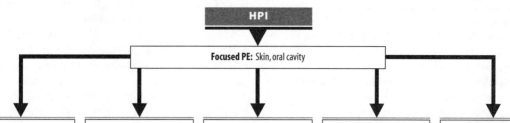

HPI

Focused PE: Skin, oral cavity

DISCOID LUPUS ERYTHEMATOSUS
Signs and symptoms
- Oral lesions on the tongue, buccal mucosa, and palate
- Erythematous areas with white spots and radiating white striae
- Lesions on the face, neck, ears, and scalp

DX: Immunofluorescent staining of skin biopsy

TX: Avoidance of sun exposure, excessive heat, cold, or trauma; medication (topical corticosteroid, antimalarials [if widespread])

F/U: Reevaluation 1 to 2 times per month

ERYTHEMA MULTIFORME
Signs and symptoms
- Sudden onset of vesicles and bullae on the lips and buccal mucosa
- Erythematous macules and papules on the hands, arms, feet, legs, face, and neck
- Lymphadenopathy
- Fever
- Malaise
- Throat and chest pain

DX: PE, Nikolsky's sign

TX: Treatment of underlying cause, moist compresses to skin lesions, medications (analgesics, antipyretics, I.V. corticosteroids [in severe cases])

F/U: Referral to dermatologist

HERPES SIMPLEX
Signs and symptoms
- Prodromal tingling and itching
- Fever
- Pharyngitis
- Vesicles on the oral mucosa that form an erythematous base and then rupture, leaving a painful ulcer that's followed by a yellowish crust
- Submaxillary lymphadenopathy

DX: PE, labs (culture of lesion, Tzanck smear)

TX: Gentle cleaning, anesthetic mouthwash, antiviral agent

F/U: None unless lesions don't heal

SQUAMOUS CELL CANCER
Signs and symptoms
- Ulcer with an elevated indurated border (most commonly on the lower lip)
- Painless lesion

DX: History of smoking and alcohol use, oral examination, biopsy

TX: Surgery

F/U: Referrals to oncologist and surgeon

STOMATITIS
Signs and symptoms
- Recurrent painful ulcerations of the oral mucosa that are usually located on the dorsum of the tongue, gingivae, and hard palate
- Ulcers that are covered by a gray membrane and surrounded by a red halo

DX: Oral examination

TX: Mouth rinses, medication (topical or oral corticosteroids; OTC topical canker medication; for large, nonhealing ulcers, antibiotics)

F/U: None unless the condition continues

Additional differential diagnoses: actinomycosis (cervicofacial) ▪ AIDS ▪ Behçet's syndrome ▪ candidiasis ▪ coxsackie virus ▪ epulis (giant cell) ▪ gingivitis (acute necrotizing ulcerative) ▪ gonorrhea ▪ herpes zoster ▪ inflammatory fibrous hyperplasia ▪ leukoplakia or erythroplakia ▪ lichen planus ▪ mucous duct obstruction ▪ pemphigus ▪ pyogenic granuloma ▪ syphilis ▪ SLE ▪ tuberculosis (oral mucosal)

Other causes: allergic reactions to penicillin, sulfonamides, gold, quinine, streptomycin, phenytoin, aspirin, and barbiturates ▪ chemotherapeutic agents ▪ radiation therapy ▪ trauma

Murmur

Murmurs are auscultatory sounds heard within the heart chambers or major arteries. They're classified by their timing and duration in the cardiac cycle, auscultatory location, loudness, configuration, pitch, and quality.

Timing can be characterized as systolic, holosystolic (continuous throughout systole), diastolic, or continuous throughout systole and diastole; systolic and diastolic murmurs can be further characterized as early, middle, or late. Location refers to the area of maximum loudness, such as the apex, the lower left sternal border, or an intercostal space. Loudness is graded on a scale of 1 to 6, with 1 signifying the faintest audible murmur. Configuration, or shape, refers to the nature of loudness — crescendo, decrescendo, crescendo-decrescendo, decrescendo-crescendo, plateau (even), or variable (uneven). The murmur's pitch may be high or low. Its quality may be described as harsh, rumbling, blowing, scratching, buzzing, musical, or squeaking.

Murmurs can reflect accelerated blood flow through normal or abnormal valves; forward blood flow through a narrowed or irregular valve or into a dilated vessel; blood backflow through an incompetent valve, septal defect, or patent ductus arteriosus; or decreased blood viscosity. Typically the result of an organic heart disease, murmurs occasionally signal an emergency — for example, a loud holosystolic murmur after an acute myocardial infarction may signal papillary muscle rupture or ventricular septal defect. Murmurs may also result from surgical implantation of a prosthetic valve.

HISTORY

- Ask the patient if the murmur is a new discovery or if it has been known since birth or childhood.
- Ask the patient if he has experienced associated signs and symptoms, particularly palpitations, dizziness, syncope, chest pain, dyspnea, and fatigue.
- Review the patient's medical history, noting especially rheumatic fever, heart disease, or heart surgery, particularly prosthetic valve replacement.

PHYSICAL ASSESSMENT

- When you discover a murmur, try to determine its type through careful auscultation. (See *Identifying common murmurs.*) Use the bell of your stethoscope for low-pitched murmurs; the diaphragm for high-pitched murmurs.
- Perform a systematic physical assessment. Note especially the presence of cardiac arrhythmias, jugular vein distention, peripheral edema, and such pulmonary signs as dyspnea, orthopnea, and crackles.
- Palpate the liver for size and tenderness.

SPECIAL CONSIDERATIONS

Prosthetic valve replacement can cause various murmurs, depending on the location, valve composition, and method of operation.

Ⓐ *PEDIATRIC POINTERS*

- *Pathognomonic heart murmurs in infants and young children usually result from congenital heart disease, such as atrial and ventricular septal defects.*
- *Innocent murmurs, such as Still's murmur, are commonly heard in young children, but typically disappear in puberty.*

PATIENT COUNSELING

Instruct the patient on what to expect from diagnostic testing, which may include electrocardiography and echocardiography.

IDENTIFYING COMMON MURMURS

The timing and configuration of a murmur can help you identify its underlying cause. Learn to recognize the characteristics of these common murmurs.

AORTIC INSUFFICIENCY (CHRONIC)

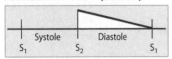

Thickened valve leaflets fail to close correctly, permitting blood backflow into the left ventricle.

AORTIC STENOSIS

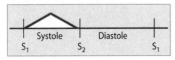

Thickened, scarred, or calcified valve leaflets impede ventricular systolic ejection.

MITRAL PROLAPSE

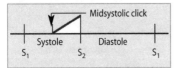

An incompetent mitral valve bulges into the left atrium because of an enlarged posterior leaflet and elongated chordae tendineae.

MITRAL INSUFFICIENCY (CHRONIC)

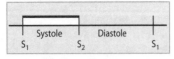

Incomplete mitral valve closure permits blood backflow into the left atrium.

MITRAL STENOSIS

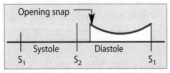

Thickened or scarred valve leaflets cause valve stenosis and restrict blood flow.

MURMUR

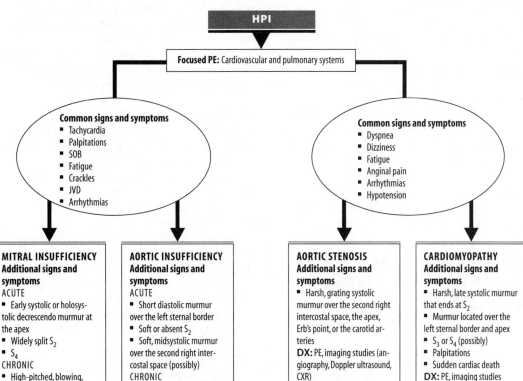

HPI

Focused PE: Cardiovascular and pulmonary systems

Common signs and symptoms
- Tachycardia
- Palpitations
- SOB
- Fatigue
- Crackles
- JVD
- Arrhythmias

Common signs and symptoms
- Dyspnea
- Dizziness
- Fatigue
- Anginal pain
- Arrhythmias
- Hypotension

MITRAL INSUFFICIENCY
Additional signs and symptoms
ACUTE
- Early systolic or holosystolic decrescendo murmur at the apex
- Widely split S_2
- S_4
CHRONIC
- High-pitched, blowing, holosystolic murmur at the apex that radiates to the axilla or back
- Weight loss
- Nocturia
DX: PE, angiography, echocardiogram
TX: Medication (antibiotics [if infection is present], anticoagulants [if atrial fibrillation is present], diuretics)
F/U: Referral to cardiologist

AORTIC INSUFFICIENCY
Additional signs and symptoms
ACUTE
- Short diastolic murmur over the left sternal border
- Soft or absent S_2
- Soft, midsystolic murmur over the second right intercostal space (possibly)
CHRONIC
- High-pitched, blowing, decrescendo diastolic murmur that's best heard over the second or third right intercostal space
DX: PE, imaging studies (ultrasound, angiography, echocardiogram), cardiac catheterization
TX: As needed (based on the severity of symptoms), medications (diuretics, digoxin)
F/U: Referral to cardiologist

AORTIC STENOSIS
Additional signs and symptoms
- Harsh, grating systolic murmur over the second right intercostal space, the apex, Erb's point, or the carotid arteries
DX: PE, imaging studies (angiography, Doppler ultrasound, CXR)
TX: Avoidance of strenuous activity, medication (diuretics, digoxin)
F/U: Reevaluation every 6 to 12 months

CARDIOMYOPATHY
Additional signs and symptoms
- Harsh, late systolic murmur that ends at S_2
- Murmur located over the left sternal border and apex
- S_3 or S_4 (possibly)
- Palpitations
- Sudden cardiac death
DX: PE, imaging studies (CXR, CT scan, MRI, angiography), echocardiogram
TX: Symptomatic treatment, oxygen therapy
F/U: Referral to cardiologist

Additional differential diagnoses: mitral prolapse ▪ mitral stenosis ▪ myxomas ▪ papillary muscle rupture ▪ tricuspid regurgitation ▪ tricuspid stenosis

Other causes: prosthetic valve replacement

Muscle atrophy

Muscle atrophy (muscle wasting) results from denervation or prolonged muscle disuse. When deprived of regular exercise, muscle fibers lose bulk and length, producing a visible loss of muscle size and contour and apparent emaciation or deformity in the affected area. Even slight atrophy usually causes some loss of motion or power.

Atrophy usually results from neuromuscular disease or injury. However, it may also stem from certain metabolic and endocrine disorders and prolonged immobility. Some muscle atrophy also occurs with aging.

HISTORY

● Ask the patient when and where he first noticed the muscle wasting and how it has progressed.

MEASURING LIMB CIRCUMFERENCE

To ensure accurate and consistent limb circumference measurements, use a consistent reference point each time and measure with the limb in full extension. The diagram here shows the correct reference points for arm and leg measurements.

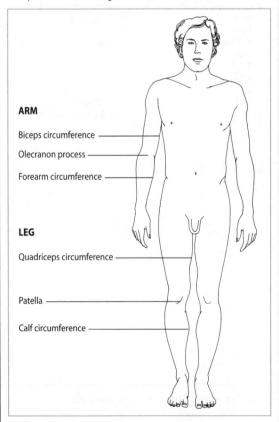

ARM

Biceps circumference

Olecranon process

Forearm circumference

LEG

Quadriceps circumference

Patella

Calf circumference

● Ask the patient about associated signs and symptoms, such as weakness, pain, loss of sensation, and recent weight loss.
● Review the patient's medical history for chronic illness or musculoskeletal or neurologic disorders, including trauma; and endocrine or metabolic disorders.
● Obtain a drug history, including prescription and over-the-counter drugs (especially steroids), herbal remedies, and recreational drugs. Also, ask the patient about alcohol intake.

PHYSICAL ASSESSMENT

● Determine the location and extent of atrophy. Visually evaluate small and large muscles. Check all major muscle groups for size, tonicity, and strength.
● Measure the circumference of all limbs, comparing sides. (See *Measuring limb circumference.*)
● Check for muscle contractures in all limbs by fully extending joints and noting pain or resistance.
● Palpate peripheral pulses for quality and rate, assessing sensory function in and around the atrophied area, and testing deep tendon reflexes.

SPECIAL CONSIDERATIONS

Prolonged steroid therapy interferes with muscle metabolism and leads to atrophy, most prominently in the limbs.

[A] PEDIATRIC POINTERS

● *In young children, profound muscle weakness and atrophy can result from muscular dystrophy.*
● *Muscle atrophy may result from cerebral palsy and poliomyelitis and from paralysis associated with meningocele and myelomeningocele.*

PATIENT COUNSELING

If the patient is immobile, encourage him to perform frequent active range-of-motion exercises. If he can't actively move a muscle, teach his family to provide active-assistive or passive exercises, and apply splints or braces to maintain muscle length.

MUSCLE ATROPHY

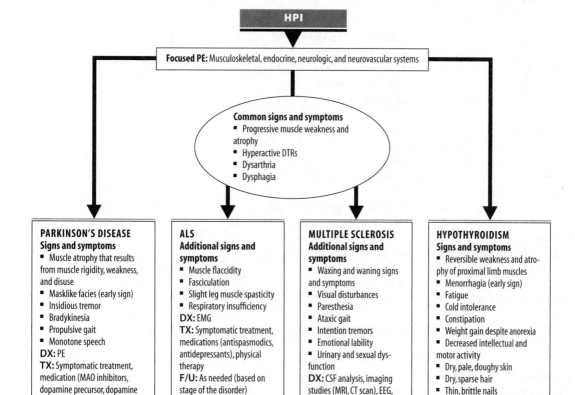

HPI

Focused PE: Musculoskeletal, endocrine, neurologic, and neurovascular systems

Common signs and symptoms
- Progressive muscle weakness and atrophy
- Hyperactive DTRs
- Dysarthria
- Dysphagia

PARKINSON'S DISEASE
Signs and symptoms
- Muscle atrophy that results from muscle rigidity, weakness, and disuse
- Masklike facies (early sign)
- Insidious tremor
- Bradykinesia
- Propulsive gait
- Monotone speech

DX: PE
TX: Symptomatic treatment, medication (MAO inhibitors, dopamine precursor, dopamine agonist, anticholinergics, antiparkinsonian agents), diet modification, physical therapy, surgery
F/U: As needed (based on the severity of the disorder)

ALS
Additional signs and symptoms
- Muscle flaccidity
- Fasciculation
- Slight leg muscle spasticity
- Respiratory insufficiency

DX: EMG
TX: Symptomatic treatment, medications (antispasmodics, antidepressants), physical therapy
F/U: As needed (based on stage of the disorder)

MULTIPLE SCLEROSIS
Additional signs and symptoms
- Waxing and waning signs and symptoms
- Visual disturbances
- Paresthesia
- Ataxic gait
- Intention tremors
- Emotional lability
- Urinary and sexual dysfunction

DX: CSF analysis, imaging studies (MRI, CT scan), EEG, evoked response testing
TX: Symptomatic treatment; medication (antispasmodics, antidepressants, cholinergics, corticosteroids); physical, speech, and occupational therapy
F/U: Referral to neurologist

HYPOTHYROIDISM
Signs and symptoms
- Reversible weakness and atrophy of proximal limb muscles
- Menorrhagia (early sign)
- Fatigue
- Cold intolerance
- Constipation
- Weight gain despite anorexia
- Decreased intellectual and motor activity
- Dry, pale, doughy skin
- Dry, sparse hair
- Thin, brittle nails

DX: PE, thyroid function studies
TX: Thyroid hormone replacement therapy, diet modification
F/U: Monitoring of thyroid function every 6 weeks until stable, then every 6 months

---

Additional differential diagnoses: burns ▪ compartment syndrome and Volkmann's ischemic contracture ▪ herniated disk ▪ hypercortisolism ▪ meniscal tear ▪ osteoarthritis ▪ peripheral nerve trauma ▪ peripheral neuropathy ▪ protein deficiency ▪ radiculopathy ▪ rheumatoid arthritis ▪ spinal cord injury ▪ stroke ▪ thyrotoxicosis

Other causes: immobility ▪ prolonged steroid therapy

Muscle flaccidity

Flaccid muscles (muscle hypotonicity) are profoundly weak and soft, with decreased resistance to movement, increased mobility, and greater than normal range of motion. The result of disrupted muscle innervation, flaccidity can be localized to a limb or muscle group or generalized over the entire body. Its onset may be acute, as in trauma, or chronic, as in neurologic disease.

➤ ALERT

If the patient's muscle flaccidity results from trauma:
- *make sure that his cervical spine is stabilized*
- *quickly determine his respiratory status, and institute emergency measures, if necessary.*

If the patient's condition permits, perform a focused assessment.

HISTORY

- Ask the patient about the onset and duration of muscle flaccidity and precipitating factors.
- Ask the patient about associated signs and symptoms, notably weakness, other muscle changes, and sensory loss or paresthesia.
- Review the patient's medical history, noting especially neurologic or viral events.

PHYSICAL ASSESSMENT

- Examine the affected muscles for atrophy, which indicates a chronic problem.
- Test muscle strength, and check deep tendon reflexes in all limbs.
- Perform a complete neurologic assessment.

SPECIAL CONSIDERATIONS

Reposition a patient with generalized flaccidity every 2 hours to protect his skin integrity. Treat isolated flaccidity by supporting the affected limb in a sling or with a splint.

Ⓐ PEDIATRIC POINTERS

- *An infant or young child with generalized flaccidity may lie in a froglike position, with his hips and knees abducted.*
- *Pediatric causes of muscle flaccidity include myelomeningocele, Lowe's disease, Werdnig-Hoffmann disease, and muscular dystrophy.*

PATIENT COUNSELING

Instruct the patient on what to expect from diagnostic testing, which may include cranial or spinal X-rays, computed tomography scan, and electromyography.

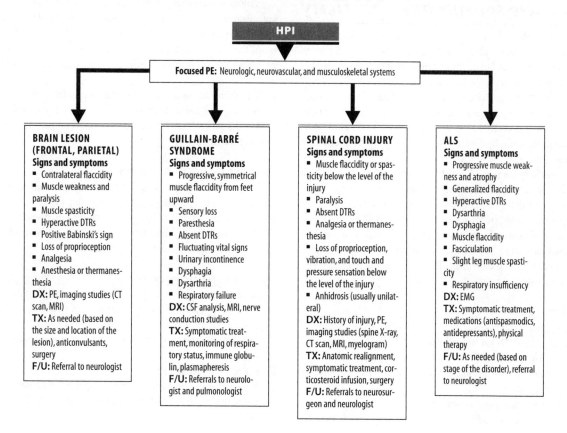

HPI

Focused PE: Neurologic, neurovascular, and musculoskeletal systems

BRAIN LESION (FRONTAL, PARIETAL)
Signs and symptoms
- Contralateral flaccidity
- Muscle weakness and paralysis
- Muscle spasticity
- Hyperactive DTRs
- Positive Babinski's sign
- Loss of proprioception
- Analgesia
- Anesthesia or thermanesthesia

DX: PE, imaging studies (CT scan, MRI)
TX: As needed (based on the size and location of the lesion), anticonvulsants, surgery
F/U: Referral to neurologist

GUILLAIN-BARRÉ SYNDROME
Signs and symptoms
- Progressive, symmetrical muscle flaccidity from feet upward
- Sensory loss
- Paresthesia
- Absent DTRs
- Fluctuating vital signs
- Urinary incontinence
- Dysphagia
- Dysarthria
- Respiratory failure

DX: CSF analysis, MRI, nerve conduction studies
TX: Symptomatic treatment, monitoring of respiratory status, immune globulin, plasmapheresis
F/U: Referrals to neurologist and pulmonologist

SPINAL CORD INJURY
Signs and symptoms
- Muscle flaccidity or spasticity below the level of the injury
- Paralysis
- Absent DTRs
- Analgesia or thermanesthesia
- Loss of proprioception, vibration, and touch and pressure sensation below the level of the injury
- Anhidrosis (usually unilateral)

DX: History of injury, PE, imaging studies (spine X-ray, CT scan, MRI, myelogram)
TX: Anatomic realignment, symptomatic treatment, corticosteroid infusion, surgery
F/U: Referrals to neurosurgeon and neurologist

ALS
Signs and symptoms
- Progressive muscle weakness and atrophy
- Generalized flaccidity
- Hyperactive DTRs
- Dysarthria
- Dysphagia
- Muscle flaccidity
- Fasciculation
- Slight leg muscle spasticity
- Respiratory insufficiency

DX: EMG
TX: Symptomatic treatment, medications (antispasmodics, antidepressants), physical therapy
F/U: As needed (based on stage of the disorder), referral to neurologist

Additional differential diagnoses: cerebellar disease ▪ Huntington's disease ▪ muscle disease ▪ peripheral nerve trauma ▪ peripheral neuropathy ▪ poliomyelitis ▪ seizure disorder

Muscle spasms and spasticity

Muscle spasms, also known as muscle cramps or muscle hypertonicity, are strong, painful contractions. They can occur in virtually any muscle, but are most common in the calf and foot. Muscle spasms typically occur from simple muscle fatigue, commonly after exercise and during pregnancy. However, they may also develop as a result of an electrolyte imbalance, a neuromuscular disorder, or the use of certain drugs. They're typically precipitated by movement, and can usually be relieved by slow stretching.

Spasticity is a state of excessive muscle tone manifested by increased resistance to stretching and heightened reflexes. It's commonly detected by evaluating a muscle's response to passive movement; a spastic muscle offers more resistance when the passive movement is performed quickly. Caused by an upper-motor-neuron lesion, spasticity usually occurs in the arm and leg muscles. Long-term spasticity results in muscle fibrosis and contractures.

 ALERT

If the patient complains of frequent or unrelieved spasms in many muscles, accompanied by paresthesia in his hands and feet:
- *quickly attempt to elicit Chvostek's and Trousseau's signs*
- *evaluate respiratory function, watching for the development of laryngospasm*
- *initiate emergency measures, if necessary.*
If the patient's condition permits, perform a focused assessment.

HISTORY

- Ask the patient about the onset, duration, and progression of muscle spasms, noting whether specific events precipitate onset.
- Ask the patient if he has experienced other muscular changes or related symptoms.
- Ask the patient when the spasms began and how long they typically last.
- Ask the patient if the spasms cause pain. If so, have him describe the pain. Does anything alleviate or aggravate the pain?
- Ask the patient about other signs and symptoms, such as weakness, sensory loss, and paresthesia.
- Ask the patient if he performed recent strenuous exercise or suffered a recent injury.
- Review the patient's medical history, especially noting degenerative or vascular disease.
- Obtain a drug history, including prescription and over-the-counter drugs, herbal remedies, and recreational drugs. (Drugs that commonly produce spasm include diuretics, corticosteroids, and estrogens.) Also, ask the patient about alcohol intake.

PHYSICAL ASSESSMENT

- Evaluate muscle strength and tone. Then, check all major muscle groups, noting whether movement precipitates spasms.
- Test the presence and quality of all peripheral pulses, and examine the limbs for color and temperature changes. Test capillary refill time and inspect for edema, especially in the involved area.
- Test reflexes and evaluate motor and sensory function in all extremities. Also, check for muscle wasting and contractures.
- Take the patient's vital signs and perform a complete neurologic examination.

SPECIAL CONSIDERATIONS

During your examination, keep in mind that generalized spasticity and trismus in a patient with a recent skin puncture or laceration indicates tetanus. If you suspect this rare disorder, look for signs of respiratory distress. If necessary, provide ventilatory support, and monitor the patient closely.

PEDIATRIC POINTERS

- *Muscle spasms rarely occur in children. However, their presence may indicate hypoparathyroidism, osteomalacia, rickets or, rarely, congenital torticollis.*
- *In children, muscle spasticity may be a sign of cerebral palsy.*

PATIENT COUNSELING

Teach the patient to help alleviate muscle spasms by slowly stretching the affected muscle in the direction opposite the contraction.

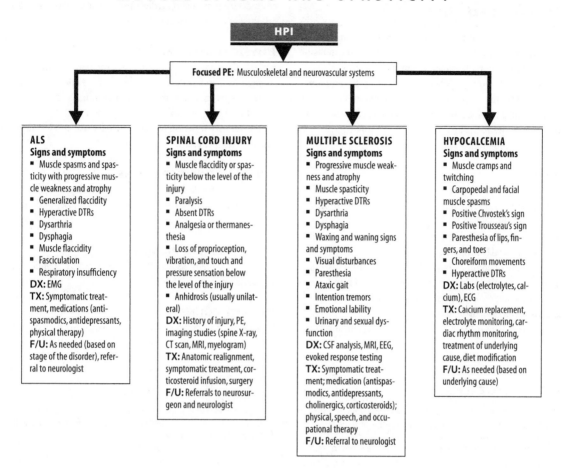

HPI

Focused PE: Musculoskeletal and neurovascular systems

ALS
Signs and symptoms
- Muscle spasms and spasticity with progressive muscle weakness and atrophy
- Generalized flaccidity
- Hyperactive DTRs
- Dysarthria
- Dysphagia
- Muscle flaccidity
- Fasciculation
- Respiratory insufficiency

DX: EMG

TX: Symptomatic treatment, medications (antispasmodics, antidepressants, physical therapy)

F/U: As needed (based on stage of the disorder), referral to neurologist

SPINAL CORD INJURY
Signs and symptoms
- Muscle flaccidity or spasticity below the level of the injury
- Paralysis
- Absent DTRs
- Analgesia or thermanesthesia
- Loss of proprioception, vibration, and touch and pressure sensation below the level of the injury
- Anhidrosis (usually unilateral)

DX: History of injury, PE, imaging studies (spine X-ray, CT scan, MRI, myelogram)

TX: Anatomic realignment, symptomatic treatment, corticosteroid infusion, surgery

F/U: Referrals to neurosurgeon and neurologist

MULTIPLE SCLEROSIS
Signs and symptoms
- Progressive muscle weakness and atrophy
- Muscle spasticity
- Hyperactive DTRs
- Dysarthria
- Dysphagia
- Waxing and waning signs and symptoms
- Visual disturbances
- Paresthesia
- Ataxic gait
- Intention tremors
- Emotional lability
- Urinary and sexual dysfunction

DX: CSF analysis, MRI, EEG, evoked response testing

TX: Symptomatic treatment; medication (antispasmodics, antidepressants, cholinergics, corticosteroids); physical, speech, and occupational therapy

F/U: Referral to neurologist

HYPOCALCEMIA
Signs and symptoms
- Muscle cramps and twitching
- Carpopedal and facial muscle spasms
- Positive Chvostek's sign
- Positive Trousseau's sign
- Paresthesia of lips, fingers, and toes
- Choreiform movements
- Hyperactive DTRs

DX: Labs (electrolytes, calcium), ECG

TX: Calcium replacement, electrolyte monitoring, cardiac rhythm monitoring, treatment of underlying cause, diet modification

F/U: As needed (based on underlying cause)

Additional differential diagnoses for muscle spasms: arterial occlusive disease ▪ dehydration ▪ fracture ▪ hypothyroidism ▪ respiratory alkalosis

Additional differential diagnoses for muscle spasticity: epidural hemorrhage ▪ stroke ▪ tetanus

Other causes for muscle spasm: corticosteroids ▪ diuretics ▪ estrogens

Muscle weakness

Muscle weakness is detected by observing and measuring the strength of an individual muscle or muscle group. It can result from a malfunction in the cerebral hemispheres, brain stem, spinal cord, nerve roots, peripheral nerves, or myoneural junctions and within the muscle itself. Muscle weakness occurs with certain neurologic, musculoskeletal, metabolic, endocrine, and cardiovascular disorders; as a response to certain drugs; and after prolonged immobilization.

HISTORY

- Ask the patient to locate his muscle weakness. Ask him if he has difficulty with specific movements, such as rising from a chair. Also, ask him when he first noticed the weakness.
- Ask the patient whether the muscle weakness worsens with exercise or as the day progresses.
- Ask the patient about associated signs and symptoms, especially muscle or joint pain, altered sensory function, and fatigue.
- Review the patient's medical history for chronic diseases, musculoskeletal or neurologic problems, and recent trauma. Also, ask the patient if there's a family history of chronic muscle weakness, especially in males.

- Obtain a drug history, including prescription and over-the-counter drugs, herbal remedies, and recreational drugs. Also, ask the patient about alcohol intake.

PHYSICAL ASSESSMENT

- Test all major muscles bilaterally. (See *Testing muscle strength.*) When testing, be sure the patient's effort is constant; if it isn't, suspect pain or other reluctance to make the effort.
- Test for range of motion at all major joints.
- Test sensory function in the involved areas, and test deep tendon reflexes bilaterally.

SPECIAL CONSIDERATIONS

Generalized muscle weakness can result from prolonged corticosteroid use, digoxin toxicity, and excessive doses of dantrolene.

A   PEDIATRIC POINTERS

Muscular dystrophy, usually the Duchenne type, is a major cause of muscle weakness in children.

PATIENT COUNSELING

Provide assistive devices, as necessary. Teach the patient and his family safety measures to protect the patient from injury.

TESTING MUSCLE STRENGTH

Obtain an overall picture of the patient's motor function by testing muscle strength in 10 selected muscle groups. Ask him to attempt normal range-of-motion movements against your resistance. If the muscle group is weak, vary the amount of resistance as necessary to permit accurate assessment. If necessary, position the patient so that his limbs don't have to resist gravity, and repeat the test.

Use the following scale to help you rate muscle strength.

0 = Total paralysis
1 = Visible or palpable contraction but no movement

2 = Full muscle movement with force of gravity eliminated
3 = Full muscle movement against gravity, but no movement against resistance

4 = Full muscle movement against gravity; partial movement against resistance
5 = Full muscle movement against gravity and resistance — normal strength

ARM MUSCLES
Biceps
With your hand on the patient's hand, ask him to flex his forearm against your resistance; watch for biceps contraction.

Deltoid muscle
With the patient's arm fully extended, place one hand over his deltoid muscle and the other on his wrist. Ask him to abduct his arm to a horizontal position against your resistance; as he does so, palpate for deltoid contraction.

Triceps
Ask the patient to abduct and hold his arm midway between flexion and extension. Hold and support his arm at the wrist, and ask him to extend it against your resistance. Watch for triceps contraction.

Dorsal interossei
Ask the patient to extend and spread his fingers, and tell him to try to resist your attempt to squeeze them together.

Forearm and hand (grip)
Ask the patient to grasp your middle and index fingers and squeeze as hard as he can.

LEG MUSCLES
Anterior tibial
With the patient's leg extended, place your hand on his foot and ask him to dorsiflex his ankle against your resistance.

Psoas
While you support his leg, ask the patient to raise his knee and then flex his hip against your resistance. Observe for psoas muscle contraction.

Extensor hallucis longus
With your finger on the patient's great toe, ask him to dorsiflex the toe against your resistance. Palpate for extensor hallucis contraction.

Quadriceps
Ask the patient to bend his knee slightly while you support his lower leg. Then ask him to extend the knee against your resistance; as he's doing so, palpate for quadriceps contraction.

Gastrocnemius
With the patient on his side, support his foot and ask him to plantarflex his ankle against your resistance. Palpate for gastrocnemius contraction.

MUSCLE WEAKNESS

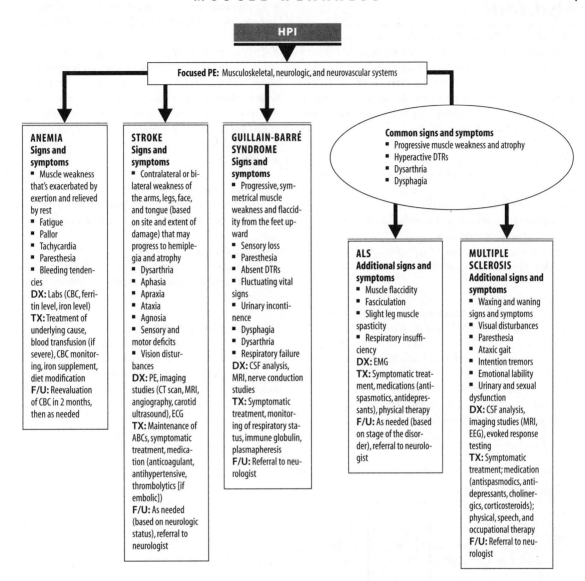

HPI

Focused PE: Musculoskeletal, neurologic, and neurovascular systems

ANEMIA
Signs and symptoms
- Muscle weakness that's exacerbated by exertion and relieved by rest
- Fatigue
- Pallor
- Tachycardia
- Paresthesia
- Bleeding tendencies

DX: Labs (CBC, ferritin level, iron level)
TX: Treatment of underlying cause, blood transfusion (if severe), CBC monitoring, iron supplement, diet modification
F/U: Reevaluation of CBC in 2 months, then as needed

STROKE
Signs and symptoms
- Contralateral or bilateral weakness of the arms, legs, face, and tongue (based on site and extent of damage) that may progress to hemiplegia and atrophy
- Dysarthria
- Aphasia
- Apraxia
- Ataxia
- Agnosia
- Sensory and motor deficits
- Vision disturbances

DX: PE, imaging studies (CT scan, MRI, angiography, carotid ultrasound), ECG
TX: Maintenance of ABCs, symptomatic treatment, medication (anticoagulant, antihypertensive, thrombolytics [if embolic])
F/U: As needed (based on neurologic status), referral to neurologist

GUILLAIN-BARRÉ SYNDROME
Signs and symptoms
- Progressive, symmetrical muscle weakness and flaccidity from the feet upward
- Sensory loss
- Paresthesia
- Absent DTRs
- Fluctuating vital signs
- Urinary incontinence
- Dysphagia
- Dysarthria
- Respiratory failure

DX: CSF analysis, MRI, nerve conduction studies
TX: Symptomatic treatment, monitoring of respiratory status, immune globulin, plasmapheresis
F/U: Referral to neurologist

Common signs and symptoms
- Progressive muscle weakness and atrophy
- Hyperactive DTRs
- Dysarthria
- Dysphagia

ALS
Additional signs and symptoms
- Muscle flaccidity
- Fasciculation
- Slight leg muscle spasticity
- Respiratory insufficiency

DX: EMG
TX: Symptomatic treatment, medications (antispasmotics, antidepressants), physical therapy
F/U: As needed (based on stage of the disorder), referral to neurologist

MULTIPLE SCLEROSIS
Additional signs and symptoms
- Waxing and waning signs and symptoms
- Visual disturbances
- Paresthesia
- Ataxic gait
- Intention tremors
- Emotional lability
- Urinary and sexual dysfunction

DX: CSF analysis, imaging studies (MRI, EEG), evoked response testing
TX: Symptomatic treatment; medication (antispasmodics, antidepressants, cholinergics, corticosteroids); physical, speech, and occupational therapy
F/U: Referral to neurologist

Additional differential diagnoses: brain tumor ▪ head trauma ▪ herniated disk ▪ Hodgkin's disease ▪ hypercortisolism ▪ hypothyroidism ▪ myasthenia gravis ▪ osteoarthritis ▪ Paget's disease ▪ Parkinson's disease ▪ peripheral nerve trauma ▪ peripheral neuropathy ▪ poliomyelitis ▪ polymyositis ▪ potassium imbalance ▪ protein deficiency ▪ rheumatoid arthritis ▪ seizure disorder ▪ spinal trauma and disease ▪ thyrotoxicosis

Other causes: aminoglycoside antibiotics (may worsen weakness in patients with myasthenia gravis) ▪ digoxin toxicity ▪ excessive doses of dantrolene ▪ immobility ▪ inactivity ▪ prolonged bed rest ▪ prolonged corticosteroid use

Mydriasis

Mydriasis—pupillary dilation caused by contraction of the dilator of the iris—is a normal response to decreased light, strong emotional stimuli, and topical administration of mydriatic and cycloplegic drugs. It can also result from an ocular or neurologic disorder, eye trauma, or a disorder that decreases level of consciousness. Mydriasis may be an adverse effect of antihistamines or other drugs.

ALERT

If mydriasis is accompanied with a change in level of consciousness:
- *quickly take the patient's vital signs*
- *assess him for other changes in neurological status, such as headache, aphasia, or hemiplegia*
- *institute emergency measures, if appropriate.*
   If the patient's condition permits, perform a focused assessment.

HISTORY

- Ask the patient about other eye problems, such as pain, blurring, diplopia, and visual field defects.
- Review the patient's medical history, noting especially eye or head trauma, glaucoma and other ocular problems, and neurologic and vascular disorders.
- Obtain a drug history, including prescription and over-the-counter drugs, herbal remedies, and recreational drugs. Also, ask the patient about alcohol intake.

PHYSICAL ASSESSMENT

- Inspect and compare the pupils' size, color, and shape—many people normally have unequal pupils. (See *Grading pupil size.*)
- Test each pupil for light reflex, consensual response, and accommodation. Perform a swinging flashlight test to evaluate a decreased response to direct light coupled with a normal consensual response (Marcus Gunn pupil).
- Check the eyes for ptosis, swelling, and ecchymosis.
- Test visual acuity in both eyes with and without correction.
- Evaluate extraocular muscle function by checking the six cardinal fields of gaze.

SPECIAL CONSIDERATIONS

Keep in mind that mydriasis appears in two ocular emergencies: acute angle-closure glaucoma and traumatic iridoplegia.

A   PEDIATRIC POINTERS

Mydriasis occurs in children as a result of ocular trauma, drug effects, Adie's syndrome and, most commonly, increased intracranial pressure.

PATIENT COUNSELING

If the patient's mydriasis is the result of mydriatic drugs received during an eye examination, explain to the patient that he'll likely experience some photophobia and loss of accommodation. Instruct him to wear dark glasses and to avoid bright light, and reassure him that the condition is only temporary.

GRADING PUPIL SIZE

To ensure accurate evaluation of pupillary size, compare the patient's pupils with the scale at right. Keep in mind that maximum constriction may be less than 1 mm and maximum dilation greater than 9 mm.

1 mm	2 mm	3 mm
4 mm	5 mm	6 mm
7 mm	8 mm	9 mm

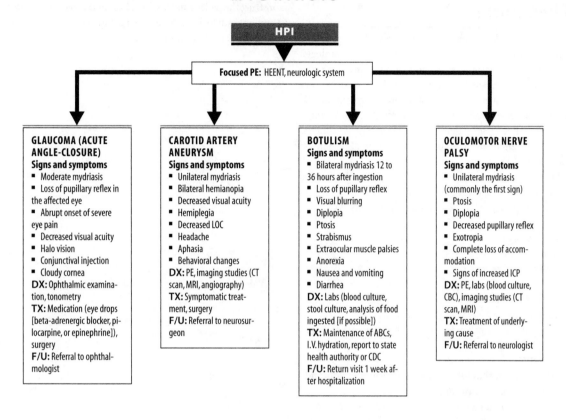

HPI

Focused PE: HEENT, neurologic system

GLAUCOMA (ACUTE ANGLE-CLOSURE)
Signs and symptoms
- Moderate mydriasis
- Loss of pupillary reflex in the affected eye
- Abrupt onset of severe eye pain
- Decreased visual acuity
- Halo vision
- Conjunctival injection
- Cloudy cornea

DX: Ophthalmic examination, tonometry
TX: Medication (eye drops [beta-adrenergic blocker, pilocarpine, or epinephrine]), surgery
F/U: Referral to ophthalmologist

CAROTID ARTERY ANEURYSM
Signs and symptoms
- Unilateral mydriasis
- Bilateral hemianopia
- Decreased visual acuity
- Hemiplegia
- Decreased LOC
- Headache
- Aphasia
- Behavioral changes

DX: PE, imaging studies (CT scan, MRI, angiography)
TX: Symptomatic treatment, surgery
F/U: Referral to neurosurgeon

BOTULISM
Signs and symptoms
- Bilateral mydriasis 12 to 36 hours after ingestion
- Loss of pupillary reflex
- Visual blurring
- Diplopia
- Ptosis
- Strabismus
- Extraocular muscle palsies
- Anorexia
- Nausea and vomiting
- Diarrhea

DX: Labs (blood culture, stool culture, analysis of food ingested [if possible])
TX: Maintenance of ABCs, I.V. hydration, report to state health authority or CDC
F/U: Return visit 1 week after hospitalization

OCULOMOTOR NERVE PALSY
Signs and symptoms
- Unilateral mydriasis (commonly the first sign)
- Ptosis
- Diplopia
- Decreased pupillary reflex
- Exotropia
- Complete loss of accommodation
- Signs of increased ICP

DX: PE, labs (blood culture, CBC), imaging studies (CT scan, MRI)
TX: Treatment of underlying cause
F/U: Referral to neurologist

Additional differential diagnoses: Adie's syndrome ▪ aortic arch syndrome ▪ brain stem infarction ▪ traumatic iridoplegia

Other causes: anesthesia induction ▪ anticholinergics ▪ antihistamines ▪ barbiturate overdose ▪ estrogens ▪ ocular surgery ▪ sympathomimetics ▪ topical mydriatics and cycloplegics ▪ tricyclic antidepressants

Myoclonus

Myoclonus—sudden, shocklike contractions of a single muscle or muscle group—can occur as a result of various neurologic disorders and commonly heralds onset of a seizure. These contractions may be isolated or repetitive, rhythmic or arrhythmic, symmetrical or asymmetrical, synchronous or asynchronous, and generalized or focal. They may be precipitated by bright flickering lights, a loud sound, or unexpected physical contact. One type, intention myoclonus, is evoked by intentional muscle movement.

Myoclonus occurs normally just before falling asleep and as a part of the natural startle reaction. It also occurs with some poisonings and, rarely, as a complication of hemodialysis.

 ALERT

If you observe myoclonus:
- *check for seizure activity*
- *take the patient's vital signs*
- *evaluate respiratory function*
- *institute emergency measures, if necessary.*
  If the patient's condition permits, perform a focused assessment.

HISTORY
- Ask the patient about the frequency, severity, location, and circumstances of the myoclonus.
- Ask the patient if he has ever had a seizure. If so, ask him whether myoclonus preceded it. Is the myoclonus ever precipitated by a sensory stimulus?
- Review the patient's medical history.
- Obtain a drug history, including prescription and over-the-counter drugs, herbal remedies, and recreational drugs. Also, ask the patient about alcohol intake.

PHYSICAL ASSESSMENT
- Evaluate the patient's level of consciousness and mental status.
- Perform a complete neurologic assessment.
- Check for muscle rigidity and wasting, and test deep tendon reflexes.

SPECIAL CONSIDERATIONS
If the patient's myoclonus is progressive, institute seizure precautions.

 PEDIATRIC POINTERS

Although myoclonus is relatively uncommon in infants and children, it can result from subacute sclerosing panencephalitis, severe meningitis, progressive poliodystrophy, childhood myoclonic epilepsy, or encephalopathy such as Reye's syndrome.

PATIENT COUNSELING
Instruct the patient and his family about the need for safety precautions. Advise them to remove potentially harmful objects from the patient's environment.

MYOCLONUS

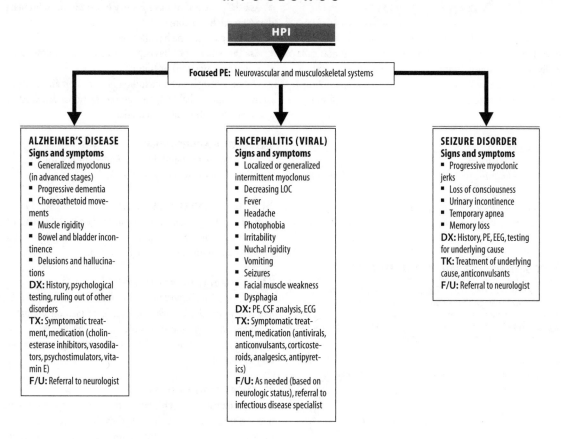

HPI

Focused PE: Neurovascular and musculoskeletal systems

ALZHEIMER'S DISEASE
Signs and symptoms
- Generalized myoclonus (in advanced stages)
- Progressive dementia
- Choreoathetoid movements
- Muscle rigidity
- Bowel and bladder incontinence
- Delusions and hallucinations

DX: History, psychological testing, ruling out of other disorders
TX: Symptomatic treatment, medication (cholinesterase inhibitors, vasodilators, psychostimulators, vitamin E)
F/U: Referral to neurologist

ENCEPHALITIS (VIRAL)
Signs and symptoms
- Localized or generalized intermittent myoclonus
- Decreasing LOC
- Fever
- Headache
- Photophobia
- Irritability
- Nuchal rigidity
- Vomiting
- Seizures
- Facial muscle weakness
- Dysphagia

DX: PE, CSF analysis, ECG
TX: Symptomatic treatment, medication (antivirals, anticonvulsants, corticosteroids, analgesics, antipyretics)
F/U: As needed (based on neurologic status), referral to infectious disease specialist

SEIZURE DISORDER
Signs and symptoms
- Progressive myoclonic jerks
- Loss of consciousness
- Urinary incontinence
- Temporary apnea
- Memory loss

DX: History, PE, EEG, testing for underlying cause
TK: Treatment of underlying cause, anticonvulsants
F/U: Referral to neurologist

Additional differential diagnoses: Creutzfeldt-Jakob disease ▪ encephalopathy

Other causes: delirium tremens ▪ drug withdrawal ▪ poisoning

N Nasal flaring

Nasal flaring is abnormal dilation of the nostrils. Although it usually occurs during inspiration, it may occasionally occur during expiration or throughout the respiratory cycle. Nasal flaring indicates respiratory dysfunction, ranging from mild difficulty to potentially life-threatening respiratory distress.

➤ A*LERT*

If you note nasal flaring:
- *quickly evaluate the patient's respiratory status and check for airway obstruction*
- *institute emergency measures, as necessary.*
  If the patient's condition permits, perform a focused assessment.

RECOGNIZING RESPIRATORY DISTRESS IN INFANTS

Because infants can't verbalize their symptoms, you'll need to teach parents how to recognize the signs of infant respiratory distress. Using these illustrations, show them how to evaluate nasal flaring. This sign, along with retractions and grunting on expiration, is graded to measure the severity of respiratory distress.

GRADE 0
The infant breathes normally, with no nasal flaring.

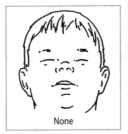
None

GRADE 1
The infant shows some signs of respiratory distress, including slightly flared nostrils and a slightly visible rib cage on inspiration. Instruct the parents to watch the infant closely and to begin measures to help him breathe more easily.

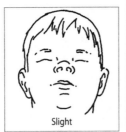
Slight

GRADE 2
The infant has pronounced respiratory distress. His nostrils flare widely, his rib cage is quite visible on exhalation, and he grunts as he exhales. Tell the parents to call his physician immediately and to continue measures to make breathing easier.

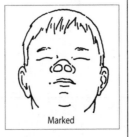
Marked

HISTORY
- Ask the patient if he has a history of cardiac or pulmonary disorders such as asthma.
- Ask the patient if he has allergies.
- Ask the patient if he has experienced a recent illness (such as a respiratory infection) or trauma.
- Obtain a drug history, including prescription and over-the-counter drugs, herbal remedies, and recreational drugs. Also, ask the patient about alcohol intake.

PHYSICAL ASSESSMENT
- Auscultate the patient's lungs for adventitious sounds.
- Obtain a pulse oximetry reading.

SPECIAL CONSIDERATIONS
To help ease breathing, place the patient in a high Fowler's position. If he's at risk for aspirating secretions, place him in a modified Trendelenburg or side-lying position.

 PEDIATRIC POINTERS
Nasal flaring is an important sign of respiratory distress in infants and very young children who can't verbalize their discomfort. Common causes include airway obstruction, hyaline membrane disease, croup, and acute epiglottiditis. (See Recognizing respiratory distress in infants.*)*

PATIENT COUNSELING
Instruct the patient and his family on what to expect from diagnostic testing, which may include chest X-rays, lung scan, pulmonary arteriography, sputum culture, complete blood count, arterial blood gas analysis, and electrocardiography.

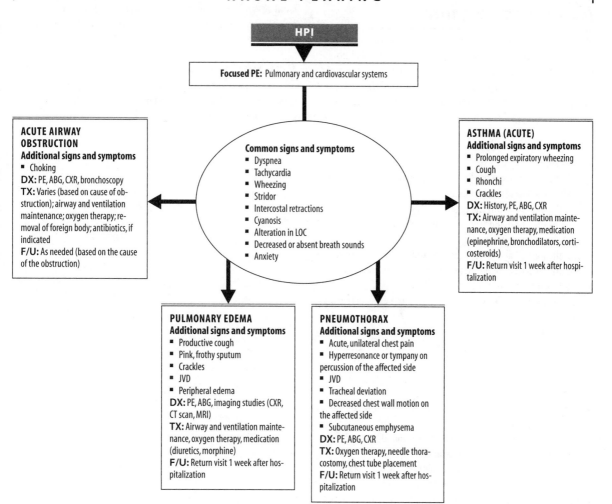

HPI

Focused PE: Pulmonary and cardiovascular systems

Common signs and symptoms
- Dyspnea
- Tachycardia
- Wheezing
- Stridor
- Intercostal retractions
- Cyanosis
- Alteration in LOC
- Decreased or absent breath sounds
- Anxiety

ACUTE AIRWAY OBSTRUCTION
Additional signs and symptoms
- Choking

DX: PE, ABG, CXR, bronchoscopy
TX: Varies (based on cause of obstruction); airway and ventilation maintenance; oxygen therapy; removal of foreign body; antibiotics, if indicated
F/U: As needed (based on the cause of the obstruction)

ASTHMA (ACUTE)
Additional signs and symptoms
- Prolonged expiratory wheezing
- Cough
- Rhonchi
- Crackles

DX: History, PE, ABG, CXR
TX: Airway and ventilation maintenance, oxygen therapy, medication (epinephrine, bronchodilators, corticosteroids)
F/U: Return visit 1 week after hospitalization

PULMONARY EDEMA
Additional signs and symptoms
- Productive cough
- Pink, frothy sputum
- Crackles
- JVD
- Peripheral edema

DX: PE, ABG, imaging studies (CXR, CT scan, MRI)
TX: Airway and ventilation maintenance, oxygen therapy, medication (diuretics, morphine)
F/U: Return visit 1 week after hospitalization

PNEUMOTHORAX
Additional signs and symptoms
- Acute, unilateral chest pain
- Hyperresonance or tympany on percussion of the affected side
- JVD
- Tracheal deviation
- Decreased chest wall motion on the affected side
- Subcutaneous emphysema

DX: PE, ABG, CXR
TX: Oxygen therapy, needle thoracostomy, chest tube placement
F/U: Return visit 1 week after hospitalization

Additional differential diagnoses: anaphylaxis ▪ ARDS ▪ COPD ▪ pneumonia (bacterial) ▪ pulmonary embolus

Other causes: deep breathing ▪ PFT such as vital capacity testing

Nasal obstruction

Nasal obstruction may result from an inflammatory, neoplastic, endocrine, or metabolic disorder or from a structural abnormality or traumatic injury. It may cause discomfort, alter a person's sense of taste and smell, and cause voice changes. Although a frequent and typically benign symptom, nasal obstruction may herald certain life-threatening disorders, such as a basilar skull fracture or malignant tumor.

HISTORY
- Ask the patient when he first noticed the nasal obstruction. Did it begin suddenly or gradually?
- Ask the patient about the obstruction's characteristics, including its duration and frequency. Is it intermittent or persistent? Unilateral or bilateral?
- Ask the patient about the presence and character of drainage.
- Ask the patient if he has nasal or sinus pain or headaches.
- Ask the patient about recent travel.
- Review the patient's medical history, noting especially trauma and surgery.
- Obtain a drug history, including prescription and over-the-counter drugs, herbal remedies, and recreational drugs. Also, ask the patient about alcohol intake.

PHYSICAL ASSESSMENT
- Examine the nose; assess airflow and the condition of the turbinates and nasal septum.
- Evaluate the orbits for evidence of dystopia, decreased vision, excess tearing, or abnormal appearance.
- Palpate the frontal and maxillary sinuses for tenderness.
- Examine the ears for signs of middle ear effusions.
- Inspect the oral cavity, pharynx, nasopharynx, and larynx to detect inflammation, ulceration, excessive mucosal dryness, and neurologic deficits.
- Palpate the neck for adenopathy.

SPECIAL CONSIDERATIONS
Topical nasal vasoconstrictors may cause rebound rhinorrhea and nasal obstruction if used longer than 5 days. Antihypertensives may cause nasal congestion as well.

[A] PEDIATRIC POINTERS
- *Acute nasal obstruction in children can result from the common cold.*
- *In infants and children, especially between ages 3 and 6, chronic nasal obstruction typically results from large adenoids.*
- *In neonates, choanal atresia is the most common congenital cause of nasal obstruction, and it may be unilateral or bilateral.*
- *Cystic fibrosis may cause nasal polyps in children, resulting in nasal obstruction. However, if the child has unilateral nasal obstruction and rhinorrhea, you should assume a foreign body in the nose until proven otherwise.*

PATIENT COUNSELING
Advise the patient to increase his fluid intake, if appropriate, to thin secretions. Remind him to take an antihistamine, a decongestant, or an antipyretic, as directed.

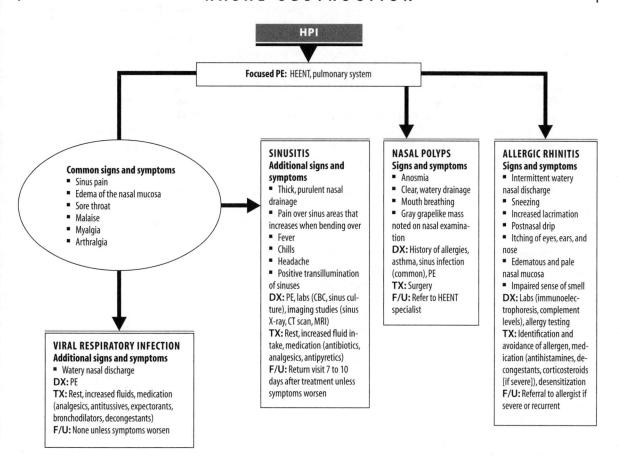

HPI

Focused PE: HEENT, pulmonary system

Common signs and symptoms
- Sinus pain
- Edema of the nasal mucosa
- Sore throat
- Malaise
- Myalgia
- Arthralgia

SINUSITIS
Additional signs and symptoms
- Thick, purulent nasal drainage
- Pain over sinus areas that increases when bending over
- Fever
- Chills
- Headache
- Positive transillumination of sinuses

DX: PE, labs (CBC, sinus culture), imaging studies (sinus X-ray, CT scan, MRI)
TX: Rest, increased fluid intake, medication (antibiotics, analgesics, antipyretics)
F/U: Return visit 7 to 10 days after treatment unless symptoms worsen

NASAL POLYPS
Signs and symptoms
- Anosmia
- Clear, watery drainage
- Mouth breathing
- Gray grapelike mass noted on nasal examination

DX: History of allergies, asthma, sinus infection (common), PE
TX: Surgery
F/U: Refer to HEENT specialist

ALLERGIC RHINITIS
Signs and symptoms
- Intermittent watery nasal discharge
- Sneezing
- Increased lacrimation
- Postnasal drip
- Itching of eyes, ears, and nose
- Edematous and pale nasal mucosa
- Impaired sense of smell

DX: Labs (immunoelectrophoresis, complement levels), allergy testing
TX: Identification and avoidance of allergen, medication (antihistamines, decongestants, corticosteroids [if severe]), desensitization
F/U: Referral to allergist if severe or recurrent

VIRAL RESPIRATORY INFECTION
Additional signs and symptoms
- Watery nasal discharge

DX: PE
TX: Rest, increased fluids, medication (analgesics, antitussives, expectorants, bronchodilators, decongestants)
F/U: None unless symptoms worsen

Additional differential diagnoses: basilar skull fracture ▪ foreign body ▪ hypothyroidism ▪ nasal deformities ▪ nasal fracture ▪ nasal tumors ▪ nasopharyngeal tumors ▪ sarcoidosis ▪ Wegener's granulomatosis

Other causes: antihypertensives ▪ rhinoplasty ▪ sinus or cranial surgery ▪ topical nasal vasoconstrictors

Nausea

Nausea, a common symptom of GI disorders, is a sensation of profound revulsion to food or of impending vomiting. Commonly accompanied by such autonomic signs as hypersalivation, diaphoresis, tachycardia, pallor, and tachypnea, it's closely associated with anorexia and vomiting.

Nausea may occur with a fluid or electrolyte imbalance, an infection, or a metabolic, endocrine, labyrinthine, or cardiac disorder. It may also be a result of drug therapy, surgery, or radiation. Common during the first trimester of pregnancy, nausea may also arise from severe pain, anxiety, alcohol intoxication, overeating, or ingestion of distasteful food or liquids.

History

- Ask the patient to describe the onset, duration, and intensity of the nausea as well as what provokes or relieves it.
- Review the patient's medical history, noting especially GI, endocrine, and metabolic disorders; recent infections; and cancer (including its treatment).
- Ask the patient about associated signs and symptoms, particularly vomiting (including color and amount), abdominal pain, anorexia and weight loss, changes in bowel habits or stool character, excessive belching or flatus, and a sensation of bloating.
- If the patient is a female of childbearing age, ask whether she is or could be pregnant.
- Ask the patient if he was recently exposed to someone with a GI disturbance.
- Obtain a drug history, including prescription and over-the-counter drugs, herbal remedies, and recreational drugs. Also, ask the patient about alcohol intake.
- Ask the patient about his diet.

Physical assessment

- Inspect the skin for jaundice, bruises, and spider angiomas, and assess skin turgor.
- Inspect the abdomen for distention, auscultate for bowel sounds and bruits, palpate for rigidity and tenderness, and test for rebound tenderness.
- Palpate and percuss the liver for enlargement.
- Assess other body systems, as appropriate.

Special considerations

Herbal remedies, such as gingko biloba and St. John's wort, have certain adverse effects, including nausea. Postoperative nausea and vomiting are common, especially after abdominal surgery.

A PEDIATRIC POINTERS

Nausea, frequently described as a stomachache, is one of the most common childhood complaints. Commonly the result of overeating, nausea can occur from any one of several disorders, ranging from acute infection to a conversion reaction caused by fear.

AGING ISSUES

Elderly patients have increased dental caries; more frequent tooth loss; decreased salivary gland function, which causes mouth dryness; reduced gastric acid output and motility; and decreased senses of taste and smell. All of these may be factors contributing to nonpathologic nausea.

PATIENT COUNSELING

Tell the patient to breathe deeply to ease nausea. Advise him to keep his room fresh and clean-smelling by providing adequate ventilation.

NAUSEA

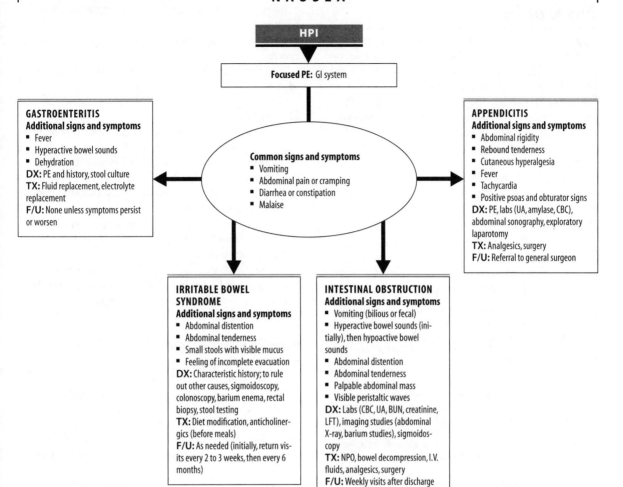

HPI

Focused PE: GI system

Common signs and symptoms
- Vomiting
- Abdominal pain or cramping
- Diarrhea or constipation
- Malaise

GASTROENTERITIS
Additional signs and symptoms
- Fever
- Hyperactive bowel sounds
- Dehydration

DX: PE and history, stool culture
TX: Fluid replacement, electrolyte replacement
F/U: None unless symptoms persist or worsen

APPENDICITIS
Additional signs and symptoms
- Abdominal rigidity
- Rebound tenderness
- Cutaneous hyperalgesia
- Fever
- Tachycardia
- Positive psoas and obturator signs

DX: PE, labs (UA, amylase, CBC), abdominal sonography, exploratory laparotomy
TX: Analgesics, surgery
F/U: Referral to general surgeon

IRRITABLE BOWEL SYNDROME
Additional signs and symptoms
- Abdominal distention
- Abdominal tenderness
- Small stools with visible mucus
- Feeling of incomplete evacuation

DX: Characteristic history; to rule out other causes, sigmoidoscopy, colonoscopy, barium enema, rectal biopsy, stool testing
TX: Diet modification, anticholinergics (before meals)
F/U: As needed (initially, return visits every 2 to 3 weeks, then every 6 months)

INTESTINAL OBSTRUCTION
Additional signs and symptoms
- Vomiting (bilious or fecal)
- Hyperactive bowel sounds (initially), then hypoactive bowel sounds
- Abdominal distention
- Abdominal tenderness
- Palpable abdominal mass
- Visible peristaltic waves

DX: Labs (CBC, UA, BUN, creatinine, LFT), imaging studies (abdominal X-ray, barium studies), sigmoidoscopy
TX: NPO, bowel decompression, I.V. fluids, analgesics, surgery
F/U: Weekly visits after discharge for 2 to 8 weeks

Additional differential diagnoses: adrenal insufficiency ▪ cholecystitis (acute) ▪ cholelithiasis ▪ diverticulitis ▪ ectopic pregnancy ▪ electrolyte imbalances ▪ gastric cancer ▪ gastritis ▪ hepatitis ▪ hyperemesis gravidarum ▪ infection ▪ inflammatory bowel disease ▪ labyrinthitis ▪ Ménière's disease ▪ mesenteric artery ischemia ▪ mesenteric venous thrombosis ▪ metabolic acidosis ▪ migraine headache ▪ motion sickness ▪ MI ▪ pancreatitis (acute) ▪ peptic ulcer ▪ peritonitis ▪ preeclampsia ▪ renal and urologic disorders ▪ thyrotoxicosis

Other causes: abdominal surgery ▪ anesthetic agents ▪ antibiotics ▪ antineoplastics ▪ digoxin or theophylline overdose ▪ estrogens ▪ ferrous sulfate ▪ ginkgo biloba ▪ levodopa ▪ opiates ▪ oral potassium chloride replacements ▪ quinidine ▪ radiation therapy ▪ St. John's wort ▪ sulfasalazine

Neck pain

Neck pain may originate from any neck structure, ranging from the meninges and cervical vertebrae to its blood vessels, muscles, and lymphatic tissue. This symptom can also be referred from other areas of the body. Its location, onset, and pattern help determine its origin and underlying causes. It usually results from trauma or a degenerative, congenital, inflammatory, metabolic, or neoplastic disorder.

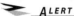 **ALERT**

If the patient's neck pain is due to trauma:
- *examine the neck for abrasions, swelling, lacerations, erythema, and ecchymoses*
- *ensure proper cervical spine immobilization, preferably with a long backboard and a hard cervical collar (See* Applying a Philadelphia collar.)

APPLYING A PHILADELPHIA COLLAR

A lightweight molded polyethylene collar designed to hold the neck straight with the chin slightly elevated and tucked in, the Philadelphia cervical collar immobilizes the cervical spine, decreases muscle spasms, and relieves some pain. It also prevents further injury and promotes healing.

When applying the collar, fit it snugly around the patient's neck and attach the Velcro fasteners or buckles at the back. Be sure to check the patient's airway and his neurovascular status to ensure that the collar isn't too tight. Also, make sure that the collar isn't placed too high in front, which can hyperextend the neck. In a patient with a neck sprain, hyperextension may cause the ligaments to heal in a shortened position; in a patient with a cervical spine fracture, it could cause serious neurologic damage.

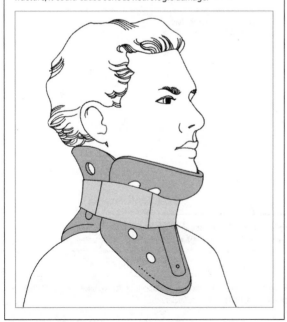

- *take his vital signs, and perform a quick neurologic evaluation*
- *assess respiratory status, and institute emergency measures, if necessary*
- *ask him (or his companion, if the patient can't answer) how the injury occurred.*

If the patient hasn't sustained trauma, perform a focused assessment.

HISTORY
- Ask the patient to describe the onset and severity of his neck pain.
- Ask the patient where in his neck he feels pain. Does anything alleviate or aggravate it?
- Ask the patient about the development of associated signs and symptoms such as headache.
- Review the patient's medical history, noting especially current and past illnesses and injuries.
- Ask the patient about his diet.
- Ask the patient if there's a family history of neck pain.
- Obtain a drug history, including prescription and over-the-counter drugs, herbal remedies, and recreational drugs. Also, ask the patient about alcohol intake.

PHYSICAL ASSESSMENT
- Inspect the neck, shoulders, and cervical spine for swelling, masses, erythema, and ecchymoses.
- Palpate the cervical spine and paracervical area, checking for muscle spasm.
- Assess active range of motion in the patient's neck by having him perform selection, extension, rotation, and lateral side bending. Note the degree of pain that these movements produce.
- Examine posture, and test muscle strength. Check the sensation in his arms, and assess his hand grasp and arm reflexes.
- Attempt to elicit Brudzinski's and Kernig's signs, and palpate the cervical lymph nodes for enlargement.

SPECIAL CONSIDERATIONS
Promote patient comfort by giving an anti-inflammatory and an analgesic, as needed.

 PEDIATRIC POINTERS
The most common causes of neck pain in children are meningitis and trauma. A rare cause is congenital torticollis.

PATIENT COUNSELING
Instruct the patient on what to expect from diagnostic testing, which may include X-rays, computed tomography scan, blood tests, and cerebrospinal fluid analysis.

NECK PAIN

HPI

Focused PE: Neurologic and musculoskeletal systems

ANKYLOSING SPONDYLITIS
Signs and symptoms
- Intermittent, moderate to severe neck pain and stiffness
- Severely restricted ROM
- Intermittent lower back pain and stiffness
- Arm pain
- Low-grade fever
- Malaise
- Anorexia
- Fatigue
- Iritis

DX: PE, HLA-B27, spine and pelvis X-rays

TX: NSAIDs, exercise program, lifestyle changes, surgery (with severe pain or joint damage)

F/U: Referral to orthopedic specialist

Common signs and symptoms
- Neck pain that restricts movement, is aggravated by movement, and causes referred pain (usually in one arm)
- Positive Lhermitte's and Spurling's signs

HERNIATED CERVICAL DISK
DX: PE, imaging studies (cervical spine X-rays, MRI, myelogram, CT scan)

TX: Rest, NSAIDs, surgery

F/U: Referral to orthopedic surgeon

CERVICAL SPONDYLOSIS
Additional signs and symptoms
- Generalized weakness in the arms and hands
- Leg weakness
- Hyperactive DTRs
- Spastic gait

DX: PE, MRI

TX: Neck brace or traction, NSAIDs, surgery

F/U: Referral to orthopedic surgeon

MENINGITIS
Signs and symptoms
- Nuchal rigidity
- Fever
- Headache
- Photophobia
- Positive Brudzinski's and Kernig's signs
- Altered LOC

DX: PE, labs (CBC with differential, blood cultures, CSF analysis), imaging studies (skull and sinus X-rays, CT scan)

TX: Seizure precautions, I.V. antibiotics (if bacterial)

F/U: As needed (dependent on the severity of the illness and complications)

CERVICAL SPINE TUMOR
Signs and symptoms
- Persistent neck pain that increases with movement and isn't relieved by rest (metastatic)
- Mild to moderate pain along a specific nerve root (primary)
- Paresthesia
- Arm and leg weakness that progresses to atrophy and paralysis

DX: PE, imaging studies (cervical spine X-ray, CT scan, MRI)

TX: Medication (analgesics, chemotherapy), radiation therapy, surgery

F/U: Referrals to neurosurgeon and oncologist

Additional differential diagnoses: cervical extension injury ▪ cervical fibrositis ▪ cervical spine fracture ▪ cervical spine infection (acute) ▪ cervical stenosis ▪ esophageal trauma ▪ Hodgkin's lymphoma ▪ laryngeal cancer ▪ lymphadenitis ▪ neck sprain ▪ osteoporosis ▪ Paget's disease ▪ rheumatoid arthritis ▪ spinous process fracture ▪ subarachnoid hemorrhage ▪ thyroid trauma ▪ torticollis ▪ tracheal trauma

Nipple discharge

Nipple discharge can occur spontaneously, or it can be elicited by nipple stimulation. It's characterized by duration (intermittent or constant), extent (unilateral or bilateral), color, consistency, and composition. Its incidence increases with age and parity. This sign rarely occurs in men and in nulligravid, regularly menstruating women, where it's more likely to be pathologic. However, it's relatively common in middle-aged, parous women, who can often elicit a thick, grayish discharge — benign epithelial debris from inactive ducts. Colostrum (a thin, yellowish or milky discharge) is common in the last weeks of pregnancy.

Nipple discharge can signal serious underlying disease, particularly when accompanied by other breast changes. Significant causes include endocrine disorders, cancer, certain drugs, and blocked lactiferous ducts.

HISTORY

● Ask the patient when she first noticed the discharge, and ask her its duration, quantity, color, and consistency. Is the discharge spontaneous, or does it have to be expressed? Is it bloody?

● Ask the patient if she has noticed other nipple and breast changes, such as pain, tenderness, itching, warmth, changes in contour, or lumps. If she reports a lump, question her about its onset, location, size, and consistency.

● Review the patient's complete gynecologic history.

● Ask the patient about her normal menstrual cycle and the date of her last menses. Does she experience breast swelling and tenderness, bloating, irritability, headaches, abdominal cramping, nausea, or diarrhea before or during menses?

● Obtain a pregnancy history, noting the outcome of each as well as pregnancy-related complications. If she breast-fed, note the approximate time of her last lactation.

● Review the patient's medical history for risk factors of breast cancer, including previous or current malignancies, nulliparity or first pregnancy after age 30, early menarche, and late menopause. Also, ask the patient if there's a family history of breast cancer.

● Obtain a drug history, including prescription and over-the-counter drugs, herbal remedies, and recreational drugs. Also, ask the patient about alcohol intake.

PHYSICAL ASSESSMENT

● Elicit discharge, if possible, and note its color, consistency, amount, and odor. (See *Eliciting nipple discharge.*)

● Examine the nipples and breasts with the patient in four different positions: sitting with her arms at her sides, sitting with her arms overhead, sitting with her hands pressing on her hips, and leaning forward so her breasts are suspended. Check for nipple deviation, flattening, retraction, redness, asymmetry, thickening, excoriation, erosion, and cracking. Inspect her breasts for asymmetry, irregular contours, dimpling, erythema, and peau d'orange.

● With the patient in a supine position, palpate the breasts and axillae for lumps, giving special attention to the areolae. Note the size, location, delineation, consistency, and mobility of any lump you find.

SPECIAL CONSIDERATIONS

Nipple discharge can be caused by psychotropic agents, particularly phenothiazines and tricyclic antidepressants; some antihypertensives; hormonal contraceptives; cimetidine; metoclopramide; and verapamil.

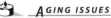
PEDIATRIC POINTERS

● *Nipple discharge in children and adolescents is rare. When it does occur, it's almost always nonpathologic, as in the bloody discharge that sometimes accompanies onset of menarche.*

● *Infants of both sexes may experience a milky breast discharge beginning 3 days after birth and lasting up to 2 weeks.*

AGING ISSUES

In postmenopausal women, breast changes are considered malignant until proven otherwise.

PATIENT COUNSELING

Advise the patient to wear a breast binder, which may reduce discharge by eliminating nipple stimulation.

ELICITING NIPPLE DISCHARGE

If the patient has a history or evidence of nipple discharge, you can attempt to elicit it during your examination. Help the patient into a supine position, and then gently squeeze her nipple between your thumb and index finger, noting discharge from the nipple. Then place your fingers on the areola, as shown, and palpate the entire areolar surface, watching for discharge from areolar ducts.

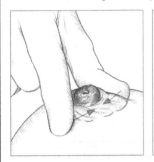
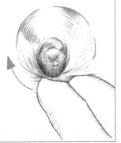

NIPPLE DISCHARGE

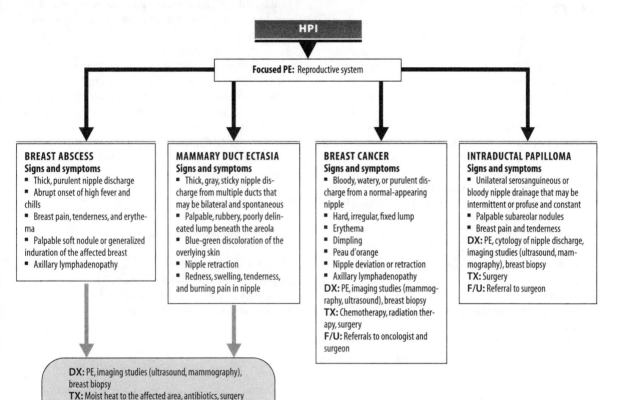

HPI

Focused PE: Reproductive system

BREAST ABSCESS
Signs and symptoms
- Thick, purulent nipple discharge
- Abrupt onset of high fever and chills
- Breast pain, tenderness, and erythema
- Palpable soft nodule or generalized induration of the affected breast
- Axillary lymphadenopathy

MAMMARY DUCT ECTASIA
Signs and symptoms
- Thick, gray, sticky nipple discharge from multiple ducts that may be bilateral and spontaneous
- Palpable, rubbery, poorly delineated lump beneath the areola
- Blue-green discoloration of the overlying skin
- Nipple retraction
- Redness, swelling, tenderness, and burning pain in nipple

BREAST CANCER
Signs and symptoms
- Bloody, watery, or purulent discharge from a normal-appearing nipple
- Hard, irregular, fixed lump
- Erythema
- Dimpling
- Peau d'orange
- Nipple deviation or retraction
- Axillary lymphadenopathy
DX: PE, imaging studies (mammography, ultrasound), breast biopsy
TX: Chemotherapy, radiation therapy, surgery
F/U: Referrals to oncologist and surgeon

INTRADUCTAL PAPILLOMA
Signs and symptoms
- Unilateral serosanguineous or bloody nipple drainage that may be intermittent or profuse and constant
- Palpable subareolar nodules
- Breast pain and tenderness
DX: PE, cytology of nipple discharge, imaging studies (ultrasound, mammography), breast biopsy
TX: Surgery
F/U: Referral to surgeon

DX: PE, imaging studies (ultrasound, mammography), breast biopsy
TX: Moist heat to the affected area, antibiotics, surgery
F/U: Reevaluation in 7 to 10 days

Additional differential diagnoses: choriocarcinoma ▪ herpes zoster ▪ hypothyroidism ▪ prolactin-secreting pituitary tumor ▪ proliferative (fibrocystic) breast disease ▪ trauma

Other causes: antihypertensives (reserpine, methyldopa) ▪ chest wall surgery ▪ cimetidine ▪ hormonal contraceptives ▪ metoclopramide ▪ psychotropic agents (particularly phenothiazines and tricyclic antidepressants) ▪ verapamil

Nocturia

Nocturia—excessive urination at night—may result from disruption of the normal diurnal pattern of urine concentration or from overstimulation of the nerves and muscles that control urination. Normally, more urine is concentrated during the night than during the day. As a result, most persons excrete three to four times more urine during the day and can sleep for 6 to 8 hours during the night without being awakened. With nocturia, the patient may awaken one or more times during the night to empty his bladder and may excrete 700 ml or more of urine.

Although nocturia usually results from a renal or lower urinary tract disorder, it may also result from a cardiovascular, endocrine, or metabolic disorder. This common sign may also result from use of a drug that induces diuresis—particularly if it's taken at night—or from ingestion of large quantities of fluids, especially caffeinated beverages or alcohol, at bedtime.

HISTORY

- Ask the patient when the nocturia began and how often it occurs.
- Ask the patient if he can identify a specific pattern or precipitating factors, such as a change in his usual pattern or in the volume of his fluid intake.
- Ask the patient to estimate the volume of urine voided.
- Ask the patient about changes in the color, odor, or consistency of his urine.
- Ask the patient about associated signs and symptoms, such as pain or burning on urination, difficulty initiating a urine stream, costovertebral angle tenderness, and flank, upper abdominal, or suprapubic pain.
- Review the patient's medical history, noting especially renal or urinary tract disorders and endocrine or metabolic disease, particularly diabetes.
- Obtain a drug history, including prescription and over-the-counter drugs, herbal remedies, and recreational drugs, noting especially drugs that increase urine output, such as diuretics, cardiac glycosides, and antihypertensives. Also, ask the patient about alcohol intake.

PHYSICAL ASSESSMENT

- Palpate and percuss the kidneys, the costovertebral angle, and the bladder.
- Carefully inspect the urinary meatus.
- Inspect a urine specimen for color, odor, and the presence of sediment.

SPECIAL CONSIDERATIONS

Monitor vital signs, intake and output, and daily weight; document the frequency of nocturia, amount, and specific gravity.

Ⓐ PEDIATRIC POINTERS

- In children, nocturia may be voluntary or involuntary. The latter is commonly known as enuresis, or bedwetting.
- With the exception of prostate disorders, causes of nocturia are generally the same for children and adults. However, children with pyelonephritis are more susceptible to sepsis; signs and symptoms include fever, irritability, and poor skin perfusion. In addition, girls may experience vaginal discharge and vulvar soreness or pruritus.

AGING ISSUES

Postmenopausal women have decreased bladder elasticity, but urine output remains constant, resulting in nocturia.

PATIENT COUNSELING

Advise the patient to plan administration of a diuretic for daytime hours, if possible. Recommend the patient reduce fluid intake (especially of caffeinated beverages) before bedtime.

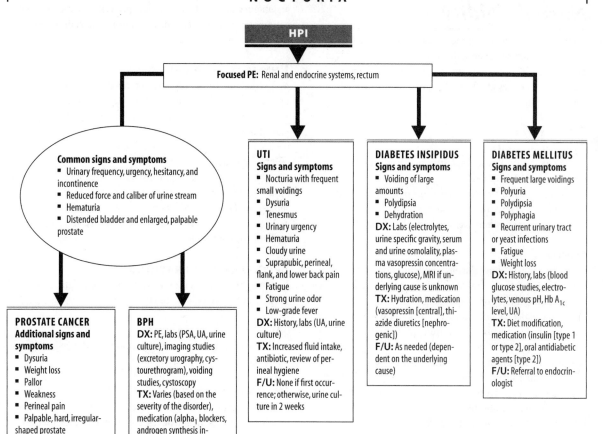

HPI

Focused PE: Renal and endocrine systems, rectum

Common signs and symptoms
- Urinary frequency, urgency, hesitancy, and incontinence
- Reduced force and caliber of urine stream
- Hematuria
- Distended bladder and enlarged, palpable prostate

UTI
Signs and symptoms
- Nocturia with frequent small voidings
- Dysuria
- Tenesmus
- Urinary urgency
- Hematuria
- Cloudy urine
- Suprapubic, perineal, flank, and lower back pain
- Fatigue
- Strong urine odor
- Low-grade fever

DX: History, labs (UA, urine culture)
TX: Increased fluid intake, antibiotic, review of perineal hygiene
F/U: None if first occurrence; otherwise, urine culture in 2 weeks

DIABETES INSIPIDUS
Signs and symptoms
- Voiding of large amounts
- Polydipsia
- Dehydration

DX: Labs (electrolytes, urine specific gravity, serum and urine osmolality, plasma vasopressin concentrations, glucose), MRI if underlying cause is unknown
TX: Hydration, medication (vasopressin [central], thiazide diuretics [nephrogenic])
F/U: As needed (dependent on the underlying cause)

DIABETES MELLITUS
Signs and symptoms
- Frequent large voidings
- Polyuria
- Polydipsia
- Polyphagia
- Recurrent urinary tract or yeast infections
- Fatigue
- Weight loss

DX: History, labs (blood glucose studies, electrolytes, venous pH, Hb A_{1c} level, UA)
TX: Diet modification, medication (insulin [type 1 or type 2], oral antidiabetic agents [type 2])
F/U: Referral to endocrinologist

PROSTATE CANCER
Additional signs and symptoms
- Dysuria
- Weight loss
- Pallor
- Weakness
- Perineal pain
- Palpable, hard, irregular-shaped prostate

DX: PE and history, labs (PSA, free PSA), ultrasound, biopsy
TX: Antineoplastic medication, surgery
F/U: Referrals to urologist and oncologist

BPH
DX: PE, labs (PSA, UA, urine culture), imaging studies (excretory urography, cystourethrogram), voiding studies, cystoscopy
TX: Varies (based on the severity of the disorder), medication (alpha$_1$ blockers, androgen synthesis inhibitor), surgery
F/U: Referral to urologist

Additional differential diagnoses: bladder neoplasm ▪ heart failure ▪ hypercalcemic nephropathy ▪ hypokalemic nephropathy ▪ pyelonephritis (acute) ▪ renal failure (chronic)

Other causes: drugs that mobilize edematous fluid or produce diuresis, such as diuretics and cardiac glycosides

Nuchal rigidity

Commonly an early sign of meningeal irritation, nuchal rigidity refers to stiffness of the neck that prevents flexion. This sign may herald life-threatening subarachnoid hemorrhage or meningitis, and may also be a late sign of cervical arthritis, in which joint mobility is gradually lost.

 ___ALERT___

After eliciting nuchal rigidity:
- *attempt to elicit Kernig's and Brudzinski's signs and evaluate level of consciousness (LOC)*
- *assess the patient for signs of increased intracranial pressure*
- *institute emergency treatment, if necessary.*
  If the patient's condition permits, perform a focused assessment.

HISTORY
- Ask the patient about the onset and duration of neck stiffness. (Ask the patient's family for information if an altered LOC prevents the patient from responding.)
- Ask the patient about associated signs and symptoms, such as headache, fever, nausea and vomiting, and motor and sensory changes. If the patient has no other signs of meningeal irritation, ask about a history of arthritis or neck trauma.
- Review the patient's medical history, noting especially hypertension, head trauma, cerebral aneurysm or arteriovenous malformation, endocarditis, recent infection (such as sinusitis or pneumonia), and recent dental work.

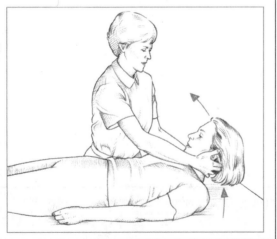

TESTING FOR NUCHAL RIGIDITY

To test for nuchal rigidity, place your hands behind the patient's neck and touch her chin to her chest, as shown here. Pain and muscle spasm will result if nuchal rigidity is present.

- Ask the patient if he can recall pulling a muscle in his neck.
- Obtain a drug history, including prescription and over-the-counter drugs, herbal remedies, and recreational drugs. Also, ask the patient about alcohol intake.

PHYSICAL ASSESSMENT
- To elicit nuchal rigidity, attempt to passively flex the patient's neck and touch his chin to his chest. (See *Testing for nuchal rigidity.*) If nuchal rigidity is present, this maneuver triggers pain and muscle spasms.

 ___ALERT___

Before testing for nuchal rigidity, make sure that no cervical spinal misalignment, such as a fracture or dislocation, exists. Severe spinal cord damage could result.
- Inspect the hands for swollen, tender joints, and palpate the neck for pain or tenderness.

SPECIAL CONSIDERATIONS
If meningeal irritation is present, monitor vital signs, intake and output, and neurologic status closely.

 PEDIATRIC POINTERS
Nuchal rigidity reliably indicates meningeal irritation in children, unless they are paralyzed or comatose.

PATIENT COUNSELING
Instruct the patient on what to expect from diagnostic testing, which may include magnetic resonance imaging, computed tomography scan, and cervical spinal X-rays.

NUCHAL RIGIDITY

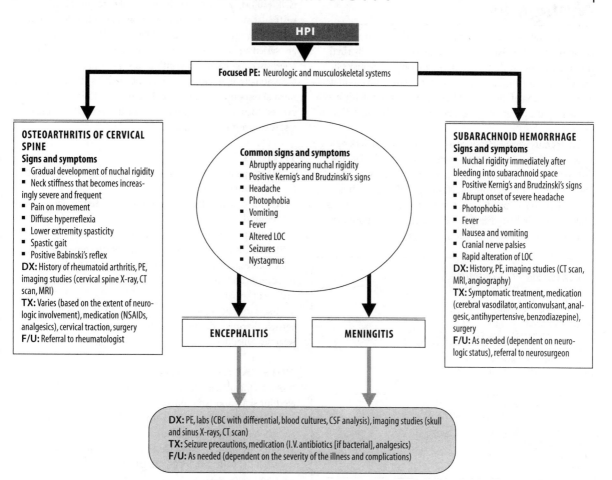

HPI

Focused PE: Neurologic and musculoskeletal systems

OSTEOARTHRITIS OF CERVICAL SPINE
Signs and symptoms
- Gradual development of nuchal rigidity
- Neck stiffness that becomes increasingly severe and frequent
- Pain on movement
- Diffuse hyperreflexia
- Lower extremity spasticity
- Spastic gait
- Positive Babinski's reflex

DX: History of rheumatoid arthritis, PE, imaging studies (cervical spine X-ray, CT scan, MRI)

TX: Varies (based on the extent of neurologic involvement), medication (NSAIDs, analgesics), cervical traction, surgery

F/U: Referral to rheumatologist

Common signs and symptoms
- Abruptly appearing nuchal rigidity
- Positive Kernig's and Brudzinski's signs
- Headache
- Photophobia
- Vomiting
- Fever
- Altered LOC
- Seizures
- Nystagmus

ENCEPHALITIS

MENINGITIS

SUBARACHNOID HEMORRHAGE
Signs and symptoms
- Nuchal rigidity immediately after bleeding into subarachnoid space
- Positive Kernig's and Brudzinski's signs
- Abrupt onset of severe headache
- Photophobia
- Fever
- Nausea and vomiting
- Cranial nerve palsies
- Rapid alteration of LOC

DX: History, PE, imaging studies (CT scan, MRI, angiography)

TX: Symptomatic treatment, medication (cerebral vasodilator, anticonvulsant, analgesic, antihypertensive, benzodiazepine), surgery

F/U: As needed (dependent on neurologic status), referral to neurosurgeon

DX: PE, labs (CBC with differential, blood cultures, CSF analysis), imaging studies (skull and sinus X-rays, CT scan)
TX: Seizure precautions, medication (I.V. antibiotics [if bacterial], analgesics)
F/U: As needed (dependent on the severity of the illness and complications)

Nystagmus

Nystagmus refers to the involuntary oscillations of one or, more commonly, both eyeballs. These oscillations are usually rhythmic and may be horizontal, vertical, or rotary. They may be transient or sustained and may occur spontaneously or on deviation or fixation of the eyes. Although nystagmus is fairly easy to identify, the patient may be unaware of it unless it affects his vision.

Nystagmus may be classified as jerk or pendular. Jerk nystagmus (convergence-retraction, downbeat, and vestibular) has a fast component and then a slow, perhaps unequal, corrective component in the opposite direction. Pendular nystagmus consists of horizontal (pendular) or vertical (seesaw) oscillations that are equal in both directions and resemble the movements of a clock's pendulum. (See *Classifying nystagmus.*)

CLASSIFYING NYSTAGMUS

JERK NYSTAGMUS

Convergence-retraction nystagmus refers to the irregular jerking of the eyes back into the orbit during upward gaze. It can indicate midbrain tegmental damage.

Downbeat nystagmus refers to the irregular downward jerking of the eyes during downward gaze. It can signal lower medullary damage.

Vestibular nystagmus, the horizontal or rotary movement of the eyes, suggests vestibular disease or cochlear dysfunction.

PENDULAR NYSTAGMUS

Horizontal, or *pendular, nystagmus* refers to oscillations of equal velocity around a center point. It can indicate congenital loss of visual acuity or multiple sclerosis.

Vertical, or *seesaw, nystagmus* is the rapid seesaw movement of the eyes: one eye appears to rise while the other appears to fall. It suggests an optic chiasm lesion.

Nystagmus is considered a supranuclear ocular palsy — that is, it results from pathology in the visual perceptual area, vestibular system, cerebellum, or brain stem rather than in the extraocular muscles or in cranial nerve III, IV, or VI. Its causes are varied and include brain stem or cerebellar lesions, multiple sclerosis, encephalitis, labyrinthine disease, and drug toxicity. Occasionally, nystagmus is entirely normal; it's also considered a normal response in the unconscious patient during the doll's eye test (oculocephalic stimulation) or the cold caloric water test (oculovestibular stimulation).

HISTORY

- Ask the patient whether he's aware of his nystagmus and, if he is, how long he has had it.
- Ask the patient if the nystagmus occurs intermittently or continuously.
- Ask the patient if the nystagmus affects his vision.
- Review the patient's medical history, noting especially recent infection (especially of the ear or respiratory tract), head trauma, cancer, and stroke. Also, ask the patient if there's a family history of stroke.
- Assess the patient for associated signs and symptoms, such as vertigo, dizziness, tinnitus, nausea or vomiting, numbness, weakness, bladder dysfunction, and fever.

PHYSICAL ASSESSMENT

- Assess the patient's level of consciousness and vital signs. Be alert for signs and symptoms of increased intracranial pressure, such as pupillary changes, drowsiness, elevated systolic pressure, and altered respiratory pattern.
- Assess nystagmus fully by testing extraocular muscle function. Ask the patient to focus straight ahead and then to follow your finger up, down, and in an "X" across his face. Note when nystagmus occurs as well as its velocity and direction.
- Test reflexes, motor and sensory function, and the cranial nerves.

SPECIAL CONSIDERATIONS

Jerk nystagmus may result from barbiturate, phenytoin, or carbamazepine toxicity or from alcohol intoxication.

🅰 PEDIATRIC POINTERS

In children, pendular nystagmus may be idiopathic or it may result from early impaired vision associated with optic atrophy, albinism, congenital cataracts, or severe astigmatism.

PATIENT COUNSELING

Instruct the patient on what to expect from diagnostic testing, which may include electronystagmography and cerebral computed tomography scan.

NYSTAGMUS

HPI

Focused PE: HEENT, neurologic system

BRAIN TUMOR
Signs and symptoms (dependent on size, type, and location of tumor)
- Insidious onset of jerk nystagmus (with tumors of the brain stem and cerebellum)
- Localized or general headache
- Intermittent deep pain that's more intense in the morning
- Associated personality changes
- Altered LOC
- Increased pain with Valsalva's maneuver
- Seizures
- Neurologic changes

DX: PE, imaging studies (CT scan, MRI, angiography), biopsy
TX: Symptomatic treatment, chemotherapy, radiation therapy, surgery
F/U: Referrals to neurosurgeon and oncologist

STROKE
Signs and symptoms
- Sudden horizontal or vertical jerk nystagmus that may be gaze dependent (with strokes involving the posterior inferior cerebellar artery)
- Dysphagia
- Dysarthria
- Sensory and motor loss
- Ipsilateral Horner's syndrome
- Ataxia
- Vertigo

DX: History, PE, imaging studies (CT scan, duplex carotid ultrasound, angiography)
TX: Maintenance of ABCs, symptomatic treatment, medication (platelet aggregation inhibitors, thrombolytics [if embolic])
F/U: As needed (dependent on neurologic status), referral to neurologist

ENCEPHALITIS
Signs and symptoms
- Abruptly appearing nuchal rigidity
- Jerk nystagmus
- Positive Kernig's and Brudzinski's signs
- Headache
- Photophobia
- Vomiting
- Fever
- Altered LOC
- Seizures

DX: PE, labs (CBC with differential, blood cultures, CSF analysis), imaging studies (skull and sinus X-rays, CT scan)
TX: Seizure precautions, medication (I.V. antibiotics [if bacterial], analgesics)
F/U: As needed (dependent on the severity of the illness and complications)

Common signs and symptoms
- Dizziness
- Vertigo
- Tinnitus
- Nausea and vomiting
- Gradual sensorineural hearing loss
- Positive Romberg's sign

LABYRINTHITIS (ACUTE)
Additional signs and symptoms
- Sudden onset of jerk nystagmus toward the unaffected ear

DX: CT scan, electronystagmography, calorie test, doll's eye test
TX: Treatment of the underlying cause, lying still in dark room during acute attack, medication (antivertigo agents, sedative-hypnotic)
F/U: Referral to otolaryngologist

MENIERE'S DISEASE
Additional signs and symptoms
- Acute attacks of jerk nystagmus that may last 10 minutes to several hours

DX: PE, otoscopy with air pressure applied to tympanic membrane, audiometry, caloric testing, MRI
TX: Medication (atropine, antiemetic-antivertigo agents, sedative-hypnotic)
F/U: Referral to otolaryngologist

Additional differential diagnoses: head trauma ▪ multiple sclerosis

Other causes: alcohol intoxication ▪ drugs (barbiturate, phenytoin, or carbamazepine toxicity)

Ocular deviation

Ocular deviation refers to abnormal eye movement that may be conjugate (both eyes move together) or dysconjugate (one eye moves differently from the other). This common sign may result from an ocular, neurologic, endocrine, or systemic disorder that interferes with the muscles, nerves, or brain centers governing eye movement. Occasionally, it signals a life-threatening disorder such as ruptured cerebral aneurysm. (See *Ocular deviation: Characteristics and causes in cranial nerve damage.*)

Normally, eye movement is directly controlled by the extraocular muscles innervated by the oculomotor, trochlear, and abducens nerves (cranial nerves III, IV, and VI). Together, these muscles and nerves direct a visual stimulus to fall on corresponding parts of the retina. Dysconjugate ocular deviation may result from unequal muscle tone (nonparalytic strabismus) or from muscle paralysis associated with cranial nerve damage (paralytic strabismus). Conjugate ocular deviation may result from disorders that affect the centers in the cerebral cortex and brain stem responsible for conjugate eye movement. Typically, such disorders cause gaze palsy—difficulty moving the eyes in one or more directions.

ALERT

If the patient displays ocular deviation:
- *quickly take his vital signs*
- *look for altered level of consciousness, pupil changes, motor or sensory dysfunction, and severe headache*
- *if possible, ask his family about behavioral changes or a history of recent head trauma*
- *institute emergency measures, if needed.*

If the patient's condition permits, perform a focused assessment.

HISTORY
- Ask the patient how long he has had the ocular deviation and if it's accompanied by double vision, eye pain, or headache.
- Ask the patient whether he has noticed associated motor or sensory changes or fever.
- Review the patient's medical history for hypertension; diabetes; allergies; thyroid, neurologic, or muscular disorders; extraocular muscle imbalance; eye or head trauma; and eye surgery.

PHYSICAL ASSESSMENT
- Observe the patient for partial or complete ptosis. Note if he spontaneously tilts his head or turns his face to compensate for ocular deviation.
- Check for eye redness or periorbital edema. Assess visual acuity; then evaluate extraocular muscle function by testing the six cardinal fields of gaze.

SPECIAL CONSIDERATIONS
If you suspect an acute neurologic disorder, take seizure precautions and monitor vital signs and neurologic status closely.

A   PEDIATRIC POINTERS
- *In children, the most common cause of ocular deviation is nonparalytic strabismus.*
- *Although severe strabismus is readily apparent, mild strabismus must be confirmed by tests for misalignment, such as the corneal light reflex test and the cover test. Testing is crucial—early corrective measures help preserve binocular vision and cosmetic appearance. Also, mild strabismus may indicate retinoblastoma, a tumor that may be asymptomatic before age 2, except for a characteristic whitish reflex in the pupil.*

PATIENT COUNSELING
Instruct the patient on what to expect from diagnostic testing, which may include blood studies, orbital and skull X-rays, and computed tomography scan.

OCULAR DEVIATION: CHARACTERISTICS AND CAUSES IN CRANIAL NERVE DAMAGE

CHARACTERISTICS	CRANIAL NERVE AND EXTRAOCULAR MUSCLES INVOLVED	PROBABLE CAUSES
Inability to focus the eye upward, downward, inward, and outward; drooping eyelid; and, except in diabetes, a dilated pupil in the affected eye	Oculomotor nerve (III); medial rectus, superior rectus, inferior rectus, and inferior oblique muscles	Cerebral aneurysm, diabetes, temporal lobe herniation from increased intracranial pressure, brain tumor
Loss of downward and outward movement in the affected eye	Trochlear nerve (IV); superior oblique muscle	Head trauma
Loss of outward movement in the affected eye	Abducens nerve (VI); lateral rectus muscle	Brain tumor

OCULAR DEVIATION

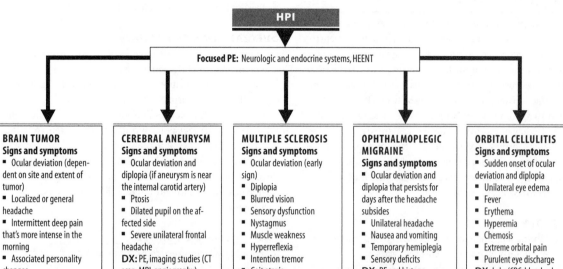

HPI

Focused PE: Neurologic and endocrine systems, HEENT

BRAIN TUMOR
Signs and symptoms
- Ocular deviation (dependent on site and extent of tumor)
- Localized or general headache
- Intermittent deep pain that's more intense in the morning
- Associated personality changes
- Changes in LOC
- Increased pain with Valsalva's maneuver

DX: PE, imaging studies (CT scan, MRI, arteriography)
TX: Medication (analgesics, anticonvulsants, osmotic diuretics, chemotherapy), radiation therapy, surgery
F/U: Referrals to neurosurgeon and oncologist

CEREBRAL ANEURYSM
Signs and symptoms
- Ocular deviation and diplopia (if aneurysm is near the internal carotid artery)
- Ptosis
- Dilated pupil on the affected side
- Severe unilateral frontal headache

DX: PE, imaging studies (CT scan, MRI, angiography)
TX: Medication (cerebral vasodilator, analgesics), surgery
F/U: Referral to neurosurgeon

MULTIPLE SCLEROSIS
Signs and symptoms
- Ocular deviation (early sign)
- Diplopia
- Blurred vision
- Sensory dysfunction
- Nystagmus
- Muscle weakness
- Hyperreflexia
- Intention tremor
- Gait ataxia

DX: PE, CSF analysis, MRI, EEG, evoked response studies
TX: Symptomatic treatment, medication (antispasmotics, antidepressants, corticosteroids)
F/U: Referral to neurologist

OPHTHALMOPLEGIC MIGRAINE
Signs and symptoms
- Ocular deviation and diplopia that persists for days after the headache subsides
- Unilateral headache
- Nausea and vomiting
- Temporary hemiplegia
- Sensory deficits

DX: PE and history
TX: Identification and avoidance of trigger, medication (5-HT$_1$ serotonin receptor agonist, ergotamines, barbiturates, analgesics, NSAIDs)
F/U: Referral to headache clinic if symptoms persist or worsen

ORBITAL CELLULITIS
Signs and symptoms
- Sudden onset of ocular deviation and diplopia
- Unilateral eye edema
- Fever
- Erythema
- Hyperemia
- Chemosis
- Extreme orbital pain
- Purulent eye discharge

DX: Labs (CBC, blood culture, throat and eye culture), imaging studies (orbit and sinus X-rays, CT scan)
TX: I.V. antibiotics, surgery
F/U: Referral to ophthalmologist

Additional differential diagnoses: cavernous sinus thrombosis ▪ diabetes mellitus ▪ encephalitis ▪ head trauma ▪ myasthenia gravis ▪ orbital blowout fracture ▪ orbital tumor ▪ stroke ▪ thyrotoxicosis

Oligomenorrhea

In most women, menstrual bleeding occurs every 28 days, plus or minus 4 days. Although some variation is normal, menstrual bleeding at intervals of greater than 36 days may indicate oligomenorrhea—abnormally infrequent menstrual bleeding characterized by three to six menstrual cycles per year. When menstrual bleeding does occur, it's usually profuse, prolonged (up to 10 days), and laden with clots and tissue. Occasionally, scant bleeding or spotting occurs between these heavy menses.

Oligomenorrhea may develop suddenly, or it may follow a period of gradually lengthening cycles. Although oligomenorrhea may alternate with normal menstrual bleeding, it can progress to secondary amenorrhea.

HISTORY

- Ask the patient when menarche occurred and whether she has ever experienced normal menstrual cycles.
- Ask the patient to describe the pattern of bleeding as well as how many days the bleeding lasts and how frequently it occurs.
- Ask the patient if she has been having symptoms of ovulatory bleeding or mild, cramping abdominal pain 14 days before she bleeds. Ask her if the bleeding is accompanied by premenstrual signs and symptoms, such as breast tenderness, irritability, bloating, weight gain, nausea, diarrhea, or cramping pain.
- Check for a history of infertility. Does the patient have children or is she trying to conceive?
- Ask the patient about her method of birth control.
- Review the patient's medical history for gynecologic disorders such as ovarian cysts. If the patient is breast-feeding, has she experienced problems with milk production? If she hasn't been breast-feeding recently, has she noticed milk leaking from her breasts?
- Ask the patient about recent weight gain or loss. Is the patient less than 80% of her ideal weight? If so, does she claim that she's overweight? Ask her whether she's exercising more vigorously than usual.
- Screen the patient for a metabolic disorder by asking about excessive thirst, frequent urination, and fatigue. Ask the patient if she has been jittery or had palpitations. Also, ask about headache, dizziness, and impaired peripheral vision.
- Obtain a drug history, including prescription and over-the-counter drugs, herbal remedies, and recreational drugs. Also, ask the patient about alcohol intake.

PHYSICAL ASSESSMENT

- Take the patient's vital signs, and weigh her.
- Check for increased facial hair growth, sparse body hair, male distribution of fat and muscle, acne, and clitoral enlargement.
- Note if the skin is abnormally dry or moist, and check hair texture.
- Be alert for signs of psychological or physical stress.

SPECIAL CONSIDERATIONS

Oligomenorrhea is common in infertile, early postmenarchal, and perimenopausal women because it's associated with anovulation. Usually, anovulation reflects abnormalities of the hormones that govern normal endometrial function.

Oligomenorrhea may result from an ovarian, hypothalamic, pituitary, or other metabolic disorder, or it may stem from the effects of certain drugs. It may also result from emotional or physical stress, such as sudden weight change, debilitating illness, or rigorous physical training. Oligomenorrhea in the perimenopausal woman usually indicates impending onset of menopause.

🅰 *PEDIATRIC POINTERS*

- *Teenage girls may experience oligomenorrhea associated with immature hormonal function.*
- *Prolonged oligomenorrhea or the development of amenorrhea may signal congenital adrenal hyperplasia or Turner's syndrome.*

PATIENT COUNSELING

Ask the patient to record her basal body temperature daily to determine if she's having ovulatory cycles. Remind the patient that she may become pregnant even though she isn't menstruating normally. Discuss contraceptive measures as appropriate.

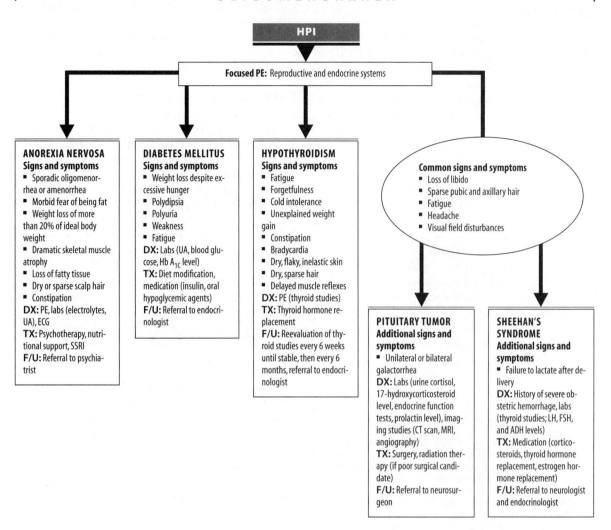

HPI

Focused PE: Reproductive and endocrine systems

ANOREXIA NERVOSA
Signs and symptoms
- Sporadic oligomenorrhea or amenorrhea
- Morbid fear of being fat
- Weight loss of more than 20% of ideal body weight
- Dramatic skeletal muscle atrophy
- Loss of fatty tissue
- Dry or sparse scalp hair
- Constipation

DX: PE, labs (electrolytes, UA), ECG
TX: Psychotherapy, nutritional support, SSRI
F/U: Referral to psychiatrist

DIABETES MELLITUS
Signs and symptoms
- Weight loss despite excessive hunger
- Polydipsia
- Polyuria
- Weakness
- Fatigue

DX: Labs (UA, blood glucose, Hb A_{1C} level)
TX: Diet modification, medication (insulin, oral hypoglycemic agents)
F/U: Referral to endocrinologist

HYPOTHYROIDISM
Signs and symptoms
- Fatigue
- Forgetfulness
- Cold intolerance
- Unexplained weight gain
- Constipation
- Bradycardia
- Dry, flaky, inelastic skin
- Dry, sparse hair
- Delayed muscle reflexes

DX: PE (thyroid studies)
TX: Thyroid hormone replacement
F/U: Reevaluation of thyroid studies every 6 weeks until stable, then every 6 months, referral to endocrinologist

Common signs and symptoms
- Loss of libido
- Sparse pubic and axillary hair
- Fatigue
- Headache
- Visual field disturbances

PITUITARY TUMOR
Additional signs and symptoms
- Unilateral or bilateral galactorrhea

DX: Labs (urine cortisol, 17-hydroxycorticosteroid level, endocrine function tests, prolactin level), imaging studies (CT scan, MRI, angiography)
TX: Surgery, radiation therapy (if poor surgical candidate)
F/U: Referral to neurosurgeon

SHEEHAN'S SYNDROME
Additional signs and symptoms
- Failure to lactate after delivery

DX: History of severe obstetric hemorrhage, labs (thyroid studies; LH, FSH, and ADH levels)
TX: Medication (corticosteroids, thyroid hormone replacement, estrogen hormone replacement)
F/U: Referral to neurologist and endocrinologist

Additional differential diagnoses: adrenal hyperplasia ▪ hypothyroidism ▪ polycystic ovary disease ▪ thyrotoxicosis

Other causes: amphetamines ▪ antihypertensives ▪ drugs that increase androgen levels (corticosteroids, corticotropin, anabolic steroids, danazol, injectable and implanted contraceptives) ▪ phenothiazine derivatives

Oliguria

A cardinal sign of renal and urinary tract disorders, oliguria is clinically defined as urine output of less than 400 ml per 24 hours. Typically, this sign occurs abruptly and may herald serious—possibly life-threatening—hemodynamic instability. Its causes can be classified as prerenal (decreased renal blood flow), intrarenal (intrinsic renal damage), or postrenal (urinary tract obstruction); the pathophysiology differs for each classification. (See *Causes of oliguria*.)

HISTORY

- Ask the patient about his usual daily voiding pattern, including frequency and amount. Ask when he first noticed changes in this pattern or in the color, odor, or consistency of his urine. Ask him if he experiences pain or burning on urination.
- Note the patient's normal daily fluid intake.
- Ask the patient if has had recent episodes of diarrhea or vomiting that might cause fluid loss. Explore associated complaints, especially fatigue, loss of appetite, thirst, dyspnea, chest pain, or recent weight gain.
- Review the patient's medical history for renal or cardiovascular disorders, recent traumatic injury or surgery associated with significant blood loss, and recent blood transfusions.

- Ask the patient if he has been exposed to nephrotoxic agents, such as heavy metals, organic solvents, anesthetics, or radiographic contrast media.
- Obtain a drug history, including prescription and over-the-counter drugs, herbal remedies, and recreational drugs. Also, ask the patient about alcohol intake.

PHYSICAL ASSESSMENT

- Take the patient's vital signs, and weigh him.
- Assess the patient's overall appearance for edema.
- Palpate both kidneys for tenderness and enlargement, and percuss for costovertebral angle tenderness. Inspect the flank area for edema or erythema.
- Auscultate the heart and lungs for abnormal sounds and the flank area for renal artery bruits.
- Obtain a urine sample, and check for abnormal color, odor, or sediment. Use reagent strips to test for glucose, protein, and blood. Measure specific gravity.

SPECIAL CONSIDERATIONS

Oliguria may result from drugs that cause decreased renal perfusion (diuretics), nephrotoxicity (aminoglycosides and chemotherapeutic agents), urine retention (adrenergic and anticholinergic agents), or urinary obstruction associated with precipitation of urinary crystals (sulfonamides and acyclovir).

A   PEDIATRIC POINTERS

- *In the neonate, oliguria may result from edema or dehydration. Major causes include congenital heart disease, respiratory distress syndrome, sepsis, congenital hydronephrosis, acute tubular necrosis, and renal vein thrombosis.*
- *Common causes of oliguria in children between ages 1 and 5 are acute poststreptococcal glomerulonephritis and hemolytic-uremic syndrome. After age 5, causes of oliguria are similar to those in adults.*

A   AGING ISSUES

In elderly patients, oliguria may result from gradual progression of an underlying disorder or from overall poor muscle tone secondary to inactivity, poor fluid intake, or infrequent voiding attempts.

PATIENT COUNSELING

Depending on the cause of the oliguria, tell the patient to restrict fluids to between 600 and 1,000 ml more than the patient's urine output for the previous day. Explain to the patient that he needs to follow a diet low in sodium, potassium, and protein.

CAUSES OF OLIGURIA

Oliguria associated with a prerenal or postrenal cause is usually reversible with treatment; it may lead to intrarenal damage if untreated. However, oliguria associated with an intrarenal cause is usually more persistent and may be irreversible.

PRERENAL CAUSES

- Bilateral renal artery occlusion
- Bilateral renal vein occlusion
- Cirrhosis
- Heart failure
- Hypovolemia
- Sepsis

INTRARENAL CAUSES

- Acute glomerulonephritis
- Acute pyelonephritis
- Acute tubular necrosis
- Chronic renal failure
- Toxemia of pregnancy

POSTRENAL CAUSES

- Benign prostatic hyperplasia
- Bladder neoplasm
- Calculi
- Retroperitoneal fibrosis
- Urethral stricture

OLIGURIA

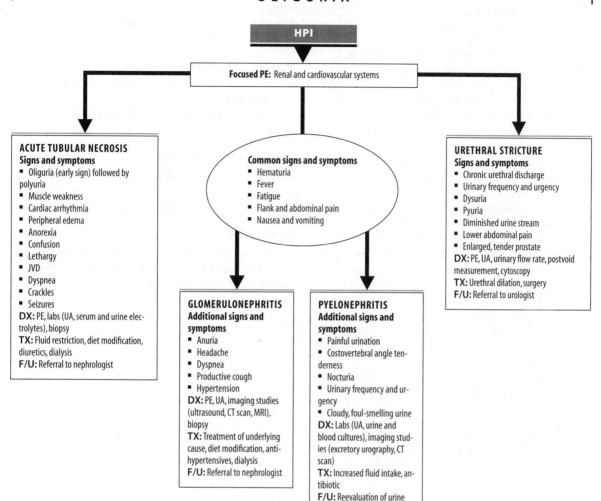

HPI

Focused PE: Renal and cardiovascular systems

ACUTE TUBULAR NECROSIS
Signs and symptoms
- Oliguria (early sign) followed by polyuria
- Muscle weakness
- Cardiac arrhythmia
- Peripheral edema
- Anorexia
- Confusion
- Lethargy
- JVD
- Dyspnea
- Crackles
- Seizures

DX: PE, labs (UA, serum and urine electrolytes), biopsy
TX: Fluid restriction, diet modification, diuretics, dialysis
F/U: Referral to nephrologist

Common signs and symptoms
- Hematuria
- Fever
- Fatigue
- Flank and abdominal pain
- Nausea and vomiting

URETHRAL STRICTURE
Signs and symptoms
- Chronic urethral discharge
- Urinary frequency and urgency
- Dysuria
- Pyuria
- Diminished urine stream
- Lower abdominal pain
- Enlarged, tender prostate

DX: PE, UA, urinary flow rate, postvoid measurement, cytoscopy
TX: Urethral dilation, surgery
F/U: Referral to urologist

GLOMERULONEPHRITIS
Additional signs and symptoms
- Anuria
- Headache
- Dyspnea
- Productive cough
- Hypertension

DX: PE, UA, imaging studies (ultrasound, CT scan, MRI), biopsy
TX: Treatment of underlying cause, diet modification, antihypertensives, dialysis
F/U: Referral to nephrologist

PYELONEPHRITIS
Additional signs and symptoms
- Painful urination
- Costovertebral angle tenderness
- Nocturia
- Urinary frequency and urgency
- Cloudy, foul-smelling urine

DX: Labs (UA, urine and blood cultures), imaging studies (excretory urography, CT scan)
TX: Increased fluid intake, antibiotic
F/U: Reevaluation of urine culture in 2, 6, and 12 weeks

Additional differential diagnoses: bladder neoplasm ▪ BPH ▪ calculi ▪ cirrhosis ▪ heart failure ▪ hypovolemia ▪ renal artery occlusion (bilateral) ▪ renal failure (chronic) ▪ renal vein occlusion (bilateral) ▪ retroperitoneal fibrosis ▪ sepsis ▪ toxemia of pregnancy

Other causes: contrast media ▪ drugs that cause decreased renal perfusion (diuretics), nephrotoxicity (most notably, aminoglycosides and chemotherapeutic agents), urine retention (adrenergic and anticholinergic agents), or urinary obstruction associated with precipitation of urinary crystals (sulfonamides and acyclovir)

Opisthotonos

A sign of severe meningeal irritation, opisthotonos is character-ized by a strongly arched, rigid back; a hyperextended neck; heels that are bent back; and arms and hands that are flexed at the joints. Usually, this posture occurs spontaneously as well as continuously; however, it may be aggravated by movement. Be-cause it immobilizes the spine, opisthotonos presumably repre-sents a protective reflex that alleviates pain associated with meningeal irritation.

Usually caused by meningitis, opisthotonos may also result from subarachnoid hemorrhage, Arnold-Chiari syndrome, or tetanus. Occasionally, it occurs with achondroplastic dwarfism, although not necessarily as an indicator of meningeal irritation.

Opisthotonos is far more common in children—especially infants—than in adults. It's also more exaggerated in children because of nervous system immaturity. (See *Opisthotonos: Sign of meningeal irritation.*)

ALERT

If the patient is stuporous or comatose:
- *quickly take his vital signs*
- *take seizure precautions; if meningitis is suspected, institute res-piratory isolation*
- *initiate emergency measures, if necessary.*
  If the patient's condition permits, perform a focused assessment.

HISTORY
- Review the patient's medical history for cerebral aneurysm, arteriovenous malformation, and hypertension.

- Note recent infections that may have spread to the nervous system.
- Explore associated signs and symptoms, such as headache, chills, and vomiting.

PHYSICAL ASSESSMENT
- Evaluate level of consciousness, and test sensorimotor and cranial nerve function.
- Check for Brudzinski's and Kernig's signs and for nuchal rigidity.

SPECIAL CONSIDERATIONS
Phenothiazines and other antipsychotics may cause opistho-tonos, usually as part of an acute dystonic reaction. This can usually be treated with I.V. diphenhydramine.

PATIENT COUNSELING
Instruct the patient on what to expect from diagnostic testing, which may include lumbar puncture, computed tomography scan, and magnetic resonance imaging.

OPISTHOTONOS: SIGN OF MENINGEAL IRRITATION

With opisthotonos, the back is severely arched and the neck hyper-extended. The heels bend back on the legs, and the arms and hands flex rigidly at the joints, as shown.

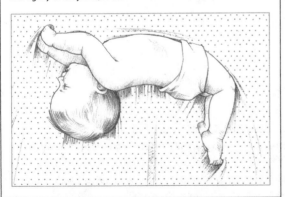

OPISTHOTONOS

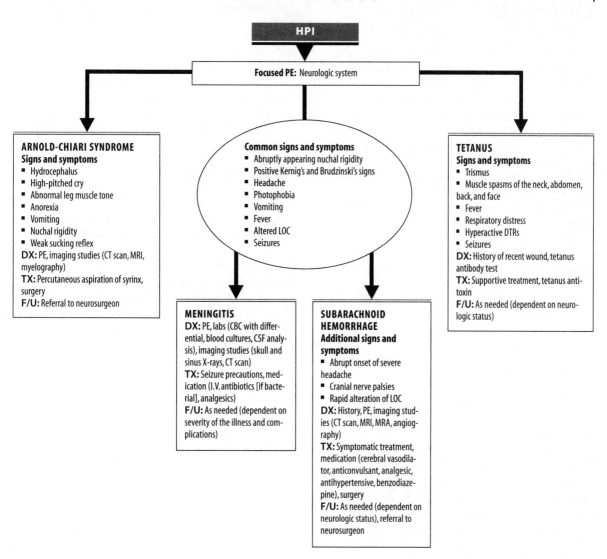

HPI

Focused PE: Neurologic system

ARNOLD-CHIARI SYNDROME
Signs and symptoms
- Hydrocephalus
- High-pitched cry
- Abnormal leg muscle tone
- Anorexia
- Vomiting
- Nuchal rigidity
- Weak sucking reflex

DX: PE, imaging studies (CT scan, MRI, myelography)
TX: Percutaneous aspiration of syrinx, surgery
F/U: Referral to neurosurgeon

Common signs and symptoms
- Abruptly appearing nuchal rigidity
- Positive Kernig's and Brudzinski's signs
- Headache
- Photophobia
- Vomiting
- Fever
- Altered LOC
- Seizures

TETANUS
Signs and symptoms
- Trismus
- Muscle spasms of the neck, abdomen, back, and face
- Fever
- Respiratory distress
- Hyperactive DTRs
- Seizures

DX: History of recent wound, tetanus antibody test
TX: Supportive treatment, tetanus antitoxin
F/U: As needed (dependent on neurologic status)

MENINGITIS
DX: PE, labs (CBC with differential, blood cultures, CSF analysis), imaging studies (skull and sinus X-rays, CT scan)
TX: Seizure precautions, medication (I.V. antibiotics [if bacterial], analgesics)
F/U: As needed (dependent on severity of the illness and complications)

SUBARACHNOID HEMORRHAGE
Additional signs and symptoms
- Abrupt onset of severe headache
- Cranial nerve palsies
- Rapid alteration of LOC

DX: History, PE, imaging studies (CT scan, MRI, MRA, angiography)
TX: Symptomatic treatment, medication (cerebral vasodilator, anticonvulsant, analgesic, antihypertensive, benzodiazepine), surgery
F/U: As needed (dependent on neurologic status), referral to neurosurgeon

Other causes: antipsychotics such as phenothiazines

Orthostatic hypotension

With orthostatic hypotension, also known as *postural hypotension*, the patient's blood pressure drops 15 to 20 mm Hg or more—with or without an increase in the heart rate of at least 20 beats/minute—when he rises from a supine position to a sitting or standing position. (Blood pressure should be measured 5 minutes after the patient has changed his position.) This common sign indicates failure of compensatory vasomotor responses to adjust to position changes. It's typically associated with light-headedness, syncope, or blurred vision, and it may occur in a hypotensive, normotensive, or hypertensive patient. Although frequently a nonpathologic sign in elderly people, orthostatic hypotension may result from prolonged bed rest, fluid and electrolyte imbalance, an endocrine or systemic disorder, or the effects of certain drugs.

To detect orthostatic hypotension, take and compare blood pressure readings with the patient in supine, sitting, and standing positions.

 ALERT

If you detect orthostatic hypotension:
- *quickly check for tachycardia, altered level of consciousness, and pale, clammy skin (If these signs are present, suspect hypovolemic shock.)*
- *institute emergency measures, if necessary.*
  If the patient's condition permits, perform a focused assessment.

HISTORY
- Ask the patient whether he frequently experiences dizziness, weakness, or fainting when he changes position.
- Ask the patient about associated signs and symptoms, particularly fatigue, orthopnea, impotence, nausea, headache, abdominal or chest discomfort, and GI bleeding.
- Obtain a drug history, including prescription and over-the-counter drugs, herbal remedies, and recreational drugs. Also, ask the patient about alcohol intake.

PHYSICAL ASSESSMENT
- Check the patient's skin turgor.
- Palpate peripheral pulses, and auscultate the heart and lungs.
- Test muscle strength, and observe the patient's gait for unsteadiness.

SPECIAL CONSIDERATIONS
Always keep the patient's safety in mind. Never leave him unattended while he's sitting or walking; evaluate his need for assistive devices, such as a cane or walker.

 PEDIATRIC POINTERS
- *Because normal blood pressure is lower in children than in adults, familiarize yourself with normal age-specific values to detect orthostatic hypotension. From birth to age 3 months, normal systolic pressure is 40 to 80 mm Hg; from ages 3 months to 1 year, 80 to 100 mm Hg; and from ages 1 to 12, 100 mm Hg plus 2 mm Hg for every year over age 1. Diastolic blood pressure is first heard at about age 4; it's normally 60 mm Hg at this age and gradually increases to 70 mm Hg by age 12.*
- *The causes of orthostatic hypotension in children are the same as those in adults.*

 AGING ISSUES

Elderly patients commonly experience autonomic dysfunction, which can present as orthostatic hypotension. Postprandial hypotension occurs 45 to 60 minutes after a meal and has been documented in up to one-third of nursing home residents.

PATIENT COUNSELING
Patients with conditions that can lead to autonomic dysfunction (such as diabetes mellitus) should be made aware of the acute drop in blood pressure that can occur with positional changes. Such patients need to avoid volume depletion and perform positional changes gradually instead of suddenly.

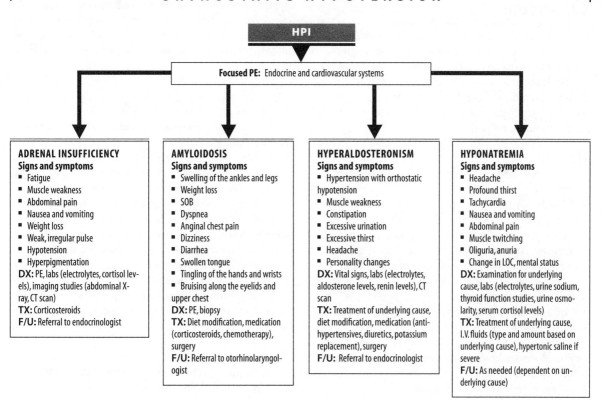

HPI

Focused PE: Endocrine and cardiovascular systems

ADRENAL INSUFFICIENCY
Signs and symptoms
- Fatigue
- Muscle weakness
- Abdominal pain
- Nausea and vomiting
- Weight loss
- Weak, irregular pulse
- Hypotension
- Hyperpigmentation

DX: PE, labs (electrolytes, cortisol levels), imaging studies (abdominal X-ray, CT scan)
TX: Corticosteroids
F/U: Referral to endocrinologist

AMYLOIDOSIS
Signs and symptoms
- Swelling of the ankles and legs
- Weight loss
- SOB
- Dyspnea
- Anginal chest pain
- Dizziness
- Diarrhea
- Swollen tongue
- Tingling of the hands and wrists
- Bruising along the eyelids and upper chest

DX: PE, biopsy
TX: Diet modification, medication (corticosteroids, chemotherapy), surgery
F/U: Referral to otorhinolaryngologist

HYPERALDOSTERONISM
Signs and symptoms
- Hypertension with orthostatic hypotension
- Muscle weakness
- Constipation
- Excessive urination
- Excessive thirst
- Headache
- Personality changes

DX: Vital signs, labs (electrolytes, aldosterone levels, renin levels), CT scan
TX: Treatment of underlying cause, diet modification, medication (antihypertensives, diuretics, potassium replacement), surgery
F/U: Referral to endocrinologist

HYPONATREMIA
Signs and symptoms
- Headache
- Profound thirst
- Tachycardia
- Nausea and vomiting
- Abdominal pain
- Muscle twitching
- Oliguria, anuria
- Change in LOC, mental status

DX: Examination for underlying cause, labs (electrolytes, urine sodium, thyroid function studies, urine osmolarity, serum cortisol levels)
TX: Treatment of underlying cause, I.V. fluids (type and amount based on underlying cause), hypertonic saline if severe
F/U: As needed (dependent on underlying cause)

Additional differential diagnoses: alcoholism ▪ diabetic autonomic neuropathy ▪ hypovolemia ▪ pheochromocytoma ▪ Shy-Drager syndrome

Other causes: antihypertensives ▪ diuretics (in large doses) ▪ levodopa ▪ MAO inhibitors ▪ morphine ▪ nitrates ▪ phenothiazines ▪ prolonged bed rest (24 hours or longer) ▪ spinal anesthesia ▪ sympathectomy ▪ tricyclic antidepressants

Otorrhea

Otorrhea — drainage from the ear — may be bloody (otorrhagia), purulent, clear, or serosanguineous. Its onset, duration, and severity provide clues to the underlying cause. This sign may result from a disorder that affects the external ear canal or the middle ear, including an allergy, infection, neoplasm, trauma, or collagen disease. Otorrhea may occur alone or with other symptoms such as ear pain.

HISTORY

- Ask the patient when the otorrhea began. Ask him how he recognized it.
- Ask the patient if he cleaned the drainage from deep within the ear canal or if he wiped it from the auricle.
- Ask the patient to describe the color, consistency, and odor of the drainage. Is it clear, purulent, or bloody? Ask him if it occurs in one or both ears and if it's continuous or intermittent.
- If the patient wears cotton in his ear to absorb the drainage, ask how often he changes it.
- Explore associated otologic symptoms, especially pain. Ask about vertigo and tinnitus.
- Review the patient's medical history for recent upper respiratory tract infection, head trauma, cancer, dermatitis, and immunosuppressant therapy.
- Ask the patient how he cleans his ears.
- Ask the patient if he's an avid swimmer.

PHYSICAL ASSESSMENT

If the patient's symptoms are unilateral, examine the uninvolved ear first.

- Inspect the external ear, and apply pressure on the tragus and mastoid area to elicit tenderness.
- Insert an otoscope, using the largest speculum that will comfortably fit into the ear canal. If necessary, clean cerumen, pus, or other debris from the canal. Check for edema, erythema, crusts, or polyps. Inspect the tympanic membrane, which should look like a shiny, pearl-gray cone. Note color changes, perforation, absence of the normal light reflex (a cone of light appearing toward the bottom of the drum), or a bulging membrane.
- Test hearing acuity. Have the patient occlude one ear while you whisper some common two-syllable words toward the unoccluded ear. Stand behind him so he can't read your lips, and ask him to repeat what he heard. Perform the test on the other ear using different words. Then use a tuning fork to perform Weber's test and the Rinne test.
- Palpate the neck and preauricular, parotid, and postauricular (mastoid) areas for lymphadenopathy. Test the function of cranial nerves VII, IX, X, and XI.

SPECIAL CONSIDERATIONS

Apply a warm, moist compress or heating pad to the patient's ear to relieve inflammation and pain. Use cotton wicks to gently clean the drainage or to apply topical drugs. Keep eardrops at room temperature; instillation of cold eardrops may cause vertigo.

🅰 PEDIATRIC POINTERS

- *When you examine or clean a child's ear, remember that the auditory canal lies horizontally and that the pinna must be pulled downward and backward.*
- *Restrain a child during an ear procedure by having him sit on a parent's lap with the ear to be examined facing you. Have him put one arm around the parent's waist and the other arm down at his side and then ask the parent to hold the child in place. Alternatively, if you're alone with the child, you can have him lie on his abdomen with his arms at his sides and his head turned so the affected ear faces the ceiling. Bend over him, restraining his upper body with your elbows and upper arms.*
- *Otitis media is the most common cause of otorrhea in infants and young children. Children are also likely to insert foreign bodies into their ears, resulting in infection, pain, and purulent discharge.*

PATIENT COUNSELING

Advise the patient with chronic ear problems to avoid forceful nose blowing when he has an upper respiratory tract infection so that infected secretions aren't channeled into the middle ear. Instruct him to blow his nose with his mouth open. Also, remind him to cleanse his ears with a washcloth only and not to put anything in his ear (such as a hairpin or a cotton-tipped applicator) that may cause injury.

OTORRHEA

HPI

Focused PE: HEENT

BASILAR SKULL FRACTURE
Signs and symptoms
- Clear watery otorrhea or bloody drainage
- Hearing loss
- CSF or bloody rhinorrhea
- Periorbital ecchymosis
- Positive Battle's sign
- Cranial nerve palsies
- Altered LOC
- Headache

DX: PE, history of head trauma, imaging studies (skull X-ray, CT scan)

TX: Symptomatic treatment, medication (antibiotics, analgesics, anti-inflammatory agents), surgery

F/U: As needed (dependent on the extent of injury or complications), referral to neurosurgeon

MASTOIDITIS
Signs and symptoms
- Thick, purulent, yellow otorrhea that becomes increasingly profuse
- Low-grade fever
- Dull, aching tenderness in the mastoid area
- Postauricular erythema and edema
- Conductive hearing loss

DX: Ear examination, culture of ear drainage, imaging studies (skull X-ray, CT scan)

TX: Medication (antibiotics, analgesics), surgery

F/U: Referral to otorhinolaryngologist

OTITIS MEDIA (ACUTE)

Common signs and symptoms
- Bloody, purulent otorrhea (with tympanic rupture)
- Appearance of otorrhea, which usually signals ear pain relief
- Conductive hearing loss
- Bulging or ruptured tympanic membrane

Additional common signs and symptoms
- Sore throat
- Nasal discharge
- Cough
- Headache

ACUTE SUPPURATIVE OTITIS MEDIA

DX: Ear examination, culture of ear drainage
TX: Local warmth, medication (analgesics, antibiotics, antipyretics), myringotomy, drainage tubes
F/U: Reevaluation in 48 hours, referral to otorhinolaryngologist if recurrent

MYRINGITIS (INFECTIOUS)
Additional signs and symptoms
- Serosanguineous otorrhea
- Severe ear pain
- Tenderness over the mastoid process
- Small, reddened, blood-filled blebs in the external canal and tympanic membrane

---

Additional differential diagnoses: allergy ▪ aural polyps ▪ dermatitis of the external ear canal ▪ epidural abscess ▪ otitis externa ▪ perichondritis ▪ trauma ▪ tuberculosis ▪ tumor ▪ Wegener's granulomatosis

P Q *Pallor*

Pallor is an abnormal paleness or loss of skin color, which may develop suddenly or gradually. Although generalized pallor affects the entire body, it's most apparent on the face, conjunctiva, oral mucosa, and nail beds. Localized pallor commonly affects a single limb.

How easily pallor is detected varies with skin color and the thickness and vascularity of underlying subcutaneous tissue. At times, it's merely a subtle lightening of skin color that may be difficult to detect in dark-skinned persons; sometimes, it's evident only on the conjunctiva and oral mucosa.

Pallor may result from decreased peripheral oxyhemoglobin or decreased total oxyhemoglobin. The former reflects diminished peripheral blood flow associated with peripheral vasoconstriction or arterial occlusion or with low cardiac output. (Transient peripheral vasoconstriction may occur with exposure to cold, causing nonpathologic pallor.) The latter usually results from anemia, the chief cause of pallor.

A LERT

If generalized pallor develops:
- *quickly take the patient's vital signs*
- *look for signs of shock, such as tachycardia, hypotension, oliguria, and decreased level of consciousness*
- *institute emergency measures, if appropriate.*
  If the patient's condition permits, perform a focused assessment.

HISTORY

- Review the patient's medical history for anemia or chronic disorders that might lead to pallor, such as renal failure, heart failure, ulcer disease, and diabetes. Ask the patient about a family history of anemia.
- Ask the patient about his diet, particularly his intake of green vegetables.
- Ask the patient when he first noticed the pallor and if it's constant or intermittent. Does it occur when he's exposed to the cold or under emotional stress?
- Ask the patient about associated signs and symptoms, such as dizziness, fainting, orthostasis, weakness and fatigue on exertion, chest pain, palpitations, menstrual irregularities, or loss of libido. Ask him about the occurrence of melena or about obvious signs of bleeding, such as epistaxis or hematemesis.
- If the pallor is confined to one or both legs, ask the patient whether walking is painful or if his legs feel cold or numb; if confined to his fingers, ask about tingling and numbness.

PHYSICAL ASSESSMENT

- Take the patient's vital signs. Be sure to check for orthostatic hypotension.
- Auscultate the heart for gallops and murmurs and the lungs for crackles.
- Perform an abdominal examination, especially checking for tenderness.
- Check the patient's skin temperature — cold extremities commonly occur with vasoconstriction or arterial occlusion.
- Note skin ulceration, and palpate peripheral pulses.

SPECIAL CONSIDERATIONS

When pallor results from low cardiac output, be prepared to administer blood and fluid replacements and a diuretic, a cardiotonic, or an antiarrhythmic, as ordered.

[A]   P EDIATRIC POINTERS

In children, pallor stems from the same causes as it does in adults. However, it may also stem from congenital heart defects or chronic lung disease.

PATIENT COUNSELING

If the patient has chronic generalized pallor, prepare him for blood studies and, possibly, bone marrow biopsy. If the patient has localized pallor, prepare him for arteriography to accurately determine the cause.

PALLOR

HPI

Focused PE: Cardiovascular system

ANEMIA
Signs and symptoms
- Gradual pallor
- Sallow or gray skin
- Fatigue
- Dyspnea
- Tachycardia
- Bounding pulse

DX: Labs (CBC, serum ferritin level, serum iron, TIBC)
TX: Treatment of underlying cause (based on specific type of anemia)
F/U: As needed (dependent on the cause and severity of anemia)

SHOCK
Signs and symptoms
- Cool, pale, moist skin
- Tachycardia
- Tachypnea
- Fever
- Elevated or collapsed neck veins
- Crackles
- Arrhythmias, murmurs, or gallops
- Confusion
- Oliguria

DX: PE, labs (CBC, electrolytes, ABG, UA, blood cultures), CXR, ECG
TX: Varies (based on the specific type of shock), symptomatic treatment, I.V. fluids, cardiac monitoring, vasopressors
F/U: Referral to specialist as indicated by the type of shock

RAYNAUD'S PHENOMENON
Signs and symptoms
- Pallor of fingers on exposure to cold or stress (after which fingers become cyanotic and on rewarming become red and paresthetic)
- Ulceration
- Capillary nail fold abnormalities

TX: Avoidance of triggers to vasospasm, smoking-cessation program, medication (calcium channel blockers, vasodilators, platelet aggregation inhibitor)
F/U: As needed (dependent on the severity of the phenomenon)

ARTERIAL OCCLUSION (ACUTE)
Signs and symptoms
- Abrupt pallor of extremity
- Line of demarcation (with cool, cyanotic, mottled skin below and normal skin above)
- Severe pain
- Intense intermittent claudication
- Paresthesia
- Paresis
- Absent pulses and diminished capillary refill in the affected extremity

DX: PE, imaging studies (Doppler ultrasound, angiography)
TX: Medication (thrombolytics, anticoagulants, analgesics), surgery
F/U: Referral to vascular surgeon

ARTERIAL OCCLUSIVE DISEASE
Signs and symptoms
- Gradual pallor of extremity
- Increased pallor with elevation
- Intermittent claudication
- Weakness in the affected extremity
- Cool skin
- Diminished pulses in the affected extremity
- Ulceration or gangrene in the affected extremity

DX: History of arteriosclerosis, imaging studies (Doppler ultrasound, angiography)
TX: Smoking-cessation program, diet modification, exercise program, medication (antiplatelet agents, vasodilators, analgesics), surgery
F/U: As needed (dependent on the severity of the disease)

Additional differential diagnoses: cardiac arrhythmias ▪ frostbite ▪ orthostatic hypotension ▪ shock ▪ vasopressor syncope

Palpitations

Defined as a conscious awareness of one's heartbeat, palpitations are usually felt over the precordium or in the throat or neck. The patient may describe them as pounding, jumping, turning, fluttering, or flopping or as missing or skipping beats. Palpitations may be regular or irregular, fast or slow, paroxysmal or sustained.

Although usually insignificant, this common symptom may result from a cardiac or metabolic disorder or from the effects of certain drugs. Nonpathologic palpitations may occur with a newly implanted prosthetic valve because the valve's clicking sound heightens the patient's awareness of his heartbeat. Transient palpitations may accompany emotional stress, such as fright, anger, and anxiety, or physical stress, such as exercise and fever. They can also accompany the use of stimulants, such as tobacco and caffeine.

To help characterize the palpitations, ask the patient to simulate their rhythm by tapping his finger on a hard surface. An irregular "skipped beat" rhythm points to premature ventricular contractions, whereas an episodic racing rhythm that ends abruptly suggests paroxysmal atrial tachycardia.

 ALERT
If the patient complains of palpitations:
* *ask him about dizziness and shortness of breath; then inspect for pale, clammy skin*
* *assess his vital signs for hypotension and irregular, abnormal, or rapid pulse; then if these signs are present, suspect cardiac arrhythmia*
* *institute emergency measures, if necessary.*
If the patient's condition permits, perform a focused assessment.

HISTORY
* Review the patient's medical history for a cardiovascular or pulmonary disorder (which may produce arrhythmias), hypertension, and hypoglycemia.
* Ask the patient about associated symptoms, such as weakness, fatigue, and angina.
* Obtain a drug history, including prescription and over-the-counter drugs, herbal remedies, and recreational drugs. Also, ask the patient about alcohol intake and caffeine consumption.

PHYSICAL ASSESSMENT
* Take the patient's vital signs.
* Auscultate the chest for gallops, murmurs, and abnormal breath sounds.
* Connect the patient to a cardiac monitor, or obtain an electrocardiogram.

SPECIAL CONSIDERATIONS
Herbal remedies, such as ginseng and ephedra, have adverse effects, including palpitations and an irregular heartbeat.

A   PEDIATRIC POINTERS
* *Palpitations in children commonly result from fever and congenital heart defects, such as patent ductus arteriosus and septal defects.*
* *Because young children commonly can't describe this complaint, focus your attention on objective measurements, such as cardiac monitoring, physical assessment, and laboratory tests.*

PATIENT COUNSELING
Instruct the patient on what to expect from diagnostic testing, which may include electrocardiogram and Holter monitoring.

PALPITATIONS

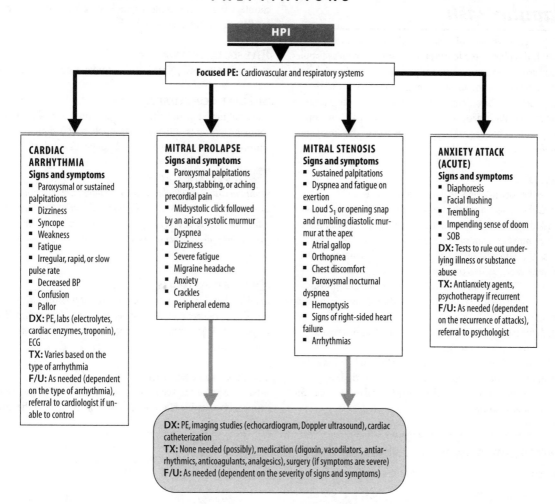

HPI

Focused PE: Cardiovascular and respiratory systems

CARDIAC ARRHYTHMIA
Signs and symptoms
- Paroxysmal or sustained palpitations
- Dizziness
- Syncope
- Weakness
- Fatigue
- Irregular, rapid, or slow pulse rate
- Decreased BP
- Confusion
- Pallor

DX: PE, labs (electrolytes, cardiac enzymes, troponin), ECG
TX: Varies based on the type of arrhythmia
F/U: As needed (dependent on the type of arrhythmia), referral to cardiologist if unable to control

MITRAL PROLAPSE
Signs and symptoms
- Paroxysmal palpitations
- Sharp, stabbing, or aching precordial pain
- Midsystolic click followed by an apical systolic murmur
- Dyspnea
- Dizziness
- Severe fatigue
- Migraine headache
- Anxiety
- Crackles
- Peripheral edema

MITRAL STENOSIS
Signs and symptoms
- Sustained palpitations
- Dyspnea and fatigue on exertion
- Loud S_1 or opening snap and rumbling diastolic murmur at the apex
- Atrial gallop
- Orthopnea
- Chest discomfort
- Paroxysmal nocturnal dyspnea
- Hemoptysis
- Signs of right-sided heart failure
- Arrhythmias

ANXIETY ATTACK (ACUTE)
Signs and symptoms
- Diaphoresis
- Facial flushing
- Trembling
- Impending sense of doom
- SOB

DX: Tests to rule out underlying illness or substance abuse
TX: Antianxiety agents, psychotherapy if recurrent
F/U: As needed (dependent on the recurrence of attacks), referral to psychologist

DX: PE, imaging studies (echocardiogram, Doppler ultrasound), cardiac catheterization
TX: None needed (possibly), medication (digoxin, vasodilators, antiarrhythmics, anticoagulants, analgesics), surgery (if symptoms are severe)
F/U: As needed (dependent on the severity of signs and symptoms)

Additional differential diagnoses: anemia ▪ hypertension ▪ hypocalcemia ▪ hypoglycemia ▪ pheochromocytoma ▪ thyrotoxicosis

Other causes: drugs that precipitate cardiac arrhythmias or increase cardiac output (cardiac glycosides, sympathomimetics, cocaine, ganglionic blockers, atropine) ▪ herbal drugs, such as ginseng and ephedra

Papular rash

A papular rash consists of small, raised, circumscribed—and possibly discolored (red to purple)—lesions known as papules. It may erupt anywhere on the body in various configurations, and it may be acute or chronic. Papular rashes characterize many cutaneous disorders; they may also result from allergy or from an infectious, neoplastic, or systemic disorder. (To compare papules with other skin lesions, see *Recognizing common skin lesions.*)

HISTORY

- Ask the patient when he first noticed the rash.
- Ask the patient if anything makes the rash better or worse.
- Ask the patient if he has noticed changes in the rash. Is it itchy or burning, painful or tender?
- Ask the patient about associated signs and symptoms, such as fever, headache, shortness of breath, and GI distress.
- Review the patient's medical history for allergies, previous rashes or skin disorders, infections, childhood diseases, and cancer.
- Ask the patient about his sexual history. Has he ever had a sexually transmitted disease?
- Ask the patient if he has recently been bitten by an insect or rodent or exposed to anyone with an infectious disease.
- Ask the patient about travel and food histories, pets, and environmental exposures.

- Obtain a drug history, including prescription and over-the-counter drugs, herbal remedies, and recreational drugs. Also, ask the patient about alcohol intake.

PHYSICAL ASSESSMENT

- Examine the rash. Note its color, configuration, and location.

SPECIAL CONSIDERATIONS

Transient maculopapular rashes, usually on the trunk, may accompany reactions to many drugs. Apply cool compresses or an antipruritic lotion to the rash for the patient's comfort.

🄰 PEDIATRIC POINTERS

Common causes of papular rashes in children are infectious diseases, such as molluscum contagiosum and scarlet fever; scabies; insect bites; allergies and drug reactions; and miliaria, which occurs in three forms depending on the depth of sweat gland involvement.

AGING ISSUES

In bedridden elderly patients, the first sign of pressure ulcers is usually an erythematous area, sometimes with firm papules. If not properly managed, these lesions progress to deep ulcers and can lead to death.

PATIENT COUNSELING

Advise the patient to keep his skin clean and dry; to wear loose fitting, nonirritating clothing; and to avoid scratching the rash.

RECOGNIZING COMMON SKIN LESIONS

MACULE

A small (usually less than 1 cm in diameter), flat blemish or discoloration that can be brown, tan, red, or white and has the same texture as the surrounding skin

VESICLE

A small (less than 0.5 cm in diameter), thin-walled, raised blister containing clear, serous, purulent, or bloody fluid

WHEAL

A slightly raised, firm lesion of variable size and shape that's surrounded by edema (skin may be red or pale)

PAPULE

A small, solid, raised lesion less than 1 cm in diameter with red to purple skin discoloration

BULLA

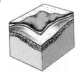

A raised, thin-walled blister that's greater than 0.5 cm in diameter and contains clear or serous fluid

PUSTULE

A circumscribed, pus- or lymph-filled, elevated lesion that varies in diameter and may be firm or soft and white or yellow

NODULE

A small, firm, circumscribed, elevated lesion approximately 1 to 2 cm in diameter with possible skin discoloration

TUMOR

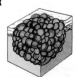

A solid, raised mass that's usually larger than 2 cm in diameter with possible skin discoloration

PAPULAR RASH

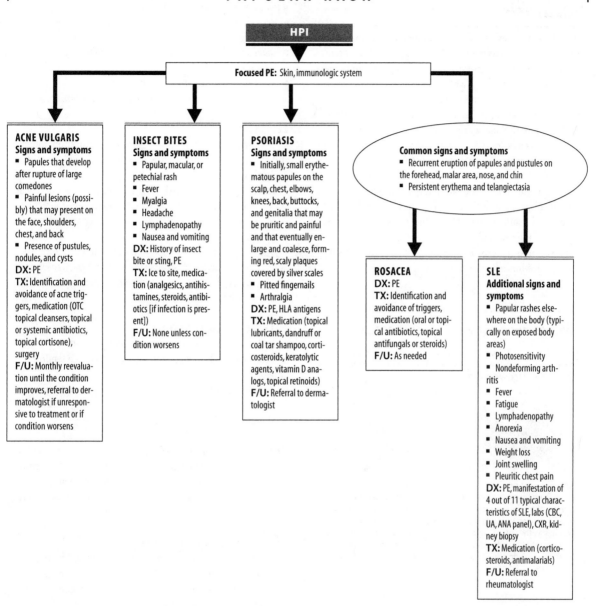

HPI

Focused PE: Skin, immunologic system

ACNE VULGARIS
Signs and symptoms
- Papules that develop after rupture of large comedones
- Painful lesions (possibly) that may present on the face, shoulders, chest, and back
- Presence of pustules, nodules, and cysts

DX: PE

TX: Identification and avoidance of acne triggers, medication (OTC topical cleansers, topical or systemic antibiotics, topical cortisone), surgery

F/U: Monthly reevaluation until the condition improves, referral to dermatologist if unresponsive to treatment or if condition worsens

INSECT BITES
Signs and symptoms
- Papular, macular, or petechial rash
- Fever
- Myalgia
- Headache
- Lymphadenopathy
- Nausea and vomiting

DX: History of insect bite or sting, PE

TX: Ice to site, medication (analgesics, antihistamines, steroids, antibiotics [if infection is present])

F/U: None unless condition worsens

PSORIASIS
Signs and symptoms
- Initially, small erythematous papules on the scalp, chest, elbows, knees, back, buttocks, and genitalia that may be pruritic and painful and that eventually enlarge and coalesce, forming red, scaly plaques covered by silver scales
- Pitted fingernails
- Arthralgia

DX: PE, HLA antigens

TX: Medication (topical lubricants, dandruff or coal tar shampoo, corticosteroids, keratolytic agents, vitamin D analogs, topical retinoids)

F/U: Referral to dermatologist

Common signs and symptoms
- Recurrent eruption of papules and pustules on the forehead, malar area, nose, and chin
- Persistent erythema and telangiectasia

ROSACEA
DX: PE

TX: Identification and avoidance of triggers, medication (oral or topical antibiotics, topical antifungals or steroids)

F/U: As needed

SLE
Additional signs and symptoms
- Papular rashes elsewhere on the body (typically on exposed body areas)
- Photosensitivity
- Nondeforming arthritis
- Fever
- Fatigue
- Lymphadenopathy
- Anorexia
- Nausea and vomiting
- Weight loss
- Joint swelling
- Pleuritic chest pain

DX: PE, manifestation of 4 out of 11 typical characteristics of SLE, labs (CBC, UA, ANA panel), CXR, kidney biopsy

TX: Medication (corticosteroids, antimalarials)

F/U: Referral to rheumatologist

Additional differential diagnoses: dermatitis (perioral) ▪ dermatomyositis ▪ erythema chronicum migrans ▪ follicular mucinosis ▪ Fox-Fordyce disease ▪ gonococcemia ▪ granuloma annulare ▪ HIV infection ▪ leprosy ▪ lichen amyloidosis ▪ lichen planus ▪ mononucleosis (infectious) ▪ mycosis fungoides ▪ necrotizing vasculitis ▪ parapsoriasis (chronic) ▪ pityriasis rosea ▪ pityriasis rubra pilaris ▪ polymorphic light eruption ▪ rat bite fever ▪ sarcoidosis ▪ seborrheic keratosis ▪ syphilis ▪ syringoma

Other causes: allopurinol ▪ antibiotics (tetracycline, ampicillin, cephalosporins, sulfonamides) ▪ benzodiazepines (diazepam) ▪ gold salts ▪ isoniazid ▪ lithium ▪ phenylbutazone ▪ salicylates

Paralysis

Paralysis—the total loss of voluntary motor function—results from severe cortical or pyramidal tract damage. It can occur with a cerebrovascular disorder, degenerative neuromuscular disease, trauma, tumors, or a central nervous system infection. Acute paralysis may be an early indicator of such life-threatening disorders as Guillain-Barré syndrome. Paralysis may also be caused by a psychological disorder.

Paralysis can be local or widespread, symmetrical or asymmetrical, transient or permanent, and spastic or flaccid. It's commonly classified according to location and severity as paraplegia (sometimes transient paralysis of the legs), quadriplegia (permanent paralysis of the arms, legs, and body below the level of the spinal lesion), or hemiplegia (unilateral paralysis of varying severity and permanence). Incomplete paralysis with profound weakness (paresis) may precede total paralysis in some patients. (See *Understanding spinal cord syndromes.*)

UNDERSTANDING SPINAL CORD SYNDROMES

When a patient's spinal cord is incompletely severed, he experiences partial motor and sensory loss. Most incomplete cord lesions fit into one of the syndromes described below.

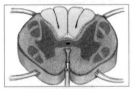

Anterior cord syndrome, usually resulting from a flexion injury, causes motor paralysis and loss of pain and temperature sensation below the level of injury. Touch, proprioception, and vibration sensation are usually preserved

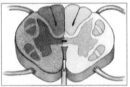

Brown-Séquard's syndrome can result from flexion, rotation, or penetration injury. It's characterized by unilateral motor paralysis ipsilateral to the injury and loss of pain and temperature sensation contralateral to the injury.

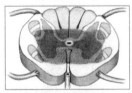

Central cord syndrome is caused by hyperextension or flexion injury. Motor loss is variable and greater in the arms than in the legs; sensory loss is usually slight.

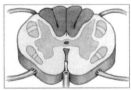

Posterior cord syndrome, produced by a cervical hyperextension injury, causes only a loss of proprioception and light touch sensation. Motor function remains intact.

If paralysis has developed suddenly:
- *determine the patient's level of consciousness, and assess vital signs*
- *make sure that the patient's neck is immobilized, especially if trauma is suspected*
- *institute emergency measures, if necessary.*
  If the patient's condition permits, perform a focused assessment.

HISTORY

- Ask the patient or family about the onset, duration, intensity, and progression of the paralysis as well as the events preceding its development.
- Review the patient's medical history for incidence of degenerative neurologic or neuromuscular disease, recent infectious illness, sexually transmitted disease, cancer, recent injury, and hypertension.
- Ask the patient about associated signs and symptoms, such as fever, headache, visual disturbances, dysphagia, nausea and vomiting, bowel or bladder dysfunction, muscle pain or weakness, and fatigue.

PHYSICAL ASSESSMENT

- Perform a complete neurologic examination, testing cranial nerve, motor, and sensory function as well as deep tendon reflexes.
- Assess strength in all major muscle groups, noting muscle atrophy.
- Document all findings to serve as a baseline.

SPECIAL CONSIDERATIONS

Because a paralyzed patient is particularly susceptible to complications of prolonged immobility, provide frequent position changes, meticulous skin care, and frequent chest physiotherapy.

🄰 PEDIATRIC POINTERS

Besides the obvious causes—trauma, infection, and tumors—children may develop paralysis from a hereditary or congenital disorder, such as Tay-Sachs disease, Werdnig-Hoffmann disease, spina bifida, or cerebral palsy.

PATIENT COUNSELING

Instruct the patient on what to expect from diagnostic testing, which may include computed tomography scan and magnetic resonance imaging. Arrange for physical, speech, occupational, or psychological therapy as appropriate.

PARALYSIS

HPI

Focused PE: Neurovascular system

TIA
Signs and symptoms
- Transient unilateral paralysis
- Visual disturbances
- Dizziness
- Aphasia
- Dysarthria
- Decreased LOC
- Carotid bruit

DX: PE, imaging studies (carotid ultrasound, CT scan), ECG

TX: Diet modification, exercise program, reduction of risk factors for stroke, medication (anticoagulants, platelet inhibitors, antihypertensives antiarrhythmics), surgery (if carotid stenosis is the cause)

F/U: Referrals to neurologist or neurosurgeon

GUILLAIN-BARRÉ SYNDROME
Signs and symptoms
- Progressive, symmetrical muscle flaccidity and paralysis from the feet upward
- Sensory loss
- Paresthesia
- Absent DTRs
- Fluctuating vital signs
- Urinary incontinence
- Dysphagia
- Dysarthria
- Respiratory failure

DX: CSF analysis, MRI, nerve conduction studies

TX: Symptomatic treatment, monitoring of respiratory status, immune globulin, plasmapheresis

F/U: Referral to neurologist

CONVERSION DISORDER
Signs and symptoms
- Hysterical paralysis (loss of voluntary movement with no obvious physical cause) that can affect any muscle group
- Paralysis that appears and disappears unpredictably
- History of a recent psychological conflict

DX: PE to rule out a physical cause, psychological evaluation

TX: Psychological counseling

F/U: Referral to psychologist

SPINAL CORD INJURY
Signs and symptoms
- Flaccid paralysis
- Loss of sensation below the level of the injury
- Reflex inactivity (temporary)
- Urinary and fecal retention
- Flexor and extensor spasms of legs

DX: History of spinal trauma, PE, imaging studies (spinal X-rays, CT scan, MRI)

TX: Immobilization of the spine, I.V. steroids, surgery

F/U: Referral to neurosurgeon, referral to psychological counseling and support, rehabilitation as appropriate

...MAY LEAD TO...

STROKE
- Contralateral paresis or paralysis
- Decreased LOC (lethargy to coma)
- Behavioral changes
- Headache
- Visual disturbances
- Aphasia
- Weakness
- Dysphagia
- Memory loss

DX: PE, imaging studies (CT scan, MRI, angiography), ECG

TX: Symptomatic treatment, medication (platelet aggregation inhibitors, thrombolytics [if embolic])

F/U: As needed (dependent on neurologic status), referral to rehabilitation program

---

Additional differential diagnoses: ALS ▪ Bell's palsy ▪ botulism ▪ brain abscess ▪ brain tumor ▪ encephalitis ▪ head trauma ▪ migraine headache ▪ multiple sclerosis ▪ myasthenia gravis ▪ neurosyphilis ▪ Parkinson's disease ▪ peripheral nerve trauma ▪ peripheral neuropathy ▪ poliomyelitis ▪ rabies ▪ seizure disorders ▪ spinal cord tumors ▪ subarachnoid hemorrhage ▪ syringomyelia ▪ thoracic aortic aneurysm ▪ West Nile encephalitis

Other causes: electroconvulsive therapy ▪ neuromuscular blocking agents (pancuronium, curare)

Paresthesia

Paresthesia is an abnormal sensation or combination of sensations—commonly described as numbness, prickling, or tingling—felt along peripheral nerve pathways. These sensations aren't generally painful; unpleasant or painful sensations are termed *dysesthesias*. Paresthesia may develop suddenly or gradually and may be transient or permanent.

A common symptom of many neurologic disorders, paresthesia may also result from a systemic disorder or the effects or a particular drug. The symptom may indicate damage or irritation of the parietal lobe, thalamus, spinothalamic tract, or spinal or peripheral nerves—the neural circuit that transmits and interprets sensory stimuli.

HISTORY

- Ask the patient when the abnormal sensations began, and ask him to describe the character and distribution of the sensations.
- Ask the patient about associated signs and symptoms, such as sensory loss and paresis or paralysis.
- Review the patient's medical history for neurologic, cardiovascular, metabolic, renal, or chronic inflammatory disorders, such as arthritis or lupus; or a recent traumatic injury or invasive procedure that may have damaged peripheral nerves.

PHYSICAL ASSESSMENT

- Assess the patient's level of consciousness and cranial nerve function.
- Test muscle strength and deep tendon reflexes in limbs affected by paresthesia.
- Systematically evaluate light touch, pain, temperature, vibration, and position sensation. (See *Testing for analgesia.*)
- Inspect the skin for color and temperature. Palpate pulses.

TESTING FOR ANALGESIA

By carefully and systematically testing your patient's sensitivity to pain, you can determine whether his nerve damage has a segmental or peripheral distribution and help locate the causative lesion.

Tell the patient to relax, and explain that you're going to lightly touch areas of his skin with a small pin. Have him close his eyes. Apply the pin firmly enough to produce pain without breaking the skin. (Practice on yourself first to learn how to apply the correct pressure.)

Starting with the patient's head and face, move down his body, pricking his skin on alternating sides. Have the patient report when he feels pain. Use the blunt end of the pin occasionally, and vary your test pattern to gauge the accuracy of his response.

Document your findings thoroughly, noting areas of lost pain sensation either on a dermatome chart or on peripheral nerve diagrams (if available).

SPECIAL CONSIDERATIONS

Chemotherapeutic agents, chloroquine, D-penicillamine, isoniazid, nitrofurantoin, parenteral gold therapy, and phenytoin may produce transient paresthesia that disappears when the drug is discontinued.

[A] PEDIATRIC POINTERS

Children may experience paresthesia associated with the same causes as adults. However, they usually can't describe this symptom. Nevertheless, hereditary polyneuropathies are usually first recognized in childhood.

PATIENT COUNSELING

Because paresthesia is commonly accompanied by patchy sensory loss, teach the patient safety measures.

PARESTHESIA

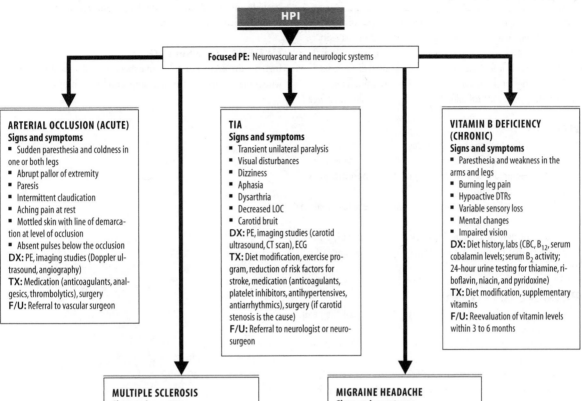

HPI

Focused PE: Neurovascular and neurologic systems

ARTERIAL OCCLUSION (ACUTE)
Signs and symptoms
- Sudden paresthesia and coldness in one or both legs
- Abrupt pallor of extremity
- Paresis
- Intermittent claudication
- Aching pain at rest
- Mottled skin with line of demarcation at level of occlusion
- Absent pulses below the occlusion

DX: PE, imaging studies (Doppler ultrasound, angiography)
TX: Medication (anticoagulants, analgesics, thrombolytics), surgery
F/U: Referral to vascular surgeon

TIA
Signs and symptoms
- Transient unilateral paralysis
- Visual disturbances
- Dizziness
- Aphasia
- Dysarthria
- Decreased LOC
- Carotid bruit

DX: PE, imaging studies (carotid ultrasound, CT scan), ECG
TX: Diet modification, exercise program, reduction of risk factors for stroke, medication (anticoagulants, platelet inhibitors, antihypertensives, antiarrhythmics), surgery (if carotid stenosis is the cause)
F/U: Referral to neurologist or neurosurgeon

VITAMIN B DEFICIENCY (CHRONIC)
Signs and symptoms
- Paresthesia and weakness in the arms and legs
- Burning leg pain
- Hypoactive DTRs
- Variable sensory loss
- Mental changes
- Impaired vision

DX: Diet history, labs (CBC, B_{12}, serum cobalamin levels; serum B_2 activity; 24-hour urine testing for thiamine, riboflavin, niacin, and pyridoxine)
TX: Diet modification, supplementary vitamins
F/U: Reevaluation of vitamin levels within 3 to 6 months

MULTIPLE SCLEROSIS
Signs and symptoms
- Progressive muscle weakness and atrophy
- Muscle spasticity
- Hyperactive DTRs
- Dysarthria
- Dysphagia
- Waxing and waning signs and symptoms
- Visual disturbances
- Ataxic gait
- Diplopia
- Intention tremors
- Emotional lability
- Urinary and sexual dysfunction

DX: CSF analysis, MRI, EEG, evoked response testing
TX: Symptomatic treatment; medication (antispasmotics, antidepressants, cholinergics, corticosteroids); physical, speech, and occupational therapy
F/U: Referral to neurologist

MIGRAINE HEADACHE
Signs and symptoms
- Paresthesia of the lips, face, and hands
- Light flashes
- Aura
- Severe, throbbing, unilateral headache
- Dizziness
- Photophobia
- Nausea and vomiting

DX: History of headache, PE
TX: Rest during headache, cold compresses, medication (serotonin agonists, ergotamines, antiemetics, analgesics), lifestyle or diet modification (if the precipitant is identified)
F/U: Referral to headache clinic if uncontrolled, referral to neurologist

---

Additional differential diagnoses: arteriosclerosis obliterans ▪ arthritis ▪ brain tumor ▪ Buerger's disease ▪ diabetes mellitus ▪ Guillain-Barré syndrome ▪ head trauma ▪ heavy metal or solvent poisoning ▪ herniated disk ▪ herpes zoster ▪ hyperventilation syndrome ▪ hypocalcemia ▪ peripheral nerve trauma ▪ peripheral neuropathy ▪ rabies ▪ Raynaud's disease ▪ seizure disorders ▪ SLE ▪ spinal cord injury ▪ spinal cord tumors ▪ stroke ▪ tabes dorsalis ▪ thoracic outlet syndrome

Other causes: chemotherapeutic agents (vincristine, vinblastine, procarbazine) ▪ chloroquine ▪ isoniazid ▪ nitrofurantoin ▪ parenteral gold therapy ▪ phenytoin ▪ radiation therapy

Peau d'orange

Usually a late sign of breast cancer, peau d'orange (orange peel skin) is the edematous thickening and pitting of breast skin. This slowly developing sign can also occur with breast or axillary lymph node infection, erysipelas, or Graves' disease. Its striking orange peel appearance stems from lymphatic edema around deepened hair follicles. (See *Recognizing peau d'orange*.)

HISTORY

- Ask the patient when she first detected the peau d'orange. Ask if she has noticed lumps, pain, or other breast changes.
- Ask the patient about associated signs and symptoms, such as malaise, achiness, and weight loss.
- Ask the patient if she's lactating or if she has recently weaned her infant.
- Review the patient's medical history, noting especially axillary surgery that might have impaired lymphatic drainage of a breast.

PHYSICAL ASSESSMENT

- Observe the patient's breasts. Estimate the extent of the peau d'orange, and check for erythema.
- Assess the nipples for discharge, deviation, retraction, dimpling, and cracking.
- Gently palpate the area of peau d'orange, noting warmth or induration. Then palpate the entire breast, noting fixed or mobile lumps, and the axillary lymph nodes, noting enlargement.
- Take the patient's vital signs, noting increased temperature.

SPECIAL CONSIDERATIONS

Because peau d'orange usually signals advanced breast cancer, provide emotional support for the patient. Encourage her to express her fears and concerns.

PATIENT COUNSELING

Instruct the patient on what to expect from diagnostic testing, which may include mammography and breast biopsy.

RECOGNIZING PEAU D'ORANGE

With peau d'orange, the skin appears to be pitted (as shown). This condition usually indicates late-stage breast cancer.

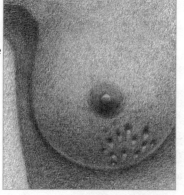

PEAU D'ORANGE

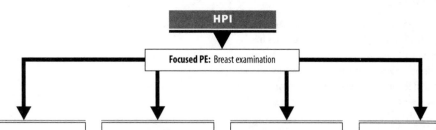

HPI

Focused PE: Breast examination

BREAST ABSCESS
Signs and symptoms
- Thick, purulent nipple discharge
- Abrupt onset of high fever and chills
- Breast pain, tenderness, and erythema
- Palpable soft nodule or generalized induration of the affected breast
- Axillary lymphadenopathy

DX: PE, mammography, breast biopsy

TX: Moist heat to the affected area, medication (antibiotics, analgesics), surgery

F/U: Reevaluation in 7 to 10 days

BREAST CANCER
Signs and symptoms
- Bloody, watery, or purulent discharge from a normal-appearing nipple
- Hard, irregular, fixed lump
- Erythema
- Dimpling
- Nipple deviation or retraction
- Axillary lymphadenopathy

DX: PE, imaging studies (mammography, ultrasound), breast biopsy

TX: Chemotherapy, radiation therapy, surgery

F/U: Referrals to oncologist and surgeon

ERYSIPELAS
Signs and symptoms
- Well-demarcated erythematous elevated area (commonly with peau d'orange texture)
- Pain
- Warmth
- Fever and chills
- Fatigue

DX: PE, labs (CBC, ESR, blood cultures), biopsy

TX: Warm, moist compresses; medication (analgesics, antipyretics, antibiotics)

F/U: Reevaluation in 48 to 72 hours, then in 7 to 10 days

GRAVES' DISEASE
Signs and symptoms
- Peau d'orange–like areas that coalesce
- Increasing appetite
- Weight loss
- Protruding eyes
- Restlessness
- Heat intolerance
- Increased swelling
- Fatigue
- Muscle cramps
- Tremor
- Frequent bowel movements
- Menstrual irregularities in women
- Goiter (possible)

DX: PE, labs (TSH, T_3, T_4, thyroid resin uptake, radioactive iodine uptake)

TX: Medication (antithyroid agents, radioactive iodine), surgery

F/U: Referral to endocrinologist

Photophobia

A common symptom, photophobia is an abnormal sensitivity to light. In many patients, photophobia simply indicates increased eye sensitivity without an underlying pathology. For example, it can stem from excessive wearing of contact lenses or the use of poorly fitted lenses. In others, this symptom can result from a systemic disorder, an ocular disorder or trauma, or the use of a particular drug.

HISTORY

- Ask your patient about the onset and severity of the photophobia. Did it follow eye trauma, a chemical splash, or exposure to the rays of a sun lamp?
- Ask the patient if he wears contact lenses. If so, how long does he keep his contact lenses in? How old are the contact lenses? If they are extended wear lenses, how often does he remove them and change them?
- Ask the patient about eye pain, and have him describe its location, duration, and intensity. Does he have a sensation of a foreign body in his eye?
- Ask the patient about associated signs and symptoms, such as increased tearing and vision changes.

PHYSICAL ASSESSMENT

- Take the patient's vital signs, and assess his neurologic status.
- Inspect the eyes' external structures for abnormalities. Examine the conjunctiva and sclera, noting especially their color. Characterize the amount and consistency of discharge, if present.
- Check pupillary reaction to light. Evaluate extraocular muscle function by testing the six cardinal fields of gaze, and test visual acuity in both eyes.

SPECIAL CONSIDERATIONS

Keep in mind that photophobia can accompany life-threatening meningitis; however, it isn't a cardinal sign of meningeal irritation.

Ⓐ PEDIATRIC POINTERS

- *Suspect photophobia in a child who squints, rubs his eyes frequently, or wears sunglasses indoors and outside.*
- *Congenital disorders (such as albinism) and certain childhood diseases (such as measles and rubella) can cause photophobia.*

PATIENT COUNSELING

Advise the patient to darken the room and close both eyes to help promote eye comfort. Dark glasses should be worn when outdoors.

PHOTOPHOBIA

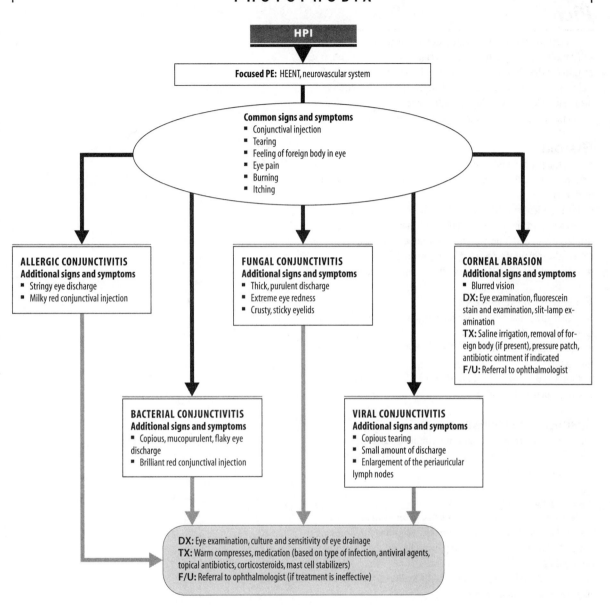

HPI

Focused PE: HEENT, neurovascular system

Common signs and symptoms
- Conjunctival injection
- Tearing
- Feeling of foreign body in eye
- Eye pain
- Burning
- Itching

ALLERGIC CONJUNCTIVITIS
Additional signs and symptoms
- Stringy eye discharge
- Milky red conjunctival injection

FUNGAL CONJUNCTIVITIS
Additional signs and symptoms
- Thick, purulent discharge
- Extreme eye redness
- Crusty, sticky eyelids

CORNEAL ABRASION
Additional signs and symptoms
- Blurred vision
DX: Eye examination, fluorescein stain and examination, slit-lamp examination
TX: Saline irrigation, removal of foreign body (if present), pressure patch, antibiotic ointment if indicated
F/U: Referral to ophthalmologist

BACTERIAL CONJUNCTIVITIS
Additional signs and symptoms
- Copious, mucopurulent, flaky eye discharge
- Brilliant red conjunctival injection

VIRAL CONJUNCTIVITIS
Additional signs and symptoms
- Copious tearing
- Small amount of discharge
- Enlargement of the periauricular lymph nodes

DX: Eye examination, culture and sensitivity of eye drainage
TX: Warm compresses, medication (based on type of infection, antiviral agents, topical antibiotics, corticosteroids, mast cell stabilizers)
F/U: Referral to ophthalmologist (if treatment is ineffective)

Additional differential diagnoses: burns ▪ corneal foreign body ▪ corneal ulcer ▪ dry eye syndrome ▪ iritis (acute) ▪ keratitis (interstitial) ▪ meningitis (acute bacterial) ▪ migraine headache ▪ scleritis ▪ sclerokeratitis ▪ trachoma ▪ uveitis

Other causes: amphetamines ▪ cocaine ▪ mydriatics (phenylephrine, atropine, scopolamine, cyclopentolate, tropicamide) ▪ ophthalmic antifungal drugs (trifluridine, vidarabine, idoxuridine)

Pica

Pica refers to the craving and ingestion of normally inedible substances, such as plaster, charcoal, clay, wool, ashes, paint, or dirt. In children, the most commonly affected group, pica typically results from nutritional deficiencies. However, in adults, pica may reflect a psychological disturbance. Depending on the substance eaten, pica can lead to poisoning and GI disorders.

HISTORY

- Ask the patient what substances he has been eating. If the patient has eaten a toxic substance (such as lead), obtain a serum lead level.
- If the patient is a child, ask the parents to describe his eating habits and nutritional history. Find out when the patient first displayed pica and if he always craves the same substance.
- Ask the patient if he has felt listless or irritable.
- If the patient is female, ask her if she may be pregnant.

PHYSICAL ASSESSMENT

- Check the patient's vital signs, especially noting bradycardia, tachycardia, or hypotension.
- Inspect the abdomen for visible peristaltic waves or other abnormalities.
- Observe the patient's hair, skin, and mucous membranes for changes, such as dryness or pallor.

SPECIAL CONSIDERATIONS

Pica is an accepted practice in some cultures, based on presumed nutritional or therapeutic properties or on religious or superstitious beliefs.

A   PEDIATRIC POINTERS

- *Many older homes contain lead-based paints. Children who live in older homes may be at risk for lead poisoning from eating chipped paint or even from sucking their fingers if the lead paint has infiltrated house dust.*
- *Inner-city children and children living in older homes should be monitored for serum lead levels.*

PATIENT COUNSELING

Teach the patient about lead poisoning, and if he lives in an older home, advise him to investigate whether the paint is lead based.

PICA

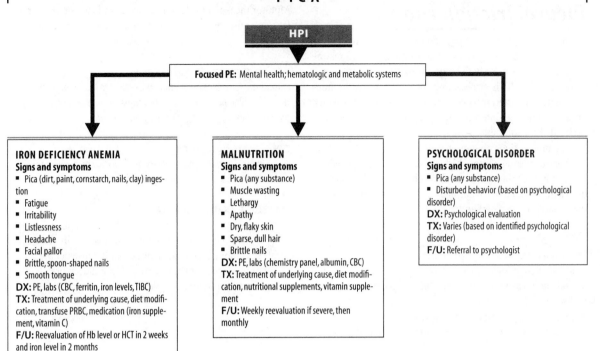

HPI

Focused PE: Mental health; hematologic and metabolic systems

IRON DEFICIENCY ANEMIA
Signs and symptoms
- Pica (dirt, paint, cornstarch, nails, clay) ingestion
- Fatigue
- Irritability
- Listlessness
- Headache
- Facial pallor
- Brittle, spoon-shaped nails
- Smooth tongue

DX: PE, labs (CBC, ferritin, iron levels, TIBC)
TX: Treatment of underlying cause, diet modification, transfuse PRBC, medication (iron supplement, vitamin C)
F/U: Reevaluation of Hb level or HCT in 2 weeks and iron level in 2 months

MALNUTRITION
Signs and symptoms
- Pica (any substance)
- Muscle wasting
- Lethargy
- Apathy
- Dry, flaky skin
- Sparse, dull hair
- Brittle nails

DX: PE, labs (chemistry panel, albumin, CBC)
TX: Treatment of underlying cause, diet modification, nutritional supplements, vitamin supplement
F/U: Weekly reevaluation if severe, then monthly

PSYCHOLOGICAL DISORDER
Signs and symptoms
- Pica (any substance)
- Disturbed behavior (based on psychological disorder)

DX: Psychological evaluation
TX: Varies (based on identified psychological disorder)
F/U: Referral to psychologist

Other causes: cultural beliefs (pica is an accepted practice in some cultures based on presumed nutritional or therapeutic properties or on religious or superstitious beliefs) ▪ pregnancy

Pleural friction rub

Commonly resulting from a pulmonary disorder or trauma, this loud, coarse, and grating, creaking, or squeaking sound may be auscultated over one or both lungs during late inspiration or early expiration. It's heard best over the low axillae or the anterior, lateral, or posterior bases of the lung fields with the patient upright. Sometimes intermittent, it may resemble crackles or a pericardial friction rub.

A pleural friction rub indicates inflammation of the visceral and parietal pleural lining, which causes congestion and edema. The resultant fibrinous exudate covers both pleural surfaces, displacing the fluid that's normally between them and causing the surfaces to rub together.

➤ ALERT
When you detect a pleural friction rub:
- *quickly look for signs of respiratory distress*
- *find out whether the patient has had chest pain; if so, ask him to describe its location and severity*
- *institute emergency measures, if necessary.*
  If the patient's condition permits, perform a focused assessment.

HISTORY
- If the patient complains of chest pain, ask him how long he has had the pain and about its characteristics. Does it radiate to his shoulder, neck, or upper abdomen? Does it worsen with breathing, movement, coughing, or sneezing?
- Ask the patient if he has experienced fever.
- Review the patient's medical history for rheumatoid arthritis, respiratory or cardiovascular disorders, recent trauma, asbestos exposure, and radiation therapy.
- If the patient smokes, obtain a history in pack-years.

PHYSICAL ASSESSMENT
- Take the patient's vital signs, noting his level of consciousness.
- Observe the patient's skin color.
- Auscultate the patient's chest with him sitting upright and breathing deeply and slowly through his mouth. Listen for absent or diminished breath sounds, noting their location and timing in the respiratory cycle. Note the work of breathing. Explore whether the pain abates if he splints his chest, holds his breath, or exerts pressure or lies on the affected side.
- Check for clubbing and pedal edema.
- Palpate for decreased chest motion, and percuss for flatness or dullness.

SPECIAL CONSIDERATIONS
Monitor the patient's respiratory status and vital signs. Administer an antitussive if the patient has a dry, persistent cough, as ordered.

 PEDIATRIC POINTERS
Auscultate for a pleural friction rub — an early sign of pleurisy — in a child who has grunting respirations, reports chest pain, or protects his chest by holding it or lying on one side.

⬡ AGING ISSUES
In an elderly patient, the intensity of pleuritic chest pain may mimic that of cardiac-related chest pain.

PATIENT COUNSELING
Because pleuritic pain commonly accompanies a pleural friction rub, teach the patient splinting maneuvers to increase his comfort. Although coughing may be painful, instruct the patient not to suppress it because coughing and deep breathing help prevent respiratory complications.

PLEURAL FRICTION RUB

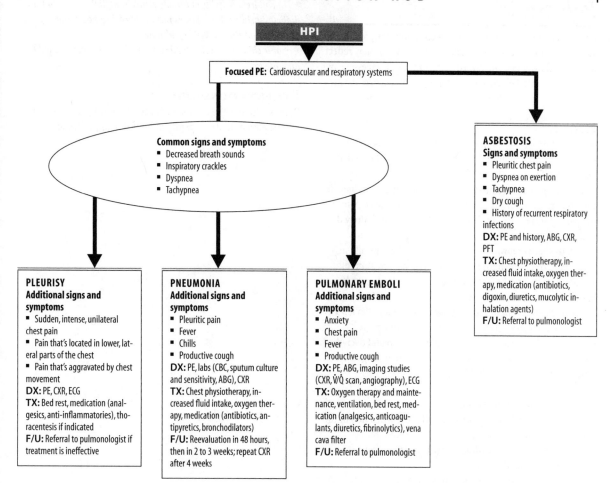

HPI

Focused PE: Cardiovascular and respiratory systems

Common signs and symptoms
- Decreased breath sounds
- Inspiratory crackles
- Dyspnea
- Tachypnea

ASBESTOSIS
Signs and symptoms
- Pleuritic chest pain
- Dyspnea on exertion
- Tachypnea
- Dry cough
- History of recurrent respiratory infections

DX: PE and history, ABG, CXR, PFT
TX: Chest physiotherapy, increased fluid intake, oxygen therapy, medication (antibiotics, digoxin, diuretics, mucolytic inhalation agents)
F/U: Referral to pulmonologist

PLEURISY
Additional signs and symptoms
- Sudden, intense, unilateral chest pain
- Pain that's located in lower, lateral parts of the chest
- Pain that's aggravated by chest movement

DX: PE, CXR, ECG
TX: Bed rest, medication (analgesics, anti-inflammatories), thoracentesis if indicated
F/U: Referral to pulmonologist if treatment is ineffective

PNEUMONIA
Additional signs and symptoms
- Pleuritic pain
- Fever
- Chills
- Productive cough

DX: PE, labs (CBC, sputum culture and sensitivity, ABG), CXR
TX: Chest physiotherapy, increased fluid intake, oxygen therapy, medication (antibiotics, antipyretics, bronchodilators)
F/U: Reevaluation in 48 hours, then in 2 to 3 weeks; repeat CXR after 4 weeks

PULMONARY EMBOLI
Additional signs and symptoms
- Anxiety
- Chest pain
- Fever
- Productive cough

DX: PE, ABG, imaging studies (CXR, V̇/Q̇ scan, angiography), ECG
TX: Oxygen therapy and maintenance, ventilation, bed rest, medication (analgesics, anticoagulants, diuretics, fibrinolytics), vena cava filter
F/U: Referral to pulmonologist

Additional differential diagnoses: lung cancer ▪ rheumatoid arthritis ▪ SLE ▪ tuberculosis (pulmonary)

Other causes: radiation therapy ▪ thoracic surgery

Polydipsia

Polydipsia refers to excessive thirst, a common symptom associated with endocrine disorders and certain drugs. It may reflect decreased fluid intake, increased urine output, or excessive loss of water and salt. Polydipsia is also a common occurrence in psychiatric patients, especially those who are psychotic.

HISTORY

● Ask the patient when he first noticed the increased thirst. Find out how much fluid the patient drinks each day and at what time of the day the thirst occurs.
● Review the patient's medical history for diabetes, kidney disease, recurrent infection, and psychological disorders. Also, ask the patient if there's a family history of diabetes or kidney disease.
● Ask the patient how often and how much he typically urinates. Find out if the need to urinate awakens him at night.
● Ask the patient if he has had a recent lifestyle change. If so, have these changes upset him?
● Ask the patient about recent weight loss or gain. Review his exercise and dietary habits. (See *Water intoxication.*)
● Obtain a drug history, including prescription and over-the-counter drugs, herbal remedies, and recreational drugs. Also, ask the patient about alcohol intake.

PHYSICAL ASSESSMENT

● Take the patient's blood pressure and pulse when he's in the supine and standing positions.
● Check for signs of dehydration, such as dry mucous membranes and decreased skin turgor.
● Check for signs of bleeding, noting edema, if present.

SPECIAL CONSIDERATIONS

Carefully monitor the patient's fluid balance. Weigh the patient at the same time and in the same type of clothes each day.

WATER INTOXICATION

Water intoxication, which can occur after ingestion of large amounts of water, causes cerebral swelling and fluid build-up in the lungs. Many athletes (such as marathon runners, cyclists, and hikers) consume large amounts of water to prevent dehydration. However, this over-consumption can cause blood plasma to increase, resulting in dilution of the sodium content of the blood. The athlete also loses sodium to sweat.

Water intoxication may also be a lethal consequence of the ingestion of the street drug called "ecstasy," which induces syndrome of inappropriate antidiuretic hormone secretion.

● *In children, polydipsia usually stems from diabetes insipidus or diabetes mellitus. Rare causes include pheochromocytoma, neuroblastoma, and Prader-Willi syndrome.*
● *Some children develop habitual polydipsia that's unrelated to any disease.*

PATIENT COUNSELING

Because thirst is the body's way of compensating for water loss, tell the patient to drink plenty of liquids, if appropriate.

POLYDIPSIA

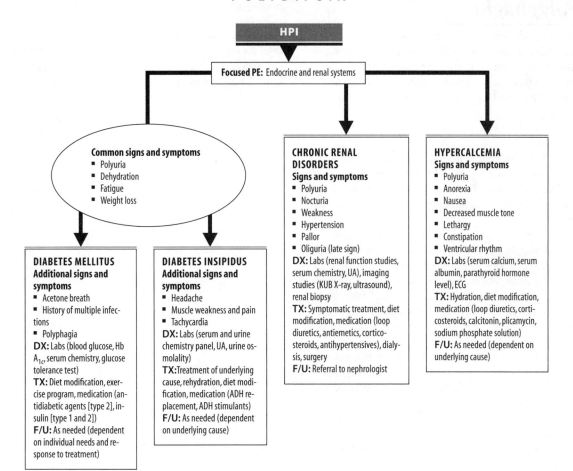

HPI

Focused PE: Endocrine and renal systems

Common signs and symptoms
- Polyuria
- Dehydration
- Fatigue
- Weight loss

DIABETES MELLITUS
Additional signs and symptoms
- Acetone breath
- History of multiple infections
- Polyphagia

DX: Labs (blood glucose, Hb A$_{1c}$, serum chemistry, glucose tolerance test)
TX: Diet modification, exercise program, medication (antidiabetic agents [type 2], insulin [type 1 and 2])
F/U: As needed (dependent on individual needs and response to treatment)

DIABETES INSIPIDUS
Additional signs and symptoms
- Headache
- Muscle weakness and pain
- Tachycardia

DX: Labs (serum and urine chemistry panel, UA, urine osmolality)
TX: Treatment of underlying cause, rehydration, diet modification, medication (ADH replacement, ADH stimulants)
F/U: As needed (dependent on underlying cause)

CHRONIC RENAL DISORDERS
Signs and symptoms
- Polyuria
- Nocturia
- Weakness
- Hypertension
- Pallor
- Oliguria (late sign)

DX: Labs (renal function studies, serum chemistry, UA), imaging studies (KUB X-ray, ultrasound), renal biopsy
TX: Symptomatic treatment, diet modification, medication (loop diuretics, antiemetics, corticosteroids, antihypertensives), dialysis, surgery
F/U: Referral to nephrologist

HYPERCALCEMIA
Signs and symptoms
- Polyuria
- Anorexia
- Nausea
- Decreased muscle tone
- Lethargy
- Constipation
- Ventricular rhythm

DX: Labs (serum calcium, serum albumin, parathyroid hormone level), ECG
TX: Hydration, diet modification, medication (loop diuretics, corticosteroids, calcitonin, plicamycin, sodium phosphate solution)
F/U: As needed (dependent on underlying cause)

Additional differential diagnoses: hypokalemia ▪ psychogenic polydipsia ▪ Sheehan's syndrome ▪ sickle cell anemia ▪ thyrotoxicosis

Other causes: anticholinergics ▪ demeclocycline ▪ diuretics ▪ phenothiazines

Polyphagia

Polyphagia, also known as *hyperphagia*, refers to voracious or excessive eating before satiety. This common symptom can be persistent or intermittent, resulting primarily from an endocrine or psychological disorder or the use of certain drugs. Depending on the underlying cause, polyphagia may cause weight gain.

History

● Ask the patient what he has had to eat and drink within the last 24 hours. (If he easily recalls this information, ask about the previous 2 days' intake for a broader view of his dietary habits.) Note the frequency of meals and the amount and types of food eaten.

● Ask the patient whether his eating or exercising habits have changed recently. Has he always had a large appetite? Does his overeating alternate with periods of anorexia?

● Ask the patient about conditions that may trigger overeating, such as stress, depression, or menstruation (if the patient is female). Does the patient actually feel hungry or does he eat simply because food is available? Does he ever vomit or have a headache after overeating?

● Ask the patient about associated signs and symptoms, such as changes in weight, fatigue, nervousness, excitability, heat intolerance, dizziness, or palpitations. Has the patient experienced diarrhea or increased thirst or urination?

● Review the patient's medical history, noting especially diabetes mellitus and thyroid disease.

● Obtain a drug history, including prescription and over-the-counter drugs, herbal remedies, and recreational drugs, including the use of laxatives or enemas. Also, ask the patient about alcohol intake.

Physical assessment

● Weigh the patient. Ask him if his current weight is different from his previous weight. Is it higher or lower?

● Inspect the skin to detect dryness or poor turgor.

● Palpate the thyroid for enlargement, noting edema, if present.

Special considerations

Corticosteroids and cyproheptadine may increase appetite, causing weight gain.

Ⓐ PEDIATRIC POINTERS

● *In children, polyphagia commonly results from juvenile diabetes.*

● *In infants ages 6 to 18 months, polyphagia can result from malabsorptive disorders such as celiac disease.*

● *Polyphagia may occur normally in a child who's experiencing a sudden growth spurt.*

Patient counseling

Offer the patient with polyphagia emotional support, and help him understand its underlying cause. Refer the patient and his family for psychological counseling, as appropriate.

POLYPHAGIA

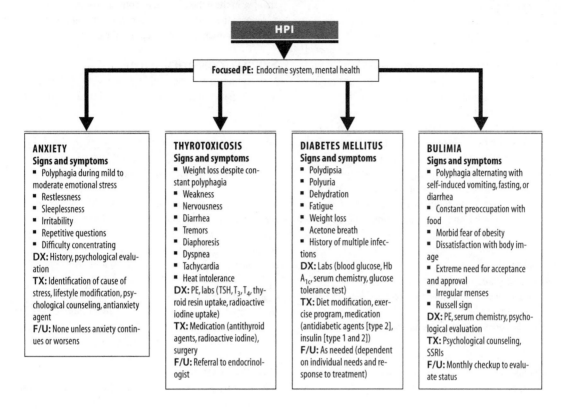

HPI

Focused PE: Endocrine system, mental health

ANXIETY
Signs and symptoms
- Polyphagia during mild to moderate emotional stress
- Restlessness
- Sleeplessness
- Irritability
- Repetitive questions
- Difficulty concentrating

DX: History, psychological evaluation

TX: Identification of cause of stress, lifestyle modification, psychological counseling, antianxiety agent

F/U: None unless anxiety continues or worsens

THYROTOXICOSIS
Signs and symptoms
- Weight loss despite constant polyphagia
- Weakness
- Nervousness
- Diarrhea
- Tremors
- Diaphoresis
- Dyspnea
- Tachycardia
- Heat intolerance

DX: PE, labs (TSH, T_3, T_4, thyroid resin uptake, radioactive iodine uptake)

TX: Medication (antithyroid agents, radioactive iodine), surgery

F/U: Referral to endocrinologist

DIABETES MELLITUS
Signs and symptoms
- Polydipsia
- Polyuria
- Dehydration
- Fatigue
- Weight loss
- Acetone breath
- History of multiple infections

DX: Labs (blood glucose, Hb A_{1c}, serum chemistry, glucose tolerance test)

TX: Diet modification, exercise program, medication (antidiabetic agents [type 2], insulin [type 1 and 2])

F/U: As needed (dependent on individual needs and response to treatment)

BULIMIA
Signs and symptoms
- Polyphagia alternating with self-induced vomiting, fasting, or diarrhea
- Constant preoccupation with food
- Morbid fear of obesity
- Dissatisfaction with body image
- Extreme need for acceptance and approval
- Irregular menses
- Russell sign

DX: PE, serum chemistry, psychological evaluation

TX: Psychological counseling, SSRIs

F/U: Monthly checkup to evaluate status

Additional differential diagnoses: migraine headache ▪ premenstrual syndrome

Other causes: corticosteroids ▪ cyproheptadine

Polyuria

A relatively common sign, polyuria is the daily production and excretion of more than 3,000 ml of urine. It's usually reported by the patient as increased urination, especially when it occurs at night. Polyuria is aggravated by overhydration, consumption of caffeine or alcohol, and excessive ingestion of salt, glucose, or other hyperosmolar substances.

Polyuria may result from the use of particular drugs (such as diuretics) or from a psychological, neurologic, or renal disorder. It can reflect central nervous system dysfunction that diminishes or suppresses the secretion of antidiuretic hormone (ADH), which regulates fluid balance. Alternatively, when ADH levels are normal, it can reflect renal impairment. In both of these pathophysiologic mechanisms, the renal tubules fail to reabsorb sufficient water, causing polyuria.

 ALERT

If the patient complains of polyuria:
- *check the patient's vital signs, noting decreased blood pressure or increased heart rate*
- *evaluate the patient's level of consciousness*
- *check for cool, clammy skin*
- *institute emergency measures, if appropriate.*
  If the patient doesn't display signs of hypovolemia, perform a focused assessment.

HISTORY

- Explore the frequency and pattern of the polyuria. Ask the patient when it began and how long it has lasted. Also, ask him if it was precipitated by a certain event.
- Ask the patient to describe the pattern and amount of his daily fluid intake.
- Review the patient's medical history for visual deficits, headaches, or head trauma, which may precede diabetes insipidus; urinary tract obstruction or infection; diabetes mellitus; renal disorders; chronic hypokalemia or hypercalcemia; and psychiatric disorders.
- Ask the patient what medications he's taking, including dosages and schedules.
- Ask the patient if he's unusually tired or thirsty.
- Ask the patient if he has recently lost more than 5% of his body weight.

PHYSICAL ASSESSMENT

- Evaluate fluid status first. Take vital signs, especially noting an increased body temperature, tachycardia, or orthostatic hypotension.
- Check for dry skin and mucous membranes, decreased skin turgor and elasticity, and reduced perspiration.

- Perform a neurologic examination, noting especially changes in the patient's level of consciousness.
- Palpate the bladder and inspect the urethral meatus. Obtain a urine specimen, and check its specific gravity.

SPECIAL CONSIDERATIONS

Maintaining an adequate fluid balance is your primary concern when the patient has polyuria. Monitor intake and output and weight.

 PEDIATRIC POINTERS

- *The major causes of polyuria in children are congenital nephrogenic diabetes insipidus, medullary cystic disease, polycystic renal disease, and distal renal tubular acidosis.*
- *Because a child's fluid balance is more delicate than an adult's, check his urine specific gravity at each voiding, and be alert for signs of dehydration, such as decreased body weight, decreased skin turgor, dry mucous membranes, decreased urine output, absence of tears when crying, and pale, mottled, or gray skin.*

 AGING ISSUES

In elderly patients, chronic pyelonephritis is commonly associated with a lymphoproliferative disorder. The possibility of associated malignant disease must be investigated.

PATIENT COUNSELING

Advise the patient to decrease his intake of caffeine, alcohol, salt, and sugar, and to avoid drinking fluids right before bedtime.

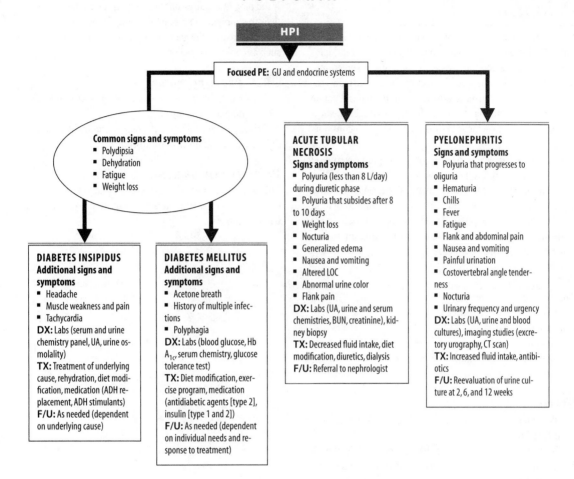

HPI

Focused PE: GU and endocrine systems

Common signs and symptoms
- Polydipsia
- Dehydration
- Fatigue
- Weight loss

DIABETES INSIPIDUS
Additional signs and symptoms
- Headache
- Muscle weakness and pain
- Tachycardia

DX: Labs (serum and urine chemistry panel, UA, urine osmolality)
TX: Treatment of underlying cause, rehydration, diet modification, medication (ADH replacement, ADH stimulants)
F/U: As needed (dependent on underlying cause)

DIABETES MELLITUS
Additional signs and symptoms
- Acetone breath
- History of multiple infections
- Polyphagia

DX: Labs (blood glucose, Hb A_{1c}, serum chemistry, glucose tolerance test)
TX: Diet modification, exercise program, medication (antidiabetic agents [type 2], insulin [type 1 and 2])
F/U: As needed (dependent on individual needs and response to treatment)

ACUTE TUBULAR NECROSIS
Signs and symptoms
- Polyuria (less than 8 L/day) during diuretic phase
- Polyuria that subsides after 8 to 10 days
- Weight loss
- Nocturia
- Generalized edema
- Nausea and vomiting
- Altered LOC
- Abnormal urine color
- Flank pain

DX: Labs (UA, urine and serum chemistries, BUN, creatinine), kidney biopsy
TX: Decreased fluid intake, diet modification, diuretics, dialysis
F/U: Referral to nephrologist

PYELONEPHRITIS
Signs and symptoms
- Polyuria that progresses to oliguria
- Hematuria
- Chills
- Fever
- Fatigue
- Flank and abdominal pain
- Nausea and vomiting
- Painful urination
- Costovertebral angle tenderness
- Nocturia
- Urinary frequency and urgency

DX: Labs (UA, urine and blood cultures), imaging studies (excretory urography, CT scan)
TX: Increased fluid intake, antibiotics
F/U: Reevaluation of urine culture at 2, 6, and 12 weeks

Additional differential diagnoses: hypercalcemia ▪ hypokalemia ▪ postobstructive uropathy ▪ psychogenic polydipsia ▪ Sheehan's syndrome ▪ sickle cell anemia

Other causes: cardiotonics ▪ contrast media ▪ demeclocycline ▪ diuretics ▪ lithium ▪ methoxyflurane ▪ phenytoin ▪ propoxyphene ▪ vitamin D

Priapism

A urologic emergency, priapism is a persistent, painful erection that's unrelated to sexual excitation. This relatively rare sign may begin during sleep and appear to be a normal erection; however, it may last for several hours or days. It's usually accompanied by a severe, constant, dull aching in the penis. Despite the pain, the patient may be too embarrassed to seek medical help and may try to achieve detumescence through continued sexual activity.

Priapism occurs when the veins of the corpora cavernosa fail to drain correctly, resulting in persistent engorgement of the tissues. Without prompt treatment, penile ischemia and thrombosis occur. In about one-half of all cases, priapism is idiopathic and develops without apparent predisposing factors. Secondary priapism may result from a blood disorder, neoplasm, trauma, or the use of a particular drug.

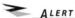 **ALERT**

If the patient has priapism:
- *apply ice packs to his penis*
- *administer an analgesic*
- *insert an indwelling catheter to relieve urine retention.*

  When the patient's condition permits, perform a focused assessment.

HISTORY

- Ask the patient when the priapism began. Ask him if it's continuous or intermittent.
- Ask the patient whether he has had a prolonged erection in the past. If so, what did he do to relieve it? How long did he remain detumescent?
- Ask the patient if he experiences pain or tenderness when he urinates.
- Ask the patient if he has noticed changes in sexual function.
- Review the patient's medical history. If there's a history of sickle cell anemia, ask the patient about factors that could precipitate a crisis, such as dehydration and infection. Also, ask the patient if he has recently suffered genital trauma.
- Obtain a drug history, including prescription and over-the-counter drugs, herbal remedies, and recreational drugs. Also, ask the patient about alcohol intake.

PHYSICAL ASSESSMENT

- Examine the patient's penis, noting its color and temperature. Check for loss of sensation, and look for signs of infection, such as redness or drainage.
- Take the patient's vital signs, particularly noting fever.

SPECIAL CONSIDERATIONS

If the patient requires surgery, keep his penis flaccid postoperatively by applying a pressure dressing. At least once every 30 minutes, inspect the glans for signs of vascular compromise, such as coolness or pallor.

 PEDIATRIC POINTERS

- *In neonates, priapism can result from hypoxia but is usually resolved with oxygen therapy.*
- *Priapism is more likely to develop in children with sickle cell disease than in adults with the disease.*

PATIENT COUNSELING

Encourage patients with sickle cell anemia to report episodes of priapism. Quick treatment is necessary to preserve normal sexual function.

PRIAPISM

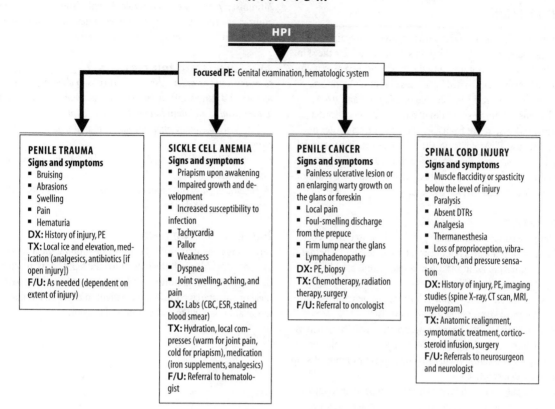

HPI

Focused PE: Genital examination, hematologic system

PENILE TRAUMA
Signs and symptoms
- Bruising
- Abrasions
- Swelling
- Pain
- Hematuria

DX: History of injury, PE
TX: Local ice and elevation, medication (analgesics, antibiotics [if open injury])
F/U: As needed (dependent on extent of injury)

SICKLE CELL ANEMIA
Signs and symptoms
- Priapism upon awakening
- Impaired growth and development
- Increased susceptibility to infection
- Tachycardia
- Pallor
- Weakness
- Dyspnea
- Joint swelling, aching, and pain

DX: Labs (CBC, ESR, stained blood smear)
TX: Hydration, local compresses (warm for joint pain, cold for priapism), medication (iron supplements, analgesics)
F/U: Referral to hematologist

PENILE CANCER
Signs and symptoms
- Painless ulcerative lesion or an enlarging warty growth on the glans or foreskin
- Local pain
- Foul-smelling discharge from the prepuce
- Firm lump near the glans
- Lymphadenopathy

DX: PE, biopsy
TX: Chemotherapy, radiation therapy, surgery
F/U: Referral to oncologist

SPINAL CORD INJURY
Signs and symptoms
- Muscle flaccidity or spasticity below the level of injury
- Paralysis
- Absent DTRs
- Analgesia
- Thermanesthesia
- Loss of proprioception, vibration, touch, and pressure sensation

DX: History of injury, PE, imaging studies (spine X-ray, CT scan, MRI, myelogram)
TX: Anatomic realignment, symptomatic treatment, corticosteroid infusion, surgery
F/U: Referrals to neurosurgeon and neurologist

Other causes: androgenic steroids ▪ anticoagulants ▪ antihypertensives ▪ intracorporeal injection of papaverine ▪ phenothiazines ▪ thioridazine ▪ trazodone

Pruritus

Commonly provoking scratching as an attempt to gain relief, pruritus is an unpleasant itching sensation that affects the skin, certain mucous membranes, and the eyes. Most severe at night, pruritus may be exacerbated by increased skin temperature, poor skin turgor, local vasodilation, dermatoses, and stress.

The most common symptom of a dermatologic disorder, pruritus may also result from a local or systemic disorder or from drug use. Physiologic pruritus (such as pruritic urticarial papules and plaques of pregnancy) may occur in primigravidas late in the third trimester. Pruritus can also stem from emotional upset or contact with skin irritants.

HISTORY
● Have the patient describe the pruritus, its onset, frequency, and intensity. If the pruritus occurs at night, ask him whether it prevents him from falling asleep or awakens him after he falls asleep. Locate the pruritic area.
● Ask the patient if the itching is localized or generalized. When is it most severe? How long does it last?
● Ask the patient if the pruritus occurs after activities, such as physical exertion, bathing, or makeup or perfume application. Has the patient recently changed medications or brands of soap or laundry detergent?
● Ask the patient how he cleans his skin. In particular, look for excessive bathing, harsh soaps, contact allergy, and excessively hot water.
● Ask the patient about occupational exposure to known skin irritants, such as fiberglass insulation or chemicals.
● Ask the patient if he has recently traveled abroad.
● Ask the patient if anyone else in his house has reported itching. Does he have pets?
● Ask the patient if stress, fear, depression, or illness seems to aggravate the itching.
● Ask the patient about his general health. Does he have related symptoms?
● Review the patient's medical history for skin disorders.
● Obtain a drug history, including prescription and over-the-counter drugs, herbal remedies, and recreational drugs. Also, ask the patient about alcohol intake.

PHYSICAL ASSESSMENT
● Note the color of the patient's skin. Check sclerae for jaundice.
● Examine the patient for signs of scratching, such as excoriation, purpura, scabs, scars, or lichenification.
● Look for primary lesions to help confirm dermatoses.
● Palpate the abdomen for tenderness.

SPECIAL CONSIDERATIONS
Administer a topical corticosteroid, an antihistamine, or a tranquilizer, as ordered. If the patient doesn't have a localized infection or skin lesions, suspect a systemic disease.

A   PEDIATRIC POINTERS
● *Many adult disorders also cause pruritus in children, but they may affect different parts of the body. For example, scabies may affect the head of an infant but not that of an adult.*
● *Pityriasis rosea may affect the face, hands, and feet of adolescents.*
● *Some childhood diseases, such as measles and chickenpox, can cause pruritus.*
● *Hepatic diseases can produce pruritus in children as bile salts accumulate on the skin.*

PATIENT COUNSELING
Advise the patient to avoid scratching or rubbing the itchy areas. To ease itching, tell the patient to take tepid baths, using little soap and rinsing thoroughly. Recommend a soothing oatmeal or cornstarch bath. Tell the patient to apply an emollient lotion after bathing to soften and cool the skin.

PRURITUS

HPI

Focused PE: Skin, immunologic system, abdomen

BILIARY DISEASE
Signs and symptoms
- Jaundice
- RUQ pain
- Epigastric burning
- Clay-colored stools
- Fever
- Chills
- Flatus
- Belching

DX: PE, CBC, imaging studies (abdominal X-ray, ultrasound, CT scan, oral cholecystogram, gall bladder radionuclide scan)
TX: Varies based on specific illness, diet modification, analgesics, surgery
F/U: Referral to gastroenterologist

HERPES ZOSTER
Signs and symptoms
- Fever
- Malaise
- Paresthesia
- Hyperesthesia
- Deep pain on the trunk, arms, and legs in dermatome distribution
- Skin eruptions (macules that vesiculate)

DX: PE
TX: Symptomatic treatment, medication (analgesics, antianxiety agents, antipruritics, antiviral agents)
F/U: Reevaluation in 10 days

Common signs and symptoms
- Pruritus in the area of infestation
- Urticaria (from scratching)

PITYRIASIS ROSEA
Signs and symptoms
- Mild to severe pruritus that's aggravated by a hot bath or shower
- Erythematous herald patch anywhere on the body
- Red-brown patches with an erythematous border and trailing scales
- Lesions that may be macular, vesicular, or urticarial

DX: Skin examination
TX: Symptomatic treatment, medication (antipyretics, topical or systemic corticosteroids), oatmeal baths
F/U: None unless the condition persists longer than 6 weeks

PEDICULOSIS CAPITIS
Additional signs and symptoms
- Matted, foul-smelling lusterless hair
- Occipital and cervical lymphadenopathy
- Oval, gray white nits on the hair shafts

PEDICULOSIS PUBIS
Additional signs and symptoms
- Erythematous papules in the pubic hair and the hair around the anus, abdomen, or thighs

DX: Close examination of hair
TX: Isolation from others until treated, use of fine-tooth comb on hair after treated, pediculicide shampoo, cleaning of articles that have possibly had contact in hot water
F/U: None necessary unless recurrent

Additional differential diagnoses: anemia (iron deficiency) ▪ conjunctivitis ▪ dermatitis ▪ diabetes ▪ enterobiasis ▪ hemorrhoids ▪ herpes zoster ▪ Hodgkin's disease ▪ leukemia (chronic lymphocytic) ▪ lichen planus ▪ lichen simplex chronicus ▪ liver failure ▪ mastocytosis ▪ multiple myeloma ▪ mycosis fungoides ▪ myringitis (chronic) ▪ polycythemia vera ▪ psoriasis ▪ psychogenic pruritus ▪ renal failure (chronic) ▪ scabies ▪ thyrotoxicosis ▪ tinea pedis ▪ urticaria ▪ vaginitis

Other causes: bedbug bites ▪ drug hypersensitivity ▪ ingestion of fruit pulp from ginkgo tree

Ptosis

Ptosis is the excessive drooping of one or both upper eyelids. This sign can be constant, progressive, or intermittent as well as unilateral or bilateral. When it's unilateral, it's easy to detect by comparing the eyelids' relative positions. When it's bilateral or mild, it's difficult to detect — the eyelids may be abnormally low, covering the upper part of the iris or even part of the pupil instead of overlapping the iris slightly. Other clues include a furrowed forehead or a tipped-back head — signs that the patient is compensating to see under his drooping lids. With severe ptosis, the patient may not be able to raise his eyelids voluntarily. Because ptosis can resemble enophthalmos, exophthalmometry may be required.

Ptosis can be classified as congenital or acquired. Classification is important for proper treatment. Congenital ptosis results from levator muscle underdevelopment or a disorder of the third cranial (oculomotor) nerve. Acquired ptosis may result from trauma to or inflammation of these muscles and nerves, use of a particular drug, a systemic disease, an intracranial lesion, or a life-threatening aneurysm. However, the most common cause is advanced age, which reduces muscle elasticity and produces senile ptosis.

HISTORY

- Ask the patient when he first noticed his drooping eyelid and whether it has worsened or improved.
- Ask the patient if he has recently suffered a traumatic eye injury.
- Ask the patient if he has experienced eye pain or headache, and determine its location and severity.
- Ask the patient if he has experienced vision changes. If so, have him describe the changes.
- Ask the patient if he wears corrective lenses or contact lenses.
- Obtain a drug history, including prescription and over-the-counter drugs, herbal remedies, and recreational drugs, noting especially chemotherapeutic agents. Also, ask the patient about alcohol intake.

PHYSICAL ASSESSMENT

- Assess the degree of ptosis, and check for eyelid edema, exophthalmos, deviation, and conjunctival injection.
- Evaluate extraocular muscle function by testing the six cardinal fields of gaze.
- Carefully examine the pupil's size, color, shape, and reaction to light, and test visual acuity. Is convergence, photosensitivity, or photophobia present?

SPECIAL CONSIDERATIONS

Keep in mind that ptosis occasionally indicates a life-threatening condition. For example, sudden unilateral ptosis can herald a cerebral aneurysm.

🄰 PEDIATRIC POINTERS

- Astigmatism and myopia may be associated with childhood ptosis.
- Parents typically discover congenital ptosis when their child is an infant. Usually, the ptosis is unilateral, constant, and accompanied by lagophthalmos, which causes the infant to sleep with his eyes open. If this occurs, teach proper eye care to prevent drying.

PATIENT COUNSELING

Instruct the patient on what to expect from diagnostic testing, which may include the Tensilon test and slit-lamp examination.

P T O S I S

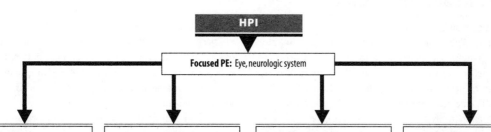

HPI

Focused PE: Eye, neurologic system

HORNER'S SYNDROME
Signs and symptoms
- Moderate unilateral ptosis that almost disappears when the eye is opened widely
- Unilateral miosis
- Ipsilateral anhidrosis of the face and neck
- Transient conjunctivitis
- Vascular headache on the affected side
- Vertigo

DX: Eye examination, pharmacologic testing of the pupil
TX: Treatment of underlying cause
F/U: As needed (dependent on underlying cause)

LACRIMAL GLAND TUMOR
Signs and symptoms
- Mild to severe ptosis (based on tumor size and location)
- Brow elevation
- Exophthalmos
- Eye deviation
- Eye pain

DX: Eye examination, imaging studies (CT scan, MRI)
TX: Radiation therapy, surgery
F/U: Referrals to ophthalmologist and oncologist

MYOTONIC DYSTROPHY
Signs and symptoms
- Mild to severe bilateral ptosis
- Distinctive cataracts with iridescent dots in the cortex
- Miosis
- Diplopia
- Decreased tearing
- Facial weakness
- Slack jaw
- Muscular and testicular atrophy

DX: History and PE, DNA analysis, EMG, ECG, muscle biopsy
TX: Symptomatic treatment, physical and speech therapy, diet modification, antiarrhythmics
F/U: As needed (dependent on the severity of symptoms)

PARRY-ROMBERG SYNDROME
Signs and symptoms
- Unilateral ptosis
- Facial hemiatrophy
- Miosis
- Sluggish pupil
- Enophthalmos
- Different colored irises
- Ocular muscle paralysis
- Nystagmus
- Muscle atrophy

DX: PE
TX: Symptomatic treatment, speech therapy, surgery
F/U: Referral to neurologist

Additional differential diagnoses: alcoholism ▪ botulism ▪ cerebral aneurysm ▪ dacryoadenitis ▪ hemangioma ▪ levator muscle maldevelopment ▪ multiple sclerosis ▪ myasthenia gravis ▪ ocular muscle dystrophy ▪ ocular trauma ▪ Parinaud's syndrome ▪ subdural hematoma (chronic)

Other causes: lead poisoning ▪ vinca alkaloids

Pulse, absent or weak

An absent or a weak pulse may be generalized or may affect only one extremity. When generalized, this sign is an important indicator of such life-threatening conditions as shock and arrhythmia. Localized loss or weakness of a pulse that's normally present and strong may indicate acute arterial occlusion, which could require emergency surgery. However, the pressure of palpation may temporarily diminish or obliterate superficial pulses, such as the posterior tibial or the dorsal pedal. Thus, bilateral weakness or absence of these pulses doesn't necessarily indicate underlying pathology. (See *Evaluating peripheral pulses.*)

ALERT

If you can't detect a pulse:
- *check the patient's level of consciousness; if he's unconscious, institute emergency measures*
- *quickly palpate the remaining arterial pulses to distinguish between localized or generalized loss or weakness*
- *quickly check other vital signs, and evaluate cardiopulmonary status.*

If the patient's condition is localized, perform a focused assessment.

HISTORY

- Review the patient's history for cardiac disease, venous insufficiency, and claudication or pain in the extremity.

- Ask the patient if he's experiencing pain in the extremity. If so, ask him if it's continuos or intermittent.

PHYSICAL ASSESSMENT

- Check the pulses in both extremities. Note the color and temperature of the extremity. Check for capillary refill.
- Perform an abdominal examination to evaluate the presence of an abdominal aortic aneurysm or renal stenosis through the detection of bruits.
- Based on your findings, proceed with a more complete examination and interventions.

SPECIAL CONSIDERATIONS

If the pulse is absent in an extremity, don't elevate the extremity. Anticipate preparing the patient for emergency embolectomy or peripheral angioplasty.

A̲ PEDIATRIC POINTERS

- *Radial, dorsal pedal, and posterior tibial pulses aren't easily palpable in infants and small children, so be careful not to mistake these normally hard-to-find pulses for weak or absent pulses. Instead, palpate the brachial, popliteal, or femoral pulses to evaluate arterial circulation to the extremities.*
- *In children and young adults, weak or absent femoral and more distal pulses may indicate coarctation of the aorta.*

PATIENT COUNSELING

Instruct the patient on what to expect from diagnostic testing, which may include arteriography, aortography, and Doppler ultrasonography. If the patient is to have surgery, explain what he can expect postoperatively.

EVALUATING PERIPHERAL PULSES

The rate, amplitude, and symmetry of peripheral pulses provide important clues to cardiac function and the quality of peripheral perfusion. To gather these clues, palpate peripheral pulses lightly with the pads of your index, middle, and ring fingers, as space permits.

Rate
Count all pulses for at least 30 seconds (60 seconds when recording vital signs). The normal rate is between 60 and 100 beats/minute.

Amplitude
Palpate the blood vessel during ventricular systole. Describe pulse amplitude by using a scale such as this:
    4+ = bounding
    3+ = normal
    2+ = difficult to palpate
    1+ = weak, thready
    0 = absent.
    Use a stick figure to easily document the location and amplitude of all pulses.

Symmetry
Simultaneously palpate pulses (except the carotid pulse) on both sides of the patient's body, and note inequality. Always assess peripheral pulses methodically, moving from the arms to the legs.

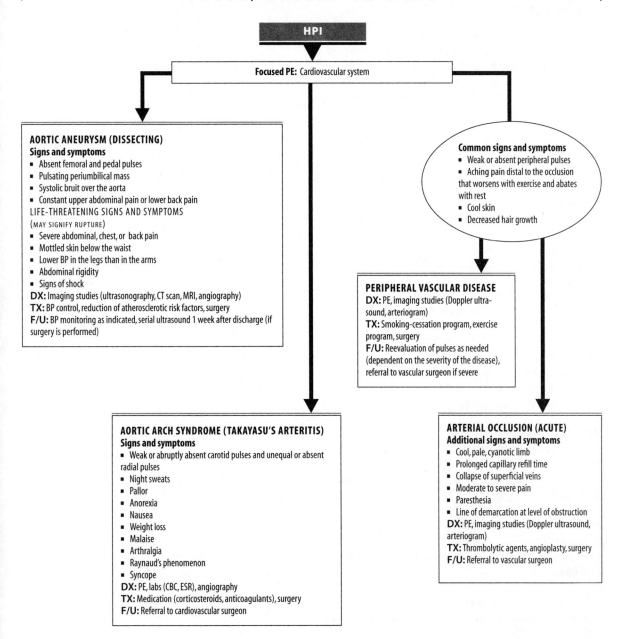

HPI

Focused PE: Cardiovascular system

AORTIC ANEURYSM (DISSECTING)
Signs and symptoms
- Absent femoral and pedal pulses
- Pulsating periumbilical mass
- Systolic bruit over the aorta
- Constant upper abdominal pain or lower back pain

LIFE-THREATENING SIGNS AND SYMPTOMS
(MAY SIGNIFY RUPTURE)
- Severe abdominal, chest, or back pain
- Mottled skin below the waist
- Lower BP in the legs than in the arms
- Abdominal rigidity
- Signs of shock

DX: Imaging studies (ultrasonography, CT scan, MRI, angiography)
TX: BP control, reduction of atherosclerotic risk factors, surgery
F/U: BP monitoring as indicated, serial ultrasound 1 week after discharge (if surgery is performed)

Common signs and symptoms
- Weak or absent peripheral pulses
- Aching pain distal to the occlusion that worsens with exercise and abates with rest
- Cool skin
- Decreased hair growth

PERIPHERAL VASCULAR DISEASE
DX: PE, imaging studies (Doppler ultrasound, arteriogram)
TX: Smoking-cessation program, exercise program, surgery
F/U: Reevaluation of pulses as needed (dependent on the severity of the disease), referral to vascular surgeon if severe

AORTIC ARCH SYNDROME (TAKAYASU'S ARTERITIS)
Signs and symptoms
- Weak or abruptly absent carotid pulses and unequal or absent radial pulses
- Night sweats
- Pallor
- Anorexia
- Nausea
- Weight loss
- Malaise
- Arthralgia
- Raynaud's phenomenon
- Syncope

DX: PE, labs (CBC, ESR), angiography
TX: Medication (corticosteroids, anticoagulants), surgery
F/U: Referral to cardiovascular surgeon

ARTERIAL OCCLUSION (ACUTE)
Additional signs and symptoms
- Cool, pale, cyanotic limb
- Prolonged capillary refill time
- Collapse of superficial veins
- Moderate to severe pain
- Paresthesia
- Line of demarcation at level of obstruction

DX: PE, imaging studies (Doppler ultrasound, arteriogram)
TX: Thrombolytic agents, angioplasty, surgery
F/U: Referral to vascular surgeon

Additional differential diagnoses: aortic bifurcation occlusion (acute) ▪ aortic stenosis ▪ arrhythmias ▪ cardiac tamponade ▪ coarctation of the aorta ▪ pulmonary embolism ▪ shock ▪ thoracic outlet syndrome

Other causes: arteriovenous shunts for dialysis

Pulse, bounding

Produced by large waves of pressure as blood ejects from the left ventricle with each contraction, a bounding pulse is strong and easily palpable and may be visible over superficial peripheral arteries. It's characterized by regular, recurrent expansion and contraction of the arterial walls, and it isn't obliterated by the pressure of palpation. A healthy person develops a bounding pulse during exercise, pregnancy, and periods of anxiety. However, this sign also results from fever and certain endocrine, hematologic, and cardiovascular disorders that increase the basal metabolic rate.

HISTORY

● Ask the patient if he noticed the bounding pulse. If he did, ask how long it has been present and if it's been continuous or intermittent.
● Ask the patient if he has noticed palpitations.
● If the patient is female, ask if she's pregnant.
● Ask the patient if he's experiencing fever, feelings of anxiety or stress, weakness, fatigue, shortness of breath, or other health changes.
● Review the patient's medical history for hyperthyroidism, anemia, and cardiovascular disorders.
● Obtain a drug history, including prescription and over-the-counter drugs, herbal remedies, and recreational drugs. Also, ask the patient about alcohol intake.

PHYSICAL ASSESSMENT

● When you detect a bounding pulse, check the patient's other vital signs.
● Auscultate the heart and lungs for abnormal sounds, rates, and rhythms.

SPECIAL CONSIDERATIONS

If a bounding pulse is accompanied by a rapid or irregular heartbeat, connect the patient to a cardiac monitor for further evaluation.

⒜ PEDIATRIC POINTERS

● *A bounding pulse can be normal in infants or children because arteries lie close to the skin surface.*
● *A bounding pulse can result from a patent ductus arteriosus if the left-to-right shunt is large.*

PATIENT COUNSELING

Instruct the patient on what to expect from diagnostic testing, which may include electrocardiography and radiology studies.

PULSE, BOUNDING

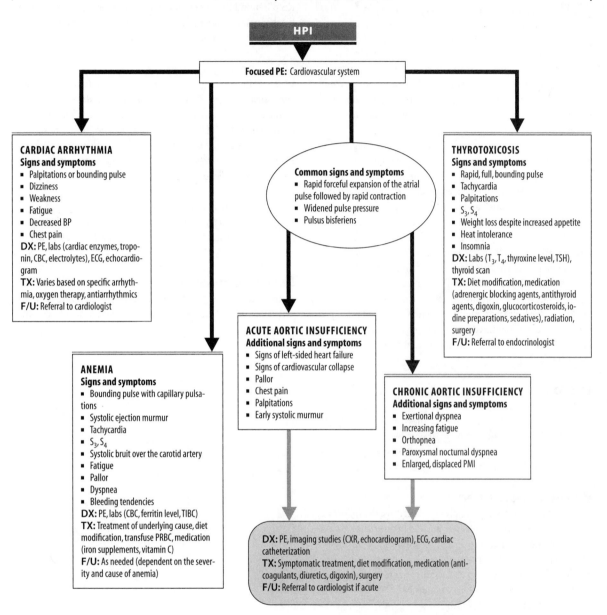

HPI

Focused PE: Cardiovascular system

CARDIAC ARRHYTHMIA
Signs and symptoms
- Palpitations or bounding pulse
- Dizziness
- Weakness
- Fatigue
- Decreased BP
- Chest pain

DX: PE, labs (cardiac enzymes, troponin, CBC, electrolytes), ECG, echocardiogram
TX: Varies based on specific arrhythmia, oxygen therapy, antiarrhythmics
F/U: Referral to cardiologist

Common signs and symptoms
- Rapid forceful expansion of the atrial pulse followed by rapid contraction
- Widened pulse pressure
- Pulsus bisferiens

THYROTOXICOSIS
Signs and symptoms
- Rapid, full, bounding pulse
- Tachycardia
- Palpitations
- S_3, S_4
- Weight loss despite increased appetite
- Heat intolerance
- Insomnia

DX: Labs (T_3, T_4, thyroxine level, TSH), thyroid scan
TX: Diet modification, medication (adrenergic blocking agents, antithyroid agents, digoxin, glucocorticosteroids, iodine preparations, sedatives), radiation, surgery
F/U: Referral to endocrinologist

ANEMIA
Signs and symptoms
- Bounding pulse with capillary pulsations
- Systolic ejection murmur
- Tachycardia
- S_3, S_4
- Systolic bruit over the carotid artery
- Fatigue
- Pallor
- Dyspnea
- Bleeding tendencies

DX: PE, labs (CBC, ferritin level, TIBC)
TX: Treatment of underlying cause, diet modification, transfuse PRBC, medication (iron supplements, vitamin C)
F/U: As needed (dependent on the severity and cause of anemia)

ACUTE AORTIC INSUFFICIENCY
Additional signs and symptoms
- Signs of left-sided heart failure
- Signs of cardiovascular collapse
- Pallor
- Chest pain
- Palpitations
- Early systolic murmur

CHRONIC AORTIC INSUFFICIENCY
Additional signs and symptoms
- Exertional dyspnea
- Increasing fatigue
- Orthopnea
- Paroxysmal nocturnal dyspnea
- Enlarged, displaced PMI

DX: PE, imaging studies (CXR, echocardiogram), ECG, cardiac catheterization
TX: Symptomatic treatment, diet modification, medication (anticoagulants, diuretics, digoxin), surgery
F/U: Referral to cardiologist if acute

Additional differential diagnosis: febrile disorder

Pulse pressure, abnormal

Pulse pressure—the difference between systolic and diastolic blood pressures—is measured by sphygmomanometry or intra-arterial monitoring. Normally, systolic pressure exceeds diastolic pressure by about 40 mm Hg. Narrowed pressure—a difference of less than 30 mm Hg—occurs when peripheral vascular resistance increases, cardiac output declines, or intravascular volume markedly decreases.

In conditions that cause mechanical obstruction (such as aortic stenosis), pulse pressure is directly related to the severity of the underlying condition. Usually a late sign, narrowed pulse pressure alone doesn't signal an emergency, even though it commonly occurs with shock and other life-threatening disorders.

Widened pulse pressure—a difference of more than 50 mm Hg—commonly occurs as a physiologic response to fever, hot weather, exercise, anxiety, anemia, or pregnancy. It can also result from a neurologic disorder—especially life-threatening increased intracranial pressure (ICP)—or from a cardiovascular disorder such as aortic insufficiency, which causes backflow of blood into the heart with each contraction. Widened pulse pressure can be easily identified by monitoring arterial blood pressure and is commonly detected during routine sphygmomanometric recordings.

HISTORY

- Review the patient's medical history for chest pain, dizziness, syncope, shortness of breath, and weakness. Also, review the patient's past blood pressure readings, if possible.
- Obtain a drug history, including prescription and over-the-counter drugs, herbal remedies, and recreational drugs.

PHYSICAL ASSESSMENT

If you detect a narrowed pulse pressure, perform the following:
- Check for signs of heart failure, such as hypotension, tachycardia, dyspnea, jugular vein distention, pulmonary crackles, and decreased urine output.
- Check for changes in skin temperature or color, strength of peripheral pulses, and level of consciousness.
- Auscultate the heart for murmurs.

If you detect a widened pulse pressure, perform the following:
- Check for signs of increased ICP. Perform a thorough neurologic examination, which will serve as a baseline for subsequent changes.
- Check cranial nerve function—especially in cranial nerves III, IV, and VI.
- Assess pupillary reactions, reflexes, and muscle tone.
- Check for edema, and auscultate for murmurs.

SPECIAL CONSIDERATIONS

Keep in mind that increasing ICP is commonly signaled by subtle changes in a patient's condition, rather than the abrupt development of any one sign or symptom.

 PEDIATRIC POINTERS

- *In children, narrowed pulse pressure can result from congenital aortic stenosis or from a disorder that affects adults.*
- *Increased ICP causes widened pulse pressure in children. Patent ductus arteriosus (PDA) can also cause widened pulse pressure, but this sign may not be evident at birth. The older child with PDA experiences exertional dyspnea, with pulse pressure that widens even further on exertion.*

AGING ISSUES

Recently, widened pulse pressure has been found to be a more powerful predictor of cardiovascular events in elderly patients than either increased systolic or diastolic blood pressure.

PATIENT COUNSELING

Instruct the patient on what to expect from diagnostic testing, which may include echocardiography and electrocardiography.

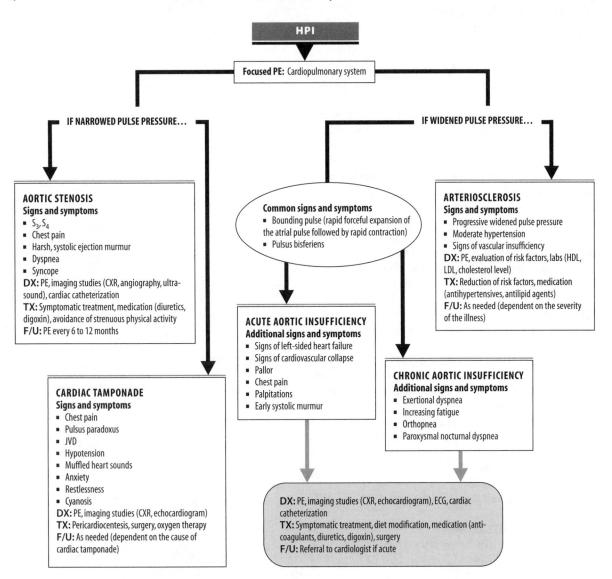

HPI

Focused PE: Cardiopulmonary system

IF NARROWED PULSE PRESSURE...

IF WIDENED PULSE PRESSURE...

AORTIC STENOSIS
Signs and symptoms
- S_3, S_4
- Chest pain
- Harsh, systolic ejection murmur
- Dyspnea
- Syncope

DX: PE, imaging studies (CXR, angiography, ultrasound), cardiac catheterization
TX: Symptomatic treatment, medication (diuretics, digoxin), avoidance of strenuous physical activity
F/U: PE every 6 to 12 months

Common signs and symptoms
- Bounding pulse (rapid forceful expansion of the atrial pulse followed by rapid contraction)
- Pulsus bisferiens

ARTERIOSCLEROSIS
Signs and symptoms
- Progressive widened pulse pressure
- Moderate hypertension
- Signs of vascular insufficiency

DX: PE, evaluation of risk factors, labs (HDL, LDL, cholesterol level)
TX: Reduction of risk factors, medication (antihypertensives, antilipid agents)
F/U: As needed (dependent on the severity of the illness)

ACUTE AORTIC INSUFFICIENCY
Additional signs and symptoms
- Signs of left-sided heart failure
- Signs of cardiovascular collapse
- Pallor
- Chest pain
- Palpitations
- Early systolic murmur

CHRONIC AORTIC INSUFFICIENCY
Additional signs and symptoms
- Exertional dyspnea
- Increasing fatigue
- Orthopnea
- Paroxysmal nocturnal dyspnea

CARDIAC TAMPONADE
Signs and symptoms
- Chest pain
- Pulsus paradoxus
- JVD
- Hypotension
- Muffled heart sounds
- Anxiety
- Restlessness
- Cyanosis

DX: PE, imaging studies (CXR, echocardiogram)
TX: Pericardiocentesis, surgery, oxygen therapy
F/U: As needed (dependent on the cause of cardiac tamponade)

DX: PE, imaging studies (CXR, echocardiogram), ECG, cardiac catheterization
TX: Symptomatic treatment, diet modification, medication (anticoagulants, diuretics, digoxin), surgery
F/U: Referral to cardiologist if acute

Additional differential diagnoses for narrowed pulse pressure: heart failure ▪ shock

Additional differential diagnoses for widened pulse pressure: febrile disorders ▪ increased ICP

Pulsus bisferiens

A bisferiens pulse is a hyperdynamic, double-beating pulse characterized by two systolic peaks separated by a midsystolic dip. Both peaks may be equal or either may be larger; however, the first peak is typically taller or more forceful than the second. The first peak (percussion wave) is believed to be the pulse pressure; the second (tidal wave), reverberation from the periphery. Pulsus bisferiens occurs in conditions such as aortic insufficiency (the most common organic cause of pulsus bisferiens), in which a large volume of blood is rapidly ejected from the left ventricle. The pulse can be palpated in peripheral arteries or observed on an arterial pressure wave recording.

To detect pulsus bisferiens, lightly palpate the carotid, brachial, radial, or femoral artery. (The pulse is easiest to palpate at the carotid artery.) At the same time, listen to the patient's heart sounds to determine whether the two palpable peaks occur during systole. If they do, you'll feel the double pulse between the first and second heart sounds.

HISTORY

- Review the patient's medical history for cardiac disorders or other illnesses.
- Ask the patient about associated signs and symptoms, such as dyspnea, chest pain, or fatigue. If the patient has experienced associated signs and symptoms, ask how long he has had these symptoms and whether they change with activity or rest.
- Obtain a drug history, including prescription and over-the-counter drugs, herbal remedies, and recreational drugs.

PHYSICAL ASSESSMENT

- Take the patient's vital signs.
- Auscultate for abnormal heart or lung sounds.

SPECIAL CONSIDERATIONS

When obtaining the patient's pulse at the carotid artery, use caution; pressure on the carotid artery can cause the patient's heart rate to decrease.

A PEDIATRIC POINTERS

Pulsus bisferiens may be palpated in children with a large patent ductus arteriosus and in those with congenital aortic stenosis and insufficiency.

PATIENT COUNSELING

Instruct the patient on what to expect from diagnostic testing, which may include electrocardiogram, chest X-ray, cardiac catheterization, and angiography.

PULSUS BISFERIENS

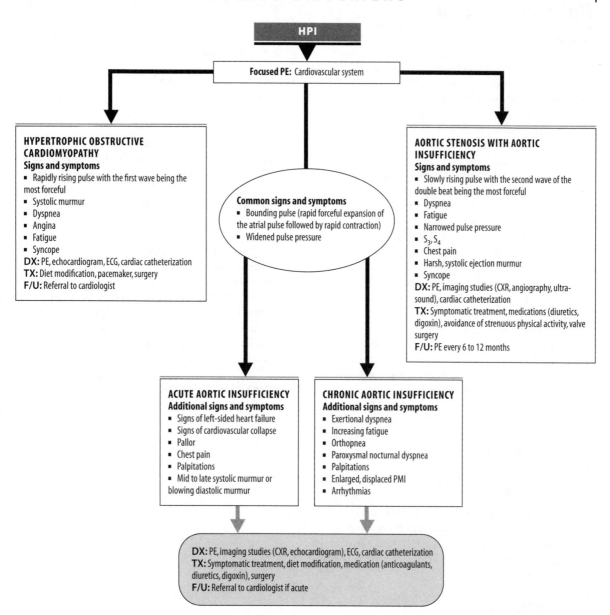

HPI

Focused PE: Cardiovascular system

HYPERTROPHIC OBSTRUCTIVE CARDIOMYOPATHY
Signs and symptoms
- Rapidly rising pulse with the first wave being the most forceful
- Systolic murmur
- Dyspnea
- Angina
- Fatigue
- Syncope

DX: PE, echocardiogram, ECG, cardiac catheterization
TX: Diet modification, pacemaker, surgery
F/U: Referral to cardiologist

Common signs and symptoms
- Bounding pulse (rapid forceful expansion of the atrial pulse followed by rapid contraction)
- Widened pulse pressure

AORTIC STENOSIS WITH AORTIC INSUFFICIENCY
Signs and symptoms
- Slowly rising pulse with the second wave of the double beat being the most forceful
- Dyspnea
- Fatigue
- Narrowed pulse pressure
- S_3, S_4
- Chest pain
- Harsh, systolic ejection murmur
- Syncope

DX: PE, imaging studies (CXR, angiography, ultrasound), cardiac catheterization
TX: Symptomatic treatment, medications (diuretics, digoxin), avoidance of strenuous physical activity, valve surgery
F/U: PE every 6 to 12 months

ACUTE AORTIC INSUFFICIENCY
Additional signs and symptoms
- Signs of left-sided heart failure
- Signs of cardiovascular collapse
- Pallor
- Chest pain
- Palpitations
- Mid to late systolic murmur or blowing diastolic murmur

CHRONIC AORTIC INSUFFICIENCY
Additional signs and symptoms
- Exertional dyspnea
- Increasing fatigue
- Orthopnea
- Paroxysmal nocturnal dyspnea
- Palpitations
- Enlarged, displaced PMI
- Arrhythmias

DX: PE, imaging studies (CXR, echocardiogram), ECG, cardiac catheterization
TX: Symptomatic treatment, diet modification, medication (anticoagulants, diuretics, digoxin), surgery
F/U: Referral to cardiologist if acute

Additional differential diagnoses: high cardiac output states (such as anemia, thyrotoxicosis, fever, and exercise)

Pulsus paradoxus

Pulsus paradoxus, or paradoxical pulse, is an exaggerated decline in blood pressure during inspiration. Normally, systolic pressure falls less than 10 mm Hg during inspiration. With paradoxical pulse, however, it falls more than 10 mm Hg. When systolic pressure falls more than 20 mm Hg, the peripheral pulses may be barely palpable or may disappear during inspiration.

Pulsus paradoxus is thought to result from an exaggerated inspirational increase in negative intrathoracic pressure. Normally, systolic pressure drops during inspiration because of blood pooling in the pulmonary system. This, in turn, reduces left ventricular filling and stroke volume and transmits negative intrathoracic pressure to the aorta. Conditions associated with large intrapleural pressure swings (such as asthma) or those that reduce left-sided heart filling (such as pericardial tamponade) produce paradoxical pulse.

To accurately detect and measure paradoxical pulse, use a sphygmomanometer or an intra-arterial monitoring device. Inflate the blood pressure cuff 10 to 20 mm Hg beyond the peak systolic pressure. Then deflate the cuff at a rate of 2 mm Hg per second until you hear the first Korotkoff's sound during expiration. Note the systolic pressure. As you continue to slowly deflate the cuff, observe the patient's respiratory pattern. If a paradoxical pulse is present, the Korotkoff's sounds will disappear with inspiration and return with expiration. Continue to deflate the cuff until you hear Korotkoff's sounds during both inspiration and expiration and, again, note the systolic pressure. Subtract this reading from the first one to determine the degree of paradoxical pulse. A difference of more than 10 mm Hg is abnormal.

You can also detect paradoxical pulse by palpating the radial pulse over several cycles of slow inspiration and expiration. Marked pulse diminution during inspiration indicates paradoxical pulse. When you check for paradoxical pulse, remember that irregular heart rhythms and tachycardia cause variations in pulse amplitude and must be ruled out before a true paradoxical pulse can be identified.

➤ ALERT

When you detect paradoxical pulse:
- *quickly assess all vital signs*
- *check for additional signs and symptoms of cardiac tamponade, such as dyspnea, tachypnea, diaphoresis, jugular vein distention, tachycardia, narrowed pulse pressure, and hypotension*
- *institute emergency measures, if necessary.*
  If the patient's condition permits, perform a focused assessment.

HISTORY
- Review the patient's medical history for chronic cardiac or pulmonary disease.
- Ask the patient about associated signs and symptoms, such as cough or chest pain.

PHYSICAL ASSESSMENT
- Take the patient's vital signs.
- Auscultate for abnormal breath sounds.

SPECIAL CONSIDERATIONS
An increase in the degree of paradox may indicate recurring or worsening cardiac tamponade or impending respiratory arrest in severe chronic obstructive pulmonary disease. Vigorous respiratory treatment, such as chest physiotherapy, may avert the need for endotracheal intubation.

A   PEDIATRIC POINTERS
- *Paradoxical pulse commonly occurs in children with chronic pulmonary disease, especially during an acute asthma attack.*
- *Children with pericarditis may develop paradoxical pulse due to cardiac tamponade; however, this disorder more commonly affects adults. A paradoxical pulse greater than 20 mm Hg is a reliable indicator of cardiac tamponade in children; a change of 10 to 20 mm Hg is equivocal.*

PATIENT COUNSELING
Instruct the patient on what to expect from diagnostic testing, which may include echocardiogram and electrocardiogram.

PULSUS PARADOXUS

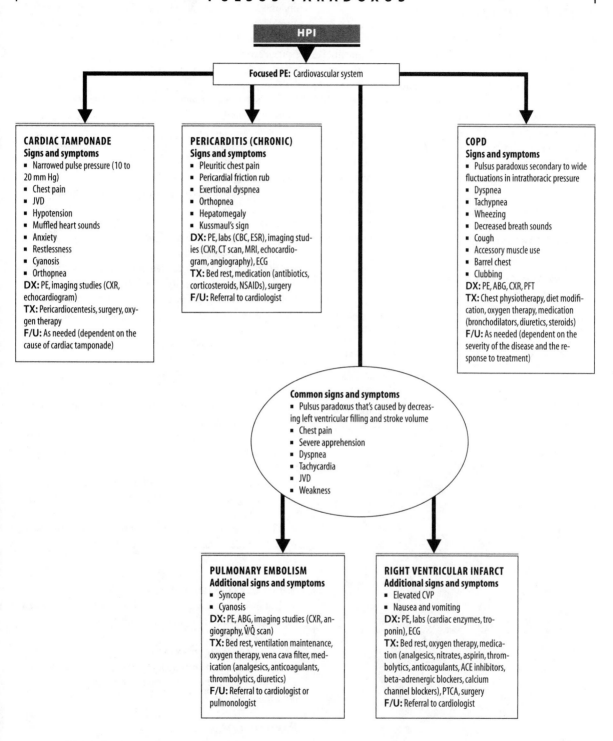

HPI

Focused PE: Cardiovascular system

CARDIAC TAMPONADE
Signs and symptoms
- Narrowed pulse pressure (10 to 20 mm Hg)
- Chest pain
- JVD
- Hypotension
- Muffled heart sounds
- Anxiety
- Restlessness
- Cyanosis
- Orthopnea

DX: PE, imaging studies (CXR, echocardiogram)
TX: Pericardiocentesis, surgery, oxygen therapy
F/U: As needed (dependent on the cause of cardiac tamponade)

PERICARDITIS (CHRONIC)
Signs and symptoms
- Pleuritic chest pain
- Pericardial friction rub
- Exertional dyspnea
- Orthopnea
- Hepatomegaly
- Kussmaul's sign

DX: PE, labs (CBC, ESR), imaging studies (CXR, CT scan, MRI, echocardiogram, angiography), ECG
TX: Bed rest, medication (antibiotics, corticosteroids, NSAIDs), surgery
F/U: Referral to cardiologist

COPD
Signs and symptoms
- Pulsus paradoxus secondary to wide fluctuations in intrathoracic pressure
- Dyspnea
- Tachypnea
- Wheezing
- Decreased breath sounds
- Cough
- Accessory muscle use
- Barrel chest
- Clubbing

DX: PE, ABG, CXR, PFT
TX: Chest physiotherapy, diet modification, oxygen therapy, medication (bronchodilators, diuretics, steroids)
F/U: As needed (dependent on the severity of the disease and the response to treatment)

Common signs and symptoms
- Pulsus paradoxus that's caused by decreasing left ventricular filling and stroke volume
- Chest pain
- Severe apprehension
- Dyspnea
- Tachycardia
- JVD
- Weakness

PULMONARY EMBOLISM
Additional signs and symptoms
- Syncope
- Cyanosis

DX: PE, ABG, imaging studies (CXR, angiography, V̇/Q̇ scan)
TX: Bed rest, ventilation maintenance, oxygen therapy, vena cava filter, medication (analgesics, anticoagulants, thrombolytics, diuretics)
F/U: Referral to cardiologist or pulmonologist

RIGHT VENTRICULAR INFARCT
Additional signs and symptoms
- Elevated CVP
- Nausea and vomiting

DX: PE, labs (cardiac enzymes, troponin), ECG
TX: Bed rest, oxygen therapy, medication (analgesics, nitrates, aspirin, thrombolytics, anticoagulants, ACE inhibitors, beta-adrenergic blockers, calcium channel blockers), PTCA, surgery
F/U: Referral to cardiologist

Pupils, nonreactive

Nonreactive (fixed) pupils fail to constrict in response to light or fail to dilate when the light is removed. The development of a unilateral or bilateral nonreactive response indicates an important change in the patient's condition and may signal a life-threatening emergency and, possibly, brain death. It also occurs with the use of certain optic drugs.

To evaluate pupillary reaction to light, first test the patient's direct light reflex. Darken the room, and cover one of the patient's eyes while you hold open the opposite eyelid. Using a bright penlight, bring the light toward the patient from the side and shine it directly into his opened eye. If normal, the pupil will promptly constrict. Next, test the consensual light reflex. Hold the patient's eyelids open and shine the light into one eye while watching the pupil of the opposite eye. If normal, both pupils will promptly constrict. Repeat both procedures in the opposite eye. A unilateral or bilateral nonreactive response indicates dysfunction of cranial nerves II and III, which mediate the pupillary light reflex. (See *Innervation of direct and consensual light reflexes.*)

ALERT

If the patient is unconscious and develops unilateral or bilateral nonreactive pupils:

- *quickly assess all vital signs*
- *be alert for decerebrate or decorticate posture, bradycardia, elevated systolic blood pressure, and other untoward changes in the patient's condition.*

If the patient is conscious, perform a focused assessment.

HISTORY

- Ask the patient what type of eyedrops he's using, if any, and when they were last instilled.
- Ask the patient if he's experiencing pain and, if so, ask him to describe its location, intensity, and duration.
- Obtain a drug history, including prescription and over-the-counter drugs, herbal remedies, and recreational drugs.

PHYSICAL ASSESSMENT

- Take the patient's vital signs.
- Assess extraocular movement to evaluate cranial nerves III, IV, and VI.
- Assess the patient for photosensitivity and photophobia. Check both eyes for visual acuity.
- Test the pupillary reaction to accommodation. Then, hold a penlight at the side of each eye, and examine the cornea and iris for abnormalities.
- Estimate intraocular pressure (IOP) by placing your second and third fingers over the patient's closed eyelid. If the eyeball feels rock hard, suspect elevated IOP.
- After the examination, be sure to cover the affected eye with a protective metal shield, but don't let the shield rest on the globe.

SPECIAL CONSIDERATIONS

Instillation of a topical mydriatic or a cycloplegic may induce a temporarily nonreactive pupil in the affected eye.

A   PEDIATRIC POINTERS

Children have nonreactive pupils for the same reasons as adults. The most common cause is oculomotor nerve palsy from increased intracranial pressure.

PATIENT COUNSELING

If the patient is unconscious, tell his family that the patient's eyes will be kept closed (possibly using tape) to prevent corneal exposure.

INNERVATION OF DIRECT AND CONSENSUAL LIGHT REFLEXES

Two reactions — direct and consensual — constitute the pupillary light reflex. Normally, when a light is shined directly onto the retina of one eye, the parasympathetic nerves are stimulated to cause brisk constriction of that pupil — the direct light reflex. The pupil of the opposite eye also constricts — the consensual light reflex.

The optic nerve (CN II) mediates the afferent arc of this reflex from each eye, whereas the oculomotor nerve (CN III) mediates the efferent arc to both eyes. A nonreactive or sluggish response in one or both pupils indicates dysfunction of these cranial nerves, usually due to degenerative disease of the central nervous system.

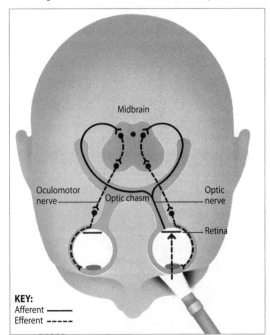

Midbrain

Oculomotor nerve

Optic chasm

Optic nerve

Retina

KEY:
Afferent ———
Efferent - - - - -

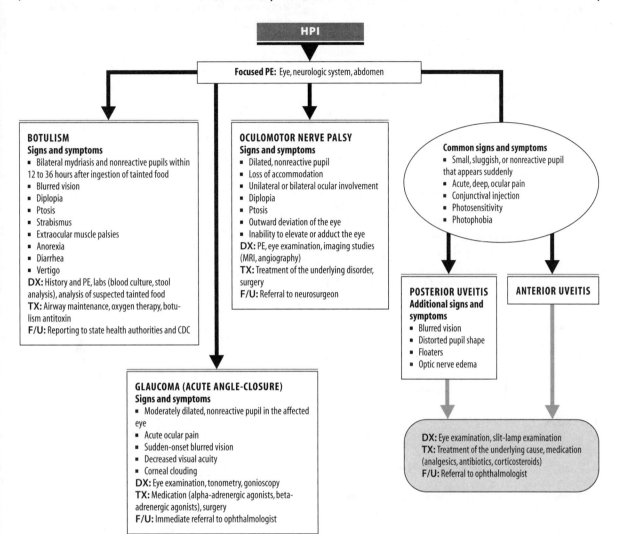

HPI

Focused PE: Eye, neurologic system, abdomen

BOTULISM
Signs and symptoms
- Bilateral mydriasis and nonreactive pupils within 12 to 36 hours after ingestion of tainted food
- Blurred vision
- Diplopia
- Ptosis
- Strabismus
- Extraocular muscle palsies
- Anorexia
- Diarrhea
- Vertigo

DX: History and PE, labs (blood culture, stool analysis), analysis of suspected tainted food
TX: Airway maintenance, oxygen therapy, botulism antitoxin
F/U: Reporting to state health authorities and CDC

OCULOMOTOR NERVE PALSY
Signs and symptoms
- Dilated, nonreactive pupil
- Loss of accommodation
- Unilateral or bilateral ocular involvement
- Diplopia
- Ptosis
- Outward deviation of the eye
- Inability to elevate or adduct the eye

DX: PE, eye examination, imaging studies (MRI, angiography)
TX: Treatment of the underlying disorder, surgery
F/U: Referral to neurosurgeon

Common signs and symptoms
- Small, sluggish, or nonreactive pupil that appears suddenly
- Acute, deep, ocular pain
- Conjunctival injection
- Photosensitivity
- Photophobia

POSTERIOR UVEITIS
Additional signs and symptoms
- Blurred vision
- Distorted pupil shape
- Floaters
- Optic nerve edema

ANTERIOR UVEITIS

GLAUCOMA (ACUTE ANGLE-CLOSURE)
Signs and symptoms
- Moderately dilated, nonreactive pupil in the affected eye
- Acute ocular pain
- Sudden-onset blurred vision
- Decreased visual acuity
- Corneal clouding

DX: Eye examination, tonometry, gonioscopy
TX: Medication (alpha-adrenergic agonists, beta-adrenergic agonists), surgery
F/U: Immediate referral to ophthalmologist

DX: Eye examination, slit-lamp examination
TX: Treatment of the underlying cause, medication (analgesics, antibiotics, corticosteroids)
F/U: Referral to ophthalmologist

Additional differential diagnoses: Adie's syndrome ▪ encephalitis ▪ familial amyloid polyneuropathy ▪ iris disease (degenerative or inflammatory) ▪ midbrain lesions ▪ ocular trauma ▪ Wernicke's disease

Other causes: atropine poisoning ▪ opiates (heroin, morphine) ▪ topical mydriatics and cycloplegics

Pupils, sluggish

A sluggish pupillary reaction is an abnormally slow pupillary response to light. It can occur in one pupil or both, unlike the normal reaction, which is always bilateral. A sluggish reaction accompanies degenerative disease of the central nervous system and diabetic neuropathy. It can occur normally in elderly people, whose pupils become smaller and less responsive with age.

To assess pupillary reaction to light, first test the patient's direct light reflex. Darken the room, and cover one of the patient's eyes while you hold open the opposite eyelid. Using a bright penlight, bring the light toward the patient from the side and shine it directly into his uncovered eye. If normal, the pupil will promptly constrict. Next, test the consensual light reflex. Hold both of the patient's eyelids open, and shine the light into one eye while watching the pupil of the opposite eye. If normal, both pupils will promptly constrict. Repeat both procedures to test light reflexes in the opposite eye. A sluggish reaction in one or both pupils indicates dysfunction of cranial nerves II and III, which mediate the pupillary light reflex.

HISTORY

● Ask the patient what type of eyedrops he's using, if any, and when they were last instilled.
● Ask the patient if he's experiencing pain and, if so, ask him to describe its location, intensity, and duration.

PHYSICAL ASSESSMENT

● Test visual acuity in both eyes, using the Snellen chart.
● Assess extraocular movements.
● Determine whether the patient suffers from photosensitivity or photophobia.
● Test the pupillary reaction to accommodation; the pupils should constrict equally as the patient shifts his glance from a distant to a near object.
● Hold a penlight at the side of each eye and examine the cornea and iris for irregularities, scars, and foreign bodies. Estimate intraocular pressure (IOP) by placing your fingers over the patient's closed eyelid. If the eyeball feels rock hard, suspect elevated IOP.
● Obtain a drug history, including prescription and over-the-counter drugs, herbal remedies, and recreational drugs.

SPECIAL CONSIDERATIONS

A sluggish pupillary reaction isn't diagnostically significant, although it occurs with various disorders.

Ⓐ PEDIATRIC POINTERS

Children experience sluggish pupillary reactions for the same reasons as adults.

PATIENT COUNSELING

Refer the patient to an opthalmologist if increased IOP is suspected.

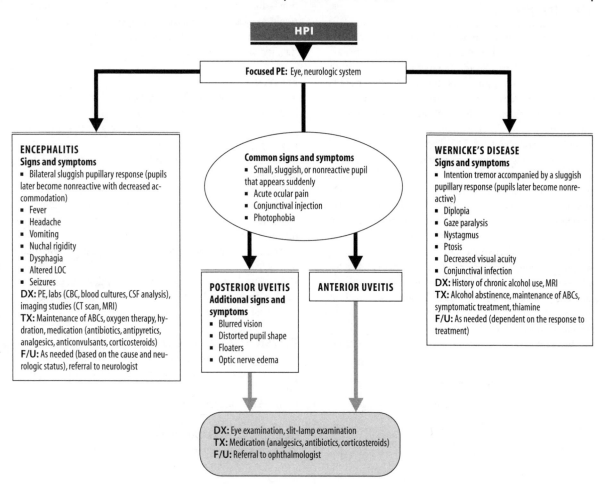

HPI

Focused PE: Eye, neurologic system

ENCEPHALITIS
Signs and symptoms
- Bilateral sluggish pupillary response (pupils later become nonreactive with decreased accommodation)
- Fever
- Headache
- Vomiting
- Nuchal rigidity
- Dysphagia
- Altered LOC
- Seizures

DX: PE, labs (CBC, blood cultures, CSF analysis), imaging studies (CT scan, MRI)
TX: Maintenance of ABCs, oxygen therapy, hydration, medication (antibiotics, antipyretics, analgesics, anticonvulsants, corticosteroids)
F/U: As needed (based on the cause and neurologic status), referral to neurologist

Common signs and symptoms
- Small, sluggish, or nonreactive pupil that appears suddenly
- Acute ocular pain
- Conjunctival injection
- Photophobia

POSTERIOR UVEITIS
Additional signs and symptoms
- Blurred vision
- Distorted pupil shape
- Floaters
- Optic nerve edema

ANTERIOR UVEITIS

WERNICKE'S DISEASE
Signs and symptoms
- Intention tremor accompanied by a sluggish pupillary response (pupils later become nonreactive)
- Diplopia
- Gaze paralysis
- Nystagmus
- Ptosis
- Decreased visual acuity
- Conjunctival infection

DX: History of chronic alcohol use, MRI
TX: Alcohol abstinence, maintenance of ABCs, symptomatic treatment, thiamine
F/U: As needed (dependent on the response to treatment)

DX: Eye examination, slit-lamp examination
TX: Medication (analgesics, antibiotics, corticosteroids)
F/U: Referral to ophthalmologist

Additional differential diagnoses: Adie's syndrome ▪ diabetic neuropathy ▪ familial amyloid polyneuropathy ▪ herpes zoster ▪ multiple sclerosis ▪ myotonic dystrophy ▪ tertiary syphilis

Purpura

Purpura is the extravasation of red blood cells from the blood vessels into the skin, subcutaneous tissue, or mucous membranes. It's characterized by discoloration — usually purplish or brownish red — that's easily visible through the epidermis. Purpuric lesions include petechiae, ecchymoses, and hematomas. (See *Identifying purpuric lesions.*) Purpura differs from erythema in that it doesn't blanch with pressure because it involves blood in the tissues, not just dilated vessels.

Purpura can result from damage to the endothelium of small blood vessels, a coagulation defect, ineffective perivascular support, capillary fragility and permeability, or a combination of these factors. These faulty hemostatic factors, in turn, can result from thrombocytopenia or another hematologic disorder, an invasive procedure, or the use of an anticoagulant.

Additional causes are nonpathologic. Purpura can be a consequence of aging, when loss of collagen decreases connective tissue support of upper skin blood vessels. In the elderly or cachectic person, skin atrophy and inelasticity and loss of subcutaneous fat increase susceptibility to minor trauma, causing purpura to appear along the veins of the forearms, hands, legs, and feet. Prolonged coughing or vomiting can produce crops of petechiae in loose face and neck tissue. Violent muscle contraction — for example, in seizures or weight lifting — sometimes results in localized ecchymoses from increased intraluminal pressure and rupture. High fever, which increases capillary fragility, can also produce purpura.

HISTORY

- Ask the patient when he first noticed the lesion and whether he has noticed other lesions on his body.
- Ask the patient if he has any known allergies. If so, ask him if he's recently been exposed to them.
- Ask the patient if he or his family have a history of bleeding disorders or easy bruising.
- Ask the patient about recent trauma or transfusions and the development of associated signs, such as epistaxis, bleeding gums, hematuria, vaginal bleeding, and hematochezia. If the patient is female, ask about heavy menstrual flow.
- Ask the patient about systemic complaints such as fever that may suggest infection.
- Obtain a drug history, including prescription and over-the-counter drugs, herbal remedies, and recreational drugs. Also, ask the patient about alcohol intake.

PHYSICAL ASSESSMENT

- Inspect the patient's entire skin surface to determine the type, size, location, distribution, and severity of purpuric lesions.
- Inspect the mucous membranes.

SPECIAL CONSIDERATIONS

Procedures that disrupt circulation, coagulation, or platelet activity or production may cause purpura.

PEDIATRIC POINTERS

- *Causes of purpura in infants include thrombocytopenia, vitamin K deficiency, and infantile scurvy.*
- *The most common type of purpura in children is allergic purpura. Others include trauma, hemophilia, autoimmune hemolytic anemia, Gaucher's disease, thrombasthenia, congenital factor deficiencies, Wiskott-Aldrich syndrome, acute idiopathic thrombocytopenic purpura, von Willebrand's disease, and the rare but life-threatening purpura fulminans, which usually follows bacterial or viral infection.*
- *When you assess a child with purpura, be alert for signs of possible child abuse.*

PATIENT COUNSELING

Tell the patient with purpura not to use cosmetic fade creams or other products in an attempt to reduce pigmentation. Reassure him that purpuric lesions aren't permanent and will fade if the underlying cause can be successfully treated.

IDENTIFYING PURPURIC LESIONS

Purpuric lesions fall into three categories: petechiae, ecchymoses, and hematomas.

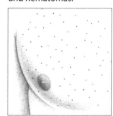

PETECHIAE
Petechiae are painless, round, pinpoint lesions, 1 to 3 mm in diameter. Caused by extravasation of red blood cells into cutaneous tissue, these red or brown lesions usually arise on dependent portions of the body. They appear and fade in crops and can group to form ecchymoses.

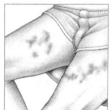

ECCHYMOSES
Ecchymoses, another form of blood extravasation, are larger than petechiae. These purple, blue, or yellow-green bruises vary in size and shape and can arise anywhere on the body as a result of trauma. Ecchymoses usually appear on the arms and legs of patients with a bleeding disorder.

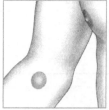

HEMATOMAS
Hematomas are palpable ecchymoses that are painful and swollen. Usually the result of trauma, superficial hematomas are red, whereas deep hematomas are blue. Many hematomas exceed 1 cm in diameter, but their size varies widely.

PURPURA

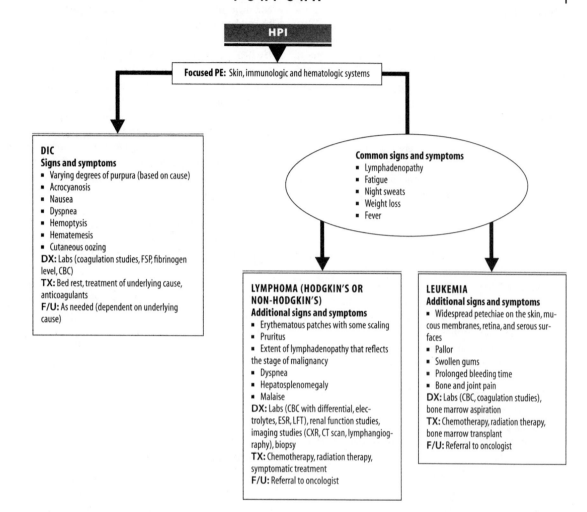

HPI

Focused PE: Skin, immunologic and hematologic systems

DIC
Signs and symptoms
- Varying degrees of purpura (based on cause)
- Acrocyanosis
- Nausea
- Dyspnea
- Hemoptysis
- Hematemesis
- Cutaneous oozing

DX: Labs (coagulation studies, FSP, fibrinogen level, CBC)
TX: Bed rest, treatment of underlying cause, anticoagulants
F/U: As needed (dependent on underlying cause)

Common signs and symptoms
- Lymphadenopathy
- Fatigue
- Night sweats
- Weight loss
- Fever

LYMPHOMA (HODGKIN'S OR NON-HODGKIN'S)
Additional signs and symptoms
- Erythematous patches with some scaling
- Pruritus
- Extent of lymphadenopathy that reflects the stage of malignancy
- Dyspnea
- Hepatosplenomegaly
- Malaise

DX: Labs (CBC with differential, electrolytes, ESR, LFT), renal function studies, imaging studies (CXR, CT scan, lymphangiography), biopsy
TX: Chemotherapy, radiation therapy, symptomatic treatment
F/U: Referral to oncologist

LEUKEMIA
Additional signs and symptoms
- Widespread petechiae on the skin, mucous membranes, retina, and serous surfaces
- Pallor
- Swollen gums
- Prolonged bleeding time
- Bone and joint pain

DX: Labs (CBC, coagulation studies), bone marrow aspiration
TX: Chemotherapy, radiation therapy, bone marrow transplant
F/U: Referral to oncologist

Additional differential diagnoses: amyloidosis ▪ autoerythrocyte sensitivity ▪ coagulopathy ▪ dermatoses (pigmented) ▪ dysproteinemias ▪ easy bruising syndrome ▪ Ehlers-Danlos syndrome ▪ liver disease ▪ myeloproliferative disorders ▪ nutritional deficiencies ▪ septicemia ▪ stasis ▪ SLE ▪ thrombotic thrombocytopenic purpura ▪ trauma

Other causes: anticoagulants ▪ antiplatelet agents ▪ invasive procedures (venipuncture, arterial catheterization) ▪ NSAIDs ▪ procedures that disrupt circulation, coagulation, or platelet activity or production (pulmonary and cardiac surgery, radiation therapy, chemotherapy, hemodialysis, multiple blood transfusions with platelet-poor blood, use of plasma expanders)

Pustular rash

A pustular rash is made up of crops of pustules — vesicles and bullae that fill with purulent exudate. These lesions vary greatly in size and shape and can be generalized or localized to the hair follicles or sweat glands. (See *Identifying a pustule.*) Pustules can result from skin or systemic disorders, the use of certain drugs, or exposure to skin irritants. For example, people who have been swimming in salt water commonly develop a papulopustular rash under the bathing suit or elsewhere on the body from irritation by sea organisms. Although many pustular lesions are sterile, a pustular rash usually indicates infection. Any vesicular eruption, or even acute contact dermatitis, can become pustular if secondary infection occurs.

HISTORY

● Ask the patient to describe the appearance, location, and onset of the first pustular lesion. Ask him if another type of skin lesion preceded the pustule and how the lesions spread.
● Obtain a drug history, including prescription and over-the-counter drugs, herbal remedies, and recreational drugs. Also, ask the patient about alcohol intake.
● Ask the patient if he has applied a topical medication to his rash. If so, ask him to name the medication. When did he last apply it?
● Ask the patient if there's a family history of skin disorders.

PHYSICAL ASSESSMENT

● Examine the entire skin surface, noting whether it's dry, oily, moist, or greasy.

● Record the exact location and distribution of the skin lesions and their color, shape, and size. Note if the rash is linear or follows a dermatome.

SPECIAL CONSIDERATIONS

Observe wound and skin isolation procedures until infection is ruled out by a Gram stain or culture and sensitivity test of the pustule's contents.

Ⓐ ▶ PEDIATRIC POINTERS

Among the various disorders that produce pustular rash in children are varicella, erythema toxicum neonatorum, candidiasis, impetigo, infantile acropustulosis, and acrodermatitis enteropathica. (See Recognizing impetigo.)

PATIENT COUNSELING

Instruct the patient to keep his toiletry articles and linens separate from those of other family members.

IDENTIFYING A PUSTULE

A pustule is a raised, circumscribed lesion that's usually less than 1 cm in diameter and contains purulent material, which makes it a yellow-white color.

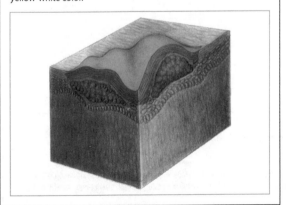

RECOGNIZING IMPETIGO

In impetigo, when vesicles break, crusts form from the exudate. This infection is especially contagious among young children.

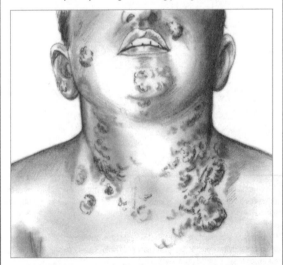

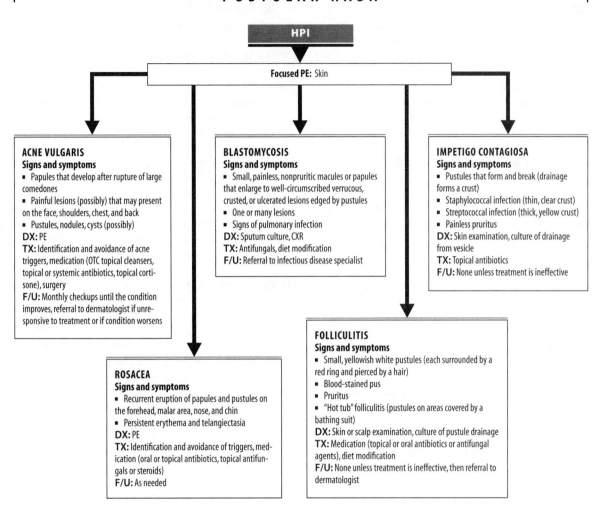

HPI

Focused PE: Skin

ACNE VULGARIS
Signs and symptoms
- Papules that develop after rupture of large comedones
- Painful lesions (possibly) that may present on the face, shoulders, chest, and back
- Pustules, nodules, cysts (possibly)
DX: PE
TX: Identification and avoidance of acne triggers, medication (OTC topical cleansers, topical or systemic antibiotics, topical cortisone), surgery
F/U: Monthly checkups until the condition improves, referral to dermatologist if unresponsive to treatment or if condition worsens

BLASTOMYCOSIS
Signs and symptoms
- Small, painless, nonpruritic macules or papules that enlarge to well-circumscribed verrucous, crusted, or ulcerated lesions edged by pustules
- One or many lesions
- Signs of pulmonary infection
DX: Sputum culture, CXR
TX: Antifungals, diet modification
F/U: Referral to infectious disease specialist

IMPETIGO CONTAGIOSA
Signs and symptoms
- Pustules that form and break (drainage forms a crust)
- Staphylococcal infection (thin, clear crust)
- Streptococcal infection (thick, yellow crust)
- Painless pruritus
DX: Skin examination, culture of drainage from vesicle
TX: Topical antibiotics
F/U: None unless treatment is ineffective

ROSACEA
Signs and symptoms
- Recurrent eruption of papules and pustules on the forehead, malar area, nose, and chin
- Persistent erythema and telangiectasia
DX: PE
TX: Identification and avoidance of triggers, medication (oral or topical antibiotics, topical antifungals or steroids)
F/U: As needed

FOLLICULITIS
Signs and symptoms
- Small, yellowish white pustules (each surrounded by a red ring and pierced by a hair)
- Blood-stained pus
- Pruritus
- "Hot tub" folliculitis (pustules on areas covered by a bathing suit)
DX: Skin or scalp examination, culture of pustule drainage
TX: Medication (topical or oral antibiotics or antifungal agents), diet modification
F/U: None unless treatment is ineffective, then referral to dermatologist

---

Additional differential diagnoses: furunculosis ▪ gonococcemia ▪ nummular or annular dermatitis ▪ pompholyx ▪ pustular miliaria ▪ pustular psoriasis ▪ scabies

Other causes: anabolic steroids ▪ androgens ▪ bromides ▪ corticosteroids ▪ corticotropin ▪ dactinomycin ▪ hormonal contraceptives ▪ iodides ▪ isoniazid ▪ lithium ▪ phenobarbital ▪ phenytoin ▪ trimethadione

Pyrosis

Caused by reflux of gastric contents into the esophagus, pyrosis (heartburn) is a substernal burning sensation that rises in the chest and may radiate to the neck or throat. It's frequently accompanied by regurgitation, which also results from gastric reflux. Because increased intra-abdominal pressure contributes to reflux, pyrosis commonly occurs with pregnancy, ascites, or obesity. It also accompanies various GI disorders, connective tissue diseases, and the use of certain drugs. Pyrosis usually develops after meals or when the patient lies down (especially on his right side), bends over, lifts heavy objects, or exercises vigorously. It typically worsens with swallowing and improves when the patient sits upright or takes an antacid. People age 50 and older are at greater risk for complications of pyrosis due to esophageal sphincter weakness.

HISTORY

● Ask the patient whether he has experienced heartburn before. Do certain foods or beverages trigger it? Does stress or fatigue aggravate his discomfort? Does it occur at a particular time of day?

● Ask the patient where the pain is located and if it radiates to other areas.

● Ask the patient what relieves the pain.

● Ask the patient if movement, a certain body position, or ingestion of very hot or cold liquids worsen or help relieve the heartburn.

● Ask the patient if he regurgitates sour- or bitter-tasting fluids. (See *Regurgitation: Mechanism and causes.*)

● Ask the patient about associated signs and symptoms.

PHYSICAL ASSESSMENT

● Take the patient's vital signs.

● Perform a complete cardiovascular and GI assessment.

SPECIAL CONSIDERATIONS

A patient experiencing a myocardial infarction (MI) may mistake chest pain for pyrosis. However, other signs and symptoms—such as dyspnea, tachycardia, palpitations, nausea, and vomiting—will help distinguish MI from pyrosis, along with laboratory studies and an electrocardiogram.

 PEDIATRIC POINTERS

A child may have difficulty distinguishing esophageal pain from pyrosis. To gain information, help the child describe the sensation.

AGING ISSUES

Elderly patients with peptic ulcer disease commonly present with nonspecific abdominal discomfort or weight loss.

PATIENT COUNSELING

Instruct the patient on what to expect from diagnostic testing, which may include upper GI series, gastroesophageal reflux scanning, and esophageal motility and acidity studies. After the causative disorder is determined, teach the patient how to avoid a recurrence of pyrosis. Advise him to eat frequent small meals, to sit upright after a meal, and to avoid lying down for at least 2 hours after eating.

REGURGITATION: MECHANISM AND CAUSES

When gastric reflux moves up the esophagus and passes through the upper esophageal sphincter, regurgitation occurs. Unlike vomiting, regurgitation is effortless and unaccompanied by nausea. It usually happens when the patient is lying down or bending over and often accompanies pyrosis. Aspiration of regurgitated gastric contents can lead to recurrent pulmonary infections.

In adults, regurgitation usually results from esophageal disorders such as achalasia. However, it can also occur when the gag reflex is absent, as in bulbar palsy, or when the patient has an overfilled stomach or esophagus.

In infants, regurgitation can signal pyloric stenosis or dysphagia lusoria. Usually, however, infants "spit up" because their esophageal sphincters aren't fully developed during the first year of life. To help reduce regurgitation in an infant, teach the parents to handle the infant gently during feeding and to burp him frequently. After feeding, they should place the infant on his right side or on his stomach with his head slightly elevated to avoid gravitational regurgitation and to help prevent aspiration.

PYROSIS

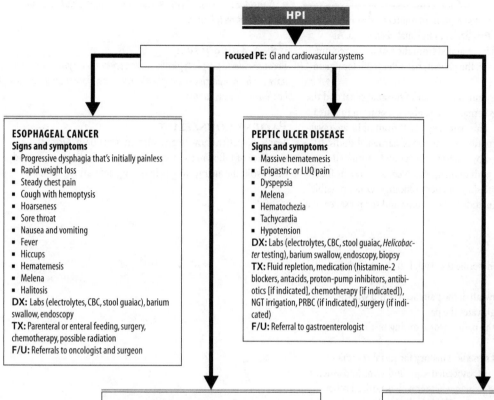

HPI

Focused PE: GI and cardiovascular systems

ESOPHAGEAL CANCER
Signs and symptoms
- Progressive dysphagia that's initially painless
- Rapid weight loss
- Steady chest pain
- Cough with hemoptysis
- Hoarseness
- Sore throat
- Nausea and vomiting
- Fever
- Hiccups
- Hematemesis
- Melena
- Halitosis

DX: Labs (electrolytes, CBC, stool guaiac), barium swallow, endoscopy

TX: Parenteral or enteral feeding, surgery, chemotherapy, possible radiation

F/U: Referrals to oncologist and surgeon

PEPTIC ULCER DISEASE
Signs and symptoms
- Massive hematemesis
- Epigastric or LUQ pain
- Dyspepsia
- Melena
- Hematochezia
- Tachycardia
- Hypotension

DX: Labs (electrolytes, CBC, stool guaiac, *Helicobacter* testing), barium swallow, endoscopy, biopsy

TX: Fluid repletion, medication (histamine-2 blockers, antacids, proton-pump inhibitors, antibiotics [if indicated], chemotherapy [if indicated]), NGT irrigation, PRBC (if indicated), surgery (if indicated)

F/U: Referral to gastroenterologist

GASTROESOPHAGEAL REFLUX DISEASE
Signs and symptoms
- Dysphagia (late sign)
- Pyrosis that's aggravated by strenuous exercise, bending over, or lying down
- Acid regurgitation
- Effortless vomiting
- Dyspepsia
- Dry, nocturnal cough
- Hypersalivation
- Substernal chest pain

DX: Labs (electrolytes, CBC, stool guaiac), barium swallow, ECG, endoscopy

TX: Dietary modification, medication (H_2 receptor antagonist, sucralfate, proton-pump inhibitor), smoking cessation program

F/U: Return visit within 2 weeks, then every 6 to 12 weeks

HIATAL HERNIA
Signs and symptoms
- Eructation after eating
- Pyrosis that worsens when lying down
- Regurgitation of sour-tasting fluid
- Abdominal distention
- Dull, substernal or epigastric pain
- Dysphagia
- Nausea
- Cough

DX: History, imaging studies (barium swallow, CT scan), endoscopy

TX: Diet modification, repositioning (sleeping with HOB elevated and avoiding lying down after meals), medication (antacids, histamine-2 blockers)

F/U: None unless symptoms worsen

Additional differential diagnoses: esophageal diverticula or stenosis ▪ gastritis ▪ obesity ▪ scleroderma

Other causes: acetohexamide ▪ anticholinergic agents ▪ aspirin ▪ drugs with anticholinergic effects ▪ lypressin ▪ NSAIDs ▪ tolbutamide

R Rectal pain

A common symptom of anorectal disorders, rectal pain is discomfort that arises in the anal-rectal area. Although the anal canal is separated from the rest of the rectum by the internal sphincter, the patient may refer to all local pain as rectal pain.

Because the mucocutaneous border of the anal canal and the perianal skin contains somatic nerve fibers, lesions in this area are especially painful. This pain may result from or be aggravated by diarrhea, constipation, or passage of hardened stools. It may also be aggravated by intense pruritus and continued scratching associated with drainage of mucous, blood, or fecal matter that irritates the skin and nerve endings. Other possible causes of rectal pain include rectal trauma and the presence of a foreign object.

HISTORY

- Ask the patient to describe the pain. Is it sharp or dull? Is it burning or knifelike?
- Ask the patient how often the pain occurs and whether anything alleviates or aggravates the pain.
- Ask the patient if the pain is worse during or immediately after defecation.
- Review the patient's medical history for rectal trauma.
- Ask the patient about associated signs and symptoms such as bleeding. Also, ask the patient whether he has noticed other drainage, such as mucous or pus, and whether he's experiencing constipation or diarrhea.

PHYSICAL ASSESSMENT

- Inspect the anal area for rectal bleeding, and abnormal drainage such as pus, foreign objects, or protrusions, such as skin tags or thrombosed hemorrhoids.
- Observe the area for inflammation and other lesions. A rectal examination may be necessary.

SPECIAL CONSIDERATIONS

If rectal pain results from prolapsed hemorrhoids, apply cold compresses to help shrink protruding hemorrhoids, avoid thrombosis, and reduce pain.

A PEDIATRIC POINTERS

- *Observe a child with rectal pain for associated bleeding, drainage, and signs and symptoms of infection (fever and irritability).*
- *Acute anal fissure is a common cause of rectal pain and bleeding in children, whose fear of provoking the pain may lead to constipation.*

- *Infants who seem to have pain on defecation should be evaluated for congenital anomalies of the rectum.*
- *Consider the possibility of sexual abuse in all children who complain of rectal pain.*

AGING ISSUES

Because elderly people typically underreport their symptoms and have an increased risk of neoplastic disorders, they should always be thoroughly evaluated.

PATIENT COUNSELING

Teach the patient how to give himself a sitz bath. Stress the importance of following a proper diet to maintain soft stools and thus avoid the aggravating pain during defecation.

RECTAL PAIN

HPI

Focused PE: GI system

RECTAL CANCER
Signs and symptoms
- Rectal bleeding
- Tenesmus
- Hard, nontender mass

DX: Rectal examination, air contrast barium study, colonoscopy, flexible sigmoidoscopy
TX: Medication (analgesics, chemotherapy), radiation therapy, surgery
F/U: Referrals to gastroenterologist and oncologist

Common signs and symptoms
- Rectal pain during defecation
- Blood on surface of stool
- Blood on toilet tissue or wipes
- Visible fissure
- Constipation

HEMORRHOIDS
Signs and symptoms
- Rectal pain that may worsen during defecation and abate after it
- Severe itching
- Internal hemorrhoids that may also produce mild, intermittent bleeding

DX: Rectal examination, stool guaiac, sigmoidoscopy, anoscopy, proctoscopy
TX: Increased fluid intake, diet modification, medication (corticosteroid creams, stool softeners), cryosurgery
F/U: Referral to colorectal surgeon if treatment is ineffective

ANAL FISSURE
DX: Rectal examination
TX: Warm sitz baths, diet modification, medication (stool softeners, anesthetic ointment)
F/U: None unless condition worsens

Additional common signs and symptoms
- Constant, throbbing local pain that's exacerbated by sitting or walking
- Fever
- Malaise
- Anal swelling
- Inflammation
- Purulent drainage
- Local tenderness

PERIRECTAL ABSCESS

ANORECTAL FISTULA
Additional signs and symptoms
- Pruritus
- Drainage of pus, blood, mucus, and stool from rectum

DX: Rectal examination, proctosigmoidoscopy
TX: Warm sitz baths, medication (analgesics, antibiotics), surgical incision and drainage
F/U: Referral to proctologist

Additional differential diagnoses: cryptitis ▪ proctalgia fugax ▪ prostatic abscess ▪ rectal prolapse ▪ rectal ulcer

Respirations, abnormal

Characterized by a deep, low-pitched grunting sound at the end of each breath, *grunting respirations* are a chief sign of respiratory distress in infants and children. They may be soft and heard only on auscultation or loud and clearly audible without a stethoscope. Typically, the intensity of grunting respirations reflects the severity of respiratory distress.

Grunting respirations indicate intrathoracic disease with lower respiratory involvement. Though most common in children, they sometimes occur in adults who are in severe respiratory distress. Whether they occur in children or adults, grunting respirations demand immediate medical attention.

Respirations are shallow when a diminished volume of air enters the lungs during inspiration. The patient with *shallow respirations* usually breathes at an accelerated rate. However, as he tires or as his muscles weaken, this compensatory increase in respirations diminishes, leading to inadequate gas exchange and such signs and symptoms as dyspnea, cyanosis, confusion, agitation, loss of consciousness, and tachycardia.

Shallow respirations may develop suddenly or gradually and may last briefly or become chronic. They're a key sign of respiratory distress and neurologic deterioration.

Characterized by a harsh, rattling, or snoring sound, *stertorous respirations* usually result from the vibration of relaxed oropharyngeal structures during sleep or coma, causing partial airway obstruction. Less commonly, these respirations result from retained mucus in the upper airway.

Stertorous respirations normally occur in about 10% of individuals, especially middle-aged, obese men. They may be aggravated by alcohol or sedative use before bed, which increases oropharyngeal flaccidity, and by sleeping in the supine position, which allows the relaxed tongue to slip back into the airway. The major pathologic causes of stertorous respirations are obstructive sleep apnea and life-threatening upper airway obstruction associated with an oropharyngeal tumor or with uvular or palatal edema. Obstruction may also occur during the postictal phase of a generalized seizure when mucous secretions or a relaxed tongue blocks the airway.

⇥ ALERT

If the patient exhibits abnormal respirations:
- *check for signs and symptoms of associated respiratory distress, including wheezing, tachypnea, accessory muscle use; retractions; nasal flaring; and tachycardia*
- *institute emergency measures, if necessary.*

If the patient isn't in severe respiratory distress, perform a focused assessment.

HISTORY
- Ask the patient when his abnormal respirations began, how long they last, and what makes them better or worse.
- Ask the patient if he smokes. If so, ask him how many packs he smokes in a year.
- Review the patient's medical history for chronic illness, surgery, trauma, asthma, allergies, heart failure or vascular disease, chronic respiratory disease or infection, or neurologic or neuromuscular disease.
- Obtain a drug history, including prescription and over-the-counter drugs, herbal remedies, and recreational drugs. Also, ask the patient about alcohol intake.

PHYSICAL ASSESSMENT
- Inspect the chest for deformities or abnormal movements, such as intercostal retractions.
- Palpate for expansion and diaphragmatic tactile fremitus, and percuss for hyperresonance or dullness.
- Auscultate the lungs, especially the lower lobes. Note diminished or abnormal sounds, such as crackles or sibilant rhonchi, which may indicate mucus or fluid buildup.
- Characterize the color, amount, and consistency of discharge or sputum, if present.
- Inspect the extremities for cyanosis and digital clubbing. Note peripheral edema, if present.

SPECIAL CONSIDERATIONS
Position the patient as nearly upright as possible to ease his breathing, and continue to monitor his respiratory status closely.

Ⓐ PEDIATRIC POINTERS
- *In children, shallow respirations commonly indicate a life-threatening condition. Airway obstruction can occur rapidly.*
- *Causes of shallow respirations in infants and children include idiopathic (infant) respiratory distress syndrome, acute epiglottiditis, diphtheria, aspiration of a foreign body, croup, acute bronchiolitis, cystic fibrosis, and bacterial pneumonia.*
- *In children, the most common cause of stertorous respirations is nasal or pharyngeal obstruction secondary to tonsillar or adenoid hypertrophy or the presence of a foreign body.*

⬟ AGING ISSUES
Stiffness or deformity of the chest wall associated with aging may cause shallow respirations.

PATIENT COUNSELING
Teach the patient to cough and deep-breathe to clear secretions and to counteract possible hypoventilation.

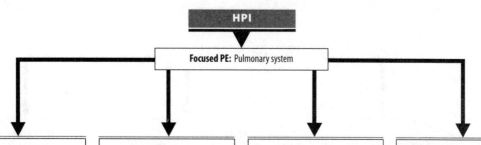

HPI

Focused PE: Pulmonary system

ASTHMA
Signs and symptoms
- Acute dyspneic attacks
- Audible or auscultated wheezing
- Dry cough
- Hyperpnea
- Chest tightness
- Accessory muscle use
- Nasal flaring
- Intercostal and supraclavicular retractions
- Tachypnea
- Tachycardia
- Diaphoresis
- Prolonged expiration
- Flushing or cyanosis
- Apprehension

DX: Labs (CBC, ABG, allergy skin testing), CXR, PFT

TX: Avoidance of allergens, tobacco, and beta-adrenergic blockers; medication (inhaled beta$_2$-agonists, inhaled corticosteroids [nedocromil or cromolyn if < age 12], leukotriene receptor agonist [possibly], corticosteroids during infections and exacerbations), peak expiratory flow monitoring

F/U: For acute exacerbation, return visit within 24 hours, then every 3 to 5 days, then every 1 to 3 months; referral to pulmonologist if treatment is ineffective

HEART FAILURE
Signs and symptoms
- Grunting respirations (late sign)
- Increasing pulmonary edema
- Productive cough
- Crackles
- Chest wall retractions

DX: Labs (CBC, cardiac enzymes), imaging studies (CXR, echocardiogram), ECG

TX: Medication (ACE inhibitors, diuretics, carvedilol [possibly], digoxin to improve ejection fraction and exercise tolerance [possibly])

DX: Imaging studies (echocardiography, CXR), ECG

F/U: Return visit within 1 week after discharge, at 4 weeks, and then every 3 months; referral to cardiologist if chronic

PNEUMONIA
Signs and symptoms
- High-grade fever
- Tachypnea
- Productive cough
- Anorexia
- Lethargy
- Decreased breath sounds
- Scattered crackles
- Sibilant rhonchi
- Severe dyspnea
- Substernal and subcostal retractions
- Nasal flaring
- Cyanosis

DX: PE, labs (sputum gram stain, CBC, ABG), CXR

TX: Medication (analgesics, antipyretics, antibiotics), oxygen therapy, chest physiotherapy

F/U: Reevaluation in 7 to 10 days unless the condition worsens

RESPIRATORY DISTRESS SYNDROME
Signs and symptoms
- Audible expiratory grunting
- Intercostal, subcostal, or substernal retractions
- Nasal flaring
- Tachycardia
- Tachypnea
- Signs of severe respiratory distress
- Harsh, diminished breath sounds
- Crackles

DX: ABG, CXR, PFT

TX: Oxygen therapy, treatment of underlying cause, symptomatic treatment, lung surfactant (infants)

F/U: Referral to pulmonologist

Other causes: abdominal pain ▪ hiccups ▪ tracheal obstruction or trauma

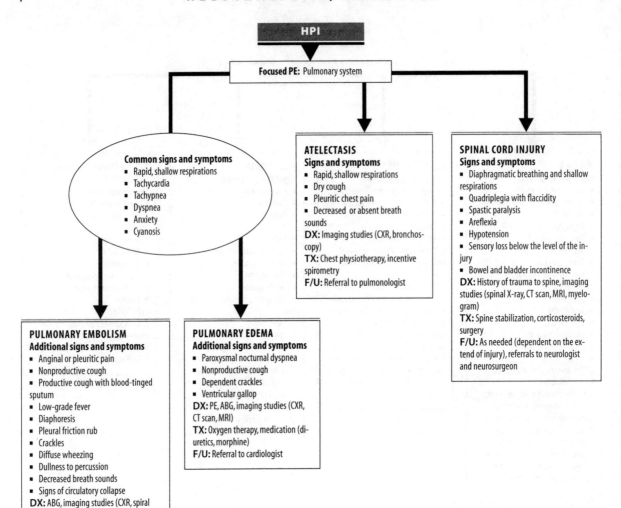

HPI

Focused PE: Pulmonary system

Common signs and symptoms
- Rapid, shallow respirations
- Tachycardia
- Tachypnea
- Dyspnea
- Anxiety
- Cyanosis

ATELECTASIS
Signs and symptoms
- Rapid, shallow respirations
- Dry cough
- Pleuritic chest pain
- Decreased or absent breath sounds

DX: Imaging studies (CXR, bronchoscopy)
TX: Chest physiotherapy, incentive spirometry
F/U: Referral to pulmonologist

SPINAL CORD INJURY
Signs and symptoms
- Diaphragmatic breathing and shallow respirations
- Quadriplegia with flaccidity
- Spastic paralysis
- Areflexia
- Hypotension
- Sensory loss below the level of the injury
- Bowel and bladder incontinence

DX: History of trauma to spine, imaging studies (spinal X-ray, CT scan, MRI, myelogram)
TX: Spine stabilization, corticosteroids, surgery
F/U: As needed (dependent on the extend of injury), referrals to neurologist and neurosurgeon

PULMONARY EMBOLISM
Additional signs and symptoms
- Anginal or pleuritic pain
- Nonproductive cough
- Productive cough with blood-tinged sputum
- Low-grade fever
- Diaphoresis
- Pleural friction rub
- Crackles
- Diffuse wheezing
- Dullness to percussion
- Decreased breath sounds
- Signs of circulatory collapse

DX: ABG, imaging studies (CXR, spiral chest CT, V̇/Q̇ scan, angiogram), PFT
TX: Medication (analgesics, anticoagulants, thrombolytic therapy)
F/U: Referral to pulmonologist

PULMONARY EDEMA
Additional signs and symptoms
- Paroxysmal nocturnal dyspnea
- Nonproductive cough
- Dependent crackles
- Ventricular gallop

DX: PE, ABG, imaging studies (CXR, CT scan, MRI)
TX: Oxygen therapy, medication (diuretics, morphine)
F/U: Referral to cardiologist

Additional differential diagnoses: ARDS ▪ ALS ▪ asthma ▪ botulism ▪ bronchiectasis ▪ chronic bronchitis ▪ coma ▪ emphysema ▪ flail chest ▪ Guillain-Barré syndrome ▪ kyphoscoliosis ▪ multiple sclerosis ▪ muscular dystrophy ▪ myasthenia gravis ▪ obesity ▪ Parkinson's disease ▪ pleural effusion ▪ pneumonia ▪ pneumothorax ▪ tetanus ▪ upper airway obstruction

Other causes: abdominal or thoracic surgery (due to postoperative pain) ▪ drugs (narcotics, sedatives and hypnotics, tranquilizers, neuromuscular blockers, magnesium sulfate, anesthetics)

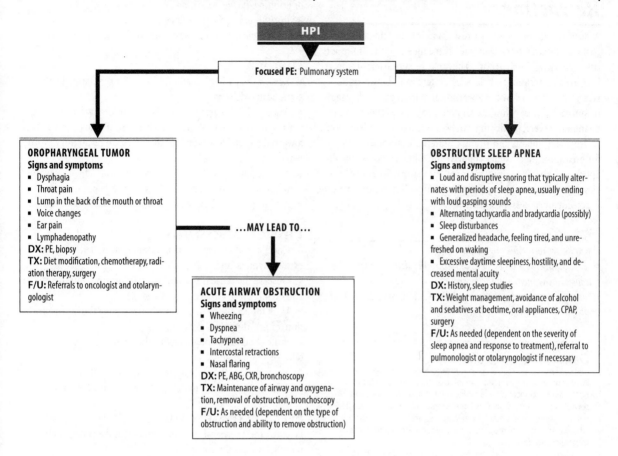

HPI

Focused PE: Pulmonary system

OROPHARYNGEAL TUMOR
Signs and symptoms
- Dysphagia
- Throat pain
- Lump in the back of the mouth or throat
- Voice changes
- Ear pain
- Lymphadenopathy

DX: PE, biopsy
TX: Diet modification, chemotherapy, radiation therapy, surgery
F/U: Referrals to oncologist and otolaryngologist

...MAY LEAD TO...

ACUTE AIRWAY OBSTRUCTION
Signs and symptoms
- Wheezing
- Dyspnea
- Tachypnea
- Intercostal retractions
- Nasal flaring

DX: PE, ABG, CXR, bronchoscopy
TX: Maintenance of airway and oxygenation, removal of obstruction, bronchoscopy
F/U: As needed (dependent on the type of obstruction and ability to remove obstruction)

OBSTRUCTIVE SLEEP APNEA
Signs and symptoms
- Loud and disruptive snoring that typically alternates with periods of sleep apnea, usually ending with loud gasping sounds
- Alternating tachycardia and bradycardia (possibly)
- Sleep disturbances
- Generalized headache, feeling tired, and unrefreshed on waking
- Excessive daytime sleepiness, hostility, and decreased mental acuity

DX: History, sleep studies
TX: Weight management, avoidance of alcohol and sedatives at bedtime, oral appliances, CPAP, surgery
F/U: As needed (dependent on the severity of sleep apnea and response to treatment), referral to pulmonologist or otolaryngologist if necessary

Additional differential diagnoses: obstructive hypoventilation syndrome ▪ stroke

Other causes: endotracheal surgery, intubation, or suction

Retractions

A cardinal sign of respiratory distress in infants and children, costal and sternal retractions are visible indentations of the soft tissue covering the chest wall. They may be suprasternal (directly above the sternum and clavicles), intercostal (between the ribs), subcostal (below the lower costal margin of the rib cage), or substernal (just below the xiphoid process). Retractions may be mild or severe, producing barely visible to deep indentations.

Normally, infants and young children use abdominal muscles for breathing, unlike older children and adults, who use the diaphragm. When breathing requires extra effort, accessory muscles assist respiration, especially inspiration. Retractions typically accompany accessory muscle use.

ALERT

If you detect retractions in a child:
- *check quickly for other signs of respiratory distress, such as cyanosis, tachypnea, and tachycardia*
- *observe the retractions, noting their location, rate, depth, and quality*

OBSERVING RETRACTIONS

When you observe retractions in infants and children, be sure to note their exact location — an important clue to the cause and severity of respiratory distress. For example, subcostal and substernal retractions usually result from lower respiratory tract disorders, whereas suprasternal retractions usually result from upper respiratory tract disorders.

Mild intercostal retractions alone may be normal. However, intercostal retractions accompanied by subcostal and substernal retractions may indicate moderate respiratory distress. Deep suprasternal retractions typically indicate severe distress.

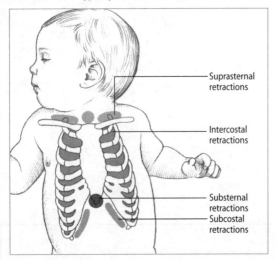

Suprasternal retractions

Intercostal retractions

Substernal retractions

Subcostal retractions

- *look for accessory muscle use, nasal flaring during inspiration, or grunting during expiration*
- *institute emergency measures, if necessary.*
  If the patient's condition permits, perform a focused assessment.

HISTORY
- Review the patient's medical history for premature birth or complicated delivery.
- Ask the child's parents if he has shown recent signs of an upper respiratory tract infection, such as a runny nose, cough, or a low-grade fever. How often has the child had respiratory problems over the past year?
- Ask the parents if the child has been in contact with anyone who has had a cold, the flu, or other respiratory ailments.
- Ask the parents about a family history of allergies or asthma.

PHYSICAL ASSESSMENT
- Check for other signs of respiratory distress, such as cyanosis, tachypnea, and tachycardia.
- Observe the retractions, noting their location, rate, depth, and quality. (See *Observing retractions*.)
- Look for accessory muscle use, nasal flaring during inspiration, or grunting during expiration.
- If the child has a cough, record the color, consistency, and odor of sputum, if present.
- Note whether the child appears restless or lethargic.
- Auscultate the lungs to detect abnormal breath sounds.

SPECIAL CONSIDERATIONS
Perform chest physical therapy with postural drainage to help mobilize and drain excess lung secretions.

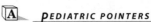
PEDIATRIC POINTERS
When examining a child for retractions, know that crying may accentuate the retractions.

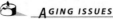
AGING ISSUES
Although retractions may occur at any age, they're more difficult to assess in an older patient who's obese or in a patient who has chronic chest wall stiffness or deformity.

PATIENT COUNSELING
Instruct the parents on what to expect from diagnostic testing, which may include chest X-rays and arterial blood gas analysis.

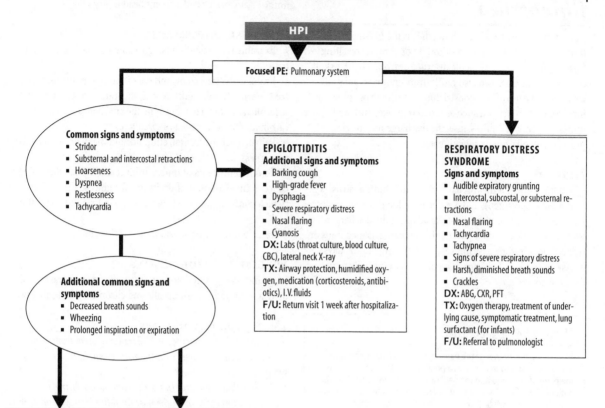

HPI

Focused PE: Pulmonary system

Common signs and symptoms
- Stridor
- Substernal and intercostal retractions
- Hoarseness
- Dyspnea
- Restlessness
- Tachycardia

Additional common signs and symptoms
- Decreased breath sounds
- Wheezing
- Prolonged inspiration or expiration

EPIGLOTTIDITIS
Additional signs and symptoms
- Barking cough
- High-grade fever
- Dysphagia
- Severe respiratory distress
- Nasal flaring
- Cyanosis

DX: Labs (throat culture, blood culture, CBC), lateral neck X-ray
TX: Airway protection, humidified oxygen, medication (corticosteroids, antibiotics), I.V. fluids
F/U: Return visit 1 week after hospitalization

RESPIRATORY DISTRESS SYNDROME
Signs and symptoms
- Audible expiratory grunting
- Intercostal, subcostal, or substernal retractions
- Nasal flaring
- Tachycardia
- Tachypnea
- Signs of severe respiratory distress
- Harsh, diminished breath sounds
- Crackles

DX: ABG, CXR, PFT
TX: Oxygen therapy, treatment of underlying cause, symptomatic treatment, lung surfactant (for infants)
F/U: Referral to pulmonologist

LARYNGOTRACHEO-BRONCHITIS (ACUTE)
Additional signs and symptoms
- Infrequent barking cough
- Low-grade to moderate fever
- Runny nose
- Poor appetite
- Shallow, rapid respirations
- Red epiglottis

DX: Auscultation of the lungs, throat examination, neck X-ray
TX: Warm or cool humidified air, oxygen therapy, antibiotics
F/U: Return visit 1 week after treatment is started (unless condition worsens) or 1 week after hospitalization

SPASMODIC CROUP
Additional signs and symptoms
- Barking cough that occurs while sleeping
- Nasal flaring
- Cyanosis
- Anxious, frantic appearance
- Absence of fever

DX: History of repeated episodes, auscultation of the lungs (decreased breath sounds, wheezing, prolonged inspiration or expiration), no signs of infection
TX: Oxygen therapy, humidified air
F/U: Referral to an allergist

Additional differential diagnoses: asthmatic attack ▪ bronchiolitis ▪ exacerbated COPD ▪ heart failure ▪ pneumonia (bacterial) ▪ rib fracture ▪ sepsis ▪ tracheal obstruction ▪ unstable sternum

Rhinorrhea

Common but rarely serious, rhinorrhea is the free discharge of thin nasal mucus. It can be self-limiting or chronic, resulting from a nasal, sinus, or systemic disorder or from a basilar skull fracture. Rhinorrhea can also result from sinus or cranial surgery, excessive use of vasoconstricting nose drops or sprays, or inhalation of an irritant, such as tobacco smoke, dust, and fumes. Depending on the cause, the discharge may be clear, purulent, bloody, or serosanguineous.

HISTORY
- Ask the patient if the discharge runs from both nostrils, is intermittent or persistent, and if it began suddenly or gradually. Does the position of the patient's head affect the discharge?
- Ask the patient to characterize the discharge. Is it copious or scanty? Does it worsen or improve with the time of the day?
- Ask the patient if he's using medications, especially nose drops or sprays.

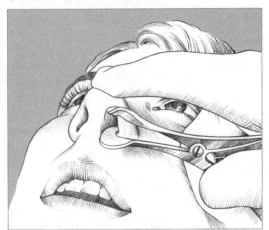

USING A NASAL SPECULUM

To visualize the interior of the nares, you'll need a nasal speculum and a good light source such as a penlight. Hold the speculum in the palm of one hand and the penlight in the other hand. Have the patient tilt his head back slightly and rest it against a wall or other firm support, if possible. Insert the speculum blades about ½" (1.3 cm) into the nasal vestibule, as shown.

Place your index finger on the tip of the patient's nose for stability. Carefully open the speculum blades. Shine the light source in the direction of the nares. Now, inspect the nares, as shown. The mucosa should be deep pink. Note discharge, masses, lesions, or mucosal swellings, if present. Check the nasal septum for perforation, bleeding, or crusting. Bluish turbinates suggest allergy. A rounded, elongated projection suggests a polyp.

- Ask the patient if he has been exposed to nasal irritants at home or at work or had a recent head injury.

PHYSICAL ASSESSMENT
- Examine the patient's nose, checking airflow from each nostril.
- Evaluate the size, color, and condition of the turbinate mucosa (normally pale pink). Note if the mucosa is red, unusually pale, blue, or gray. Then examine the area beneath each turbinate. (See *Using a nasal speculum*.)
- Palpate over the frontal, ethmoid, and maxillary sinuses for tenderness.
- To differentiate nasal mucus from cerebrospinal fluid (CSF), collect a small amount of drainage on a glucose test strip. If CSF (which contains glucose) is present, the test result will be abnormal.
- Use a nonirritating substance to test for anosmia.

SPECIAL CONSIDERATIONS
Pregnancy causes physiologic changes that may aggravate rhinorrhea, resulting in eosinophilia and chronic irritable airways.

PEDIATRIC POINTERS
- *Be aware that rhinorrhea in children may stem from choanal atresia, allergic or chronic rhinitis, acute ethmoiditis, or congenital syphilis.*
- *Assume that unilateral rhinorrhea and nasal obstruction is caused by a foreign body in the nose until this is proven otherwise.*

AGING ISSUES
Elderly patients may suffer increased adverse reactions to medications used to treat rhinorrhea.

PATIENT COUNSELING
Warn the patient to avoid using over-the-counter nasal sprays for longer than 5 days.

RHINORRHEA

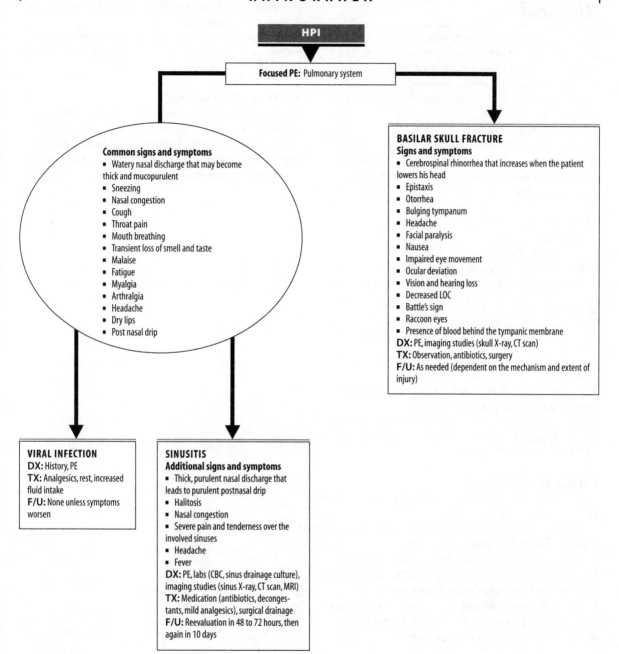

HPI

Focused PE: Pulmonary system

Common signs and symptoms
- Watery nasal discharge that may become thick and mucopurulent
- Sneezing
- Nasal congestion
- Cough
- Throat pain
- Mouth breathing
- Transient loss of smell and taste
- Malaise
- Fatigue
- Myalgia
- Arthralgia
- Headache
- Dry lips
- Post nasal drip

BASILAR SKULL FRACTURE
Signs and symptoms
- Cerebrospinal rhinorrhea that increases when the patient lowers his head
- Epistaxis
- Otorrhea
- Bulging tympanum
- Headache
- Facial paralysis
- Nausea
- Impaired eye movement
- Ocular deviation
- Vision and hearing loss
- Decreased LOC
- Battle's sign
- Raccoon eyes
- Presence of blood behind the tympanic membrane
DX: PE, imaging studies (skull X-ray, CT scan)
TX: Observation, antibiotics, surgery
F/U: As needed (dependent on the mechanism and extent of injury)

VIRAL INFECTION
DX: History, PE
TX: Analgesics, rest, increased fluid intake
F/U: None unless symptoms worsen

SINUSITIS
Additional signs and symptoms
- Thick, purulent nasal discharge that leads to purulent postnasal drip
- Halitosis
- Nasal congestion
- Severe pain and tenderness over the involved sinuses
- Headache
- Fever
DX: PE, labs (CBC, sinus drainage culture), imaging studies (sinus X-ray, CT scan, MRI)
TX: Medication (antibiotics, decongestants, mild analgesics), surgical drainage
F/U: Reevaluation in 48 to 72 hours, then again in 10 days

Additional differential diagnoses: headache (cluster) ▪ mucormycosis ▪ nasal or sinus tumors ▪ rhinitis ▪ rhinoscleroma ▪ Wegener's granulomatosis

Other causes: nasal sprays or drops containing vasoconstrictors ▪ sinus or cranial surgery

Rhonchi

Rhonchi are continuous adventitious breath sounds detected by auscultation. They're usually louder and lower pitched than crackles — more like a hoarse moan or a deep snore — though they may be described as rattling, sonorous, bubbling, rumbling, or musical. However, sibilant rhonchi, or wheezes, are high pitched.

Rhonchi are heard over large airways such as the trachea. They occur in patients with pulmonary disorders when air flows through passages that have been narrowed by secretions, a tumor or foreign body, bronchospasm, or mucosal thickening. The resulting vibration of airway walls produces the rhonchi.

 ALERT

If you auscultate rhonchi:
- *take the patient's vital signs*
- *be alert for signs of respiratory distress.*
  If the patient's condition permits, perform a focused assessment.

HISTORY
- Ask the patient if he smokes. If so, obtain a history in pack-years.
- Ask the patient if he has recently lost weight or felt tired or weak.
- Review the patient's medical history, noting especially if he has asthma or another pulmonary disorder.
- Obtain a drug history, including prescription and over-the-counter drugs, herbal remedies, and recreational drugs. Also, ask the patient about alcohol intake.

PHYSICAL ASSESSMENT
- Characterize the patient's respirations as rapid or slow, shallow or deep, and regular or irregular.
- Inspect the chest, noting the use of accessory muscles. Note if the patient is audibly wheezing or gurgling.
- Auscultate for other abnormal breath sounds, such as crackles and a pleural friction rub. If you detect these sounds, note their location. Note diminished or absent breath sounds.
- Percuss the chest. If the patient has a cough, note its frequency and characterize its sound. If it's productive, examine the sputum for color, odor, consistency, and blood.

SPECIAL CONSIDERATIONS
Keep in mind that thick or excessive secretions, bronchospasm, or inflammation of mucous membranes may lead to airway obstruction. If necessary, suction the patient and keep equipment available for inserting an airway. Keep a bronchodilator available to treat bronchospasm.

 PEDIATRIC POINTERS
- *Rhonchi in children can result from bacterial pneumonia, cystic fibrosis, or croup syndrome.*
- *Because a respiratory tract disorder may begin abruptly and progress rapidly in an infant or a child, observe the patient closely for signs of airway obstruction.*

PATIENT COUNSELING
If appropriate, encourage increased activity to promote drainage of secretions. Teach deep-breathing and coughing techniques. Encourage the patient to drink plenty of fluids to help liquefy secretions and prevent dehydration. Advise him not to suppress a moist cough in most cases.

HPI

Focused PE: Pulmonary system

ARDS
Signs and symptoms
- Crackles
- Rapid, shallow respirations
- Dyspnea
- Intercostal and suprasternal retractions
- Diaphoresis
- Fluid accumulation

DX: PE, ABG, CXR
TX: Oxygen therapy, treatment of underlying cause
F/U: Referral to pulmonologist

Common signs and symptoms
- Wheezing
- Exertional dyspnea
- Barrel chest
- Tachypnea
- Clubbing
- Decreased breath sounds

Common signs and symptoms
- Tachycardia
- Tachypnea
- Dyspnea
- Cyanosis

BRONCHITIS
Additional signs and symptoms
ACUTE
- Chills
- Sore throat
- Low-grade fever
- Muscle and back pain
- Substernal tightness
CHRONIC
- Coarse crackles
- Prolonged expiration
- Chronic productive cough
- Increased accessory muscle use
- Cyanosis
- Fluid retention

DX: PE, ABG, CXR, PFT
TX: Smoking cessation; antibiotics, if indicated; nebulizer treatment; oxygen therapy; chest physiotherapy
F/U: Referral to pulmonologist

EMPHYSEMA
Additional signs and symptoms
- Weight loss
- Mild, chronic productive cough
- Accessory muscle use on inspiration
- Grunting expirations

DX: PE, labs (ABG, serum alpha-$_1$ antitrypsin level), CXR, PFT
TX: Smoking-cessation program, medication (diuretics, bronchodilators, corticosteroids)
F/U: Referral to pulmonologist

PNEUMONIA
Additional signs and symptoms
- Productive cough
- Shaking chills
- Fever
- Myalgia
- Headache
- Pleuritic chest pain
- Diaphoresis
- Decreased breath sounds
- Fine crackles

DX: PE, labs (CBC, ABG, sputum gram stain), CXR
TX: Antibiotics, oxygen therapy
F/U: Reevaluation after 7 days

PULMONARY EDEMA
Additional signs and symptoms
- Anxiety
- Paroxysmal nocturnal dyspnea
- Nonproductive cough
- Dependent crackles
- S_3

DX: PE, ABG, imaging studies (CXR, CT scan, MRI)
TX: Oxygen therapy, medication (diuretics, morphine)
F/U: Referral to cardiologist

Additional differential diagnoses: asthma ▪ bronchiectasis ▪ pulmonary coccidioidomycosis

Other causes: bronchoscopy ▪ foreign body aspiration ▪ PFTs ▪ respiratory therapy

Romberg's sign

A positive Romberg's sign refers to a patient's inability to maintain balance when standing erect with his feet together and his eyes closed. It indicates a vestibular or proprioceptive disorder or a disorder of the spinal tracts (the posterior columns) that carry proprioceptive information — the perception of one's position in space, of joint movements, and of pressure sensations — to the brain. Insufficient vestibular or proprioceptive information causes an inability to execute precise movements and maintain balance without visual cues.

After you've detected a positive Romberg's sign, perform a focused assessment.

HISTORY

● Ask the patient if he has noticed sensory changes, such as numbness and tingling in his limbs. If so, find out when they began.
● Ask the patient when he first noticed a problem with his balance.
● Review the patient's medical history, noting especially neurological disorders.
● Obtain a drug history, including prescription and over-the-counter drugs, herbal remedies, and recreational drugs.

PHYSICAL ASSESSMENT

● Perform neurologic screening tests. A positive Romberg's sign only indicates the presence of a defect; it doesn't pinpoint its cause or location. First, test proprioception. If the patient can maintain his balance with his eyes open, ask him to hop on one foot and then on the other. Next, ask him to do a knee bend and to walk a straight line, placing heel to toe. Lastly, ask him to walk a short distance so you can evaluate his gait.
● Test the patient's awareness of body part position by changing the position of one of his fingers, or any other joint, while his eyes are closed. Ask him to describe the change you've made.
● Test the patient's direction of movement. Ask him to close his eyes and to touch his nose with the index finger of one hand and then with the other. Ask him to repeat this movement several times, gradually increasing his speed.
● Test the accuracy of the patient's movement by having him rapidly touch each finger of one hand to the thumb.
● Test sensation in all dermatomes, using a pin or cold object. Also test two-point discrimination by touching two pins (one in each hand) to his skin simultaneously. Does he feel one or two pinpricks?
● Test and characterize the patient's deep tendon reflexes.
● To test the patient's vibratory sense, ask him to close his eyes; then apply a mildly vibrating tuning fork to his feet. If the patient doesn't feel the stimulus initially, increase the vibration,

and then test the knee or hip. This procedure can also be done to test the fingers, the elbow, and the shoulder.

SPECIAL CONSIDERATIONS

Help the patient with walking, especially in poorly lit areas. Follow safety measures.

A ▸ PEDIATRIC POINTERS

Although Romberg's sign can't be tested in children until they can stand without support and follow commands, a positive sign in children commonly results from spinal cord disease.

PATIENT COUNSELING

Encourage the patient to ask for assistance and to use visual cues to maintain his balance.

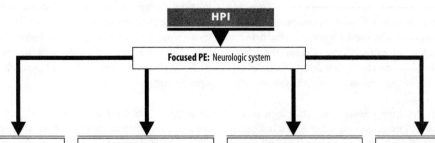

Focused PE: Neurologic system

MULTIPLE SCLEROSIS
Signs and symptoms
- Vision changes
- Diplopia
- Paresthesia
- Nystagmus
- Constipation
- Muscle weakness
- Spasticity
- Hyperreflexia
- Dysphagia
- Dysarthria
- Incontinence
- Urinary frequency and urgency
- Impotence
- Emotional instability

DX: PE, CSF analysis, MRI, EEG
TX: Medication (antispasmodics, cholinergics, antidepressants, amantadine, corticosteroids); physical, occupational, and speech therapy
F/U: Referral to neurologist

PERNICIOUS ANEMIA
Signs and symptoms
- Loss of vibratory in the lower limbs
- Gait changes
- Muscle weakness
- Impaired coordination
- Paresthesia
- Sensory loss
- Hypoactive or hyperactive DTRs
- Positive Babinski's reflex
- Fatigue
- Blurred vision
- Light-headedness

DX: Labs (CBC, vitamin B_{12} level, Schilling test, serum colbulmin), bone marrow analysis
TX: Vitamin B_{12} injections
F/U: Referral to hematologist

PERIPHERAL NERVE DISEASE
Signs and symptoms
- Impotence
- Fatigue
- Paresthesia
- Hyperesthesia
- Anesthesia of the hands and feet
- Incoordination
- Ataxia
- Burning pain in the affected area
- Progressive muscle weakness and atrophy
- Loss of vibration sense
- Hypoactive DTRs (possibly)

DX: PE, EMG, nerve conduction tests, nerve biopsy
TX: Treatment of underlying cause, analgesics
F/U: Referral to neurologist

MÉNIÈRE'S DISEASE
Signs and symptoms
- Dizziness
- Vertigo
- Tinnitus
- Nausea and vomiting
- Gradual sensorineural hearing loss
- Acute attacks of jerk nystagmus that last 10 minutes to several hours

DX: PE (otoscopy with air pressure applied to the tympanic membrane), audiometry, caloric testing, MRI
TX: Medication (atropine, antiemetic-antivertigo agents), sedative-hypnotic
F/U: Referral to otolaryngologist

Additional differential diagnoses: head trauma ▪ spinal cerebellar degeneration ▪ spinal cord disease ▪ stroke ▪ tabes dorsalis ▪ vestibular disorders

S Scotoma

A scotoma is an area of partial or complete blindness within an otherwise-normal or slightly impaired visual field. Usually located within the central 30° area of vision, the defect ranges from absolute blindness to a barely detectable loss of visual acuity. Typically, the patient can pinpoint the scotoma's location in the visual field.

A scotoma can result from a retinal, choroid, or optic nerve disorder. It can be classified as absolute, relative, or scintillating. An absolute scotoma refers to the total inability to see all sizes of test objects used in mapping the visual field. A relative scotoma, in contrast, refers to the ability to see only large test objects. A scintillating scotoma refers to the flashes or bursts of light commonly seen during a migraine headache.

HISTORY

- Review the patient's medical history for eye disorders, vision problems, and chronic systemic disorders.
- Obtain a drug history, including prescription and over-the-counter drugs (especially eyedrops), herbal remedies, and recreational drugs. Also, ask the patient about alcohol intake.

PHYSICAL ASSESSMENT

- Identify and characterize the scotoma, using such visual field tests as the tangent screen examination, the Goldmann perimeter test, and the automated perimetry test. Two other visual field tests — confrontation testing and the Amsler's grid — may also help in identifying a scotoma. (See *Locating scotomas*.)
- Test the patient's visual acuity, and inspect his pupils for size, equality, and reaction to light.

SPECIAL CONSIDERATIONS

For the patient with an arcuate scotoma associated with glaucoma, emphasize regular testing of intraocular pressure and visual fields.

A PEDIATRIC POINTERS

In young children, visual field testing is difficult and requires patience. Confrontation testing is the method of choice.

PATIENT COUNSELING

Teach the patient with a disorder involving the fovea centralis (or the area surrounding it) to periodically use the Amsler grid to detect progression of macular degeneration.

LOCATING SCOTOMAS

Scotomas, or "blind spots," are classified according to the affected area of the visual field. The normal scotoma — shown in the temporal region of the right eye — appears in black in all the illustrations

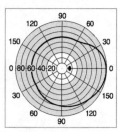

The *normally present scotoma* represents the position of the optic nerve head in the visual field. It appears between 10 and 20 degrees on this chart of the normal visual field.

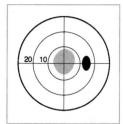

A *central scotoma* involves the point of central fixation. It's always associated with decreased visual acuity.

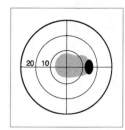

A *centrocecal scotoma* involves the point of central fixation and the area between the blind spot and the fixation point.

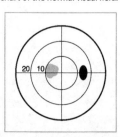

A *paracentral scotoma* affects an area of the visual field that's nasal or temporal to the point of central fixation.

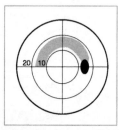

An *arcuate scotoma* arches around the fixation point, usually ending on the nasal side of the visual field.

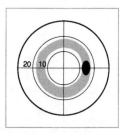

An *annular scotoma* forms a circular defect around the fixation point. It's common with retinal pigmentary degenerations.

SCOTOMA

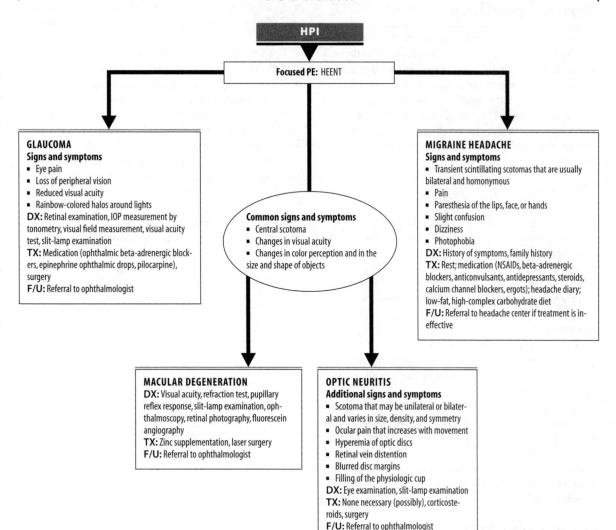

HPI

Focused PE: HEENT

GLAUCOMA
Signs and symptoms
- Eye pain
- Loss of peripheral vision
- Reduced visual acuity
- Rainbow-colored halos around lights

DX: Retinal examination, IOP measurement by tonometry, visual field measurement, visual acuity test, slit-lamp examination
TX: Medication (ophthalmic beta-adrenergic blockers, epinephrine ophthalmic drops, pilocarpine), surgery
F/U: Referral to ophthalmologist

Common signs and symptoms
- Central scotoma
- Changes in visual acuity
- Changes in color perception and in the size and shape of objects

MIGRAINE HEADACHE
Signs and symptoms
- Transient scintillating scotomas that are usually bilateral and homonymous
- Pain
- Paresthesia of the lips, face, or hands
- Slight confusion
- Dizziness
- Photophobia

DX: History of symptoms, family history
TX: Rest; medication (NSAIDs, beta-adrenergic blockers, anticonvulsants, antidepressants, steroids, calcium channel blockers, ergots); headache diary; low-fat, high-complex carbohydrate diet
F/U: Referral to headache center if treatment is ineffective

MACULAR DEGENERATION
DX: Visual acuity, refraction test, pupillary reflex response, slit-lamp examination, ophthalmoscopy, retinal photography, fluorescein angiography
TX: Zinc supplementation, laser surgery
F/U: Referral to ophthalmologist

OPTIC NEURITIS
Additional signs and symptoms
- Scotoma that may be unilateral or bilateral and varies in size, density, and symmetry
- Ocular pain that increases with movement
- Hyperemia of optic discs
- Retinal vein distention
- Blurred disc margins
- Filling of the physiologic cup

DX: Eye examination, slit-lamp examination
TX: None necessary (possibly), corticosteroids, surgery
F/U: Referral to ophthalmologist

Additional differential diagnoses: chorioretinitis ▪ retinal pigmentary degeneration

Other cause: direct visualization of solar eclipse

Scrotal swelling

Scrotal swelling occurs when a condition affecting the testicles, epididymis, or scrotal skin produces edema or a mass; the penis may or may not be involved. Scrotal swelling can affect males of any age. It can be unilateral or bilateral, painful or painless.

The sudden onset of painful scrotal swelling suggests torsion of a testicle or testicular appendages, especially in a prepubescent male. This emergency requires immediate surgery to untwist and stabilize the spermatic cord or to remove the appendage.

 ALERT

If severe pain accompanies scrotal swelling:
- *use a Doppler stethoscope to evaluate blood flow to the testicle (If it's decreased or absent, suspect testicular torsion and prepare the patient for surgery.)*
- *apply ice packs to the scrotum*
- *withhold food and fluids, until surgery is ruled out. If the patient's condition permits, perform a focused assessment.*

HISTORY
- Ask the patient when the swelling started.
- Ask the patient if the swelling is associated with pain. If so, ask him if changing his body position or level of activity affects the swelling or pain.
- Ask the patient about injuries to the scrotum, urethral discharge, cloudy urine, increased urinary frequency, and dysuria.
- Ask the patient if he's sexually active. If so, ask him when he had his last sexual contact.
- Review the patient's medical history for recent illnesses, particularly mumps, and for a history of prostate surgery or prolonged catheterization.

PHYSICAL ASSESSMENT
- Take the patient's vital signs, especially noting fever.
- Palpate the abdomen for tenderness.
- Examine the entire genital area. Assess the scrotum with the patient in a supine position and standing. Note its size and color. Is the swelling unilateral or bilateral? Are there signs of trauma or bruising?
- Gently palpate the scrotum for a cyst or a lump. Especially noting tenderness or increased firmness.
- Check the position of the testicles in the scrotum.
- Transilluminate the scrotum to distinguish a fluid-filled cyst from a solid mass. (A solid mass can't be transilluminated.)

SPECIAL CONSIDERATIONS
An effusion of blood from surgery can produce a hematocele, leading to scrotal swelling.

 PEDIATRIC POINTERS

- *A thorough physical assessment is especially important for children with scrotal swelling, who may be unable to provide history data.*
- *In infants up to age 1, a hernia or hydrocele of the spermatic cord may stem from abnormal fetal development.*
- *Scrotal swelling may stem from ammonia-related dermatitis if an infant's diapers aren't changed often enough.*
- *In prepubescent males, scrotal swelling usually results from torsion of the spermatic cord.*
- *Other disorders that can produce scrotal swelling in children include epididymitis (rare before age 10), adherence of the foreskin to the penile head, traumatic orchitis from contact sports, and mumps, which is most common after puberty.*

PATIENT COUNSELING
Encourage the patient to perform testicular self-examination at home.

SCROTAL SWELLING

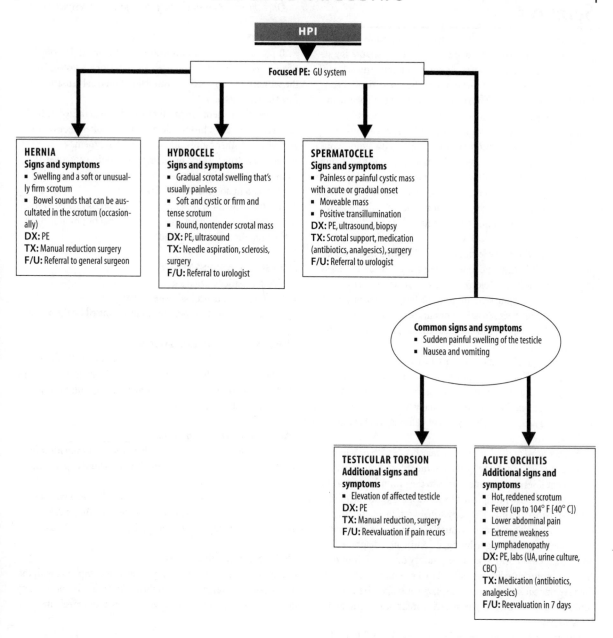

HPI

Focused PE: GU system

HERNIA
Signs and symptoms
- Swelling and a soft or unusually firm scrotum
- Bowel sounds that can be auscultated in the scrotum (occasionally)

DX: PE
TX: Manual reduction surgery
F/U: Referral to general surgeon

HYDROCELE
Signs and symptoms
- Gradual scrotal swelling that's usually painless
- Soft and cystic or firm and tense scrotum
- Round, nontender scrotal mass

DX: PE, ultrasound
TX: Needle aspiration, sclerosis, surgery
F/U: Referral to urologist

SPERMATOCELE
Signs and symptoms
- Painless or painful cystic mass with acute or gradual onset
- Moveable mass
- Positive transillumination

DX: PE, ultrasound, biopsy
TX: Scrotal support, medication (antibiotics, analgesics), surgery
F/U: Referral to urologist

Common signs and symptoms
- Sudden painful swelling of the testicle
- Nausea and vomiting

TESTICULAR TORSION
Additional signs and symptoms
- Elevation of affected testicle

DX: PE
TX: Manual reduction, surgery
F/U: Reevaluation if pain recurs

ACUTE ORCHITIS
Additional signs and symptoms
- Hot, reddened scrotum
- Fever (up to 104° F [40° C])
- Lower abdominal pain
- Extreme weakness
- Lymphadenopathy

DX: PE, labs (UA, urine culture, CBC)
TX: Medication (antibiotics, analgesics)
F/U: Reevaluation in 7 days

Additional differential diagnoses: elephantiasis of the scrotum ▪ epididymal cysts ▪ epididymal tuberculosis ▪ epididymitis ▪ fistula ▪ granuloma ▪ gumma ▪ idiopathic scrotal edema ▪ lymphoma ▪ scrotal burns ▪ scrotal trauma ▪ testicular tumor ▪ torsion of a hydatid of Morgagni

Other cause: surgery

Seizures

A simple partial seizure, also known as a *focal seizure*, may manifest in different areas of the body. A focal motor seizure is a series of unilateral clonic (muscle jerking) and tonic (muscle stiffening) movements of one part of the body. The patient's head and eyes characteristically turn away from the hemispheric focus—usually the frontal lobe near the motor strip. A tonic-clonic contraction of the trunk or extremities may follow.

A *jacksonian motor seizure* typically begins with a tonic contraction of a finger, the corner of the mouth, or one foot. Clonic movements follow, spreading to other muscles on the same side of the body, moving up the arm or leg and, eventually, involving the whole side. Alternatively, clonic movements may spread to the opposite side, becoming generalized and leading to a loss of consciousness.

A *focal somatosensory seizure* affects a localized body area on one side. Usually, this type of seizure initially causes numbness, tingling, or crawling or "electric" sensations; occasionally, it causes pain or burning sensations in the lips, fingers, or toes. A visual seizure involves sensations of darkness or of stationary or moving lights or spots, usually red at first, then blue, green, and yellow.

A *complex partial seizure* occurs when a focal seizure begins in the temporal lobe and causes a partial alteration of consciousness—usually confusion. Psychomotor seizures can occur at any age, but their incidence usually increases during adolescence and adulthood. Two-thirds of patients also have generalized seizures.

A *generalized tonic-clonic seizure* may begin with or without an aura. As seizure activity spreads to the subcortical structures, the patient loses consciousness, falls to the ground, and may utter a loud cry that's precipitated by air rushing from the lungs through the vocal cords. His body stiffens (tonic phase), then undergoes rapid, synchronous muscle jerking and hyperventilation (clonic phase). Tongue biting, incontinence, diaphoresis, profuse salivation, and signs of respiratory distress may also occur. The seizure usually stops after 2 to 5 minutes. The patient then regains consciousness but displays confusion. He may complain of headache, fatigue, muscle soreness, and arm and leg weakness.

Life-threatening *status epilepticus* is marked by prolonged seizure activity or by rapidly recurring seizures with no intervening periods of recovery. It's usually triggered by abrupt discontinuation of anticonvulsant therapy.

⊁ ALERT

If you witness a seizure:
- *check the patient's airway, breathing, and circulation*
- *institute emergency measures, if necessary*
- *protect the patient from injury.*
Once the patient is stable, perform a focused assessment.

HISTORY

- If possible, have a witness who was at the scene describe the seizure, including when it started and how long it lasted. Did the witness hear the patient complain of unusual sensations before the seizure began?
- Review the patient's medical history for generalized or focal seizures. If there is a history, determine how often they occur and whether other family members also have them.
- Obtain a drug history, including prescription and over-the-counter drugs, herbal remedies, and recreational drugs. Also, ask the patient about alcohol intake.
- Ask the patient (or his family if the patient is unable to respond) about sleep deprivation or emotional or physical stress at the time the seizure occurred.

PHYSICAL ASSESSMENT

- Take the patient's vital signs.
- Perform a full neurologic assessment.
- Assess the patient for possible injuries caused by the seizures.

SPECIAL CONSIDERATIONS

An absence seizure is a benign, generalized seizure thought to originate subcortically, usually lasting 3 to 20 seconds. This type of seizure can occur 100 or more times per day, commonly causing periods of inattention.

Ⓐ PEDIATRIC POINTERS

- *Complex partial seizures in children can result from birth injury, abuse, infection, or cancer. In about one-third of patients, their cause is unknown.*
- *Many children between the ages of 3 months and 3 years experience generalized seizures associated with fever. About 25% of febrile seizures may present as focal seizures.*

PATIENT COUNSELING

Emphasize to the patient the importance of complying with the prescribed drug regimen. Teach the patient's family about safety measures to take if the patient experiences another seizure.

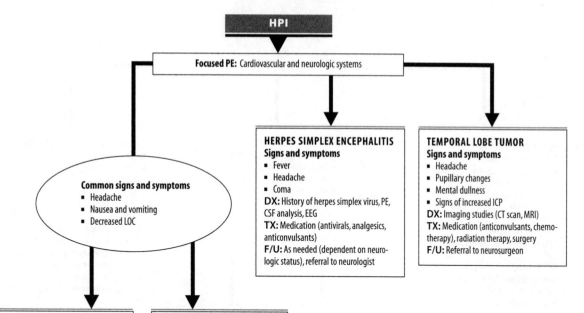

HPI

Focused PE: Cardiovascular and neurologic systems

Common signs and symptoms
- Headache
- Nausea and vomiting
- Decreased LOC

HERPES SIMPLEX ENCEPHALITIS
Signs and symptoms
- Fever
- Headache
- Coma

DX: History of herpes simplex virus, PE, CSF analysis, EEG
TX: Medication (antivirals, analgesics, anticonvulsants)
F/U: As needed (dependent on neurologic status), referral to neurologist

TEMPORAL LOBE TUMOR
Signs and symptoms
- Headache
- Pupillary changes
- Mental dullness
- Signs of increased ICP

DX: Imaging studies (CT scan, MRI)
TX: Medication (anticonvulsants, chemotherapy), radiation therapy, surgery
F/U: Referral to neurosurgeon

HEAD TRAUMA
Additional signs and symptoms
- Seizures that occur months or years after trauma
- Seizures that increase in frequency or eventually stop
- Behavior and personality changes
- Obvious wound

DX: History of trauma, PE, imaging studies (CT scan, MRI)
TX: Varies based on the extent of trauma, safety maintenance during seizure, medication (analgesics, anticonvulsants), surgery (if indicated)
F/U: As needed (dependent on the severity of trauma and neurologic status)

BRAIN ABSCESS
Additional signs and symptoms
- Central facial weakness
- Auditory receptive aphasia
- Hemiparesis
- Ocular disturbances

DX: Imaging studies (CT scan, MRI), EEG
TX: Medication (antibiotics, analgesics, anticonvulsants), surgery
F/U: Referral to neurosurgeon

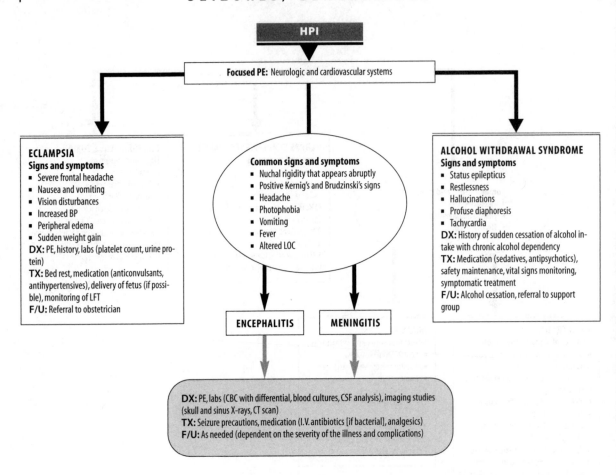

HPI

Focused PE: Neurologic and cardiovascular systems

ECLAMPSIA
Signs and symptoms
- Severe frontal headache
- Nausea and vomiting
- Vision disturbances
- Increased BP
- Peripheral edema
- Sudden weight gain

DX: PE, history, labs (platelet count, urine protein)
TX: Bed rest, medication (anticonvulsants, antihypertensives), delivery of fetus (if possible), monitoring of LFT
F/U: Referral to obstetrician

Common signs and symptoms
- Nuchal rigidity that appears abruptly
- Positive Kernig's and Brudzinski's signs
- Headache
- Photophobia
- Vomiting
- Fever
- Altered LOC

ENCEPHALITIS

MENINGITIS

ALCOHOL WITHDRAWAL SYNDROME
Signs and symptoms
- Status epilepticus
- Restlessness
- Hallucinations
- Profuse diaphoresis
- Tachycardia

DX: History of sudden cessation of alcohol intake with chronic alcohol dependency
TX: Medication (sedatives, antipsychotics), safety maintenance, vital signs monitoring, symptomatic treatment
F/U: Alcohol cessation, referral to support group

DX: PE, labs (CBC with differential, blood cultures, CSF analysis), imaging studies (skull and sinus X-rays, CT scan)
TX: Seizure precautions, medication (I.V. antibiotics [if bacterial], analgesics)
F/U: As needed (dependent on the severity of the illness and complications)

Additional differential diagnoses: brain abscess ▪ brain tumor ▪ cerebral aneurysm ▪ chronic renal failure ▪ epilepsy (idiopathic) ▪ head trauma ▪ hepatic encephalopathy ▪ hypertensive encephalopathy ▪ hypoglycemia ▪ hyponatremia ▪ hypoparathyroidism ▪ hypoxic encephalopathy ▪ multiple sclerosis ▪ neurofibromatosis ▪ porphyria (intermittent acute) ▪ sarcoidosis ▪ stroke

Other causes: amphetamines ▪ arsenic poisoning ▪ barbiturate withdrawal ▪ contrast agents ▪ isoniazid ▪ phenothiazines ▪ toxic levels of theophylline, lidocaine, meperidine, penicillin, or cimetidine ▪ tricyclic antidepressants ▪ vincristine (in patients with preexisting seizure disorders)

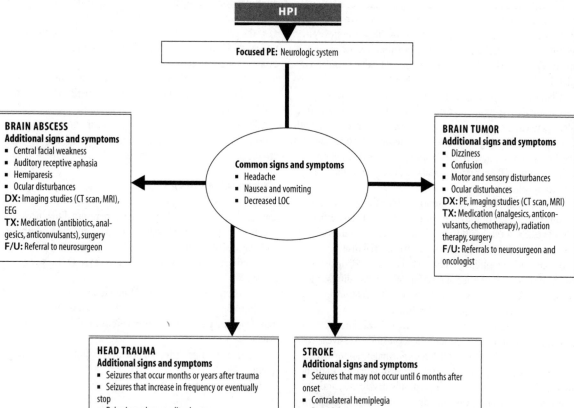

HPI

Focused PE: Neurologic system

Common signs and symptoms
- Headache
- Nausea and vomiting
- Decreased LOC

BRAIN ABSCESS
Additional signs and symptoms
- Central facial weakness
- Auditory receptive aphasia
- Hemiparesis
- Ocular disturbances

DX: Imaging studies (CT scan, MRI), EEG
TX: Medication (antibiotics, analgesics, anticonvulsants), surgery
F/U: Referral to neurosurgeon

BRAIN TUMOR
Additional signs and symptoms
- Dizziness
- Confusion
- Motor and sensory disturbances
- Ocular disturbances

DX: PE, imaging studies (CT scan, MRI)
TX: Medication (analgesics, anticonvulsants, chemotherapy), radiation therapy, surgery
F/U: Referrals to neurosurgeon and oncologist

HEAD TRAUMA
Additional signs and symptoms
- Seizures that occur months or years after trauma
- Seizures that increase in frequency or eventually stop
- Behavior and personality changes
- Obvious wound

DX: History of trauma, PE, imaging studies (CT scan, MRI)
TX: Varies based on the extent of trauma, safety maintenance during seizure, medication (analgesics, anticonvulsants), surgery (if indicated)
F/U: As needed (dependent on the severity of trauma and neurologic status)

STROKE
Additional signs and symptoms
- Seizures that may not occur until 6 months after onset
- Contralateral hemiplegia
- Dysarthria
- Dysphagia
- Ataxia
- Unilateral sensory loss
- Aphasia

DX: History of illness, imaging studies (skull X-ray, CT scan, MRI, angiography), EEG
TX: Airway stabilization, treatment of cause of injury, control of extension of injury, medication (for embolic stroke, thrombolytics; anticonvulsants; analgesics), surgery
F/U: Referral to neurologist or neurosurgeon, transfer to brain injury center

Additional differential diagnoses: multiple sclerosis ▪ neurofibromatosis ▪ sarcoidosis

Skin, abnormal

Clammy skin — moist, cool, and often pale — is a sympathetic response to stress, which triggers release of the hormones epinephrine and norepinephrine. These hormones cause cutaneous vasoconstriction and secretion of cold sweat from eccrine glands, particularly on the palms, forehead, and soles.

Clammy skin typically accompanies shock, acute hypoglycemia, anxiety reactions, arrhythmias, and heat exhaustion. It also occurs as a vasovagal reaction to severe pain associated with nausea, anorexia, epigastric distress, hyperpnea, tachypnea, weakness, confusion, tachycardia, and pupillary dilation or a combination of these findings. Marked bradycardia and syncope may follow.

Mottled skin is patchy discoloration indicating primary or secondary changes of the deep, middle, or superficial dermal blood vessels. It can result from a hematologic, immune, or connective tissue disorder; chronic occlusive arterial disease; dysproteinemias; immobility; exposure to heat or cold; or shock. Mottled skin can be a normal reaction, such as the diffuse mottling that occurs when exposure to cold causes venous stasis in cutaneous blood vessels (cutis marmorata).

Scaly skin results when cells of the uppermost skin layer (stratum corneum) desiccate and shed, causing excessive accumulation of loosely adherent flakes of normal or abnormal keratin. Scaly skin varies in texture from fine and delicate to branny, coarse, or stratified. Scales are typically dry, brittle, and shiny, but they can be greasy and dull. Their color ranges from whitish gray, yellow, or brown to a silvery sheen.

➤ ALERT

If you detect clammy skin:
- *immediately ask the patient about a history of type 1 diabetes mellitus or cardiac disorders*
- *ask the patient if he's taking medication, especially an antiarrhythmic*
- *ask the patient if he's experiencing pain, chest pressure, nausea, or epigastric distress*
- *examine the patient's pupils for dilation*
- *check for abdominal distention and increased muscle tension.*
  If you detect mottled skin:
- *ask the patient if the mottling began suddenly or gradually*
- *quickly take the patient's vital signs and assess for respiratory distress*
- *institute emergency measures, if necessary.*
  If the patient's condition permits, perform a focused assessment.

HISTORY

- Ask the patient when he first noticed a change in his skin. Ask if the change began suddenly or gradually.

- Ask the patient if he knows what precipitated the skin change.
- Ask the patient about associated symptoms, such as pain, numbness, or tingling in an extremity. If so, do they disappear with temperature changes?
- If the patient has scaly skin, ask him if he has recently used a topical skin product. Ask how often he bathes and whether he's exposed to chemicals at work.
- Ask the patient if there's a family history of skin disorders.
- Ask the patient what kinds of soap, cosmetics, skin lotion, and hair preparations he uses.
- Obtain a drug history, including prescription and over-the-counter drugs, herbal remedies, and recreational drugs. Also, ask the patient about alcohol intake.

PHYSICAL ASSESSMENT

- Observe the patient's skin color, and palpate his arms and legs for skin texture, swelling, and temperature differences between extremities. Note breaks in the skin, muscle appearance, and hair distribution.
- Examine the entire skin surface. Is it dry, oily, moist, or greasy?
- Observe the general pattern of skin lesions, and record their location, color, shape, and size. Are they thick or fine? Do they itch? Does the patient have other lesions in addition to scaly skin?
- Palpate for the presence (or absence) of pulses and for their quality.
- Assess motor and sensory function.

SPECIAL CONSIDERATIONS

Patients with chronic conditions, such as systemic lupus erythematosus, periarteritis nodosa, and cryoglobulinemia, may develop mottled skin when they have a flare-up of their disorder.

[A] PEDIATRIC POINTERS

- *A common cause of mottled skin in children is systemic vasoconstriction from shock.*
- *In children, scaly skin may stem from infantile eczema, pityriasis rosea, epidermolytic hyperkeratosis, psoriasis, various forms of ichthyosis, atopic dermatitis, a viral infection, or an acute transient dermatitis.*
- *Desquamation may follow a febrile illness.*

AGING ISSUES

Elderly patients develop clammy or mottled skin easily because of decreased tissue perfusion.

PATIENT COUNSELING

Instruct the patient to avoid tight clothing and overexposure to cold or heating devices, such as hot-water bottles and heating pads.

SKIN, CLAMMY

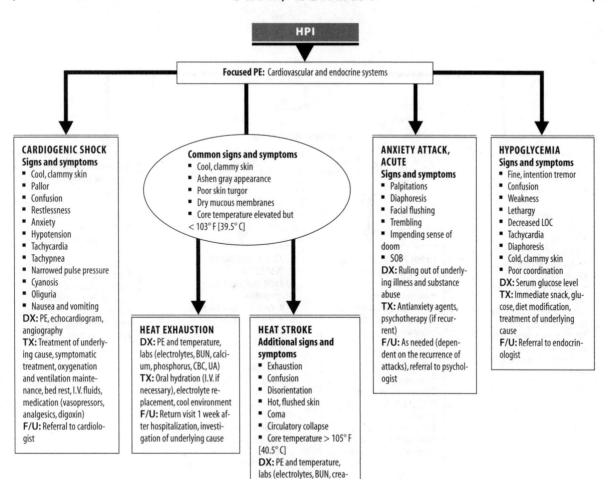

HPI

Focused PE: Cardiovascular and endocrine systems

CARDIOGENIC SHOCK
Signs and symptoms
- Cool, clammy skin
- Pallor
- Confusion
- Restlessness
- Anxiety
- Hypotension
- Tachycardia
- Tachypnea
- Narrowed pulse pressure
- Cyanosis
- Oliguria
- Nausea and vomiting

DX: PE, echocardiogram, angiography
TX: Treatment of underlying cause, symptomatic treatment, oxygenation and ventilation maintenance, bed rest, I.V. fluids, medication (vasopressors, analgesics, digoxin)
F/U: Referral to cardiologist

Common signs and symptoms
- Cool, clammy skin
- Ashen gray appearance
- Poor skin turgor
- Dry mucous membranes
- Core temperature elevated but < 103° F [39.5° C]

HEAT EXHAUSTION
DX: PE and temperature, labs (electrolytes, BUN, calcium, phosphorus, CBC, UA)
TX: Oral hydration (I.V. if necessary), electrolyte replacement, cool environment
F/U: Return visit 1 week after hospitalization, investigation of underlying cause

HEAT STROKE
Additional signs and symptoms
- Exhaustion
- Confusion
- Disorientation
- Hot, flushed skin
- Coma
- Circulatory collapse
- Core temperature > 105° F [40.5° C]

DX: PE and temperature, labs (electrolytes, BUN, creatinine)
TX: I.V. hydration, careful electrolyte monitoring, airway and ventilation maintenance, hemodynamic monitoring, rapid cooling with ice packs, cooling blanket
F/U: Return visit 1 week after hospitalization, investigation of underlying cause

ANXIETY ATTACK, ACUTE
Signs and symptoms
- Palpitations
- Diaphoresis
- Facial flushing
- Trembling
- Impending sense of doom
- SOB

DX: Ruling out of underlying illness and substance abuse
TX: Antianxiety agents, psychotherapy (if recurrent)
F/U: As needed (dependent on the recurrence of attacks), referral to psychologist

HYPOGLYCEMIA
Signs and symptoms
- Fine, intention tremor
- Confusion
- Weakness
- Lethargy
- Decreased LOC
- Tachycardia
- Diaphoresis
- Cold, clammy skin
- Poor coordination

DX: Serum glucose level
TX: Immediate snack, glucose, diet modification, treatment of underlying cause
F/U: Referral to endocrinologist

Additional differential diagnoses: arrhythmias ▪ hypovolemic shock ▪ septic shock

SKIN, MOTTLED

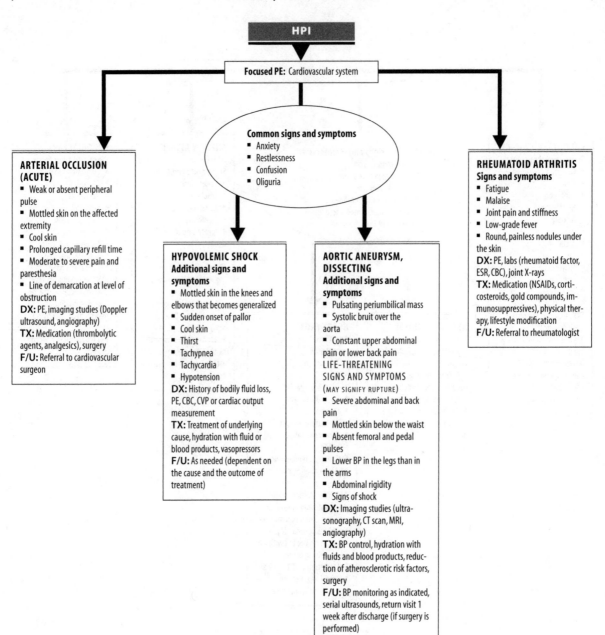

HPI

Focused PE: Cardiovascular system

Common signs and symptoms
- Anxiety
- Restlessness
- Confusion
- Oliguria

ARTERIAL OCCLUSION (ACUTE)
- Weak or absent peripheral pulse
- Mottled skin on the affected extremity
- Cool skin
- Prolonged capillary refill time
- Moderate to severe pain and paresthesia
- Line of demarcation at level of obstruction

DX: PE, imaging studies (Doppler ultrasound, angiography)
TX: Medication (thrombolytic agents, analgesics), surgery
F/U: Referral to cardiovascular surgeon

HYPOVOLEMIC SHOCK
Additional signs and symptoms
- Mottled skin in the knees and elbows that becomes generalized
- Sudden onset of pallor
- Cool skin
- Thirst
- Tachypnea
- Tachycardia
- Hypotension

DX: History of bodily fluid loss, PE, CBC, CVP or cardiac output measurement
TX: Treatment of underlying cause, hydration with fluid or blood products, vasopressors
F/U: As needed (dependent on the cause and the outcome of treatment)

AORTIC ANEURYSM, DISSECTING
Additional signs and symptoms
- Pulsating periumbilical mass
- Systolic bruit over the aorta
- Constant upper abdominal pain or lower back pain

LIFE-THREATENING SIGNS AND SYMPTOMS (MAY SIGNIFY RUPTURE)
- Severe abdominal and back pain
- Mottled skin below the waist
- Absent femoral and pedal pulses
- Lower BP in the legs than in the arms
- Abdominal rigidity
- Signs of shock

DX: Imaging studies (ultrasonography, CT scan, MRI, angiography)
TX: BP control, hydration with fluids and blood products, reduction of atherosclerotic risk factors, surgery
F/U: BP monitoring as indicated, serial ultrasounds, return visit 1 week after discharge (if surgery is performed)

RHEUMATOID ARTHRITIS
Signs and symptoms
- Fatigue
- Malaise
- Joint pain and stiffness
- Low-grade fever
- Round, painless nodules under the skin

DX: PE, labs (rheumatoid factor, ESR, CBC), joint X-rays
TX: Medication (NSAIDs, corticosteroids, gold compounds, immunosuppressives), physical therapy, lifestyle modification
F/U: Referral to rheumatologist

Additional differential diagnoses: acrocyanosis ▪ arteriosclerosis obliterans ▪ Buerger's disease ▪ livedo reticularis (idiopathic or primary) ▪ periarteritis nodosa ▪ polycythemia vera ▪ SLE

Other causes: immobility ▪ thermal exposure

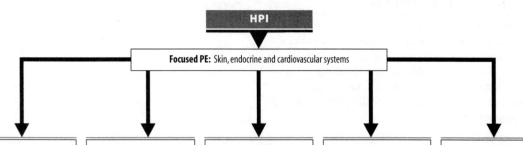

SEBORRHEIC DERMATITIS
Signs and symptoms
MILD
- Fine, dry, white or yellow scales on inflamed base
MODERATE
- Dull, red plaques with thick white or yellow scales in a diffuse distribution
- Pruritus
DX: Skin examination
TX: Medicated shampoo, medication (topical corticosteroids, ketoconazole, selenium)
F/U: None unless signs and symptoms worsen

NUMMULAR DERMATITIS
Signs and symptoms
- Round, pustular lesions
- Purulent exudate
- Encrustation and scaling
- Pruritus
DX: Skin examination, personal and family history
TX: Symptomatic treatment, medication (antipruritics, topical tar lotions, topical corticosteroids)
F/U: Referral to dermatologist

PITYRIASIS ROSEA
Signs and symptoms
- Mild to severe pruritus that's aggravated by a hot bath or shower
- Erythematous herald patch anywhere on the body
- Red-brown patches with erythematous borders and trailing scales
- Lesions that may be macular, vesicular, or urticarial
DX: Skin examination
TX: Symptomatic treatment, medication (antipyretics, antihistamines, topical or systemic corticosteroids), oatmeal baths
F/U: None unless the condition persists longer than 6 weeks

PSORIASIS
Signs and symptoms
- Initially small erythematous papules on the scalp, chest, elbows, knees, back, buttocks, and genitalia that may be pruritic and painful and eventually enlarge and coalesce, forming red, scaly plaques covered by silver scales
- Pitted fingernails
- Arthralgia
DX: PE, HLAs
TX: Medication (topical lubricants, dandruff or coal tar shampoo, corticosteroids, keratolytic agents, vitamin D analogs, topical retinoids)
F/U: Referral to dermatologist

TINEA VERSICOLOR
Signs and symptoms
- Macular, hyperpigmented, scaly patches of varying size and shapes
- Lesions that usually affect the upper trunk, arms, and lower abdomen
DX: Skin examination, potassium preparation of scales
TX: Tar preparation shampoo, topical antifungal
F/U: None unless treatment is ineffective

Additional differential diagnoses: Bowen's disease • dermatophytosis • discoid lupus erythematosus • lichen planus • lymphoma • parapsoriasis (chronic) • syphilis (secondary) • SLE • tinea coporis • tinea pedis

Other causes: drugs, such as penicillins, sulfonamides, barbiturates, quinidine, diazepam, phenytoin, and isoniazid

Stools, clay-colored

Normally, bile pigments give the stool its characteristic brown color. However, hepatocellular degeneration or biliary obstruction may interfere with the formation or release of these pigments into the intestine, resulting in clay-colored stools. These stools are commonly associated with jaundice and dark urine. Pale, putty-colored stools usually result from a hepatic, gallbladder, or pancreatic disorder.

HISTORY

- Ask the patient when he first noticed clay-colored stools.
- Ask the patient about associated signs and symptoms, such as abdominal pain, nausea and vomiting, fatigue, anorexia, weight loss, and dark urine.
- Ask the patient if he has trouble digesting fatty foods or heavy meals or if he bruises easily.
- Review the patient's medical history for gallbladder, hepatic, or pancreatic disorders; biliary surgery; and recent barium studies.
- Ask the patient about antacid use, and note a history of alcoholism or exposure to other hepatotoxic substances.

PHYSICAL ASSESSMENT

- Assess the patient's general appearance, take his vital signs, and check his skin and eyes for jaundice.
- Examine the abdomen; inspect the area for distention, and auscultate for hypoactive bowel sounds. Percuss and palpate for masses and rebound tenderness.
- Obtain urine and stool specimens for laboratory analysis.

SPECIAL CONSIDERATIONS

Biliary surgery may cause bile duct stricture, resulting in clay-colored stools.

PEDIATRIC POINTERS

Clay-colored stools may occur in infants with biliary atresia.

AGING ISSUES

Because elderly patients with cholelithiasis are at greater risk for developing complications if the condition isn't treated, surgery should be considered early on for treatment of persistent systems.

PATIENT COUNSELING

Instruct the patient on what to expect from diagnostic testing, which may include liver enzyme and serum bilirubin levels, sonograms, computed tomography scan, and stool analysis.

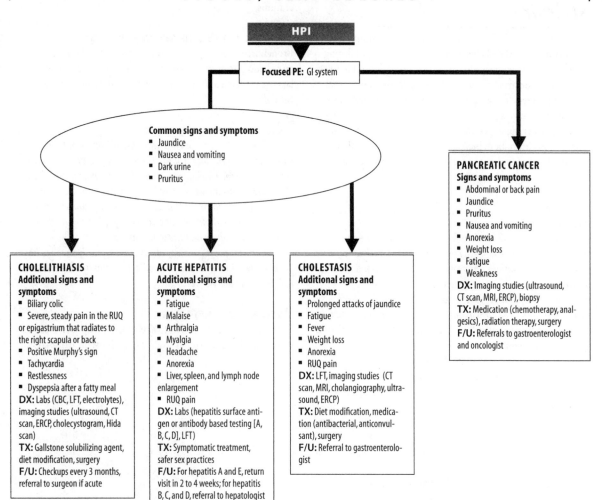

HPI

Focused PE: GI system

Common signs and symptoms
- Jaundice
- Nausea and vomiting
- Dark urine
- Pruritus

CHOLELITHIASIS
Additional signs and symptoms
- Biliary colic
- Severe, steady pain in the RUQ or epigastrium that radiates to the right scapula or back
- Positive Murphy's sign
- Tachycardia
- Restlessness
- Dyspepsia after a fatty meal

DX: Labs (CBC, LFT, electrolytes), imaging studies (ultrasound, CT scan, ERCP, cholecystogram, Hida scan)
TX: Gallstone solubilizing agent, diet modification, surgery
F/U: Checkups every 3 months, referral to surgeon if acute

ACUTE HEPATITIS
Additional signs and symptoms
- Fatigue
- Malaise
- Arthralgia
- Myalgia
- Headache
- Anorexia
- Liver, spleen, and lymph node enlargement
- RUQ pain

DX: Labs (hepatitis surface antigen or antibody based testing [A, B, C, D], LFT)
TX: Symptomatic treatment, safer sex practices
F/U: For hepatitis A and E, return visit in 2 to 4 weeks; for hepatitis B, C, and D, referral to hepatologist or gastroenterologist

CHOLESTASIS
Additional signs and symptoms
- Prolonged attacks of jaundice
- Fatigue
- Fever
- Weight loss
- Anorexia
- RUQ pain

DX: LFT, imaging studies (CT scan, MRI, cholangiography, ultrasound, ERCP)
TX: Diet modification, medication (antibacterial, anticonvulsant), surgery
F/U: Referral to gastroenterologist

PANCREATIC CANCER
Signs and symptoms
- Abdominal or back pain
- Jaundice
- Pruritus
- Nausea and vomiting
- Anorexia
- Weight loss
- Fatigue
- Weakness

DX: Imaging studies (ultrasound, CT scan, MRI, ERCP), biopsy
TX: Medication (chemotherapy, analgesics), radiation therapy, surgery
F/U: Referrals to gastroenterologist and oncologist

Additional differential diagnoses: bile duct cancer ▪ biliary cirrhosis ▪ cholangitis (sclerosing) ▪ hepatic cancer ▪ pancreatitis (acute)

Other cause: biliary surgery

Stridor

A loud, harsh, musical respiratory sound, stridor results from an obstruction in the trachea or larynx. Usually heard during inspiration, this sign may also occur during expiration in severe upper airway obstruction. It may begin as low-pitched "croaking" and progress to high-pitched "crowing" as respirations become more vigorous.

Life-threatening upper airway obstruction can stem from foreign-body aspiration, increased secretions, intraluminal tumor, localized edema or muscle spasms, or external compression by a tumor or aneurysm.

⬦ ALERT

If you hear stridor:
- *quickly examine the patient for other signs and symptoms of partial airway obstruction — choking or gagging, tachypnea, dyspnea, shallow respirations, intercostal retractions, nasal flaring, tachycardia, cyanosis, and diaphoresis.*
- *be aware that abrupt cessation of stridor signals complete obstruction in which the patient has inspiratory chest movement but absent breath sounds; unable to talk, he quickly becomes lethargic and loses consciousness*
- *institute emergency measures, if necessary.*
  If the patient's condition permits, perform a focused assessment.

HISTORY

- Ask the patient or a family member when the stridor began and if he has had it before.
- Ask the patient if he has an upper respiratory tract infection. If he does, how long has he had it?
- Ask the patient if he has recently been exposed to smoke or noxious fumes or gases.
- Review the patient's medical history for allergies, tumors, and respiratory and vascular disorders.
- If the patient is a child, ask the patient if the child could have ingested a foreign body.
- Ask the patient about associated signs and symptoms, such as pain or a cough.

PHYSICAL ASSESSMENT

- Examine the patient's mouth for excessive secretions, foreign matter, inflammation, and swelling.
- Assess his neck for swelling, masses, subcutaneous crepitation, and scars.
- Observe his chest for delayed, decreased, or asymmetrical chest expansion. Auscultate for wheezes, rhonchi, crackles, rubs, and other abnormal breath sounds. Percuss for dullness, tympany, or flatness.

- Note burns or signs of trauma, such as ecchymoses and lacerations.

SPECIAL CONSIDERATIONS

Bronchoscopy or laryngoscopy may precipitate laryngospasm and stridor. After prolonged intubation, the patient may exhibit laryngeal edema and stridor when the endotracheal tube is removed.

PEDIATRIC POINTERS

- *Stridor is a major sign of airway obstruction in children. When you hear this sign, you must intervene quickly to prevent total airway obstruction. This emergency can happen more rapidly in a child because his airway is narrower than an adult's airway.*
- *Causes of stridor include foreign-body aspiration, croup syndrome, laryngeal diphtheria, pertussis, retropharyngeal abscess, and congenital abnormalities of the larynx.*
- *Therapy for partial airway obstruction typically involves hot or cold steam in a mist tent or hood, parenteral fluids and electrolytes, and plenty of rest.*

PATIENT COUNSELING

Instruct the patient on what to expect from diagnostic testing, which may include arterial blood gas analysis, bronchoscopy, and chest X-rays.

STRIDOR

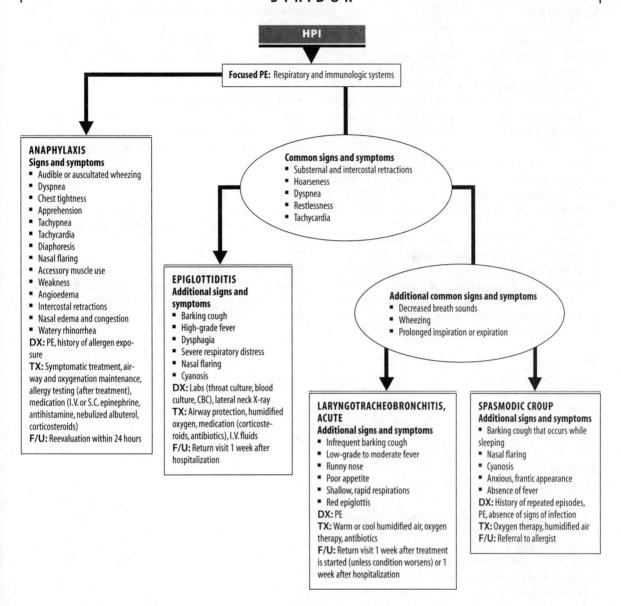

HPI

Focused PE: Respiratory and immunologic systems

ANAPHYLAXIS
Signs and symptoms
- Audible or auscultated wheezing
- Dyspnea
- Chest tightness
- Apprehension
- Tachypnea
- Tachycardia
- Diaphoresis
- Nasal flaring
- Accessory muscle use
- Weakness
- Angioedema
- Intercostal retractions
- Nasal edema and congestion
- Watery rhinorrhea

DX: PE, history of allergen exposure
TX: Symptomatic treatment, airway and oxygenation maintenance, allergy testing (after treatment), medication (I.V. or S.C. epinephrine, antihistamine, nebulized albuterol, corticosteroids)
F/U: Reevaluation within 24 hours

Common signs and symptoms
- Substernal and intercostal retractions
- Hoarseness
- Dyspnea
- Restlessness
- Tachycardia

EPIGLOTTIDITIS
Additional signs and symptoms
- Barking cough
- High-grade fever
- Dysphagia
- Severe respiratory distress
- Nasal flaring
- Cyanosis

DX: Labs (throat culture, blood culture, CBC), lateral neck X-ray
TX: Airway protection, humidified oxygen, medication (corticosteroids, antibiotics), I.V. fluids
F/U: Return visit 1 week after hospitalization

Additional common signs and symptoms
- Decreased breath sounds
- Wheezing
- Prolonged inspiration or expiration

LARYNGOTRACHEOBRONCHITIS, ACUTE
Additional signs and symptoms
- Infrequent barking cough
- Low-grade to moderate fever
- Runny nose
- Poor appetite
- Shallow, rapid respirations
- Red epiglottis

DX: PE
TX: Warm or cool humidified air, oxygen therapy, antibiotics
F/U: Return visit 1 week after treatment is started (unless condition worsens) or 1 week after hospitalization

SPASMODIC CROUP
Additional signs and symptoms
- Barking cough that occurs while sleeping
- Nasal flaring
- Cyanosis
- Anxious, frantic appearance
- Absence of fever

DX: History of repeated episodes, PE, absence of signs of infection
TX: Oxygen therapy, humidified air
F/U: Referral to allergist

Additional differential diagnoses: airway trauma ▪ hypocalcemia ▪ inhalation injury ▪ laryngeal tumor ▪ mediastinal tumor ▪ retrosternal thyroid ▪ thoracic aortic aneurysm

Other causes: bronchoscopy ▪ foreign body aspiration ▪ laryngoscopy ▪ neck surgery ▪ prolonged intubation

Syncope

A common neurologic sign, syncope (fainting) refers to transient loss of consciousness associated with impaired cerebral blood supply. It usually occurs abruptly and lasts for seconds to minutes. Typically, the patient lies motionless with his skeletal muscles relaxed but sphincter muscles controlled. However, the depth of unconsciousness varies—some patients can hear voices or see blurred outlines; others are unaware of their surroundings.

In many ways, syncope simulates death: The patient is strikingly pale with a slow, weak pulse, hypotension, and almost imperceptible breathing. If severe hypotension lasts for 20 seconds or longer, the patient may also develop convulsive, tonic-clonic movements.

Syncope may result from a cardiac or cerebrovascular disorder, hypoxemia, or postural changes in the presence of autonomic dysfunction. It may also follow vigorous coughing (tussive syncope) and emotional stress, injury, shock, or pain (vasovagal syncope, or common fainting). Hysterical syncope may also follow emotional stress but isn't accompanied by other vasodepressor effects.

 ALERT

If you see a patient faint:
- *ensure a patent airway and take his vital signs*
- *institute emergency measures, if necessary.*

If a patient reports a fainting episode, perform a focused assessment.

HISTORY
- Gather information from the patient and any witnesses to the episode.
- Ask the patient if he felt weak, light-headed, nauseous, or diaphoretic just before he fainted. Ask him if he got up quickly from a chair or from lying down.
- Ask witnesses if the patient experienced muscle spams or incontinence during the fainting episode.
- Ask witnesses how long the patient was unconscious.
- Ask the patient if he was alert or confused or if he had a headache when he regained consciousness.
- Review the patient's medical history for diabetes mellitus, cardiac disorders, and prior fainting episodes. If the patient has had prior fainting episodes, find out their occurrence.
- Ask the patient if he experienced palpitations prior to the syncopal episode.
- Ask the patient if he is on a weight-loss diet. If so, ask him the type of diet and how long he has been on it.
- Obtain a drug history, including prescription and over-the-counter drugs, herbal remedies, and recreational drugs.

PHYSICAL ASSESSMENT
- Examine the patient for injuries that may have occurred during his fall.
- Take the patient's vital signs. If an irregular heartbeat is detected, obtain an electrocardiogram or place the patient on a cardiac monitor.

SPECIAL CONSIDERATIONS
Quinidine may cause syncope—and possibly sudden death—associated with ventricular fibrillation. Prazosin may cause severe orthostatic hypotension and syncope, usually after the first dose.

 PEDIATRIC POINTERS

Syncope is much less common in children than in adults. It may result from a cardiac or neurologic disorder, allergy, or emotional stress.

PATIENT COUNSELING
Advise the patient to pace his activities, to rise slowly from a recumbent position, to avoid standing still for a prolonged time, and to sit or lie down as soon as he feels faint.

SYNCOPE

HPI

Focused PE: Cardiovascular, respiratory, and hematologic systems

AORTIC ARCH SYNDROME (TAKAYASU'S ARTERITIS)
Signs and symptoms
- Weak or abruptly absent carotid pulses and unequal or absent radial pulses
- Night sweats
- Pallor
- Anorexia
- Nausea
- Weight loss
- Arthralgia
- Raynaud's phenomenon

DX: PE, labs (CBC, ESR), angiography

TX: Medication (corticosteroids, anticoagulants), surgery

F/U: Referral to cardiovascular surgeon

CARDIAC ARRHYTHMIA
Signs and symptoms
- Paroxysmal or sustained palpitations
- Dizziness
- Weakness
- Fatigue
- Irregular, rapid, or slow pulse rate
- Normal or decreased BP
- Confusion
- Pallor

DX: PE, labs (electrolytes, cardiac enzymes), ECG, Holter monitor

TX: Varies based on type of arrhythmia

F/U: As needed (dependent on type of arrhythmia), referral to cardiologist if uncontrollable

TIA
Signs and symptoms (temporary)
- Decreased LOC
- Confusion
- Unilateral hemiparesis
- Homonymous hemianopia (usually on the right side)
- Paresthesia
- Slurred speech
- Loss of sensation

DX: History of illness, imaging studies (carotid ultrasound, MRI, MRA, CT scan, echocardiogram, angiography)

TX: Airway stabilization, reduction of risk factors for stroke, surgery

F/U: Referral to neurologist or neurosurgeon

ORTHOSTATIC HYPOTENSION
Signs and symptoms
- Syncope after rising quickly
- BP drop of 10 to 20 mm Hg with position change
- Tachycardia
- Pallor
- Dizziness
- Blurred vision
- Nausea
- Diaphoresis

DX: History, vital signs

TX: Treatment of underlying cause, fluid replacement

F/U: As needed (based on reoccurrence)

Additional differential diagnoses: aortic stenosis ▪ carotid sinus hypersensitivity ▪ hypoxemia ▪ vagal glossopharyngeal neuralgia

Other causes: drugs, such as quinidine, prazosin, griseofulvin, levodopa, and indomethacin

T Tachycardia

Easily detected by counting the apical, carotid, or radial pulse, tachycardia is a heart rate greater than 100 beats/minute. The patient with tachycardia usually complains of palpitations or of a "racing" heart. (See *What happens in tachycardia.*) This common sign normally occurs in response to emotional or physical stress, such as excitement, exercise, pain, and fever. It may also result from the use of stimulants, such as caffeine and tobacco. However, tachycardia may be an early sign of a life-threatening disorder, such as cardiogenic, hypovolemic, or septic shock. It may also result from cardiovascular, respiratory, or metabolic disorders and from the effects of certain drugs, tests, and treatments.

 ALERT

After detecting tachycardia:
- *obtain an electrocardiogram or place the patient on a cardiac monitor to evaluate the heart rhythm*
- *take the patient's other vital signs, and determine his level of consciousness.*

   If the patient's condition permits, perform a focused assessment.

HISTORY
- Ask the patient if he has had palpitations before. If so, how were they treated?
- Ask the patient about associated signs and symptoms, such as shortness of breath, feeling weak or fatigued, or chest pain.
- Review the patient's medical history for trauma, diabetes, and cardiac, pulmonary, or thyroid disorders.
- Obtain a drug history, including prescription and over-the-counter drugs, herbal remedies, and recreational drugs. Also, ask the patient about alcohol intake.

PHYSICAL ASSESSMENT
- Inspect the skin for pallor or cyanosis.
- Assess pulses, noting peripheral edema.
- Auscultate the heart and lungs for abnormal sounds or rhythms.

SPECIAL CONSIDERATIONS
Various drugs such as diet pills affect the nervous system, circulatory system, or heart muscle, resulting in tachycardia.

[A] *PEDIATRIC POINTERS*
- *When examining a child for tachycardia, recognize that normal heart rates for children are higher than those for adults.*
- *In children, tachycardia may result from any one of the many adult causes described above.*

PATIENT COUNSELING
Instruct the patient on what to expect from diagnostic testing, which may include blood work, pulmonary function studies, and electrocardiography.

WHAT HAPPENS IN TACHYCARDIA

Tachycardia represents the heart's effort to deliver more oxygen to body tissues by increasing the rate at which blood passes through the vessels. This sign can reflect overstimulation within the sinoatrial node, the atrium, the atrioventricular node, or the ventricles.

Because heart rate affects cardiac output (cardiac output = heart rate × stroke volume), tachycardia can lower cardiac output by reducing ventricular filling time and stroke volume (the output of each ventricle at every contraction). As cardiac output plummets, arterial pressure and peripheral perfusion decrease. Tachycardia further aggravates myocardial ischemia by increasing the heart's demand for oxygen while reducing the duration of diastole—the period of greatest coronary flow.

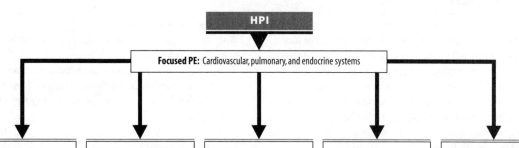

TACHYCARDIA

HPI

Focused PE: Cardiovascular, pulmonary, and endocrine systems

CARDIAC ARRHYTHMIA
Signs and symptoms
- Palpitations
- Chest pain
- SOB
- Diaphoresis
- Hypotension
- Dizziness
- Weakness
- Fatigue

DX: PE, ECG, electrophysiology study, labs (serum chemistry, digoxin level, cardiac enzymes, troponin)
TX: Varies based on the type of arrhythmia and the underlying cause, antiarrhythmic if needed, cardioversion
F/U: Referral to cardiologist if treatment is ineffective

ANXIETY
Signs and symptoms
- Intermittent, sharp, stabbing pain behind the breast bone
- Precordial tenderness
- Palpitations
- Fatigue
- Headache
- Insomnia
- Nausea and vomiting
- Breathlessness
- Tachypnea
- Diarrhea
- Tremors

DX: Labs (CBC, UA, thyroid studies), psychological testing
TX: Medication (based on the type of anxiety disorder; benzodiazepines, SSRIs, azapirones, TCAs), psychological counseling, exercise program
F/U: Regular office visits, referral to psychologist

HHNS
Signs and symptoms
- Rapidly deteriorating LOC
- Hypotension
- Seizure disorder
- Oliguria
- Dehydration

DX: Labs (serum electrolytes, ABG)
TX: I.V. normal saline solution infusion, I.V. insulin, frequent blood glucose monitoring
F/U: Referral to endocrinologist

THYROTOXICOSIS
Signs and symptoms
- Ptosis
- Progressive exophthalmus
- Increased tearing
- Visual changes
- Lid edema
- Lid lag
- Photophobia
- Enlarged thyroid
- Nervousness
- Heat intolerance
- Weight loss
- Tremors
- Palpitation
- Dyspnea

DX: PE, thyroid function studies, thyroid scan
TX: Medication (antithyroid therapy, radioiodine, beta-adrenergic blockers)
F/U: Thyroid function testing 6 weeks after treatment is initiated, then biannually if at euthyroid state

ANEMIA
Signs and symptoms
- Fatigue
- Weakness
- Pallor
- Dyspnea
- Postural hypotension
- Atrial gallop

DX: PE, CBC
TX: Treatment of underlying cause, medication (iron supplements, PRBC if indicated), diet modification
F/U: Regular checkups

Additional differential diagnoses: adrenocortical insufficiency ▪ ARDS ▪ alcohol withdrawal syndrome ▪ anaphylactic shock ▪ aortic insufficiency ▪ aortic stenosis ▪ cardiac contusion ▪ cardiac tamponade ▪ cardiogenic shock ▪ COPD ▪ diabetic ketoacidosis ▪ febrile illness ▪ heart failure ▪ hypertensive crisis ▪ hypoglycemia ▪ hyponatremia ▪ hypovolemia ▪ hypovolemic shock ▪ hypoxemia ▪ MI ▪ myocardial ischemia ▪ neurogenic shock ▪ orthostatic hypotension ▪ pheochromocytoma ▪ pneumothorax ▪ pulmonary edema ▪ pulmonary embolism ▪ septic shock

Other causes: alcohol ▪ cardiac catheterization ▪ cardiac surgery ▪ drugs (sympathomimetics, phenothiazines, anticholinergics, thyroid drugs, vasodilators, acetylcholinesterase inhibitors, nitrates, alpha-adrenergic blockers) ▪ electrophysiologic studies ▪ excessive caffeine intake ▪ pacemaker malfunction ▪ smoking

Tachypnea

A common sign of a cardiopulmonary disorder, tachypnea is an abnormally fast respiratory rate — 20 breaths/minute or more. Tachypnea may reflect the need to increase minute volume — the amount of air breathed each minute. Under these circumstances, it may be accompanied by an increase in tidal volume — the volume of air inhaled or exhaled per breath — resulting in hyperventilation. However, tachypnea may also reflect stiff lungs or overloaded ventilatory muscles, in which case tidal volume may actually be reduced.

Tachypnea may result from reduced arterial oxygen tension or arterial oxygen content, decreased perfusion, or increased oxygen demand. Heightened oxygen demand, for example, may result from fever, exertion, anxiety, and pain. It may also occur as a compensatory response to metabolic acidosis or may result from pulmonary irritation, stretch receptor stimulation, or a neurologic disorder that upsets medullary respiratory control. Generally, respirations increase by 4 breaths/minute for every 1° F (0.6° C) increase in body temperature.

▲ ALERT

After detecting tachypnea:
- *quickly evaluate cardiopulmonary status; check for cyanosis, chest pain, dyspnea, tachycardia, and hypotension*
- *administer oxygen, if appropriate*
- *institute emergency measures, if necessary.*
  If the patient's condition permits, perform a focused assessment.

HISTORY
- Ask the patient when the tachypnea began. Did it follow activity? Has he experienced tachypnea before?
- Ask the patient about associated signs and symptoms, such as diaphoresis, pain, and recent weight loss.
- Ask the patient if he's anxious about anything or has a history of anxiety attacks.
- Obtain a drug history, including prescription and over-the-counter drugs, herbal remedies, and recreational drugs. Note whether he's taking analgesics. If so, how effective are they? Also, ask the patient about alcohol intake.

PHYSICAL ASSESSMENT
- Take the patient's vital signs.
- Observe his overall behavior. Note if he seems restless.
- Auscultate the chest for abnormal heart and breath sounds. If the patient has a productive cough, record the color, amount, and consistency of sputum.
- Check for jugular vein distention, and examine the skin for pallor, cyanosis, edema, and warmth or coolness.
- Obtain a pulse oximetry reading.

SPECIAL CONSIDERATIONS
Tachypnea may result from an overdose of salicylates.

 PEDIATRIC POINTERS
- *When assessing a child for tachypnea, be aware that the normal respiratory rate varies with the child's age.*
- *If you detect tachypnea, consider these pediatric causes: congenital heart defects, meningitis, metabolic acidosis, and cystic fibrosis. Keep in mind, however, that hunger and anxiety may also cause tachypnea.*

▲ AGING ISSUES
Tachypnea can have various causes in elderly patients, and mild increases in respiratory rate may go unnoticed.

PATIENT COUNSELING
Reassure the patient that slight increases in respiratory rate may be normal. Instruct the patient on what to expect from diagnostic testing, which may include arterial blood gas analysis, chest X-rays, and an electrocardiogram.

TACHYPNEA

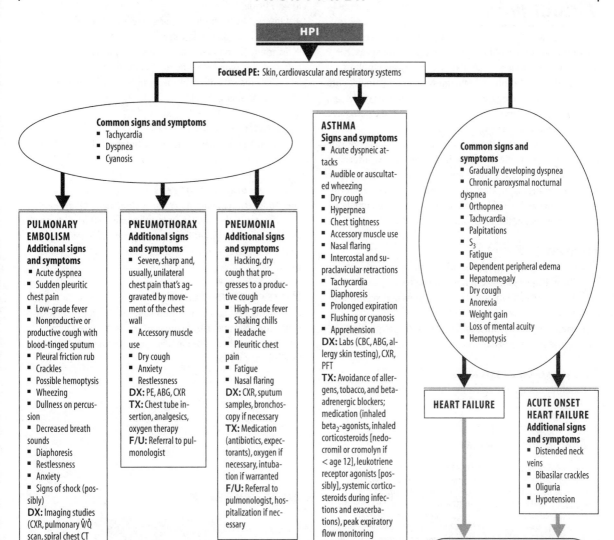

HPI

Focused PE: Skin, cardiovascular and respiratory systems

Common signs and symptoms
- Tachycardia
- Dyspnea
- Cyanosis

PULMONARY EMBOLISM
Additional signs and symptoms
- Acute dyspnea
- Sudden pleuritic chest pain
- Low-grade fever
- Nonproductive or productive cough with blood-tinged sputum
- Pleural friction rub
- Crackles
- Possible hemoptysis
- Wheezing
- Dullness on percussion
- Decreased breath sounds
- Diaphoresis
- Restlessness
- Anxiety
- Signs of shock (possibly)
DX: Imaging studies (CXR, pulmonary V̇/Q̇ scan, spiral chest CT scan, pulmonary angiography), ECG
TX: Oxygen therapy, medication (anticoagulants, thrombolytic therapy)
F/U: Return visit within first week after hospitalization

PNEUMOTHORAX
Additional signs and symptoms
- Severe, sharp and, usually, unilateral chest pain that's aggravated by movement of the chest wall
- Accessory muscle use
- Dry cough
- Anxiety
- Restlessness
DX: PE, ABG, CXR
TX: Chest tube insertion, analgesics, oxygen therapy
F/U: Referral to pulmonologist

PNEUMONIA
Additional signs and symptoms
- Hacking, dry cough that progresses to a productive cough
- High-grade fever
- Shaking chills
- Headache
- Pleuritic chest pain
- Fatigue
- Nasal flaring
DX: CXR, sputum samples, bronchoscopy if necessary
TX: Medication (antibiotics, expectorants), oxygen if necessary, intubation if warranted
F/U: Referral to pulmonologist, hospitalization if necessary

ASTHMA
Signs and symptoms
- Acute dyspneic attacks
- Audible or auscultated wheezing
- Dry cough
- Hyperpnea
- Chest tightness
- Accessory muscle use
- Nasal flaring
- Intercostal and supraclavicular retractions
- Tachycardia
- Diaphoresis
- Prolonged expiration
- Flushing or cyanosis
- Apprehension
DX: Labs (CBC, ABG, allergy skin testing), CXR, PFT
TX: Avoidance of allergens, tobacco, and beta-adrenergic blockers; medication (inhaled beta$_2$-agonists, inhaled corticosteroids [nedocromil or cromolyn if < age 12], leukotriene receptor agonists [possibly], systemic corticosteroids during infections and exacerbations), peak expiratory flow monitoring
F/U: For acute exacerbation, return visit within 24 hours, then every 3 to 5 days, and then every 1 to 3 months; referral to pulmonologist if treatment is ineffective

Common signs and symptoms
- Gradually developing dyspnea
- Chronic paroxysmal nocturnal dyspnea
- Orthopnea
- Tachycardia
- Palpitations
- S$_3$
- Fatigue
- Dependent peripheral edema
- Hepatomegaly
- Dry cough
- Anorexia
- Weight gain
- Loss of mental acuity
- Hemoptysis

HEART FAILURE

ACUTE ONSET HEART FAILURE
Additional signs and symptoms
- Distended neck veins
- Bibasilar crackles
- Oliguria
- Hypotension

DX: Labs (CBC, cardiac enzymes, troponin), imaging studies (CXR, echocardiogram), ECG
TX: Medication (ACE inhibitors, diuretics, carvedilol [possibly], digoxin [possibly])
F/U: Return visit within 1 week after discharge, at 4 weeks, and then every 3 months; referral to cardiologist if condition is chronic

---

Additional differential diagnoses: abdominal pain ▪ anaphylactic shock ▪ anemia ▪ ARDS ▪ ascites ▪ bronchiectasis ▪ bronchitis (chronic) ▪ cardiac arrhythmias ▪ cardiac tamponade ▪ cardiogenic shock ▪ chest trauma ▪ COPD ▪ emphysema ▪ febrile illness ▪ flail chest ▪ foreign body aspiration ▪ head trauma ▪ hepatic failure ▪ HHNS ▪ hypovolemic shock ▪ hypoxia ▪ interstitial fibrosis ▪ lung abscess ▪ lung, pleural, or mediastinal tumor ▪ mesothelioma (malignant) ▪ neurogenic shock ▪ pancreatitis ▪ pleural effusion ▪ pulmonary edema ▪ pulmonary hypertension ▪ septic shock

Other cause: salicylates

Throat pain

Throat pain—commonly known as a sore throat—refers to discomfort in any part of the pharynx: the nasopharynx, the oropharynx, or the hypopharynx. This common symptom ranges from a sensation of scratchiness to severe pain. It's commonly accompanied by ear pain because cranial nerves IX and X innervate the pharynx as well as the middle and external ear. (See *Anatomy of the throat.*)

Throat pain may result from infection, trauma, allergy, cancer, or certain systemic disorders. It may also follow surgery and endotracheal intubation. Nonpathologic causes include dry mucous membranes associated with mouth breathing and laryngeal irritation associated with alcohol consumption, inhalation of smoke or chemicals such as ammonia, and vocal strain.

HISTORY

● Ask the patient when he first noticed the pain, and have him describe it. Has he ever had throat pain before?
● Ask the patient about accompanying signs and symptoms, such as fever, ear pain, or dysphagia.
● Review the patient's medical history for throat problems, allergies, and systemic disorders.

PHYSICAL ASSESSMENT

● Carefully examine the pharynx, noting redness, exudate, or swelling.

● Examine the oropharynx, using a warmed metal spatula or tongue blade.
● Observe the tonsils for redness, swelling, or exudate. In addition, obtain an exudate specimen for culture.
● Examine the nose, using a nasal speculum. Also, check the patient's ears, especially if he reports ear pain.
● Palpate the patient's neck and oropharynx for nodules or lymph node enlargement.

SPECIAL CONSIDERATIONS

Provide analgesic sprays or lozenges to relieve throat pain, as ordered.

Ⓐ PEDIATRIC POINTERS

Sore throat is a common complaint in children and may result from any one of the many disorders that affect adults. Other pediatric causes of sore throat include acute epiglottitis, herpangina, scarlet fever, acute follicular tonsillitis, and retropharyngeal abscess.

PATIENT COUNSELING

If the patient is taking an antibiotic, stress the importance of completing the prescribed course of treatment, even if symptoms improve after a few days. Suggest gargling with salt water to soothe the throat.

ANATOMY OF THE THROAT

The throat, or pharynx, is divided into three areas: the nasopharynx (the soft palate and the posterior nasal cavity), the oropharynx (the area between the soft palate and the upper edge of the epiglottis), and the hypopharynx (the area between the epiglottis and the level of the cricoid cartilage). A disorder affecting any of these areas may cause throat pain. Pinpointing the causative disorder begins with accurate assessment of the throat structures illustrated here.

FRONTAL VIEW

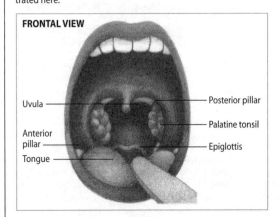

CROSS-SECTIONAL VIEW

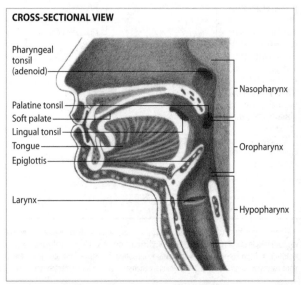

THROAT PAIN

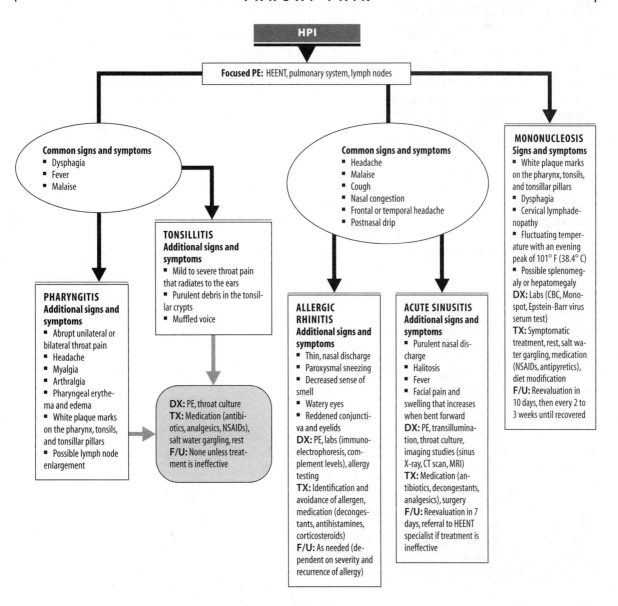

HPI

Focused PE: HEENT, pulmonary system, lymph nodes

Common signs and symptoms
- Dysphagia
- Fever
- Malaise

TONSILLITIS
Additional signs and symptoms
- Mild to severe throat pain that radiates to the ears
- Purulent debris in the tonsillar crypts
- Muffled voice

PHARYNGITIS
Additional signs and symptoms
- Abrupt unilateral or bilateral throat pain
- Headache
- Myalgia
- Arthralgia
- Pharyngeal erythema and edema
- White plaque marks on the pharynx, tonsils, and tonsillar pillars
- Possible lymph node enlargement

DX: PE, throat culture
TX: Medication (antibiotics, analgesics, NSAIDs), salt water gargling, rest
F/U: None unless treatment is ineffective

Common signs and symptoms
- Headache
- Malaise
- Cough
- Nasal congestion
- Frontal or temporal headache
- Postnasal drip

ALLERGIC RHINITIS
Additional signs and symptoms
- Thin, nasal discharge
- Paroxysmal sneezing
- Decreased sense of smell
- Watery eyes
- Reddened conjunctiva and eyelids
DX: PE, labs (immunoelectrophoresis, complement levels), allergy testing
TX: Identification and avoidance of allergen, medication (decongestants, antihistamines, corticosteroids)
F/U: As needed (dependent on severity and recurrence of allergy)

ACUTE SINUSITIS
Additional signs and symptoms
- Purulent nasal discharge
- Halitosis
- Fever
- Facial pain and swelling that increases when bent forward
DX: PE, transillumination, throat culture, imaging studies (sinus X-ray, CT scan, MRI)
TX: Medication (antibiotics, decongestants, analgesics), surgery
F/U: Reevaluation in 7 days, referral to HEENT specialist if treatment is ineffective

MONONUCLEOSIS
Signs and symptoms
- White plaque marks on the pharynx, tonsils, and tonsillar pillars
- Dysphagia
- Cervical lymphadenopathy
- Fluctuating temperature with an evening peak of 101° F (38.4° C)
- Possible splenomegaly or hepatomegaly
DX: Labs (CBC, Monospot, Epstein-Barr virus serum test)
TX: Symptomatic treatment, rest, salt water gargling, medication (NSAIDs, antipyretics), diet modification
F/U: Reevaluation in 10 days, then every 2 to 3 weeks until recovered

Additional differential diagnoses: agranulocytosis ▪ bronchitis (acute) ▪ chronic fatigue syndrome ▪ contact ulcers ▪ eagle's syndrome ▪ foreign body ▪ glossopharyngeal neuralgia ▪ herpes simplex virus ▪ influenza ▪ laryngeal cancer ▪ laryngitis (acute) ▪ necrotizing ulcerative gingivitis (acute) ▪ peritonsillar abscess ▪ pharyngomaxillary space abscess ▪ reflux laryngopharyngitis ▪ tongue cancer ▪ tonsillar cancer ▪ uvulitis ▪ viral infection

Other causes: endotracheal intubation ▪ local surgery (tonsillectomy, adenoidectomy)

Thyroid enlargement

An enlarged thyroid can result from inflammation, physiologic changes, iodine deficiency, or a thyroid tumor. Depending on the medical cause, hyperfunction or hypofunction may occur with resulting excess or deficiency, respectively, of the hormone thyroxine. If no infection is present, enlargement is usually slow and progressive. An enlarged thyroid that causes visible swelling in the front of the neck is called a goiter.

HISTORY

- Ask the patient when the thyroid enlargement began.
- Review the patient's medical history for irradiation of the thyroid or the neck, recent infections, and the use of thyroid replacement drugs.
- Ask the patient if he has a family history of thyroid disease.
- Review the patient's diet, especially food ingested prior to thyroid enlargement.

PHYSICAL ASSESSMENT

- Inspect the trachea for midline deviation.
- Palpate the thyroid gland. During palpation, be sure to note the size, shape, and consistency of the gland and the presence or absence of nodules. (See *Palpating the thyroid gland.*)
- Using the bell of a stethoscope, listen over the lateral lobes for a bruit. The bruit is commonly continuous.

SPECIAL CONSIDERATIONS

Goitrogens are drugs and substances in foods that decrease thyroxine production. Goitrogenic drugs include lithium, sulfonamides, phenylbutazone, and para-aminosalicylic acid. Foods containing goitrogens include peanuts, cabbage, soybeans, strawberries, spinach, rutabagas, and radishes.

A   *PEDIATRIC POINTERS*

Congenital goiter, a syndrome of infantile myxedema or cretinism, is characterized by mental retardation, growth failure, and other signs and symptoms of hypothyroidism. Early treatment can prevent mental retardation. Genetic counseling is important because subsequent children are at risk.

PATIENT COUNSELING

Instruct the patient to watch for signs and symptoms of hypothyroidism, such as lethargy, restlessness, dry skin, and sensitivity to the cold. After thyroidectomy or radioactive destruction of the thyroid gland, explain to the patient that lifelong thyroid hormone replacement therapy is necessary. Tell him to watch for signs and symptoms of overdose, such as nervousness and palpitations.

PALPATING THE THYROID GLAND

To palpate the thyroid gland, you'll need to stand in front of or behind the patient. Give the patient a cup of water, and have him extend his neck slightly. Place the fingers of both hands on the patient's neck, just below the cricoid cartilage and just lateral to the trachea. Tell the patient to take a sip of water and swallow. The thyroid gland should rise as he swallows. Use your fingers to palpate laterally and downward to feel the whole thyroid gland. Palpate over the midline to feel the isthmus of the thyroid.

THYROID ENLARGEMENT

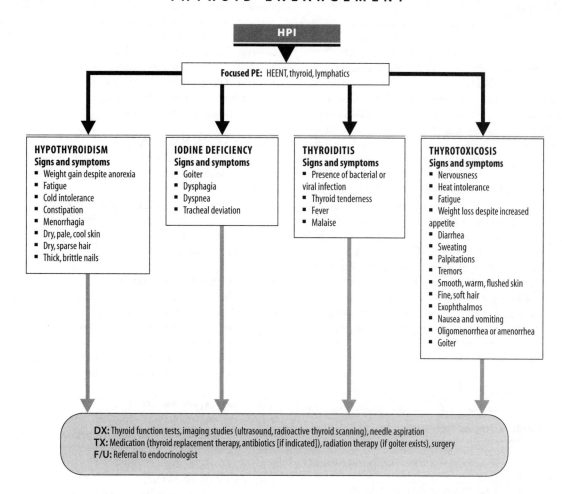

HPI

Focused PE: HEENT, thyroid, lymphatics

HYPOTHYROIDISM
Signs and symptoms
- Weight gain despite anorexia
- Fatigue
- Cold intolerance
- Constipation
- Menorrhagia
- Dry, pale, cool skin
- Dry, sparse hair
- Thick, brittle nails

IODINE DEFICIENCY
Signs and symptoms
- Goiter
- Dysphagia
- Dyspnea
- Tracheal deviation

THYROIDITIS
Signs and symptoms
- Presence of bacterial or viral infection
- Thyroid tenderness
- Fever
- Malaise

THYROTOXICOSIS
Signs and symptoms
- Nervousness
- Heat intolerance
- Fatigue
- Weight loss despite increased appetite
- Diarrhea
- Sweating
- Palpitations
- Tremors
- Smooth, warm, flushed skin
- Fine, soft hair
- Exophthalmos
- Nausea and vomiting
- Oligomenorrhea or amenorrhea
- Goiter

DX: Thyroid function tests, imaging studies (ultrasound, radioactive thyroid scanning), needle aspiration
TX: Medication (thyroid replacement therapy, antibiotics [if indicated]), radiation therapy (if goiter exists), surgery
F/U: Referral to endocrinologist

Additional differential diagnosis: tumor

Other causes: drugs (lithium, sulfonamides, phenylbutazone, para-aminosalicylic acid) ▪ foods containing goitrogens (peanuts, cabbage, soybeans, strawberries, spinach, rutabagas, radishes)

Tinnitus

Tinnitus literally means ringing in the ears, although many other abnormal sounds fall under this term. For example, tinnitus may be described as the sound of escaping air, running water, or the inside of a seashell or as a sizzling, buzzing, or humming noise. Occasionally, it's described as a roaring or musical sound. This common symptom may be unilateral or bilateral and constant or intermittent. Although the brain can adjust to or suppress constant tinnitus, intermittent tinnitus may be so disturbing that some patients contemplate suicide as their only source of relief.

Tinnitus can be classified in several ways. *Subjective tinnitus* is heard only by the patient; *objective tinnitus* is also heard by the observer who places a stethoscope near the patient's affected ear. *Tinnitus aurium* refers to noise that the patient hears in his ears; *tinnitus cerebri,* to noise that he hears in his head.

Tinnitus is usually associated with neural injury within the auditory pathway, resulting in altered, spontaneous firing of sensory auditory neurons. Commonly resulting from an ear disorder, tinnitus may also stem from a cardiovascular or systemic disorder or from the effects of a drug. Nonpathologic causes of tinnitus include acute anxiety and presbycusis. (See *Common causes of tinnitus.*)

HISTORY

- Ask the patient to describe the sound he hears, including its onset, pattern, pitch, location, and intensity.
- Ask the patient about associated signs and symptoms, such as vertigo, headache, and hearing loss.
- Ask the patient about other illnesses or disorders.
- Obtain a drug history, including prescription and over-the-counter drugs, herbal remedies, and recreational drugs. Also, ask the patient about alcohol intake.

PHYSICAL ASSESSMENT

- Using an otoscope, inspect the patient's ears and examine the tympanic membrane. To check for hearing loss, perform the Weber's and Rinne tests.
- Auscultate for bruits in the neck. Then compress the jugular or carotid artery to see if this affects the tinnitus.
- Examine the nasopharynx for masses that might cause eustachian tube dysfunction and tinnitus.

SPECIAL CONSIDERATIONS

Be aware that tinnitus usually can't be treated successfully. To help the patient tolerate this symptom, you may need to provide a vasodilator, a tranquilizer, or an anticonvulsant, or encourage the use of biofeedback and tinnitus maskers. A tinnitus masker produces a band of noise measuring about 1800 Hz, which helps block out tinnitus without interfering with hearing.

A   PEDIATRIC POINTERS

An expectant mother's use of ototoxic drugs during the third trimester of pregnancy can cause labyrinthine damage in the fetus, resulting in tinnitus.

PATIENT COUNSELING

Advise the patient to avoid exposure to excessive noise, ototoxic agents, and other factors that may cause cochlear damage. Inform him that even persons with normal hearing may experience intermittent periods of mild, high-pitched tinnitus that can last for several minutes.

COMMON CAUSES OF TINNITUS

Tinnitus usually results from disorders that affect the external, middle, or inner ear. Below are some of its more common causes and their locations.

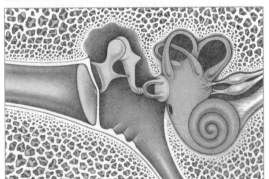

External ear
- Ear canal obstruction by cerumen or a foreign body
- Otitis externa
- Tympanic membrane perforation

Middle ear
- Ossicle dislocation
- Otitis media
- Otosclerosis

Inner ear
- Acoustic neuroma
- Atherosclerosis of the carotid artery
- Labyrinthitis
- Ménière's disease

TINNITUS

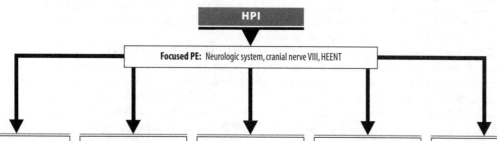

HPI

Focused PE: Neurologic system, cranial nerve VIII, HEENT

ACOUSTIC NEUROMA
Signs and symptoms
- Unilateral tinnitus
- Unilateral sensorineural hearing loss and vertigo
- Facial paralysis
- Headache
- Nausea and vomiting

DX: Otoscopic examination, CT scan
TX: Surgery
F/U: Referral to a neurologist

ATHEROSCLEROSIS OF CAROTID ARTERY
Signs and symptoms
- Constant tinnitus
- Confused, weak, and unsteady in the morning and upon arising quickly
- Possible carotid bruit

DX: Auscultation of the carotid arteries, carotid ultrasound
TX: Surgery, medication (antiplatelets, anticoagulants)
F/U: Referral to vascular surgeon or neurosurgeon

EAR CANAL OBSTRUCTION
Signs and symptoms
- Conductive hearing loss
- Ear canal itching
- Feeling of fullness or pain in the ear

DX: Otoscopic examination
TX: Removal of cerumen or obstruction
F/U: Referral to otolaryngologist

HYPERTENSION
Signs and symptoms
- Bilateral high-pitched tinnitus
- Systolic BP > 140 mm Hg, diastolic BP > 90 mm Hg
- Headache
- Retinopathy
- Fatigue
- Anxiety
- Blurred vision
- Signs and symptoms of underlying disorder (if any)

DX: History of risk factors, sustained elevated BP, test for suspected underlying disorder, labs (CBC, electrolytes, cholesterol)
TX: Treatment of underlying cause (if any); reduction of controllable risk factors; low-fat, low-salt diet; medication (diuretics, alpha-adrenergic blockers, ACE inhibitors, angiotensin II receptor blocker, calcium channel blockers, beta-adrenergic blockers)
F/U: When stable, checkups every 3 to 6 months

INTRACRANIAL ARTERIOVENOUS MALFORMATION
Signs and symptoms
- Pulsating tinnitus
- Bruit over the mastoid process

DX: CT scan
TX: Surgery
F/U: Referral to neurosurgeon

Additional differential diagnoses: anemia ▪ cervical spondylosis ▪ glomus jugulare or tympanicum tumor ▪ labyrinthitis ▪ Ménière's disease ▪ ossicle dislocation ▪ otitis externa ▪ otitis media ▪ otosclerosis ▪ palatal myoclonus ▪ tympanic membrane perforation

Other causes: alcohol ▪ drugs ▪ loud noise

Tracheal deviation

Normally, the trachea is located at the midline of the neck—except at the bifurcation, where it shifts slightly toward the right. Visible deviation from its normal position signals an underlying condition that can compromise pulmonary function and possibly cause respiratory distress. A hallmark of life-threatening tension pneumothorax, tracheal deviation occurs in disorders that produce mediastinal shift due to asymmetrical thoracic volume or pressure. A nonlesional pneumothorax can produce tracheal deviation to the ipsilateral side. (See *Detecting slight tracheal deviation*.)

 ALERT

If you detect tracheal deviation:
- *be alert for signs and symptoms of respiratory distress, such as tachypnea, dyspnea, decreased or absent breath sounds, stridor, nasal flaring, accessory muscle use, asymmetrical chest expansion, restlessness, and anxiety.*
- *place the patient in semi-Fowler's position, and give supplemental oxygen*
- *institute emergency measures, if necessary.*
    If the patient's condition permits, perform a focused assessment.

HISTORY
- Review the patient's medical history for pulmonary or cardiac disorders, trauma, and infection.

- Ask the patient if he smokes. If he does, ask him how many packs of cigarettes he smokes per year.
- Ask the patient about associated signs and symptoms, especially breathing difficulties, pain, and cough.

PHYSICAL ASSESSMENT
- Auscultate the chest, and note adventitious or absent breath sounds. Observe for asymmetrical chest expansion.
- Palpate for subcutaneous crepitation in the neck and chest.
- Obtain a pulse oximetry or arterial blood gas analysis.
- Palpate for subcutaneous crepitation in the neck and chest, a sign of tension pneumothorax.

SPECIAL CONSIDERATIONS
Because tracheal deviation usually signals a severe underlying disorder that can cause respiratory distress at any time, monitor the patient's respiratory and cardiac status constantly, and make sure that emergency equipment is readily available.

 PEDIATRIC POINTERS

Keep in mind that respiratory distress commonly develops more rapidly in children than in adults.

 AGING ISSUES

In elderly persons, tracheal deviation to the right commonly stems from an elongated, atherosclerotic aortic arch; however, this deviation isn't considered abnormal.

PATIENT COUNSELING
Instruct the patient on what to expect from diagnostic testing, which may include chest X-rays, electrocardiogram, and arterial blood gas analysis.

DETECTING SLIGHT TRACHEAL DEVIATION

Although gross tracheal deviation is visible, detection of slight deviation requires palpation and perhaps even an X-ray. Try palpation first.

With the tip of you index finger, locate the patient's trachea by palpating between the sternocleidomastoid muscles. Then compare the trachea's position with an imaginary line drawn vertically through the suprasternal notch. Any deviation from midline is usually considered abnormal.

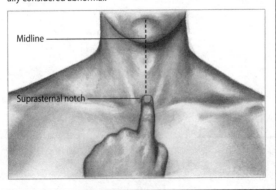

Midline

Suprasternal notch

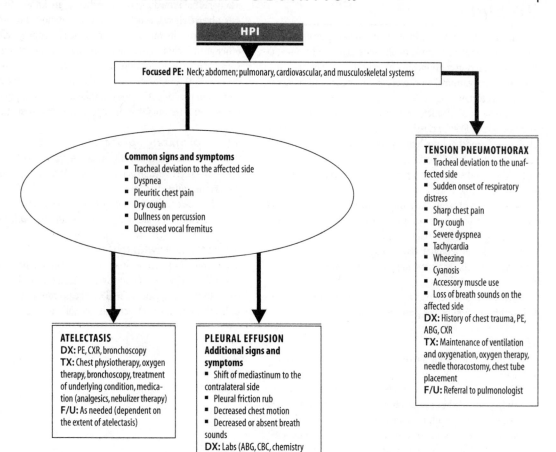

HPI

Focused PE: Neck; abdomen; pulmonary, cardiovascular, and musculoskeletal systems

Common signs and symptoms
- Tracheal deviation to the affected side
- Dyspnea
- Pleuritic chest pain
- Dry cough
- Dullness on percussion
- Decreased vocal fremitus

TENSION PNEUMOTHORAX
- Tracheal deviation to the unaffected side
- Sudden onset of respiratory distress
- Sharp chest pain
- Dry cough
- Severe dyspnea
- Tachycardia
- Wheezing
- Cyanosis
- Accessory muscle use
- Loss of breath sounds on the affected side

DX: History of chest trauma, PE, ABG, CXR
TX: Maintenance of ventilation and oxygenation, oxygen therapy, needle thoracostomy, chest tube placement
F/U: Referral to pulmonologist

ATELECTASIS
DX: PE, CXR, bronchoscopy
TX: Chest physiotherapy, oxygen therapy, bronchoscopy, treatment of underlying condition, medication (analgesics, nebulizer therapy)
F/U: As needed (dependent on the extent of atelectasis)

PLEURAL EFFUSION
Additional signs and symptoms
- Shift of mediastinum to the contralateral side
- Pleural friction rub
- Decreased chest motion
- Decreased or absent breath sounds

DX: Labs (ABG, CBC, chemistry profile, ESR, coagulation studies), CXR
TX: Pulse oximetry monitoring, chest physiotherapy, oxygen therapy, thoracentesis, chest tube placement
F/U: Referral to pulmonologist

Additional differential diagnoses: hiatal hernia ▪ kyphoscoliosis ▪ mediastinal tumor ▪ pulmonary fibrosis ▪ retrosternal thyroid ▪ thoracic aortic aneurysm

Tremors

The most common type of involuntary muscle movement, tremors are regular rhythmic oscillations that result from alternating contractions of opposing muscle groups. They're typical signs of extrapyramidal and cerebellar disorders and can also result from certain drugs.

Tremors can be characterized by their location, amplitude, and frequency. They're classified as resting, intention, or postural. *Resting tremors* occur when an extremity is at rest and subside with movement. They include the classic pill-rolling tremor of Parkinson's disease. Conversely, *intention tremors* occur only with movement and subside with rest. *Postural (or action) tremors* appear when an extremity or the trunk is actively held in a particular posture or position. A common type of postural tremor is called an essential tremor.

Tremorlike movements may also be elicited, such as asterixis—the characteristic flapping tremor seen in hepatic failure.

Stress or emotional upset tends to aggravate a tremor. Alcohol commonly diminishes postural tremors.

HISTORY

● Ask the patient about the tremor's onset. Was it sudden or gradual?
● Ask the patient about the tremor's duration and progression.
● Ask the patient about aggravating or alleviating factors. Does the tremor interfere with the patient's normal activities?
● Ask the patient about associated signs and symptoms, such as behavioral changes or memory loss. (The patient's family or friends may provide more accurate information on this.)
● Review the patient's medical history for neurologic, endocrine, and metabolic disorders, noting especially a history of seizures. Is there a family history of these disorders?
● Obtain a drug history, including prescription and over-the-counter drugs, herbal remedies, and recreational drugs. Especially note the use of phenothiazines. Also, ask the patient about alcohol intake.

PHYSICAL ASSESSMENT

● Assess the patient's overall appearance and demeanor, noting mental status.
● Test range of motion and strength in all major muscle groups, while observing the patient for chorea, athetosis, dystonia, and other involuntary movements.
● Check deep tendon reflexes and, if possible, observe the patient's gait.

SPECIAL CONSIDERATIONS

Many herbal remedies, such as ephedra, are known to have serious adverse effects, which may include tremors. Phenothiazines (particularly piperazine derivatives such as fluphenazine) and other antipsychotics may cause resting and pill-rolling tremors. Infrequently, metoclopramide and metyrosine also cause these tremors. Lithium toxicity, sympathomimetics (such as terbutaline and pseudoephedrine), amphetamines, and phenytoin can all cause tremors that disappear with dose reduction.

Ⓐ PEDIATRIC POINTERS

● *A healthy neonate may display coarse tremors with stiffening—an exaggerated hypocalcemic startle reflex—in response to noises and chills.*
● *Pediatric-specific causes of pathologic tremors include cerebral palsy, fetal alcohol syndrome, and maternal drug addiction.*

PATIENT COUNSELING

Severe intention tremors may interfere with the patient's ability to perform activities of daily living. Teach the family how to assist with these activities as well as take precautions against possible injury during such activities as walking or eating.

TREMORS

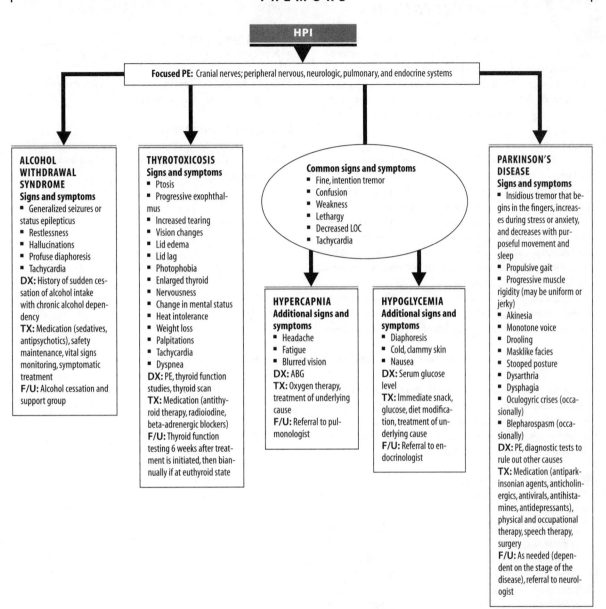

HPI

Focused PE: Cranial nerves; peripheral nervous, neurologic, pulmonary, and endocrine systems

ALCOHOL WITHDRAWAL SYNDROME
Signs and symptoms
- Generalized seizures or status epilepticus
- Restlessness
- Hallucinations
- Profuse diaphoresis
- Tachycardia

DX: History of sudden cessation of alcohol intake with chronic alcohol dependency

TX: Medication (sedatives, antipsychotics), safety maintenance, vital signs monitoring, symptomatic treatment

F/U: Alcohol cessation and support group

THYROTOXICOSIS
Signs and symptoms
- Ptosis
- Progressive exophthalmus
- Increased tearing
- Vision changes
- Lid edema
- Lid lag
- Photophobia
- Enlarged thyroid
- Nervousness
- Change in mental status
- Heat intolerance
- Weight loss
- Palpitations
- Tachycardia
- Dyspnea

DX: PE, thyroid function studies, thyroid scan

TX: Medication (antithyroid therapy, radioiodine, beta-adrenergic blockers)

F/U: Thyroid function testing 6 weeks after treatment is initiated, then biannually if at euthyroid state

Common signs and symptoms
- Fine, intention tremor
- Confusion
- Weakness
- Lethargy
- Decreased LOC
- Tachycardia

HYPERCAPNIA
Additional signs and symptoms
- Headache
- Fatigue
- Blurred vision

DX: ABG

TX: Oxygen therapy, treatment of underlying cause

F/U: Referral to pulmonologist

HYPOGLYCEMIA
Additional signs and symptoms
- Diaphoresis
- Cold, clammy skin
- Nausea

DX: Serum glucose level

TX: Immediate snack, glucose, diet modification, treatment of underlying cause

F/U: Referral to endocrinologist

PARKINSON'S DISEASE
Signs and symptoms
- Insidious tremor that begins in the fingers, increases during stress or anxiety, and decreases with purposeful movement and sleep
- Propulsive gait
- Progressive muscle rigidity (may be uniform or jerky)
- Akinesia
- Monotone voice
- Drooling
- Masklike facies
- Stooped posture
- Dysarthria
- Dysphagia
- Oculogyric crises (occasionally)
- Blepharospasm (occasionally)

DX: PE, diagnostic tests to rule out other causes

TX: Medication (antiparkinsonian agents, anticholinergics, antivirals, antihistamines, antidepressants), physical and occupational therapy, speech therapy, surgery

F/U: As needed (dependent on the stage of the disease), referral to neurologist

---

Additional differential diagnoses: alkalosis ▪ benign familial essential tumor ▪ cerebellar tumor ▪ general paresis ▪ kwashiorkor ▪ manganese toxicity ▪ multiple sclerosis ▪ porphyria ▪ thalamic syndrome ▪ Wernicke's disease ▪ West Nile encephalitis ▪ Wilson's disease

Other causes: herbal products (ephedra)

U Urinary frequency

Urinary frequency refers to increased incidence of the urge to void. Usually resulting from decreased bladder capacity, frequency is a cardinal sign of a urinary tract infection (UTI). However, it can also stem from another urologic disorder, neurologic dysfunction, or pressure on the bladder from a nearby tumor or from organ enlargement (as with pregnancy).

HISTORY

- Ask the patient about the onset and duration of his abnormal urinary frequency.
- Ask the patient how many times a day he voids. Ask him how this compares with his previous voiding pattern.
- Ask the patient about associated urinary signs and symptoms, such as dysuria, urinary urgency, urinary incontinence, hematuria, nocturia, and lower abdominal pain with urination.
- Ask the patient about neurologic symptoms, such as muscle weakness, numbness, or tingling.
- Review the patient's medical history for UTI, other urologic problems or recent urologic procedures, and neurologic disorders. With a male patient, note a history of prostatic enlargement.
- If the patient is a female of childbearing age, ask her whether she is or could be pregnant.
- Ask the patient about his typical fluid intake and if this amount has increased recently.
- Obtain a drug history, including prescription and over-the-counter drugs, herbal remedies, and recreational drugs. Also, ask the patient about alcohol intake.

PHYSICAL ASSESSMENT

- Obtain a clean-catch midstream urine sample for urinalysis, culture, and sensitivity tests.
- Palpate the suprapubic area, abdomen, and flanks, noting tenderness, if present.
- Examine the urethral meatus for redness, discharge, or swelling. In a male patient, palpate the prostate gland for enlargement or abnormalities.
- If the patient's medical history reveals symptoms or a history of a neurologic disorder, perform a neurologic examination.

SPECIAL CONSIDERATIONS

Excessive intake of coffee, tea, and other caffeine-containing beverages leads to urinary frequency.

[A] PEDIATRIC POINTERS

UTI is a common cause of urinary frequency in children, especially girls. Congenital anomalies that can cause UTI include a duplicated ureter, congenital bladder diverticulum, and an ectopic ureteral orifice.

AGING ISSUES

- *Men older than age 50 are prone to frequent non–sex-related UTIs.*
- *In postmenopausal women, decreased estrogen levels cause urinary frequency, urgency, and nocturia.*

PATIENT COUNSELING

Instruct sexually active patients in safe sex practices. Advise females to clean the genital area from front to back to reduce contamination by *Escherichia coli*.

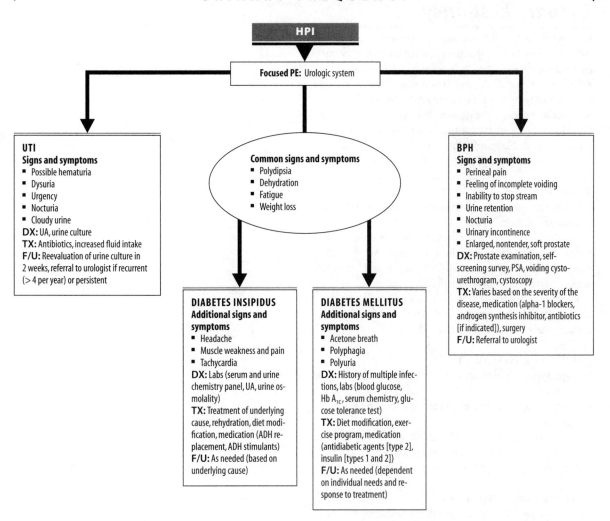

HPI

Focused PE: Urologic system

UTI
Signs and symptoms
- Possible hematuria
- Dysuria
- Urgency
- Nocturia
- Cloudy urine

DX: UA, urine culture
TX: Antibiotics, increased fluid intake
F/U: Reevaluation of urine culture in 2 weeks, referral to urologist if recurrent (> 4 per year) or persistent

Common signs and symptoms
- Polydipsia
- Dehydration
- Fatigue
- Weight loss

DIABETES INSIPIDUS
Additional signs and symptoms
- Headache
- Muscle weakness and pain
- Tachycardia

DX: Labs (serum and urine chemistry panel, UA, urine osmolality)
TX: Treatment of underlying cause, rehydration, diet modification, medication (ADH replacement, ADH stimulants)
F/U: As needed (based on underlying cause)

DIABETES MELLITUS
Additional signs and symptoms
- Acetone breath
- Polyphagia
- Polyuria

DX: History of multiple infections, labs (blood glucose, Hb A_{1c}, serum chemistry, glucose tolerance test)
TX: Diet modification, exercise program, medication (antidiabetic agents [type 2], insulin [types 1 and 2])
F/U: As needed (dependent on individual needs and response to treatment)

BPH
Signs and symptoms
- Perineal pain
- Feeling of incomplete voiding
- Inability to stop stream
- Urine retention
- Nocturia
- Urinary incontinence
- Enlarged, nontender, soft prostate

DX: Prostate examination, self-screening survey, PSA, voiding cysto-urethrogram, cystoscopy
TX: Varies based on the severity of the disease, medication (alpha-1 blockers, androgen synthesis inhibitor, antibiotics [if indicated]), surgery
F/U: Referral to urologist

Additional differential diagnoses: multiple sclerosis ▪ rectal tumor ▪ Reiter's syndrome ▪ reproductive tract tumor ▪ spinal cord lesion

Other causes: diuretics ▪ radiation therapy

Urinary hesitancy

Urinary hesitancy — difficulty starting a urine stream — can result from a urinary tract infection, a partial lower urinary tract obstruction, a neuromuscular disorder, or the use of certain drugs. Occurring at all ages and in both sexes, it's most common in older men with prostatic enlargement. It also occurs in women with tumors in the reproductive system, such as uterine fibroids or ovarian, uterine, or vaginal carcinoma. Hesitancy usually arises gradually, typically going unnoticed until urine retention causes bladder distention and discomfort.

HISTORY

● Ask the patient when he first noticed hesitancy and if he has ever had the problem before.
● Ask the patient about other urinary problems, especially reduced force or interruption of the urine stream. Ask the male patient if he has ever been treated for a prostate problem or for urinary tract infection or obstruction.
● Obtain a drug history, including prescription and over-the-counter drugs, herbal remedies, and recreational drugs. Also, ask the patient about alcohol intake.

PHYSICAL ASSESSMENT

● Inspect the urethral meatus for inflammation, discharge, and other abnormalities.
● Examine the anal sphincter, and test sensation in the perineum.
● Obtain a clean-catch sample for urinalysis.
● In a male patient, the prostate gland requires palpation. A female patient requires a gynecologic examination.

SPECIAL CONSIDERATIONS

Monitor the patient's voiding pattern, and frequently palpate for bladder distention. Apply local heat to the perineum or the abdomen to enhance muscle relaxation and aid urination.

[A] PEDIATRIC POINTERS

The most common cause of urinary obstruction in male infants is posterior strictures. Infants with this problem may have a less forceful urine stream and may also present with fever due to urinary tract infection, failure to thrive, or a palpable bladder.

PATIENT COUNSELING

Teach the patient how to perform a clean, intermittent self-catheterization. Instruct the patient on what to expect from diagnostic testing, which may include cystometrography and cystourethrography.

URINARY HESITANCY

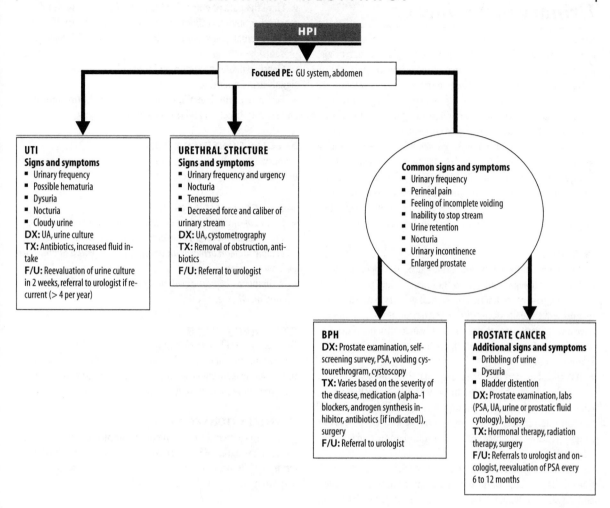

HPI

Focused PE: GU system, abdomen

UTI
Signs and symptoms
- Urinary frequency
- Possible hematuria
- Dysuria
- Nocturia
- Cloudy urine

DX: UA, urine culture
TX: Antibiotics, increased fluid intake
F/U: Reevaluation of urine culture in 2 weeks, referral to urologist if recurrent (> 4 per year)

URETHRAL STRICTURE
Signs and symptoms
- Urinary frequency and urgency
- Nocturia
- Tenesmus
- Decreased force and caliber of urinary stream

DX: UA, cystometrography
TX: Removal of obstruction, antibiotics
F/U: Referral to urologist

Common signs and symptoms
- Urinary frequency
- Perineal pain
- Feeling of incomplete voiding
- Inability to stop stream
- Urine retention
- Nocturia
- Urinary incontinence
- Enlarged prostate

BPH
DX: Prostate examination, self-screening survey, PSA, voiding cystourethrogram, cystoscopy
TX: Varies based on the severity of the disease, medication (alpha-1 blockers, androgen synthesis inhibitor, antibiotics [if indicated]), surgery
F/U: Referral to urologist

PROSTATE CANCER
Additional signs and symptoms
- Dribbling of urine
- Dysuria
- Bladder distention

DX: Prostate examination, labs (PSA, UA, urine or prostatic fluid cytology), biopsy
TX: Hormonal therapy, radiation therapy, surgery
F/U: Referrals to urologist and oncologist, reevaluation of PSA every 6 to 12 months

Additional differential diagnosis: spinal cord lesion

Other causes: drugs (anticholinergics, tricyclic antidepressants, nasal decongestants, some cold remedies, general anesthesia)

Urinary incontinence

Urinary incontinence, the uncontrollable passage of urine, can result from a bladder abnormality, a neurologic disorder, or aging. A common urologic sign, incontinence may be transient or permanent and may involve large volumes of urine or scant dribbling. It can be classified as stress, overflow, urge, or total incontinence. *Stress incontinence* refers to intermittent leakage resulting from a sudden physical strain, such as a cough, sneeze, or quick movement. *Overflow incontinence* is a dribble resulting from urine retention, which fills the bladder and prevents it from contracting with sufficient force to expel a urine stream. *Urge incontinence* refers to the inability to suppress a sudden urge to urinate. *Total incontinence* is continuous leakage resulting from the bladder's inability to retain any urine.

HISTORY

- Ask the patient when he first experienced the incontinence and whether it began suddenly or gradually.
- Ask the patient to describe his typical urinary pattern. Does incontinence usually occur during the day or at night? Does he have any urinary control, or is he totally incontinent? If he sometimes urinates with control, ask him the usual times and amounts voided.
- Ask the patient to describe his normal fluid intake.
- Ask the patient about other urinary problems, such as urinary hesitancy, frequency, and urgency; nocturia; and decreased force or interruption of the urine stream. Also, ask if he has ever sought treatment for incontinence or found a way to deal with it himself.
- Review the patient's medical history for urinary tract infection (UTI), prostate conditions, spinal injury or tumor, stroke, and surgery involving the bladder, prostate, or pelvic floor.

PHYSICAL ASSESSMENT

- Have the patient empty his bladder. Inspect the urethral meatus for obvious inflammation or anatomic defect. If the patient is a female, have her bear down, and note urine leakage, if present.
- Gently palpate the abdomen for bladder distention, which signals urine retention.
- Perform a complete neurologic assessment, noting motor and sensory function and obvious muscle atrophy.

SPECIAL CONSIDERATIONS

Urinary incontinence may occur after prostectomy as a result of urethral sphincter damage.

PEDIATRIC POINTERS

- *Causes of incontinence in children include infrequent voiding and incomplete voiding. These may also lead to UTI.*
- *Ectopic ureteral orifice is an uncommon congenital anomaly associated with incontinence.*
- *A complete diagnostic evaluation usually is necessary to rule out organic disease.*

AGING ISSUES

Diagnosing a UTI in an elderly patient can be problematic because many present only with incontinence or changes in mental status, anorexia, or malaise. Also, many elderly patients without UTIs present with dysuria, frequency, urgency, or incontinence.

PATIENT COUNSELING

Begin management of incontinence by implementing a bladder retraining program. (See *Correcting incontinence with bladder retraining.*) To prevent stress incontinence, teach exercises to help strengthen the pelvic floor muscles.

CORRECTING INCONTINENCE WITH BLADDER RETRAINING

The incontinent patient typically feels frustrated, embarrassed, and sometimes hopeless. Fortunately, though, his problems can often be corrected by bladder retraining — a program that aims to establish a regular voiding pattern. Here are some guidelines for establishing such a program:

- Assess the patient's intake pattern, voiding pattern, and behavior (for example, restlessness or talkativeness) before each voiding episode.
- Encourage the patient to use the toilet 30 minutes before he's usually incontinent. If this isn't successful, readjust the schedule. After he's able to stay dry for 2 hours, increase the time between voidings by 30 minutes each day until he achieves a 3- to 4-hour voiding schedule.
- When your patient voids, make sure that the sequence of conditioning stimuli is always the same.
- Ensure that the patient has privacy while voiding.
- Keep a record of continence and incontinence for 5 days.
- Display a positive attitude.

- Make sure that the patient is close to a bathroom or a portable toilet. Leave a light on at night.
- If your patient needs assistance getting out of his bed or chair, promptly answer his call for help.
- Acceptable alternatives to diapers include condoms for the male patient and incontinence pads, or panties, for the female patient.
- Encourage the patient to drink 2,000 to 2,500 ml of fluid each day. Less fluid doesn't prevent incontinence but does promote bladder infection. Limit his intake after 5 p.m
- Reassure the patient that episodes of incontinence don't signal a failure of the program. Encourage him to maintain a persistent, tolerant attitude.

URINARY INCONTINENCE

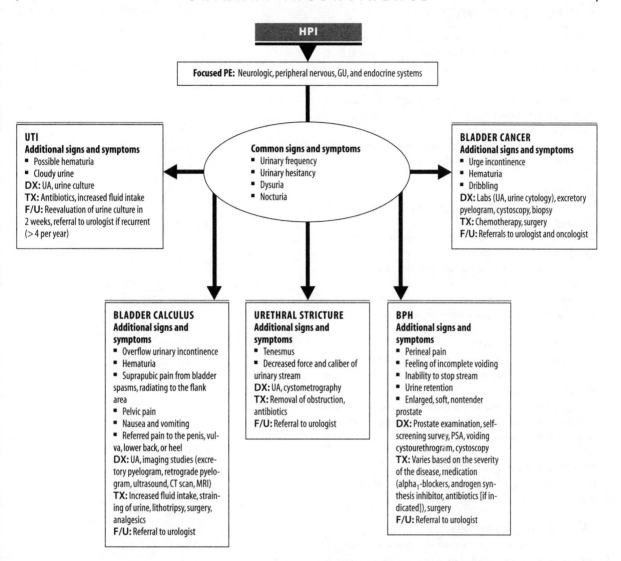

HPI

Focused PE: Neurologic, peripheral nervous, GU, and endocrine systems

Common signs and symptoms
- Urinary frequency
- Urinary hesitancy
- Dysuria
- Nocturia

UTI
Additional signs and symptoms
- Possible hematuria
- Cloudy urine

DX: UA, urine culture
TX: Antibiotics, increased fluid intake
F/U: Reevaluation of urine culture in 2 weeks, referral to urologist if recurrent (> 4 per year)

BLADDER CANCER
Additional signs and symptoms
- Urge incontinence
- Hematuria
- Dribbling

DX: Labs (UA, urine cytology), excretory pyelogram, cystoscopy, biopsy
TX: Chemotherapy, surgery
F/U: Referrals to urologist and oncologist

BLADDER CALCULUS
Additional signs and symptoms
- Overflow urinary incontinence
- Hematuria
- Suprapubic pain from bladder spasms, radiating to the flank area
- Pelvic pain
- Nausea and vomiting
- Referred pain to the penis, vulva, lower back, or heel

DX: UA, imaging studies (excretory pyelogram, retrograde pyelogram, ultrasound, CT scan, MRI)
TX: Increased fluid intake, straining of urine, lithotripsy, surgery, analgesics
F/U: Referral to urologist

URETHRAL STRICTURE
Additional signs and symptoms
- Tenesmus
- Decreased force and caliber of urinary stream

DX: UA, cystometrography
TX: Removal of obstruction, antibiotics
F/U: Referral to urologist

BPH
Additional signs and symptoms
- Perineal pain
- Feeling of incomplete voiding
- Inability to stop stream
- Urine retention
- Enlarged, soft, nontender prostate

DX: Prostate examination, self-screening survey, PSA, voiding cystourethrogram, cystoscopy
TX: Varies based on the severity of the disease, medication (alpha$_1$-blockers, androgen synthesis inhibitor, antibiotics [if indicated]), surgery
F/U: Referral to urologist

Additional differential diagnoses: Guillain-Barré syndrome ▪ multiple sclerosis ▪ spinal cord injury ▪ stroke

Other causes: aging ▪ cerebral disease ▪ cystocele ▪ multiple pregnancies ▪ retrocele ▪ surgery ▪ uterine prolapse

Urinary urgency

Urinary urgency, a classic symptom of urinary tract infection (UTI), is characterized by a sudden compelling urge to urinate that's accompanied by bladder pain. As inflammation decreases bladder capacity, discomfort results from the accumulation of even small amounts of urine. Repeated, frequent voiding in an effort to alleviate this discomfort produces urine output of only a few milliliters at each voiding.

Urgency without bladder pain may point to an upper-motor-neuron lesion that has disrupted bladder control.

HISTORY

- Ask the patient about the onset of urinary urgency and whether he has ever experienced it before.
- Ask the patient about other urologic signs and symptoms, such as dysuria and cloudy urine.
- Ask the patient about neurologic symptoms such as paresthesia.
- Review the patient's medical history for recurrent or chronic UTIs and for surgery or procedures involving the urinary tract.

PHYSICAL ASSESSMENT

- Obtain a clean-catch sample for urinalysis. Note the urine's character, color, and odor, and use a reagent strip to test for pH, glucose, and blood.
- Palpate the suprapubic area and both flanks for tenderness.
- If the patient's history or symptoms suggest neurologic dysfunction, perform a neurologic examination.

SPECIAL CONSIDERATIONS

Increase the patient's fluid intake, if appropriate, to dilute the urine and diminish the feeling of urgency.

A PEDIATRIC POINTERS

- *In young children, urinary urgency may appear as a change in toilet habits, such as a sudden onset of bed-wetting or daytime accidents in a toilet-trained child. It may also result from urethral irritation caused by bubble bath salts.*
- *Girls may experience vaginal discharge and vulvar soreness or pruritus.*

PATIENT COUNSELING

Instruct sexually active patients in safe-sex practices. Advise female patients about proper genital hygiene such as cleaning the genital area from front to back to reduce contamination from fecal bacteria. Instruct women to maintain adequate fluid intake and allow for frequent daily voiding.

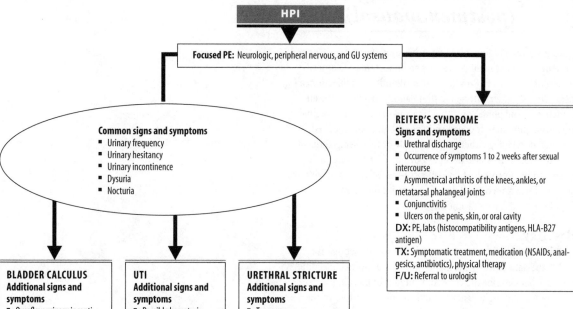

HPI

Focused PE: Neurologic, peripheral nervous, and GU systems

Common signs and symptoms
- Urinary frequency
- Urinary hesitancy
- Urinary incontinence
- Dysuria
- Nocturia

REITER'S SYNDROME
Signs and symptoms
- Urethral discharge
- Occurrence of symptoms 1 to 2 weeks after sexual intercourse
- Asymmetrical arthritis of the knees, ankles, or metatarsal phalangeal joints
- Conjunctivitis
- Ulcers on the penis, skin, or oral cavity

DX: PE, labs (histocompatibility antigens, HLA-B27 antigen)
TX: Symptomatic treatment, medication (NSAIDs, analgesics, antibiotics), physical therapy
F/U: Referral to urologist

BLADDER CALCULUS
Additional signs and symptoms
- Overflow urinary incontinence
- Hematuria
- Suprapubic pain from bladder spasms, radiating to flank area
- Pelvic pain
- Referred pain to the penis, vulva, lower back, or heel

DX: UA, imaging studies (excretory pyelogram, retrograde pyelogram, ultrasound, CT scan, MRI)
TX: Increased fluid intake, straining of urine, lithotripsy, surgery, analgesics
F/U: Referral to urologist

UTI
Additional signs and symptoms
- Possible hematuria
- Cloudy urine

DX: UA, urine culture
TX: Antibiotics, increased fluid intake
F/U: Reevaluation of urine culture in 2 weeks, referral to urologist if recurrent (> 4 per year)

URETHRAL STRICTURE
Additional signs and symptoms
- Tenesmus
- Decreased force and caliber of urinary stream

DX: UA, cystometrography
TX: Removal of obstruction, antibiotics
F/U: Referral to urologist

Additional differential diagnosis: ALS

Other cause: radiation therapy

V

Vaginal bleeding (postmenopausal)

Postmenopausal vaginal bleeding—bleeding that occurs 6 or more months after menopause—is an important indicator of gynecologic cancer. However, it can also result from infection, a local pelvic disorder, estrogenic stimulation, atrophy of the endometrium, and physiologic thinning and drying of the vaginal mucous membranes. It usually occurs as slight, brown or red spotting, developing either spontaneously or following coitus or douching, but it may also occur as oozing of fresh blood or as bright red hemorrhage. Many patients—especially those with a history of heavy menstrual flow—minimize the importance of this bleeding, delaying diagnosis.

HISTORY
- Ask the patient her current age and her age at menopause.
- Ask the patient when she first noticed the abnormal bleeding and have her describe the color and amount of bleeding
- Obtain a thorough obstetric and gynecologic history of the patient and her mother. Find out when the patient began menstruating and whether her menses were regular. If they weren't, ask her to describe the irregularities. Also her about a family history of gynecologic cancer.
- Ask the patient about her sexual and reproductive history.
- Ask the patient about associated signs and symptoms.
- Ask the patient if she's currently taking estrogen.

PHYSICAL ASSESSMENT
- Observe the external genitalia, noting the character of vaginal discharge, if present, and the appearance of the labia, vaginal rugae, and clitoris.
- Carefully inspect and palpate the patient's breasts for dimpling, color differences, and masses.
- Inspect and palpate the lymph nodes for nodules or enlargement.

SPECIAL CONSIDERATIONS
About 80% of postmenopausal vaginal bleeding is benign; endometrial atrophy is the predominant cause. Malignancy should be ruled out.

Women can decrease their risk of getting vulvar cancer by practicing safe sex and by reducing controllable risk factors, such as hypertension, obesity, diabetes, and smoking.

PATIENT COUNSELING
Instruct the patient on what to expect from diagnostic testing, such as ultrasonography, endometrial biopsy, and dilatation and fractional curettage. Tell her she may need to discontinue estrogen therapy until a diagnosis is made.

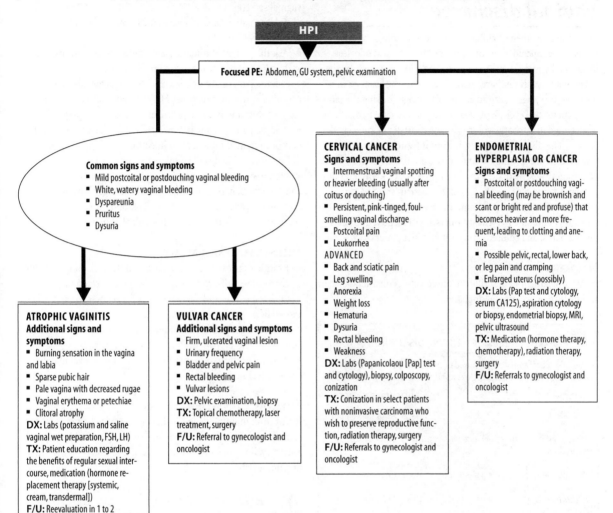

HPI

Focused PE: Abdomen, GU system, pelvic examination

Common signs and symptoms
- Mild postcoital or postdouching vaginal bleeding
- White, watery vaginal bleeding
- Dyspareunia
- Pruritus
- Dysuria

CERVICAL CANCER
Signs and symptoms
- Intermenstrual vaginal spotting or heavier bleeding (usually after coitus or douching)
- Persistent, pink-tinged, foul-smelling vaginal discharge
- Postcoital pain
- Leukorrhea
ADVANCED
- Back and sciatic pain
- Leg swelling
- Anorexia
- Weight loss
- Hematuria
- Dysuria
- Rectal bleeding
- Weakness
DX: Labs (Papanicolaou [Pap] test and cytology), biopsy, colposcopy, conization
TX: Conization in select patients with noninvasive carcinoma who wish to preserve reproductive function, radiation therapy, surgery
F/U: Referrals to gynecologist and oncologist

ENDOMETRIAL HYPERPLASIA OR CANCER
Signs and symptoms
- Postcoital or postdouching vaginal bleeding (may be brownish and scant or bright red and profuse) that becomes heavier and more frequent, leading to clotting and anemia
- Possible pelvic, rectal, lower back, or leg pain and cramping
- Enlarged uterus (possibly)
DX: Labs (Pap test and cytology, serum CA125), aspiration cytology or biopsy, endometrial biopsy, MRI, pelvic ultrasound
TX: Medication (hormone therapy, chemotherapy), radiation therapy, surgery
F/U: Referrals to gynecologist and oncologist

ATROPHIC VAGINITIS
Additional signs and symptoms
- Burning sensation in the vagina and labia
- Sparse pubic hair
- Pale vagina with decreased rugae
- Vaginal erythema or petechiae
- Clitoral atrophy
DX: Labs (potassium and saline vaginal wet preparation, FSH, LH)
TX: Patient education regarding the benefits of regular sexual intercourse, medication (hormone replacement therapy [systemic, cream, transdermal])
F/U: Reevaluation in 1 to 2 months, then every 3 to 6 months to monitor BP and adverse effects

VULVAR CANCER
Additional signs and symptoms
- Firm, ulcerated vaginal lesion
- Urinary frequency
- Bladder and pelvic pain
- Rectal bleeding
- Vulvar lesions
DX: Pelvic examination, biopsy
TX: Topical chemotherapy, laser treatment, surgery
F/U: Referral to gynecologist and oncologist

Additional differential diagnoses: cervical or endometrial polyps ▪ ovarian tumors (feminizing)

Other cause: unopposed estrogen replacement therapy

Vaginal discharge

Common in women of childbearing age, physiologic vaginal discharge is mucoid, clear or white, nonbloody, and odorless. Produced by the cervical mucosa and, to a lesser degree, by the vulvar glands, this discharge may occasionally be scant or profuse due to estrogenic stimulation and changes during the patient's menstrual cycle. However, a marked increase in discharge or a change in discharge color, odor, or consistency can signal disease. The discharge may result from infection, a sexually transmitted or reproductive tract disease, a fistula, or the effects of certain drugs. Also, the prolonged presence of a foreign body, such as a tampon or diaphragm, in the patient's vagina can cause irritation and an inflammatory exudate, as can frequent douching, feminine hygiene products, contraceptive products, bubble baths, and colored or perfumed toilet papers.

HISTORY

● Ask the patient to describe the onset, color, consistency, odor, and texture of her vaginal discharge.

IDENTIFYING CAUSES OF VAGINAL DISCHARGE

The color, consistency, amount, and odor of your patient's vaginal discharge provide important clues about the underlying disorder.

CHARACTERISTICS	POSSIBLE CAUSES
Thin, scant, watery white discharge	Atrophic vaginitis
White, curdlike, profuse discharge with yeasty, sweet odor	Candidiasis
Mucopurulent, foul-smelling discharge	Chancroid
Yellow, mucopurulent, odorless, or acrid discharge	*Chlamydia* infection
Scant, serosanguineous, or purulent discharge with foul odor	Endometritis
Thin, green or grayish white, foul-smelling discharge	*Gardnerella* vaginitis
Watery discharge	Genital herpes
Profuse, mucopurulent discharge, possibly foul smelling	Genital warts
Yellow or green, foul-smelling discharge from the cervix or occasionally from Bartholin's or Skene's ducts	Gonorrhea
Chronic, watery, bloody, or purulent discharge, possibly foul smelling	Gynecologic cancer
Frothy, greenish yellow, and profuse (or thin, white, and scant) foul-smelling discharge	Trichomoniasis

---

● Ask the patient how the discharge differs from her usual vaginal secretions.
● Ask the patient if she believes the onset is related to her menstrual cycle. If so, why?
● Ask the patient about associated signs and symptoms, such as dysuria and perineal pruritus and burning.
● Ask the patient about her sexual history. Does she have spotting after coitus or douching? Has she had recent changes in her sexual habits and hygiene practices? Could she be pregnant?
● Ask the patient if she has had vaginal discharge before or has ever been treated for a vaginal infection. If so, what treatment did she receive? Did she complete the course of medication?
● Obtain a drug history, including prescription and over-the-counter drugs, herbal remedies, and recreational drugs, especially noting antibiotics, oral estrogens, and hormonal contraceptives. Also, ask the patient about alcohol intake.

PHYSICAL ASSESSMENT

● Examine the external genitalia, and note the character of the discharge. (See *Identifying causes of vaginal discharge.*)
● Observe vulvar and vaginal tissues for redness, edema, and excoriation.
● Palpate the inguinal lymph nodes to detect tenderness or enlargement, and palpate the abdomen for tenderness.
● A pelvic examination may be required. Obtain vaginal discharge specimens for testing.

SPECIAL CONSIDERATIONS

Estrogen-containing drugs, including hormonal contraceptives, can cause increased mucoid vaginal discharge. Antibiotics, such as tetracycline, may increase the risk of a candidal vaginal infection and discharge.

[A] PEDIATRIC POINTERS

● *Female neonates who have been exposed to maternal estrogens in utero may have a white mucous vaginal discharge for the 1st month after birth; a yellow mucous discharge indicates a pathologic condition.*
● *In the older child, a purulent, foul-smelling and, possibly, bloody vaginal discharge commonly results from a foreign object placed in the vagina. The possibility of sexual abuse should be considered.*

PATIENT COUNSELING

If the patient has a vaginal infection, tell her to continue taking the prescribed medications even if the symptoms clear or she menstruates. Advise her to avoid intercourse until her symptoms clear and then have her partner use condoms until she completes her course of medication.

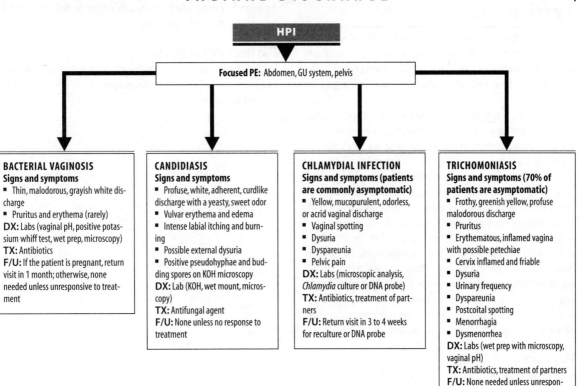

HPI

Focused PE: Abdomen, GU system, pelvis

BACTERIAL VAGINOSIS
Signs and symptoms
- Thin, malodorous, grayish white discharge
- Pruritus and erythema (rarely)

DX: Labs (vaginal pH, positive potassium whiff test, wet prep, microscopy)
TX: Antibiotics
F/U: If the patient is pregnant, return visit in 1 month; otherwise, none needed unless unresponsive to treatment

CANDIDIASIS
Signs and symptoms
- Profuse, white, adherent, curdlike discharge with a yeasty, sweet odor
- Vulvar erythema and edema
- Intense labial itching and burning
- Possible external dysuria
- Positive pseudohyphae and budding spores on KOH microscopy

DX: Lab (KOH, wet mount, microscopy)
TX: Antifungal agent
F/U: None unless no response to treatment

CHLAMYDIAL INFECTION
Signs and symptoms (patients are commonly asymptomatic)
- Yellow, mucopurulent, odorless, or acrid vaginal discharge
- Vaginal spotting
- Dysuria
- Dyspareunia
- Pelvic pain

DX: Labs (microscopic analysis, *Chlamydia* culture or DNA probe)
TX: Antibiotics, treatment of partners
F/U: Return visit in 3 to 4 weeks for reculture or DNA probe

TRICHOMONIASIS
Signs and symptoms (70% of patients are asymptomatic)
- Frothy, greenish yellow, profuse malodorous discharge
- Pruritus
- Erythematous, inflamed vagina with possible petechiae
- Cervix inflamed and friable
- Dysuria
- Urinary frequency
- Dyspareunia
- Postcoital spotting
- Menorrhagia
- Dysmenorrhea

DX: Labs (wet prep with microscopy, vaginal pH)
TX: Antibiotics, treatment of partners
F/U: None needed unless unresponsive to therapy

Additional differential diagnoses: atrophic vaginitis ▪ chancroid ▪ endometritis ▪ genital warts ▪ gonorrhea ▪ gynecologic cancer ▪ herpes simplex (genital)

Other causes: contraceptive creams and jellies ▪ drugs (such as hormonal contraceptives and antibiotics) ▪ radiation therapy

Vertigo

Vertigo is an illusion of movement in which the patient feels that he's revolving in space (subjective vertigo) or that his surroundings are revolving around him (objective vertigo). He may complain of a feeling of being pulled sideways, as though drawn by a magnet.

A common symptom, vertigo usually begins abruptly and may be temporary or permanent, mild or severe. It may worsen when the patient moves or subside when he lies down. Frequently, it's confused with dizziness—a sensation of imbalance and light-headedness that's nonspecific. However, unlike dizziness, vertigo is commonly accompanied by nausea, vomiting, nystagmus, and tinnitus or hearing loss. Although the patient's limb coordination is unaffected, vertiginous gait may occur.

Vertigo may result from a neurologic or otologic disorder that affects the equilibratory apparatus (the vestibule, semicircular canals, eighth cranial nerve, vestibular nuclei in the brain stem and their temporal lobe connections, and eyes). However, this symptom may also result from alcohol intoxication, hyperventilation, postural changes (benign postural vertigo), or the effects of certain drugs, tests, or procedures.

HISTORY

● Ask your patient to describe the onset and duration of his vertigo, being careful to distinguish this symptom from dizziness.
● Ask the patient if he feels that he's moving or that his surroundings are moving around him.
● Ask the patient how often the attacks occur and whether they follow position changes or are unpredictable.
● Ask the patient if he can walk during an attack, if he leans to one side, and if he's ever fallen.
● Ask the patient if he experiences motion sickness and if he prefers one position during an attack.
● Ask the patient if he has experienced recent head trauma, loss of hearing, nausea, vomiting, or fever.
● Obtain a drug history, including prescription and over-the-counter drugs, herbal remedies, and recreational drugs. Also, ask the patient about alcohol intake.

PHYSICAL ASSESSMENT

● Perform a neurologic assessment, focusing particularly on eighth cranial nerve function.
● Observe the patient's gait and posture for abnormalities.
● Examine the ear for signs of infection.

SPECIAL CONSIDERATIONS

High or toxic doses of certain drugs or alcohol may produce vertigo.

 PEDIATRIC POINTERS

An ear infection is a common cause of vertigo in children. Vestibular neuritis may also cause vertigo.

PATIENT COUNSELING

Instruct the patient on what to expect from diagnostic testing, which may include electronystagmography, EEG, and X-rays of the middle and inner ears.

VERTIGO

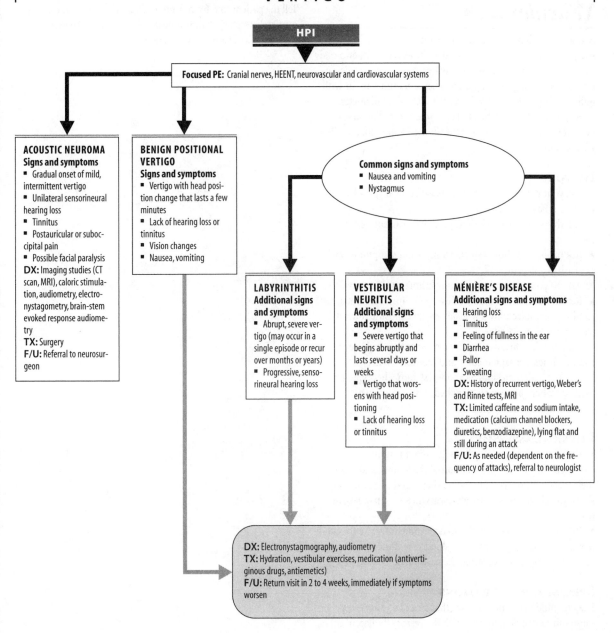

HPI

Focused PE: Cranial nerves, HEENT, neurovascular and cardiovascular systems

ACOUSTIC NEUROMA
Signs and symptoms
- Gradual onset of mild, intermittent vertigo
- Unilateral sensorineural hearing loss
- Tinnitus
- Postauricular or suboccipital pain
- Possible facial paralysis

DX: Imaging studies (CT scan, MRI), caloric stimulation, audiometry, electronystagometry, brain-stem evoked response audiometry

TX: Surgery

F/U: Referral to neurosurgeon

BENIGN POSITIONAL VERTIGO
Signs and symptoms
- Vertigo with head position change that lasts a few minutes
- Lack of hearing loss or tinnitus
- Vision changes
- Nausea, vomiting

Common signs and symptoms
- Nausea and vomiting
- Nystagmus

LABYRINTHITIS
Additional signs and symptoms
- Abrupt, severe vertigo (may occur in a single episode or recur over months or years)
- Progressive, sensorineural hearing loss

VESTIBULAR NEURITIS
Additional signs and symptoms
- Severe vertigo that begins abruptly and lasts several days or weeks
- Vertigo that worsens with head positioning
- Lack of hearing loss or tinnitus

MÉNIÈRE'S DISEASE
Additional signs and symptoms
- Hearing loss
- Tinnitus
- Feeling of fullness in the ear
- Diarrhea
- Pallor
- Sweating

DX: History of recurrent vertigo, Weber's and Rinne tests, MRI

TX: Limited caffeine and sodium intake, medication (calcium channel blockers, diuretics, benzodiazepine), lying flat and still during an attack

F/U: As needed (dependent on the frequency of attacks), referral to neurologist

DX: Electronystagmography, audiometry
TX: Hydration, vestibular exercises, medication (antivertiginous drugs, antiemetics)
F/U: Return visit in 2 to 4 weeks, immediately if symptoms worsen

---

Additional differential diagnoses: brain stem ischemia ▪ head trauma ▪ herpes zoster ▪ multiple sclerosis ▪ posterior fossa tumor ▪ seizures

Other causes: administration of overly warm or cold eardrops or irrigating solutions ▪ alcohol ▪ antibiotics ▪ aminoglycosides ▪ caloric testing ▪ ear surgery ▪ high or toxic levels of salicylates ▪ quinine and hormonal contraceptives

Vesicular rash

A vesicular rash is a scattered or linear distribution of vesicles—sharply circumscribed lesions filled with clear, cloudy, or bloody fluid. The lesions, which are usually less than 0.5 cm in diameter, may occur singly or in groups. They sometimes occur with bullae—fluid-filled lesions larger than 0.5 cm in diameter.

A vesicular rash may be mild or severe and temporary or permanent. It can result from infection, inflammation, or allergic reactions.

HISTORY
● Ask your patient when the rash began, how it spread, and whether it has appeared before.
● Ask the patient if skin lesions preceded eruption of the vesicles.
● Ask the patient about associated signs and symptoms, such as pruritus and pain.
● Ask the patient if there is a family history of skin disorders.
● Review the patient's medical history for immunizations, allergies, recent infections (especially recent exposure to viral infections), and insect bites.
● Obtain a drug history, including prescription and over-the-counter drugs, herbal remedies, and recreational drugs. If the patient has used topical medications, ask him what types he used and when they were last applied. Also, ask the patient about alcohol intake.

PHYSICAL ASSESSMENT
● Examine the skin, noting if it's dry, oily, or moist.
● Observe the general distribution of the lesions, and record their exact location. Note the color, shape, and size of the lesions, and check for crusts, scales, scars, macules, papules, or wheals.
● Palpate the vesicles or bullae to determine if they're flaccid or tense. Slide your finger across the skin to see if the outer layer of epidermis separates easily from the basal layer (Nikolsky's sign).

SPECIAL CONSIDERATIONS
Keep in mind that skin eruptions that cover large areas may cause substantial fluid loss through the vesicles, bullae, or other weeping lesions. Be sure to evaluate hydration status.

[A] *PEDIATRIC POINTERS*
Vesicular rashes in children are caused by staphylococcal infections (staphylococcal scalded skin syndrome is a life-threatening infection occurring in infants), varicella, hand-foot-and-mouth disease, and miliaria rubra.

PATIENT COUNSELING
Tell the patient to refrain from touching the lesions and to immediately wash his hands if he does touch them. Advise him to report signs of secondary infection.

VESICULAR RASH

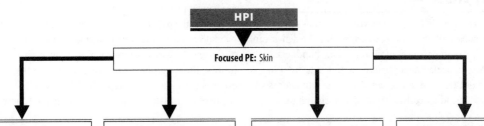

HPI

Focused PE: Skin

CONTACT DERMATITIS
Signs and symptoms
- Small vesicles on an erythematous base and edema that may ooze or scale
- Severe pruritus (possibly)

DX: Skin examination

TX: Medication (steroids [topical or systemic], antihistamine, antipruritic), cool tub baths with colloidal oatmeal, topical compresses of frozen (use for 15 to 20 minutes, three to four times per day), patient education on seeking immediate attention for SOB or chest tightness

F/U: None necessary if localized, 2 to 3 days if generalized

HERPES ZOSTER
Signs and symptoms
- Dermatomal pain, itching, and burning 4 to 5 days before eruption of vesicles
- Unilateral spread of vesicles on an erythematous base along dermatome
- Vesicles that dry and scab about 10 days after eruption
- Fever
- Headache
- Malaise
- Pruritus
- Paresthesia or hyperesthesia of involved area
- Involvement of thorax, extremities, and cranial nerves (possibly)

DX: Labs (Tzanck smear, viral antigen smear, viral culture, HIV testing)

TX: Cool compresses, medication (antivirals, NSAIDs, antidepressant, topical anesthetic)

F/U: Reevaluation in 7 to 10 days

SCABIES
Signs and symptoms
- Small, isolated serous vesicles on an erythematous base (may be at the end of a burrow)
- Burrows (gray or skin-colored ridges with a small, isolated red papule that contains the mite)
- Pustules and excoriations (possibly)
- Intense itching at night
- Rash commonly found on hands and finger webs but also occurring on the wrists, elbows, axillae, waistline, breasts, penis, and scrotum

DX: Microscopic identification of a mite or ova

TX: Medication (scabicide, antihistamine), treatment of all household members, laundering of all clothing and bedding in hot water and hot dryer cycle, cool bath with colloidal oatmeal, topical compresses wet with water kept in freezer (use for 15 to 20 minutes, three to four per day)

F/U: None unless treatment is ineffective

ERYTHEMA MULTIFORME
Signs and symptoms
- Sudden eruption of erythematous macules, papules, vesicles, and bullae
- Rash that appears on the hands, feet, arms, legs, face, and neck
- Vesiculobullous lesions that appear on mucous membranes and may rupture and ulcerate
- Thick yellow or white exudate
- Lymphadenopathy
- Pruritus

DX: Skin examination, positive Nikolsky's sign, biopsy

TX: Compresses, medication (antihistamines, analgesics, topical anesthetics)

F/U: As needed

Additional differential diagnoses: burns ▪ dermatitis herpetiformis ▪ dermatophytid ▪ herpes simplex ▪ insect bites ▪ pemphigoid (bullous) ▪ pemphigus ▪ pompholyx ▪ porphyria cutanea tarda ▪ tinea pedis ▪ toxic epidermal necrolysis

Vision loss

Vision loss—the inability to perceive visual stimuli—can be sudden or gradual and temporary or permanent. The deficit can range from a slight impairment of vision to total blindness. It can result from an ocular, neurologic, or systemic disorder or from trauma or a reaction to a certain drug. The ultimate visual outcome may depend on early, accurate diagnosis and treatment.

ALERT
Sudden vision loss can signal an ocular emergency. Don't touch the eye if the patient has perforating or penetrating ocular trauma. (See Managing sudden vision loss.*)*

If the vision loss occurred gradually, perform a focused assessment.

HISTORY
- Ask the patient if the vision loss affects one eye or both and all or only part of the visual field.
- Ask the patient if the visual loss is transient or persistent.
- Ask the patient if the visual loss developed over hours, days, or weeks.
- Ask the patient if he wears corrective lenses or contacts.

MANAGING SUDDEN VISION LOSS

Sudden vision loss can signal central retinal artery occlusion or acute angle-closure glaucoma—ocular emergencies that require immediate intervention. If your patient reports sudden vision loss, immediately notify an ophthalmologist for an emergency examination, and perform these interventions.

For a patient with suspected central retinal artery occlusion, perform light massage over his closed eyelid. Increase his carbon dioxide level by administering a set flow of oxygen and carbon dioxide through a Venturi mask, or have the patient breathe in a paper bag to retain exhaled carbon dioxide. These steps will dilate the artery and, possibly, restore blood flow to the retina.

For a patient with suspected acute angle-closure glaucoma, measure intraocular pressure with a tonometer. (You can also estimate intraocular pressure without a tonometer by placing your fingers over the patient's closed eyelid. A rock-hard eyeball usually indicates increased intraocular pressure.) Expect to administer timolol drops and I.V. acetazolamide to help decrease intraocular pressure.

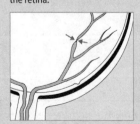 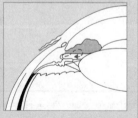

- Ask the patient if he has experienced photosensitivity.
- Ask the patient about the location, intensity, and duration of eye pain, if present.
- Review the patient's ocular history, including the date of the patient's last ocular examination and its outcome.
- Review the patient's medical history (including his family history) for eye problems and systemic disease that may lead to eye problems, such as hypertension; diabetes mellitus; thyroid, rheumatic, or vascular disease; infections; and cancer.

PHYSICAL ASSESSMENT
- Assess visual acuity, with the best available correction in each eye.
- Carefully inspect both eyes, noting edema, foreign bodies, drainage, or conjunctival or scleral redness. Observe whether lid closure is complete or incomplete, and check for ptosis.
- Using a flashlight, examine the cornea and iris for scars, irregularities, and foreign bodies. Observe the size, shape, and color of the pupils, and test direct and consensual light reflexes and the effect of accommodation.
- Evaluate extraocular muscle function by testing the six cardinal fields of gaze.

SPECIAL CONSIDERATIONS
Vision loss is extremely frightening. Be sure to orient the patient to his environment, and announce your presence each time you approach him.

PEDIATRIC POINTERS
- *Children who complain of slowly progressive vision loss may have an optic nerve glioma (a slow-growing, usually benign tumor) or retinoblastoma (a malignant tumor of the retina).*
- *Congenital rubella and syphilis may cause vision loss in infants.*
- *Retrolental fibroplasia may cause vision loss in premature infants.*
- *Other congenital causes of vision loss include Marfan syndrome, retinitis pigmentosa, and amblyopia.*

AGING ISSUES
In elderly patients, reduced visual acuity may be caused by morphologic changes in the choroid, pigment epithelium, and retina or by decreased function of the rods, cones, and other neural elements.

PATIENT COUNSELING
Instruct the patient to avoid touching the unaffected eye with items that have been in contact with the affected eye. Tell him to wash his hands often and to avoid rubbing his eyes.

VISION LOSS

HPI

Focused PE: HEENT, neurologic system

ACUTE ANGLE-CLOSURE GLAUCOMA
Signs and symptoms
- Rapid onset of unilateral inflammation, pain, and pressure of the eye
- Moderate pupil dilation
- Nonreactive pupillary response
- Cloudy cornea
- Reduced visual acuity
- Photophobia
- Perception of blue or red halos around lights
- Unilateral headache
- Nausea and vomiting
- Visual blurring that may progress to blindness

DX: Eye examination, tonometric testing
TX: Medication (topical beta-adrenergic antagonists, carbonic anhydrase inhibitors, systemic hyperosmotic agents, miotics, corticosteroids, NSAIDs)
F/U: Referral to ophthalmologist

Common signs and symptoms
- Small, sluggish or nonreactive pupil that appears suddenly
- Acute ocular pain
- Conjunctival injection
- Photophobia

ANTERIOR UVEITIS

POSTERIOR UVEITIS
Additional signs and symptoms
- Blurred vision
- Decreased visual acuity
- Distorted pupil shape
- Floaters
- Optic nerve edema

RETINAL DETACHMENT
Signs and symptoms
- Painless vision loss that may be rapid or may occur over several days
- Flashing light sensation
- Shower of floaters
- Shadow in peripheral vision
- Wavy distortion
- Decreased visual acuity

DX: Visual field testing, slit-lamp examination, ultrasonography
TX: None in certain cases, surgery
F/U: Referral to ophthalmologist

DX: Eye examination, slit-lamp examination
TX: Medication (analgesics, antibiotics, corticosteroids)
F/U: Referral to ophthalmologist

Additional differential diagnoses: Alzheimer's disease ▪ amaurosis fugax ▪ cataract ▪ concussion ▪ diabetic retinopathy ▪ endophthalmitis ▪ hereditary corneal dystrophies ▪ herpes zoster ▪ hyphema ▪ keratitis ▪ ocular trauma ▪ optic atrophy ▪ optic neuritis ▪ Paget's disease ▪ papilledema ▪ pituitary tumor ▪ retinal artery occlusion (central) ▪ retinal vein occlusion (central) ▪ senile macular degeneration ▪ Stevens-Johnson syndrome ▪ temporal arteritis ▪ trachoma ▪ vitreous hemorrhage

Other causes: cardiac glycosides ▪ chloroquine therapy ▪ ethambutol ▪ indomethacin ▪ methanol toxicity ▪ phenylbutazone ▪ quinine

Visual blurring

A common symptom, visual blurring refers to the loss of visual acuity with indistinct visual details. It may result from eye injury, a neurologic or eye disorder, or a disorder with vascular complications such as diabetes mellitus. Visual blurring may also result from mucus passing over the cornea, refractive errors, improperly fitted contact lenses, or the effects of certain drugs.

 ALERT

If your patient has visual blurring accompanied by sudden, severe eye pain, a history of trauma, or sudden vision loss, an ophthalmologic examination is needed. If the patient has a penetrating or perforating eye injury, don' t touch the eye.

If the patient's condition permits, perform a focused assessment.

HISTORY

- If the patient isn't in distress, ask him how long he has had the visual blurring and when it occurs.
- Ask the patient about associated signs and symptoms, such as pain and discharge.
- If visual blurring followed an injury, ask the patient for details of the accident and if his vision was impaired immediately after the injury.
- Review the patient's medical history.
- Obtain a drug history, including prescription and over-the-counter drugs, herbal remedies, and recreational drugs. Also, ask the patient about alcohol intake.

PHYSICAL ASSESSMENT

- Inspect the patient's eye, noting lid edema, drainage, or conjunctival or scleral redness. Also note an irregularly shaped iris, which may indicate previous trauma, and excessive blinking, which may indicate corneal damage.
- Assess for pupillary changes, and test visual acuity in both eyes. (See *Testing visual acuity.*)

SPECIAL CONSIDERATIONS

If visual blurring leads to permanent vision loss, provide emotional support, orient him to his surroundings, and provide for his safety.

[A] *PEDIATRIC POINTERS*

- *Visual blurring in children may stem from congenital syphilis, a congenital cataract, a refractive error, an eye injury or infection, or increased intracranial pressure.*
- *Test vision in school-age children as you would in adults; test children ages 3 to 6 with the Snellen chart. Test toddlers with Allen cards, each illustrated with a familiar object, such as an animal. Ask the child to cover one eye and identify the objects as you flash them. Then ask him to identify them as you gradually back away. Record the maximum distance at which he can identify at least three pictures.*

PATIENT COUNSELING

Instruct the patient on what to expect from diagnostic testing, which may include tonometry, slit-lamp examination, X-rays of the skull and orbit, and computed tomography scan. As necessary, teach the patient how to instill ophthalmic medication.

TESTING VISUAL ACUITY

Use a Snellen letter chart to test visual acuity in the literate patient older than age 6. Have the patient sit or stand 20′ (6.1 m) from the chart. Then tell him to cover his left eye and read aloud the smallest line of letters that he can see. Record the fraction assigned to that line on the chart (the numerator indicates distance from the chart; the denominator indicates the distance at which a normal eye can read the chart). Normal vision is 20/20. Repeat the test with the patient's right eye covered.

If your patient can't read the largest letter from a distance of 20′, have him approach the chart until he can read it. Then record the distance between him and the chart as the numerator of the fraction. For example, if he can see the top line of the chart at a distance of 3′ (0.9 m), record the test result as 3/200.

Use a Snellen symbol chart to test children ages 3 to 6 and illiterate patients. Follow the same procedure as for the Snellen letter chart, but ask the patient to indicate the direction of the E's fingers as you point to each symbol.

SNELLEN LETTER CHART

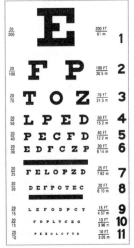

SNELLEN SYMBOL CHART

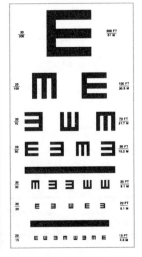

VISUAL BLURRING

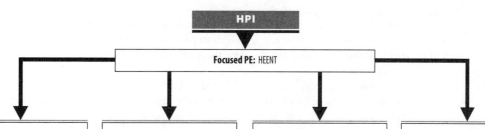

HPI

Focused PE: HEENT

BACTERIAL CONJUNCTIVITIS
Signs and symptoms
- Photophobia
- Pain
- Burning
- Tearing
- Itching
- Foreign body sensation
- Feeling of fullness around the eyes
- Erythema near the fornices
- Copious, mucopurulent, flaky drainage
- Matting of the eyelashes
- Edema of the eyelids

DX: Culture if chronic or recurrent condition
TX: Ophthalmic antibiotic
F/U: Reevaluation if there's no improvement in 24 to 48 hours or if the condition worsens, referral to ophthalmologist if recurrent

MIGRAINE HEADACHE, CLASSIC
Signs and symptoms
- Prodromal visual blurring
- Sensory or visual auras
- Severe, throbbing, usually unilateral headache
- Nausea and vomiting
- Photophobia
- Phonophobia
- Perspiration

DX: History
TX: Medication (NSAIDs, beta-adrenergic blockers, anticonvulsants, antidepressants, steroids, calcium channel blockers, ergots); headache diary; low-fat, high-complex carbohydrate diet
F/U: Referrals to ophthalmologist, neurologist, and headache center

HYPERTENSION
Signs and symptoms
- Constant morning headache that decreases in severity during the day
- Systolic BP >140 mm Hg or diastolic BP > 90 mm Hg
- Restlessness
- Nausea and vomiting
- Dizziness
- Possible epistaxis
- Fatigue
- Anxiety
- Tinnitus

DX: Labs (CBC, BUN, creatinine, electrolytes, plasma renin, uric acid), renal ultrasound, 12-lead ECG
TX: Treatment of underlying condition for secondary hypertension, medication (beta-adrenergic blockers, ACE inhibitors, calcium channel blockers), BP diary
F/U: Return visit in 1 week, then every 4 weeks until hypertension is well controlled

RETINAL DETACHMENT
Signs and symptoms
- Painless vision loss that may be rapid or may occur over several days
- Flashing light sensation
- Shower of floaters
- Shadow in peripheral vision
- Wavy distortion
- Decreased visual acuity

DX: Visual field testing, slit-lamp examination, ultrasonography
TX: None in certain cases, surgery
F/U: Referral to ophthalmologist

Additional differential diagnoses: brain tumor • cataract • concussion • conjunctivitis • corneal abrasions • corneal foreign bodies • diabetic retinopathy • dislocated lens • eye tumor • glaucoma • hereditary corneal dystrophies • hyphema • iritis • multiple sclerosis • optic neuritis • retinal vein occlusion (central) • senile macular degeneration • serous retinopathy (central) • temporal arteritis • uveitis (posterior) • vitreous hemorrhage

Other causes: anticholinergics • antihistamines • clomiphene • cycloplegics • guanethidine • phenothiazines • phenylbutazone • reserpine • thiazide diuretics

Vomiting

Vomiting is the forceful expulsion of gastric contents through the mouth. Characteristically preceded by nausea, vomiting results from a coordinated sequence of abdominal muscle contractions and reverse esophageal peristalsis.

A common sign of a GI disorder, vomiting also occurs with fluid and electrolyte imbalances; infections; and metabolic, endocrine, labyrinthine, central nervous system (CNS), and cardiac disorders. It can also result from drug therapy, surgery, or radiation.

Vomiting occurs normally during the first trimester of pregnancy, but its subsequent development may signal complications. It can also result from stress, anxiety, pain, alcohol intoxication, overeating, or ingestion of distasteful foods or liquids.

HISTORY

- Ask your patient to describe the onset, duration, and intensity of his vomiting. Try to determine what started the vomiting, what the vomitus looked like, and how often the vomiting occurred. If possible, collect, measure, and inspect the character of the vomitus. (See *Vomitus: Characteristics and causes.*)
- Ask the patient about associated signs and symptoms, particularly nausea, abdominal pain, anorexia and weight loss, changes in bowel habits or stools, excessive belching or flatus, and bloating or fullness.
- Review the patient's medical history, noting GI, endocrine, or metabolic disorders; recent infections; and cancer, including chemotherapy or radiation therapy.
- Ask the patient about his recent diet history.
- Ask the patient if he has recently been exposed to another person who was vomiting.

VOMITUS: CHARACTERISTICS AND CAUSES

When you collect a sample of the patient's vomitus, observe it carefully for clues to the underlying disorder. Here's what different types of vomitus may indicate:

- *bile-stained (greenish) vomitus* — obstruction below the pylorus, as from a duodenal lesion
- *bloody vomitus* — upper GI bleeding, as from gastritis or peptic ulcer, if bright red; as from esophageal or gastric varices, if dark red
- *brown vomitus with a fecal odor* — intestinal obstruction or infarction
- *burning, bitter-tasting vomitus* — excessive hydrochloric acid in gastric contents
- *coffee-ground vomitus* — digested blood from slowly bleeding gastric or duodenal lesion
- *undigested food* — gastric outlet obstruction, as from gastric tumor or ulcer.

- If the patient is a female of childbearing age, ask her if she is or could be pregnant. Ask her which contraceptive method she's using.
- Obtain a drug history, including prescription and over-the-counter drugs, herbal remedies, and recreational drugs. Also, ask the patient about alcohol intake.

PHYSICAL ASSESSMENT

- Inspect the abdomen for distention, and auscultate for bowel sounds and bruits. Palpate for rigidity and tenderness, and test for rebound tenderness.
- Palpate and percuss the liver for enlargement. Assess other body systems as appropriate.

SPECIAL CONSIDERATIONS

Keep in mind that projectile vomiting unaccompanied by nausea may indicate increased intracranial pressure, a life-threatening emergency. If this occurs in a patient with CNS injury, you should quickly check his vital signs. Be alert for widened pulse pressure or bradycardia.

Ⓐ PEDIATRIC POINTERS

- *In a neonate, pyloric obstruction may cause projectile vomiting, whereas Hirschsprung's disease may cause fecal vomiting.*
- *Intussusception may lead to vomiting of bile and fecal matter in an infant or toddler.*

AGING ISSUES

Although elderly patients can develop any of the disorders already mentioned, always rule out intestinal ischemia first — it's especially common in patients of this age-group and has a high mortality rate.

PATIENT COUNSELING

Advise patients to replace fluid losses to avoid dehydration. Patients suffering from migraine headaches should be advised that vomiting may be a prodromal symptom; an antimigraine drug should be taken.

VOMITING

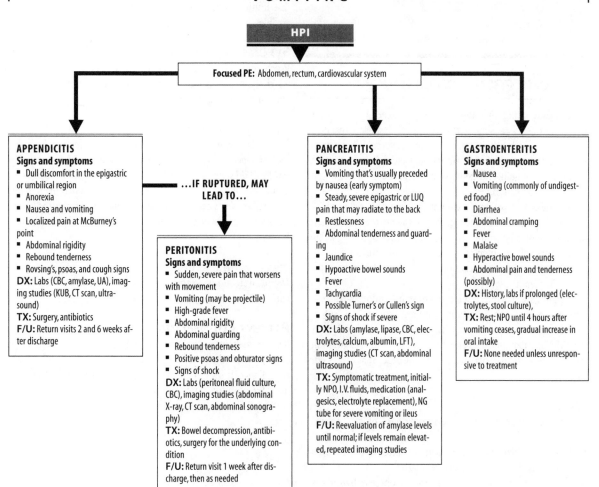

HPI

Focused PE: Abdomen, rectum, cardiovascular system

APPENDICITIS
Signs and symptoms
- Dull discomfort in the epigastric or umbilical region
- Anorexia
- Nausea and vomiting
- Localized pain at McBurney's point
- Abdominal rigidity
- Rebound tenderness
- Rovsing's, psoas, and cough signs

DX: Labs (CBC, amylase, UA), imaging studies (KUB, CT scan, ultrasound)
TX: Surgery, antibiotics
F/U: Return visits 2 and 6 weeks after discharge

...IF RUPTURED, MAY LEAD TO...

PERITONITIS
Signs and symptoms
- Sudden, severe pain that worsens with movement
- Vomiting (may be projectile)
- High-grade fever
- Abdominal rigidity
- Abdominal guarding
- Rebound tenderness
- Positive psoas and obturator signs
- Signs of shock

DX: Labs (peritoneal fluid culture, CBC), imaging studies (abdominal X-ray, CT scan, abdominal sonography)
TX: Bowel decompression, antibiotics, surgery for the underlying condition
F/U: Return visit 1 week after discharge, then as needed

PANCREATITIS
Signs and symptoms
- Vomiting that's usually preceded by nausea (early symptom)
- Steady, severe epigastric or LUQ pain that may radiate to the back
- Restlessness
- Abdominal tenderness and guarding
- Jaundice
- Hypoactive bowel sounds
- Fever
- Tachycardia
- Possible Turner's or Cullen's sign
- Signs of shock if severe

DX: Labs (amylase, lipase, CBC, electrolytes, calcium, albumin, LFT), imaging studies (CT scan, abdominal ultrasound)
TX: Symptomatic treatment, initially NPO, I.V. fluids, medication (analgesics, electrolyte replacement), NG tube for severe vomiting or ileus
F/U: Reevaluation of amylase levels until normal; if levels remain elevated, repeated imaging studies

GASTROENTERITIS
Signs and symptoms
- Nausea
- Vomiting (commonly of undigested food)
- Diarrhea
- Abdominal cramping
- Fever
- Malaise
- Hyperactive bowel sounds
- Abdominal pain and tenderness (possibly)

DX: History, labs if prolonged (electrolytes, stool culture),
TX: Rest; NPO until 4 hours after vomiting ceases, gradual increase in oral intake
F/U: None needed unless unresponsive to treatment

Additional differential diagnoses: adrenal insufficiency ▪ bulimia ▪ cholecystitis (acute) ▪ cholelithiasis ▪ cirrhosis ▪ ectopic pregnancy ▪ electrolyte imbalances ▪ food poisoning ▪ gastric cancer ▪ gastritis ▪ heart failure ▪ hepatitis ▪ hyperemesis gravidarum ▪ increased ICP ▪ infection ▪ intestinal obstruction ▪ labyrinthitis ▪ mesenteric artery ischemia ▪ mesenteric venous thrombosis ▪ metabolic acidosis ▪ MI ▪ migraine headache ▪ motion sickness ▪ peptic ulcer ▪ preeclampsia ▪ renal and urologic disorders ▪ thyrotoxicosis ▪ ulcerative colitis

Other causes: drugs (such as antineoplastic agents, opiates, ferrous sulfate, levodopa, oral potassium, chloride replacement, estrogens, sulfasalazine, antibiotics, quinidine, anesthetic agents, and overdoses of cardiac glycosides and theophylline) ▪ radiation

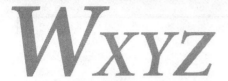

WXYZ

Weight gain, excessive

Weight gain occurs when ingested calories exceed body requirements for energy, causing increased adipose tissue storage. It can also occur when fluid retention causes edema. When weight gain results from overeating, emotional factors—most commonly anxiety, guilt, and depression—and social factors may be the primary causes.

Among elderly patients, weight gain commonly reflects a sustained food intake in the presence of the normal, progressive fall in basal metabolic rate. Among women, a progressive weight gain occurs with pregnancy, whereas a periodic weight gain usually occurs with menstruation. Weight gain also commonly occurs in menopause.

Weight gain, a primary symptom of many endocrine disorders, also occurs with conditions that limit activity, especially cardiovascular and pulmonary disorders. It can also result from drug therapy that increases appetite or causes fluid retention or from a cardiovascular, hepatic, or renal disorder that causes edema.

HISTORY

- Ask your patient about his previous patterns of weight gain and loss.
- Assess the patient's eating and activity patterns. Has his appetite increased? Does he exercise regularly?
- Ask the patient about a family history of obesity, thyroid disease, or diabetes mellitus.
- Ask the patient about associated signs and symptoms, such as visual disturbances, hoarseness, paresthesia, and increased urination and thirst.
- Ask the patient if he has become impotent. If the patient is female, ask her if she has experienced menstrual irregularities or weight gain during menstruation.
- Form an impression of the patient's mental status. Is he anxious or depressed? Does he respond slowly? Is his memory poor?
- Obtain a drug history, including prescription and over-the-counter drugs, herbal remedies, and recreational drugs. Also, ask the patient about alcohol intake.

PHYSICAL ASSESSMENT

- Measure skin-fold thickness to estimate fat reserves. Note fat distribution and the presence of localized or generalized edema and overall nutritional status.
- Inspect for other abnormalities, such as abnormal body hair distribution or hair loss and dry skin.
- Take the patient's vital signs.

SPECIAL CONSIDERATIONS

Psychological counseling may be necessary for patients with weight gain, particularly when it results from emotional problems or when weight gain alters body image.

 PEDIATRIC POINTERS

- *Weight gain in children can result from an endocrine disorder such as hypercortisolism. Other causes include inactivity caused by Prader-Willi syndrome, Werdnig-Hoffmann disease, Down syndrome, late stages of muscular dystrophy, and severe cerebral palsy.*
- *Nonpathologic causes of weight gain include poor eating habits, sedentary lifestyle, and emotional problems, especially among adolescents.*

AGING ISSUES

Desired weights (associated with lowest mortality rates) increase with age.

PATIENT COUNSELING

It's extremely important to educate the patient regarding weight control. Stress the benefits of behavior modification and dietary compliance. If the patient is obese or has a cardiopulmonary disorder, monitor exercise closely.

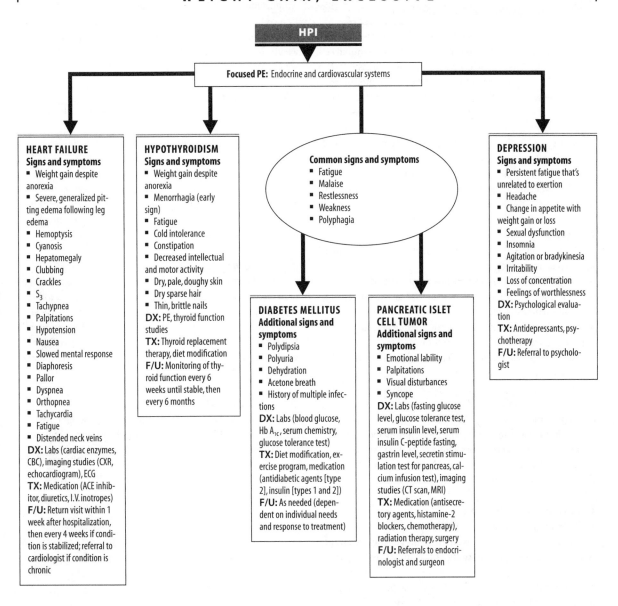

HPI

Focused PE: Endocrine and cardiovascular systems

HEART FAILURE
Signs and symptoms
- Weight gain despite anorexia
- Severe, generalized pitting edema following leg edema
- Hemoptysis
- Cyanosis
- Hepatomegaly
- Clubbing
- Crackles
- S_3
- Tachypnea
- Palpitations
- Hypotension
- Nausea
- Slowed mental response
- Diaphoresis
- Pallor
- Dyspnea
- Orthopnea
- Tachycardia
- Fatigue
- Distended neck veins

DX: Labs (cardiac enzymes, CBC), imaging studies (CXR, echocardiogram), ECG
TX: Medication (ACE inhibitor, diuretics, I.V. inotropes)
F/U: Return visit within 1 week after hospitalization, then every 4 weeks if condition is stabilized; referral to cardiologist if condition is chronic

HYPOTHYROIDISM
Signs and symptoms
- Weight gain despite anorexia
- Menorrhagia (early sign)
- Fatigue
- Cold intolerance
- Constipation
- Decreased intellectual and motor activity
- Dry, pale, doughy skin
- Dry sparse hair
- Thin, brittle nails

DX: PE, thyroid function studies
TX: Thyroid replacement therapy, diet modification
F/U: Monitoring of thyroid function every 6 weeks until stable, then every 6 months

Common signs and symptoms
- Fatigue
- Malaise
- Restlessness
- Weakness
- Polyphagia

DIABETES MELLITUS
Additional signs and symptoms
- Polydipsia
- Polyuria
- Dehydration
- Acetone breath
- History of multiple infections

DX: Labs (blood glucose, Hb A$_{1c}$, serum chemistry, glucose tolerance test)
TX: Diet modification, exercise program, medication (antidiabetic agents [type 2], insulin [types 1 and 2])
F/U: As needed (dependent on individual needs and response to treatment)

PANCREATIC ISLET CELL TUMOR
Additional signs and symptoms
- Emotional lability
- Palpitations
- Visual disturbances
- Syncope

DX: Labs (fasting glucose level, glucose tolerance test, serum insulin level, serum insulin C-peptide fasting, gastrin level, secretin stimulation test for pancreas, calcium infusion test), imaging studies (CT scan, MRI)
TX: Medication (antisecretory agents, histamine-2 blockers, chemotherapy), radiation therapy, surgery
F/U: Referrals to endocrinologist and surgeon

DEPRESSION
Signs and symptoms
- Persistent fatigue that's unrelated to exertion
- Headache
- Change in appetite with weight gain or loss
- Sexual dysfunction
- Insomnia
- Agitation or bradykinesia
- Irritability
- Loss of concentration
- Feelings of worthlessness

DX: Psychological evaluation
TX: Antidepressants, psychotherapy
F/U: Referral to psychologist

Additional differential diagnoses: acromegaly ▪ hypercortisolism ▪ hyperinsulinism ▪ hypogonadism ▪ hypothalamic dysfunction ▪ nephrotic syndrome ▪ preeclampsia ▪ Sheehan's syndrome

Other causes: corticosteroids ▪ cyproheptadine ▪ hormonal contraceptives ▪ lithium ▪ phenothiazines ▪ tricyclic antidepressants

Weight loss, excessive

Weight loss can reflect decreased food intake, decreased food absorption, increased metabolic requirements, or a combination of the three. Its causes include endocrine, neoplastic, GI, and psychiatric disorders; nutritional deficiencies; infections; and neurologic lesions that cause paralysis and dysphagia. However, weight loss may accompany a condition that prevents sufficient food intake, such as painful oral lesions, ill-fitting dentures, or loss of teeth. It may be the metabolic consequences of poverty, fad diets, excessive exercise, or certain drugs.

Weight loss may occur as a late sign in such chronic diseases as heart failure and renal disease. With these diseases, however, it's the result of anorexia.

HISTORY

- Obtain a thorough diet history. Evaluate whether the patient has been eating properly.
- Ask the patient about his previous weight and whether the recent loss was intentional. Ask him about exact weight changes (with approximate dates).
- Ask the patient about lifestyle or occupational changes that may be a source of anxiety or depression.
- Ask the patient about recent changes in bowel habits, such as diarrhea or bulky, floating stools.
- Ask the patient about other associated signs and symptoms, such as nausea, vomiting, abdominal pain, excessive thirst, excessive urination, and heat intolerance.
- Obtain a drug history, including prescription and over-the-counter drugs, herbal remedies, and recreational drugs, especially noting the use of diet pills and laxatives. Also, ask the patient about alcohol intake.

PHYSICAL ASSESSMENT

- Carefully check the patient's height and weight.
- Take the patient's vital signs and note his general appearance: Is he well nourished? Do his clothes fit? Is muscle wasting evident?
- Examine the skin for turgor and abnormal pigmentation, especially around the joints. Inspect for pallor or jaundice.
- Examine the patient's mouth, including the condition of his teeth or dentures. Look for signs of infection or irritation on the roof of the mouth, and note hyperpigmentation of the buccal mucosa.
- Check the patient's eyes for exophthalmos and his neck for swelling.
- Auscultate the lungs for adventitious sounds.
- Inspect the abdomen for signs of wasting, and palpate for masses, tenderness, and an enlarged liver.

SPECIAL CONSIDERATIONS

Amphetamine use and inappropriate dosage of thyroid preparation commonly lead to weight loss. Laxative abuse may cause a malabsorptive state that leads to weight loss. Chemotherapeutic agents may cause stomatitis, which, when severe, results in weight loss.

 PEDIATRIC POINTERS

- In infants, weight loss may be caused by failure-to-thrive syndrome.
- In children, severe weight loss may be the first indication of diabetes mellitus.
- Chronic, gradual weight loss occurs in children with marasmus—nonedematous protein-calorie malnutrition.
- Other causes of weight loss include child abuse or neglect, an infection causing a high fever, a GI disorder causing vomiting and diarrhea, or celiac disease.

AGING ISSUES

- Some elderly patients experience mild, gradual weight loss due to changes in body composition, such as loss of height and lean body mass, and lower basal metabolic rate, leading to decreased energy requirements. Rapid, unintentional weight loss, however, is highly predictive of morbidity and mortality in elderly patients.
- Nondisease causes of weight loss in elderly adults include tooth loss, difficulty chewing, and social isolation.

PATIENT COUNSELING

Refer the patient for psychological counseling if weight loss negatively affects his body image. Teach the patient about nutrition. Advise him to take daily calorie counts and monitor his weight weekly.

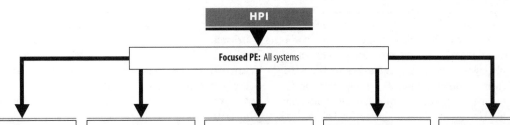

WEIGHT LOSS, EXCESSIVE

HPI

Focused PE: All systems

ADRENAL INSUFFICIENCY
Signs and symptoms
- Anorexia
- Weakness
- Fatigue
- Irritability
- Syncope
- Nausea and vomiting
- Abdominal pain
- Diarrhea or constipation
- Hyperpigmentation at the joints, beltline, palmar creases, lips, gums, tongue, and buccal mucosa
- Loss of axillary and pubic hair
- Amenorrhea

DX: Labs (CBC, BUN, creatinine, electrolytes, cortisol level, calcium, thyroid studies, adrenocorticotropic hormone stimulation test, 24-hour urinary cortisol level), imaging studies (CXR, CT scan), ECG

TX: Ventilation and circulation maintenance, medication (glucocorticoid and mineral corticoid hormone replacement therapy, electrolyte replacement), hydration, treatment of underlying condition

F/U: Referral to endocrinologist

MALIGNANCY
Signs and symptoms
- Fatigue
- Pain
- Nausea and vomiting
- Anorexia
- Abnormal bleeding
- Palpable mass (possibly)

DX: Labs (stool for occult blood, CBC with differential, UA, LFT, ESR), imaging studies (CXR, CT scan, mammogram)

TX: Varies based on the type of malignancy, diet modification, medication (analgesics, chemotherapy), radiation therapy, surgery

F/U: Referrals to oncologist and other specialist (based on type of malignancy)

DIABETES MELLITUS, TYPE 1
Signs and symptoms
- Polyphagia
- Polydipsia
- Polyuria
- Weakness
- Fatigue
- Blurred vision
- Listlessness
- Frequent infections
- Nocturnal enuresis in previously toilet-trained children
- Failure to grow

DX: Labs (serum glucose, Hb A_{1c}, postprandial serum C peptide, urine for ketones and protein)

TX: Diet modification, insulin therapy, blood glucose monitoring, teaching regarding managing hypoglycemia

F/U: Referrals to endocrinologist and diabetic counselor

ANOREXIA NERVOSA
Signs and symptoms
- Primary or secondary amenorrhea
- Emaciated appearance
- Compulsive behavior patterns
- Constipation
- Loss of scalp hair and lanugo on the face and arms
- Skeletal muscle atrophy
- Sleep disturbances

DX: Malnourished state, labs (electrolytes, CBC, renal studies, LFT, thyroid levels)

TX: Parenteral nutrition, psychological and nutritional counseling

F/U: Weekly return visits, then monthly visits if weight gain occurs; inpatient therapy if the condition doesn't improve

THYROTOXICOSIS
Signs and symptoms
- Ptosis
- Progressive exophthalmus
- Increased tearing
- Visual changes
- Lid edema
- Lid lag
- Photophobia
- Enlarged thyroid
- Nervousness
- Heat intolerance
- Tremors
- Palpitations
- Tachycardia
- Dyspnea

DX: PE, thyroid function studies, imaging studies (thyroid scan, ultrasound)

TX: Medication (antithyroid therapy, radioiodine, beta$_2$-adrenergic blockers)

F/U: Thyroid function testing 6 weeks after treatment is initiated, then biannually if at euthyroid state

---

Additional differential diagnoses: Crohn's disease ▪ cryptosporidiosis ▪ depression ▪ esophagitis ▪ gastroenteritis ▪ leukemia ▪ lymphoma ▪ pulmonary tuberculosis ▪ stomatitis ▪ thyrotoxicosis ▪ ulcerative colitis ▪ Whipple's disease

Other causes: amphetamines ▪ chemotherapeutic agents ▪ inappropriate dosages of thyroid preparations ▪ laxative abuse

Wheezing

Wheezing is an adventitious breath sound with a high-pitched, musical, squealing, creaking, or groaning quality. When wheezes (sibilant rhonchi) originate in the large airways, they can be heard by placing an unaided ear over the chest wall or at the mouth. When they originate in smaller airways, they can be heard by placing a stethoscope over the anterior or posterior chest. Unlike crackles and rhonchi, wheezes can't be cleared by coughing.

Usually, prolonged wheezing occurs during expiration when bronchi are shortened and narrowed. Causes of airway narrowing include bronchospasm; mucosal thickening or edema; partial obstruction from a tumor, foreign body, or secretions; and extrinsic pressure, as in tension pneumothorax or goiter. With airway obstruction, wheezing occurs during inspiration.

 ALERT

If you detect wheezing:
- *examine the degree of the patient's respiratory distress and level of consciousness*
- *take the patient's vital signs, noting hypotension or hypertension and an irregular, weak, rapid, or slow pulse*
- *institute emergency measures, if appropriate.*

If the patient isn't in respiratory distress, perform a focused assessment.

HISTORY

- Ask the patient if he has had wheezing before. If so, ask him what aggravated or alleviated it.
- Review the patient's medical history for asthma, allergies, and smoking; pulmonary, cardiac, or circulatory disorders; cancer; and recent surgery, illness, or trauma.
- Ask the patient about changes in appetite, weight, exercise tolerance, or sleep patterns.

- Obtain a drug history, including prescription and over-the-counter drugs, herbal remedies, and recreational drugs. Also, ask the patient about alcohol intake.
- Ask the patient about exposure to toxic fumes or respiratory irritants.
- If the patient has a cough, ask him when it starts and how often it occurs. Does he have paroxysms of coughing? Is his cough dry, sputum producing, or bloody?
- Ask the patient about chest pain. If he reports pain, determine its quality, onset, duration, intensity, and radiation. Does it increase with breathing, coughing, or certain positions?

PHYSICAL ASSESSMENT

- Examine the patient's nose and mouth for congestion, drainage, or signs of infection, such as halitosis. If he produces sputum, obtain a sample for examination.
- Check for cyanosis, pallor, clamminess, masses, tenderness, swelling, distended jugular veins, and enlarged lymph nodes.
- Inspect the chest for abnormal configuration and asymmetrical motion, and determine if the trachea is midline. Percuss for dullness or hyperresonance, and auscultate for crackles, rhonchi, or pleural friction rubs. Note absent or hypoactive breath sounds, abnormal heart sounds, gallops, or murmurs. Also note arrhythmias, bradycardia, or tachycardia. (See *Evaluating breath sounds*.)

SPECIAL CONSIDERATIONS

Ease the patient's breathing by placing him in a semi-Fowler's position and repositioning him frequently.

 PEDIATRIC POINTERS

- *Children are especially susceptible to wheezing because their small airways allow rapid obstruction.*
- *Primary causes of wheezing in children include bronchospasm, mucosal edema, and accumulation of secretions. These may occur with such disorders as cystic fibrosis, aspiration of a foreign body, acute bronchiolitis, and pulmonary hemosiderosis.*

PATIENT COUNSELING

Encourage regular deep breathing and coughing. If appropriate, encourage fluid intake to liquefy secretions and prevent dehydration; increased activity to promote drainage of secretions.

Evaluating breath sounds

Diminished or absent breath sounds indicate some interference with airflow. If pus, fluid, or air fills the pleural space, breath sounds will be quieter than normal. If a foreign body or secretions obstruct a bronchus, breath sounds will be diminished or absent over distal lung tissue. Increased thickness of the chest wall, such as with a patient who is obese or extremely muscular, may cause breath sounds to be decreased or inaudible. Absent breath sounds typically indicate loss of ventilation power.

When air passes through narrowed airways or through moisture, or when the membranes lining the chest cavity become inflamed, adventitious breath sounds will be heard. These include crackles, rhonchi, wheezes, and pleural friction rubs. Usually, these sounds indicate pulmonary disease.

WHEEZING

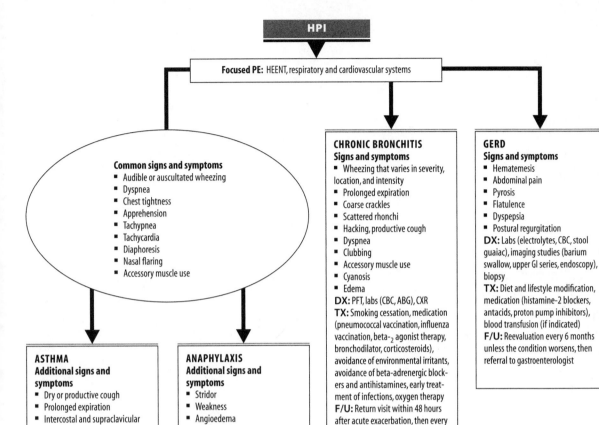

HPI

Focused PE: HEENT, respiratory and cardiovascular systems

Common signs and symptoms
- Audible or auscultated wheezing
- Dyspnea
- Chest tightness
- Apprehension
- Tachypnea
- Tachycardia
- Diaphoresis
- Nasal flaring
- Accessory muscle use

CHRONIC BRONCHITIS
Signs and symptoms
- Wheezing that varies in severity, location, and intensity
- Prolonged expiration
- Coarse crackles
- Scattered rhonchi
- Hacking, productive cough
- Dyspnea
- Clubbing
- Accessory muscle use
- Cyanosis
- Edema

DX: PFT, labs (CBC, ABG), CXR
TX: Smoking cessation, medication (pneumococcal vaccination, influenza vaccination, beta-$_2$ agonist therapy, bronchodilator, corticosteroids), avoidance of environmental irritants, avoidance of beta-adrenergic blockers and antihistamines, early treatment of infections, oxygen therapy
F/U: Return visit within 48 hours after acute exacerbation, then every 3 months

GERD
Signs and symptoms
- Hematemesis
- Abdominal pain
- Pyrosis
- Flatulence
- Dyspepsia
- Postural regurgitation

DX: Labs (electrolytes, CBC, stool guaiac), imaging studies (barium swallow, upper GI series, endoscopy), biopsy
TX: Diet and lifestyle modification, medication (histamine-2 blockers, antacids, proton pump inhibitors), blood transfusion (if indicated)
F/U: Reevaluation every 6 months unless the condition worsens, then referral to gastroenterologist

ASTHMA
Additional signs and symptoms
- Dry or productive cough
- Prolonged expiration
- Intercostal and supraclavicular retractions
- Rhonchi

DX: Allergy skin testing, PFT, labs (CBC, ABG), CXR
TX: Avoidance of allergens, tobacco, and beta-adrenergic blockers; medication (inhaled beta$_2$ agonists, inhaled corticosteroids, leukotriene receptor agonists, systemic steroids [during infections and exacerbations]), peak expiratory flow monitoring
F/U: Reevaluation in 24 hours, then every 3 to 5 days, then every 1 to 3 months

ANAPHYLAXIS
Additional signs and symptoms
- Stridor
- Weakness
- Angioedema
- Intercostal retractions
- Nasal edema and congestion
- Watery rhinorrhea

DX: PE, history of allergen exposure
TX: Symptomatic treatment, airway and oxygenation maintenance, allergy testing (after treatment), medication (I.V. or S.C. epinephrine, antihistamines, nebulized albuterol)
F/U: Reevaluation within 24 hours

Additional differential diagnoses: aspiration of a foreign body ▪ aspiration pneumonitis ▪ bronchial adenoma ▪ bronchiectasis ▪ bronchogenic carcinoma ▪ chemical pneumonitis (acute) ▪ emphysema ▪ inhalation injury ▪ pneumothorax (tension) ▪ pulmonary coccidioidomycosis ▪ pulmonary edema ▪ pulmonary embolus ▪ pulmonary tuberculosis ▪ thyroid goiter ▪ tracheobronchitis ▪ Wegener's granulomatosis

Appendices
Selected references
Index

Normal laboratory test values

HEMATOLOGY

Bleeding time
Duke: 1 to 3 minutes
Ivy: 3 to 6 minutes
Template: 3 to 6 minutes

Clot retraction
50% of size within 1 hour

Erythrocyte sedimentation rate
Males: 0 to 10 mm/hour
Females: 0 to 20 mm/hour

Fibrinogen, plasma
150 to 350 mg/dl

Fibrin split products
Screening assay: < 10 mcg/ml
Quantitative assay: < 3 mcg/ml

Hematocrit
Males: 42% to 54%
Females: 38% to 46%

Hemoglobin (Hb), total
Males: 14 to 18 g/dl
Females: 12 to 16 g/dl

Partial thromboplastin time
21 to 35 seconds

Platelet aggregation
3 to 5 minutes

Platelet count
140,000 to 400,000/μl

Prothrombin consumption time
15 to 20 seconds

Prothrombin time
10 to 14 seconds

Red blood cell (RBC) count
Males: 4.5 to 6.2 million/μl venous blood
Females: 4.2 to 5.4 million/μl venous blood

Red cell indices
Mean corpuscular volume: 84 to 99 fl/cell
Mean corpuscular Hb: 26 to 32 pg/cell
Mean corpuscular Hb concentration: 30 to 36 g/dl

Reticulocyte count
0.5% to 2% of total RBC count

Sickle cell test
Negative

Thrombin time, plasma
10 to 15 seconds

White blood cell (WBC) count, blood
4,000 to 10,000/μl

WBC differential, blood
Basophils: 0.3% to 2%
Eosinophils: 0.3% to 7%
Lymphocytes: 16.2% to 43%
Monocytes: 0.6% to 9.6%
Neutrophils: 47.6% to 76.8%

Whole blood clotting time
5 to 15 minutes

BLOOD CHEMISTRY

Acid phosphatase
0.5 to 1.9 U/ml (based on assay method)

Alanine aminotransferase
Males: 10 to 35 U/L
Females: 9 to 24 U/L

Alkaline phosphatase, serum
Chemical inhibition method:
Males: 98 to 251 U/L
Females: 81 to 312 U/L

Amylase, serum
25 to 125 U/L

Arterial blood gases
Pao_2: 75 to 100 mm Hg
$Paco_2$: 35 to 45 mm Hg
pH: 7.35 to 7.45
Sao_2: 94% to 100%
HCO_3^-: 22 to 26 mEq/L

Aspartate aminotransferase
Males: 8 to 20 U/L
Females: 5 to 40 U/L

Bilirubin, serum
Direct: < 0.5 mg/dl
Indirect: ≤ 1.1 mg/dl

Blood urea nitrogen
8 to 20 mg/dl

Calcium, serum
Ionized: 4 to 5 mg/dl
Total: 8.9 to 10.1 mg/dl

Carbon dioxide, total, blood
22 to 34 mEq/L

Catecholamines, plasma
Supine: dopamine, 0 to 30 pg/ml; epinephrine, 0 to 110 pg/ml; norepi-
    nephrine, 70 to 750 pg/ml
Standing: dopamine, 0 to 30 pg/ml; epinephrine, 0 to 140 pg/ml; norepi-
    nephrine, 200 to 1,700 pg/ml

Chloride, serum
100 to 108 mEq/L

Cholesterol, total, serum
< 200 mg/dl (desirable)

C-reactive protein, serum
< 0.8 mg/dl

Creatine kinase (CK)
Total: males, 38 to 190 U/L; females, 10 to 150 U/L
CK-BB: None
CK-MB: < 6% of total CK
CK-MM: 90% to 100% of total CK

Creatinine, serum
Males: 0.8 to 1.2 mg/dl
Females: 0.6 to 0.9 mg/dl

Free thyroxine
0.8 to 3.3 ng/dl

Free triiodothyronine
0.2 to 0.6 ng/dl

Gamma-glutamyl transferase
Males: 6 to 38 U/L
Females: younger than age 45, 4 to 27 U/L; older than age 45, 6 to 37 U/L

Glucose, fasting, plasma
70 to 110 mg/dl

Glucose, plasma, oral tolerance
Peak at 160 to 180 mg/dl 30 to 60 minutes after challenge dose

Glucose, plasma, 2-hour postprandial
< 145 mg/dl

Iron, serum
Males: 70 to 150 mcg/dl
Females: 80 to 150 mcg/dl

Lactic acid, blood
0.93 to 1.65 mEq/L

Lactic dehydrogenase (LD)
Total: 35 to 378 U/L
LD_1: 14% to 26% of total
LH_2: 29% to 39% of total
LH_3: 20% to 26% of total
LH_4: 8% to 16% of total
LH_5: 6% to 16% of total

Lipase
< 300 U/L

Lipoproteins, serum
High-density lipoprotein cholesterol:
Males: 37 to 70 mg/dl;
Females: 40 to 85 mg/dl

Low-density lipoprotein cholesterol:
Patients without coronary artery disease (CAD): < 130 mg/dl (desirable)
Patients with CAD: < 100 mg/dl (desirable)

Magnesium, serum
1.5 to 2.5 mEq/L
Atomic absorption: 1.7 to 2.1 mg/dl

Phosphates, serum
1.8 to 2.6 mEq/L
Atomic absorption: 2.5 to 4.5 mg/dl

Potassium, serum
3.8 to 5.5 mEq/L

Protein, total, serum
6.6 to 7.9 g/dl
Albumin fraction: 3.3 to 4.5 g/dl
Globulin level: Alpha$_1$ globulin, 0.1 to 0.4 g/dl; alpha$_2$ globulin, 0.5 to 1 g/dl; beta globulin, 0.7 to 1.2 g/dl; gamma globulin, 0.5 to 1.6 g/dl

Sodium, serum
135 to 145 mEq/L

Thyroxine, total, serum
5 to 13.5 mcg/dl

Triglycerides, serum
Males: 40 to 160 mg/dl
Females: 35 to 135 mg/dl

Troponin I
0 to 0.4 mcg/ml

Uric acid, serum
Males: 4.3 to 8 mg/dl
Females: 2.3 to 6 mg/dl

URINE CHEMISTRY

Amylase
10 to 80 U/hour

Bilirubin
Negative

Calcium
Males: < 275 mg/24 hours
Females: < 250 mg/24 hours

Catecholamines
dopamine: 0 to 400 µl/24 hours
epinephrine: 0 to 20 µl/24 hours
norepinephrine: 0 to 80 µl/24 hours

Creatinine
Males: 800 to 2,000 mg/24 hours
Females: 600 to 1,800 mg/24 hours

Creatinine clearance
Males: 94 to 140 ml/minute/1.73 m^2
Females: 72 to 110 ml/minute/1.73 m^2

Glucose
Negative

17-Hydroxycorticosteroids
Males: 4.5 to 12 mg/24 hours
Females: 2.5 to 10 mg/24 hours

17-Ketogenic steroids
Males: 4 to 14 mg/24 hours
Females: 2 to 12 mg/24 hours

Ketones
Negative

17-Ketosteroids
Males: 6 to 21 mg/24 hours
Females: 4 to 17 mg/24 hours

Proteins
Up to 150 mg/24 hours

Sodium
30 to 280 mEq/24 hours

Urea
Maximal clearance: 64 to 99 ml/minute

Uric acid
250 to 750 mg/24 hours

Urinalysis, routine
Color: Straw to dark yellow
Odor: Slightly aromatic
Appearance: Clear
Specific gravity: 1.005 to 1.035
pH: 4.5 to 8
Protein: None
Glucose: None
Epithelial cells: 0 to 5
Casts: None, except occasional hyaline casts
Crystals: Present
Yeast cells: None

Urine concentration
Specific gravity:
Concentrated: 1.025 to 1.030+
Dilute: 1.001 to 1.010

Urine osmolality
50 to 1,400 mOsm/kg water

Urobilinogen
Males: 0.3 to 2.1 Ehrlich U/2 hours
Females: 0.1 to 1.1 Ehrlich U/2 hours

Vanillylmandelic acid
0.7 to 6.8 mg/24 hours

MISCELLANEOUS

Cerebrospinal fluid
Pressure: 50 to 180 mm H_2O

Enzyme-linked immunosorbent assay for human immunodeficiency virus infection
Negative

HIVAGEN test
Negative

Lupus erythematosus cell preparation
Negative

Occult blood, fecal
< 2.5 ml

Rheumatoid factor, serum
Negative

Urobilinogen, fecal
50 to 300 mg/24 hours

Venereal Disease Research Laboratory test, serum
Negative

Western blot assay
Negative

Types of cardiac arrhythmias

Use a standard electrocardiogram strip, if available, to compare normal cardiac rhythm configurations with the rhythm strips depicted here. (Note the various features, causes, and treatments of these common cardiac arrhythmias.) Characteristics of normal rhythm include :

- ventricular and atrial rates of 60 to 100 beats/minute
- regular and uniform QRS complexes and P waves
- PR interval of 0.12 to 0.20 second
- QRS duration < 0.12 second
- identical atrial and ventricular rates, with a constant PR interval.

ARRHYTHMIA AND FEATURES	CAUSES	TREATMENT
Sinus arrhythmia 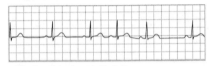 • Irregular atrial and ventricular rhythms • Normal P wave preceding each QRS complex	• Normal variation of normal sinus rhythm for athletes, children, and elderly people • Also seen in digoxin toxicity and inferior wall myocardial infarction (MI)	• No treatment necessary
Sinus tachycardia 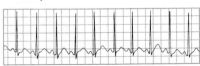 • Atrial and ventricular rhythms regular • Rate > 100 beats/minute; rarely, > 160 beats/minute • Normal P wave preceding each QRS complex	• Normal physiologic response to fever, exercise, anxiety, pain, dehydration; may also accompany shock, left-sided heart failure, cardiac tamponade, hyperthyroidism, anemia, hypovolemia, pulmonary embolism, anterior wall MI • May also occur with atropine, epinephrine, isoproterenol, quinidine, caffeine, alcohol, and nicotine use	• Correction of underlying cause • Beta-adrenergic blockers or calcium channel blocker
Sinus bradycardia 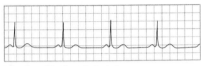 • Regular atrial and ventricular rhythms • Rate < 60 beats/minute • Normal P wave preceding each QRS complex	• Normal in a well-conditioned heart, as in an athlete • Increased intracranial pressure; increased vagal tone due to straining during defecation, vomiting, intubation, mechanical ventilation; sick sinus syndrome; hypothyroidism; inferior wall MI • May also occur with anticholinesterase, beta-adrenergic blocker, digoxin, or morphine use	• Correction of underlying cause • For low cardiac output, dizziness, weakness, altered level of consciousness (LOC), or low blood pressure: advanced cardiac life support (ACLS) protocol for administration of atropine • Temporary or permanent pacemaker • Dopamine • Epinephrine

ARRHYTHMIA AND FEATURES	CAUSES	TREATMENT

Sinoatrial (SA) arrest or block *(sinus arrest)*

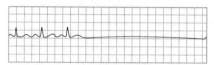

- Atrial and ventricular rhythms normal except for missing complex
- Normal P wave preceding each QRS complex
- Pause not equal to a multiple of the previous sinus rhythm

Causes
- Acute infection
- Coronary artery disease (CAD), degenerative heart disease, acute inferior wall MI
- Vagal stimulation, Valsalva's maneuver, carotid sinus massage
- Digoxin, quinidine, or salicylate toxicity
- Pesticide poisoning
- Pharyngeal irritation caused by endotracheal (ET) intubation
- Sick sinus syndrome

Treatment
- No treatment if asymptomatic
- For low cardiac output, dizziness, weakness, altered LOC, or low blood pressure: ACLS protocol for administration of atropine
- Temporary or permanent pacemaker for repeated episodes

Wandering atrial pacemaker

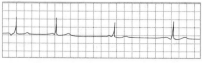

- Atrial and ventricular rhythms may vary slightly
- Irregular PR interval
- P waves irregular with changing configuration, indicating that they aren't all from SA node or single atrial focus; may appear after QRS complexes
- QRS complexes uniform in shape but irregular in rhythm

Causes
- Rheumatic carditis due to inflammation involving the SA node
- Digoxin toxicity
- Sick sinus syndrome

Treatment
- None necessary if patient is asymptomatic
- Treatment of underlying cause if patient is symptomatic

Premature atrial contraction *(PAC)*

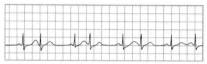

- Premature, abnormal-looking P waves that differ in configuration from normal P waves
- QRS complexes after P waves, except in very early or blocked PACs
- P wave often buried in the preceding T wave or identified in the preceding T wave

Causes
- Coronary or valvular heart disease, atrial ischemia, coronary atherosclerosis, heart failure, acute respiratory failure, chronic obstructive pulmonary disease (COPD), electrolyte imbalance, and hypoxia
- Digoxin toxicity; use of aminophylline, beta-adrenergic blockers, or caffeine
- Anxiety

Treatment
- None (usually)
- Treatment of underlying cause

Paroxysmal atrial tachycardia *(paroxysmal supraventricular tachycardia)*

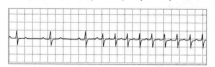

- Atrial and ventricular rhythms regular
- Heart rate > 160 beats/minute; rarely exceeds 250 beats/minute
- P waves regular but aberrant; difficult to differentiate from preceding T wave
- P wave preceding each QRS complex
- Sudden onset and termination of arrhythmia

Causes
- Intrinsic abnormality of AV conduction system
- Physical or psychological stress, hypoxia, hypokalemia, cardiomyopathy, congenital heart disease, MI, valvular disease, Wolff-Parkinson-White syndrome, cor pulmonale, hyperthyroidism, systemic hypertension
- Digoxin toxicity; use of caffeine, marijuana, or central nervous system stimulants

Treatment
- If patient is unstable: immediate cardioversion
- If patient is stable: vagal stimulation, Valsalva's maneuver, carotid sinus massage
- If cardiac function is preserved: ACLS treatment priority—calcium channel blocker, beta-adrenergic blocker, digoxin, and cardioversion; then possibly procainamide, amiodarone, or sotalol
- If ejection fraction is < 40% or the patient is in heart failure: ACLS treatment order—digoxin, amiodarone, and then diltiazem

ARRHYTHMIA AND FEATURES	CAUSES	TREATMENT

Atrial flutter

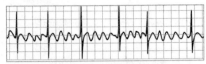

- Atrial rhythm regular; rate, 250 to 400 beats/minute
- Ventricular rate variable, depending on degree of atrioventricular (AV) block (usually 60 to 100 beats/minute)
- Sawtooth P-wave configuration possible (F waves)
- QRS complexes uniform in shape but often irregular in rate

CAUSES
- Heart failure, tricuspid or mitral valve disease, pulmonary embolism, cor pulmonale, inferior wall MI, carditis
- Digoxin toxicity

TREATMENT
- If patient is unstable with a ventricular rate > 150 beats/minute: immediate cardioversion
- If patient is stable: ACLS protocol for cardioversion and drug therapy, which may include calcium channel blockers, beta-adrenergic blockers, or antiarrhythmics
- Anticoagulation therapy, if necessary
- Radiofrequency ablation to control rhythm

Atrial fibrillation (AFIB)

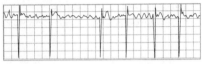

- Atrial rhythm grossly irregular; rate, > 400 beats/minute
- Ventricular rate grossly irregular
- QRS complexes of uniform configuration and duration
- PR interval indiscernible
- No P waves, or P waves that appear as erratic, irregular, baseline fibrillary waves

CAUSES
- Heart failure, COPD, thyrotoxicosis, constrictive pericarditis, ischemic heart disease, sepsis, pulmonary embolus, rheumatic heart disease, hypertension, mitral stenosis, atrial irritation, complication of coronary bypass or valve replacement surgery

TREATMENT
- If patient is unstable with a ventricular rate > 150 beats/minute: immediate cardioversion
- If patient is stable: ACLS protocol for cardioversion and drug therapy, which may include calcium channel blockers, beta-adrenergic blockers, or antiarrhythmics
- Anticoagulation therapy, if necessary
- In some patients with refractory atrial fibrillation uncontrolled by drugs, radiofrequency catheter ablation

Junctional rhythm

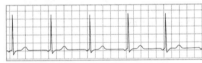

- Atrial and ventricular rhythms regular
- Atrial rate 40 to 60 beats/minute
- Ventricular rate usually 40 to 60 beats/minute (60 to 100 beats/minute is accelerated junctional rhythm)
- P waves preceding, hidden within (absent), or after QRS complex; usually inverted if visible
- PR interval (when present) < 0.12 second
- QRS complex configuration and duration normal, except in aberrant conduction

CAUSES
- Inferior wall MI or ischemia, hypoxia, vagal stimulation, sick sinus syndrome
- Acute rheumatic fever
- Valve surgery
- Digoxin toxicity

TREATMENT
- Correction of underlying cause
- Atropine for symptomatic slow rate
- Pacemaker insertion if patient is refractory to drugs
- Discontinuation of digoxin, if appropriate

Junctional contractions (junctional premature beats)

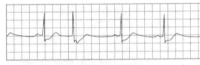

- Atrial and ventricular rhythms irregular
- P waves inverted; may precede, be hidden within, or follow QRS complexes
- PR interval < 0.12 second if P wave precedes QRS complex
- QRS complex configuration and duration normal

CAUSES
- MI or ischemia
- Digoxin toxicity and excessive caffeine or amphetamine use

TREATMENT
- Correction of underlying cause
- None (usually)

ARRHYTHMIA AND FEATURES	CAUSES	TREATMENT

Junctional tachycardia

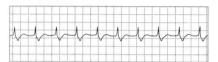

- Atrial rate > 100 beats/minute; however, P wave may be absent, hidden in QRS complex, or preceding T wave
- Ventricular rate > 100 beats/minute
- P wave inverted
- QRS complex configuration and duration normal
- Onset of rhythm often sudden, occurring in bursts

- Myocarditis, cardiomyopathy, inferior wall MI or ischemia, acute rheumatic fever, complication of valve replacement surgery
- Digoxin toxicity

- If heart function is preserved: ACLS guidelines for amiodarone, calcium channel blocker, or beta-adrenergic blocker
- If ejection fraction is < 40% or the patient is in heart failure: ACLS guidelines for amiodarone

First-degree AV block

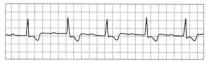

- Atrial and ventricular rhythms regular
- PR interval > 0.20 second
- P wave preceding each QRS complex
- QRS complex normal

- May be seen in a healthy person
- Inferior wall myocardial ischemia or MI, hypothyroidism, hypokalemia, hyperkalemia
- Digoxin toxicity; use of quinidine, procainamide, beta-adrenergic blockers, calcium channel blockers, or amiodarone

- Correction of underlying cause
- Possibly atropine if severe bradycardia develops
- Cautious use of digoxin, calcium channel blockers, and beta-adrenergic blockers

Second-degree AV block *Mobitz I (Wenckebach)*

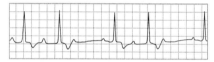

- Atrial rhythm regular
- Ventricular rhythm irregular
- Atrial rate exceeds ventricular rate
- PR interval progressively, but only slightly, longer with each cycle until QRS complex disappears (dropped beat); PR interval shorter after dropped beat

- Inferior wall MI, cardiac surgery, acute rheumatic fever, and vagal stimulation
- Digoxin toxicity; use of propranolol, quinidine, or procainamide

- Treatment of underlying cause
- Atropine or temporary pacemaker for symptomatic bradycardia
- Discontinuation of digoxin, if appropriate

Second-degree AV block *Mobitz II*

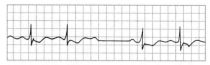

- Atrial rhythm regular
- Ventricular rhythm regular or irregular, with varying degree of block
- P-P interval constant
- QRS complexes periodically absent

- Severe CAD, anterior wall MI, acute myocarditis
- Digoxin toxicity

- Temporary or permanent pacemaker
- Atropine, dopamine, or epinephrine for symptomatic bradycardia
- Discontinuation of digoxin, if appropriate

ARRHYTHMIA AND FEATURES	CAUSES	TREATMENT

Third-degree AV block *(complete heart block)*

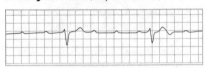

- Atrial rhythm regular
- Ventricular rhythm slow and regular
- No relation between P waves and QRS complexes
- No constant PR interval
- QRS interval normal (nodal pacemaker) or wide and bizarre (ventricular pacemaker)

- Inferior or anterior wall MI, congenital abnormality, rheumatic fever, hypoxia, postoperative complication of mitral valve replacement, Lev's disease (fibrosis and calcification that spreads from cardiac structures to the conductive tissue), Lenègre's disease (conductive tissue fibrosis)
- Digoxin toxicity

- Temporary or permanent pacemaker
- Atropine, dopamine, or epinephrine for symptomatic bradycardia

---

Premature ventricular contraction *(PVC)*

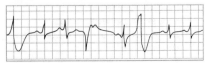

- Atrial rhythm regular
- Ventricular rhythm irregular
- QRS complex premature, usually followed by a complete compensatory pause
- QRS complex wide and distorted, usually > 0.14 second
- Premature QRS complexes occurring singly, in pairs, or in threes; alternating with normal beats; focus from one or more sites
- Ominous when clustered, multifocal, and with R wave on T pattern

- Heart failure; old or acute myocardial ischemia, MI, or contusion; myocardial irritation by ventricular catheter, such as a pacemaker; hypercapnia; hypokalemia; hypocalcemia
- Drug toxicity (cardiac glycosides, aminophylline, tricyclic antidepressants, beta-adrenergic blockers [isoproterenol or dopamine])
- Caffeine, tobacco, or alcohol use
- Psychological stress, anxiety, pain, exercise

- If symptomatic, procainamide, amiodarone, or lidocaine I.V.
- Treatment of underlying cause
- Discontinuation of drug causing toxicity
- Potassium chloride I.V. if PVC induced by hypokalemia
- Magnesium sulfate I.V. if PVC induced by hypomagnesemia

Ventricular tachycardia

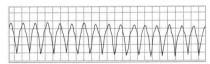

- Ventricular rate 140 to 220 beats/minute, regular or irregular
- QRS complexes wide, bizarre, and independent of P waves
- P waves not discernible
- May start and stop suddenly

- Myocardial ischemia, MI, or aneurysm; CAD; rheumatic heart disease; mitral valve prolapse; heart failure; cardiomyopathy; ventricular catheters; hypokalemia; hypercalcemia; pulmonary embolism
- Digoxin, procainamide, epinephrine, or quinidine toxicity
- Anxiety

- With pulse: if hemodynamically stable with monomorphic QRS complexes, administration of procainamide, sotalol, amiodarone, or lidocaine (follow ACLS protocol); if drugs are ineffective, cardioversion
- If polymorphic QRS complexes and normal QT interval, beta-adrenergic blockers, lidocaine, amiodarone, procainamide, or sotalol (follow ACLS protocol); if drugs are unsuccessful, cardioversion
- If polymorphic QRS and QT interval prolonged, magnesium I.V. (overdrive pacing if rhythm persists); also, isoproterenol, phenytoin, or lidocaine
- Pulseless: cardiopulmonary resuscitation (CPR); ACLS protocol for defibrillation, administration of epinephrine or vasopressin, followed by amiodarone or lidocaine and, if ineffective, magnesium sulfate or procainamide
- Implanted cardioverter defibrillator if recurrent ventricular tachycardia

ARRHYTHMIA AND FEATURES	CAUSES	TREATMENT

Ventricular fibrillation

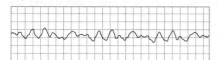

- Ventricular rhythm rapid and chaotic
- QRS complexes wide and irregular; no visible P waves

- Myocardial ischemia, MI, R-on-T phenomenon, untreated ventricular tachycardia, hypokalemia, hyperkalemia, hypercalcemia, alkalosis, electric shock, hypothermia
- Digoxin, epinephrine, or quinidine toxicity

- CPR; ACLS protocol for defibrillation, ET intubation, and administration of epinephrine or vasopressin, amiodarone, or lidocaine, and, if ineffective, magnesium sulfate or procainamide
- Implantable cardioverter-defibrillator if risk for recurrent ventricular fibrillation

Asystole

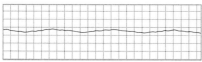

- No atrial or ventricular rate or rhythm
- No discernible P waves, QRS complexes, or T waves

- Myocardial ischemia, MI, aortic valve disease, heart failure, hypoxemia, hypokalemia, severe acidosis, electric shock, ventricular arrhythmias, AV block, pulmonary embolism, heart rupture, cardiac tamponade, hyperkalemia, electromechanical dissociation
- Cocaine overdose

- CPR; ACLS protocol for ET intubation, transcutaneous pacing, and administration of epinephrine and atropine

Resources for professionals, patients, and caregivers

GENERAL HEALTH CARE WEB SITES
- *www.healthfinder.gov*—from the U.S. government; searchable database with links to Web sites, support groups, government agencies, and not-for-profit organizations that provide health care information for patients
- *www.healthweb.org*—from a group of librarians and information professionals at academic medical centers in the midwestern United States; offers a searchable database of evaluated Web sites for patients and health care professionals
- *www.medmatrix.org*—includes journal articles, abstracts, reviews, conference highlights, and links to other major sources for health care professionals
- *www.mwsearch.com* — named Medical World Search, this site searches thousands of selected medical sites

ORGANIZATIONS
- American Academy of Family Physicians—offers handouts and other resources to patients and health care professionals, plus links to other sites: *www.aafp.org*
- Joint Commission on Accreditation of Healthcare Organizations: *www.jcaho.org*

GOVERNMENT AGENCIES
- Agency for Healthcare Research and Quality: *www.ahcpr.gov*
- Centers for Disease Control and Prevention: *www.cdc.gov*
- Centers for Medicare & Medicaid Services: *www.cms.hss.gov*
- National Center for Complementary and Alternative Medicine: *www.nccam.nih.gov*
- National Guideline Clearinghouse: *www.guideline.com*
- National Library of Medicine, Specialized Information Services (information resources and services in toxicology, environmental health, chemistry, HIV/AIDS, and specialized topics in minority health): *www.sis.nlm.nih.gov*
- U.S. Department of Health & Human Services: *www.dhhs.gov*
- U.S. Food and Drug Administration: *www.fda.gov*

LINKS TO SPANISH-LANGUAGE SITES
- Agency for Healthcare Research and Quality: *www.ahcpr.gov* (click on "Información en español")
- CANCERCare, Inc.: *www.cancercare.org* (click on "En español")
- Healthfinder: *www.healthfinder.gov* (click on "Español")
- National Cancer Institute: *www.cancer.gov/espanol*

CONDITION-SPECIFIC SITES
Aging
- American Society on Aging: *www.asaging.org*
- National Institute on Aging: *www.nia.nih.gov;* 301-496-1752
- U.S. Administration on Aging: *www.aoa.dhhs.gov*

AIDS/HIV/STDs
- Centers for Disease Control and Prevention, National Prevention Information Network: *www.cdcnpin.org/scripts/index.asp*
- HIV/AIDS Treatment Information Service; *www.sis.nlm.nih.gov/aids/aidstrea.html* ; 800-448-0440 (Spanish available); TTY, 800-243-7012
- National AIDS Hotline (24 hours): 800-342-AIDS; Spanish, 800-344-7432; TTY, 800-243-7889
- Office of AIDS Research: *www.sis.nlm.nih.gov/aids/oar.html*

Allergies and asthma
- Allergy & Asthma Disease Management Center: *www.aaaai.org/aadmc*
- Allergy & Asthma Network—Mothers of Asthmatics: *www.aanma.org;* 800-878-4403
- Allergy, Asthma & Immunology Online: *www.allergy.mcg.edu*
- American Academy of Allergy Asthma & Immunology: *www.aaaai.org;* 800-822-2762
- Global Initiative For Asthma: *www.ginasthma.com*
- Joint Council of Allergy, Asthma and Immunology: *www.jcaai.org*

- National Asthma Education and Prevention Program: *www.nhlbi.nih.gov/about/naepp*
- National Institute of Allergy and Infectious Diseases: *www.niaid.nih.gov*

Alzheimer's disease
- Agency for Healthcare Research and Quality (AHRQ) Early Alzheimer's Disease Clinical Practice Guideline — Patient and Family Guide: *www.ahcpr.gov/clinic/alzcons.htm*
- AHRQ's Recognition and Assessment Guideline: *www.ahcpr.gov/clinic/alzover.htm*
- Alzheimer's Association: *www.alz.org*; 800-272-3900
- Alzheimer's Disease Education & Referral Center: *www.alzheimers.org*; 800-438-4380
- Alzheimer Europe: *www.alzheimer-europe.org*
- AlzWell Caregiver Page: *www.alzwell.com*

Arthritis
- American Autoimmune Related Diseases Association, Inc.: *www.aarda.org*
- American College of Rheumatology: *www.rheumatology.org*
- Arthritis Foundation: *www.arthritis.org*; 800-283-7800
- National Institute of Arthritis and Musculoskeletal and Skin Diseases: *www.nih.gov/niams*

Attention deficit disorder/hyperactivity
- National Attention Deficit Disorder Association: *www.add.org*

Cancer
- American Cancer Society: *www.cancer.org*; 800-ACS-2345
- CANCERCare, Inc.: *www.cancercare.org*
- Cancer News on the Net: *www.cancernews.com*
- National Breast Cancer Awareness Month: *www.nbcam.org*
- National Cancer Institute: *www.cancer.gov*
- National Cancer Institute, Cancer Information Service: 800-4-CANCER
- National Cancer Institute, Cancer Literature Search: *www.cancer.gov/search/pubmed*
- National Cancer Institute, Cancer Trials: *www.cancer.gov/clinicaltrials*
- National Center for Chronic Disease Prevention and Health Promotion: *www.cdc.gov/nccdphp*
- National Comprehensive Cancer Network: *www.nccn.org*
- Susan G. Komen Breast Cancer Foundation: *www.komen.org*
- Y-Me National Breast Cancer Organization: *www.y-me.org*; 800-221-2141; 800-986-9505 (Español)

Cardiac
- American Heart Association: *www.americanheart.org*; 800-242-8721
- Mayo Heart Center: *www.mayohealth.org* (click on "Heart")
- National Heart, Lung, and Blood Institute: *www.nhlbi.nih.gov*
- National Stroke Association: *www.stroke.org*

Diabetes
- American Association of Diabetes Educators: *www.aadenet.org*; 800-338-3633
- American Diabetes Association: *www.diabetes.org*
- Diabetes self-care equipment for the visually impaired: Palco Labs, Inc.: *www.palcolabs.com*; 800-346-4488
- Joslin Diabetes Center: *www.joslin.harvard.edu*
- National Institute of Diabetes & Digestive & Kidney Diseases: *www.niddk.nih.gov*

Disabilities
- University of Virginia: General Resources About Disabilities: *www.curry.edschool.virginia.edu/go/cise/ose/resources/general.html*; Assistive Technology Resources, *www.curry.edschool.virginia.edu/go/cise/ose/resources/asst_tech.html*

Elder abuse
- National Center for Victims of Crime: *www.ncvc.org*
- National Center on Elder Abuse: *www.elderabusecenter.org*

Gastrointestinal
- American Liver Foundation: *www.liverfoundation.org*
- National Institute of Diabetes & Digestive & Kidney Diseases: *www.niddk.nih.gov*
- National Kidney Foundation: *www.kidney.org*; 800-622-9010

Musculoskeletal
- American College of Foot and Ankle Surgeons: *www.acfas.org*
- Amputee Coalition of America: *www.amputee-coalition.org*; 888-AMP-KNOW (267-5669)
- National Institue of Arthritis and Musculoskeletal and Skin Disorders: *www.niams.nih.gov*
- National Osteoporosis Foundation: *www.nof.org*

Neurology
- ALS Association: *www.alsa.org*; 818-880-9007
- American Brain Tumor Association: *www.abta.org*; 800-886-2282
- Association of Late-Deafened Adults, Inc.: *www.alda.org*
- EAR Foundation/Meniere's Network: *www.theearfoundation.org*
- National Association of the Deaf: *www.nad.org*

- National Federation of the Blind: *www.nfb.org*
- National Institute of Neurological Disorders and Stroke: *www.ninds.nih.gov*
- National Institute on Deafness and Other Communication Disorders: *www.nidcd.nih.gov*

Pediatrics
- Children with Diabetes: *www.childrenwithdiabetes.com*
- Cystic Fibrosis Foundation: *www.cff.org*; 800-FIGHT CF (344-4823)
- Cystic Fibrosis Mutation Data Base: *www.genet.sickkids.on.ca/cftr*
- Cystic Fibrosis USA: *www.cfusa.org*
- Down's Heart Group: *www.downs-heart.downsnet.org*
- Emory University Sickle Cell Information Center: *www.emory.edu/PEDS/SICKLE/newweb.htm*
- Families of Spinal Muscular Atrophy: *www.fsma.org*; 800-886-1762
- Growth Charts for Children with Down Syndrome: *www.growthcharts.com*
- Internet Resource for Special Children: *www.irsc.org*
- National Down Syndrome Society: *www.ndss.org*
- National Institute of Child Health & Human Development: *www.nichd.nih.gov*
- National Pediatric AIDS Network: *www.npan.org*
- Spina Bifida Association of America: *www.sbaa.org*; 800-621-3141
- United Cerebral Palsy: *www.ucpa.org*; 800-872-5827

Psychiatry
- American Psychological Association: *www.apa.org*; 800-374-2721
- Depressive and Bipolar Support Alliance: *www.dbsalliance.org*
- National Alliance for the Mentally Ill: *www.nami.org*; 800-950-NAMI (950-6264)
- National Mental Health Association: *www.nmha.org*; 800-969-6642

Respiratory
- American Heart Association (smoking cessation information): 800-242-8721
- American Lung Association: *www.lungusa.org*; 800-LUNG-USA (local affiliates answer)
- National Emphysema Foundation: *www.emphysemafoundation.org*

Skin
- National Pressure Ulcer Advisory Panel: *www.npuap.org*
- Wound Care Information Network: *www.medicaledu.com*

- Wound Care Institute, Inc.: *www.woundcare.org*; 305-919-9192
- Wound, Ostomy and Continence Nurses Society: *www.wocn.org*; 888-224-WOCN

Substance abuse
- Al-Anon & Alateen (including Spanish and French language options): *www.al-anon.alateen.org*
- Alcoholics Anonymous (including Spanish and French language options): *www.alcoholics-anonymous.org*
- Narcotics Anonymous World Services: *www.wsoinc.com*
- National Centers for Disease Control and Prevention, Tobacco Information and Prevention Source: *www.cdc.gov/tobacco*
- National Council on Alcoholism and Drug Dependence: *www.ncadd.org*; 800-NCA-CALL (622-2255)
- National Institute on Alcohol Abuse and Alcoholism: *www.niaaa.nih.gov*
- Substance Abuse & Mental Health Services Administration: *www.samhsa.gov*

Women's health
- American College of Cardiology: *www.acc.org*
- American Heart Association: *www.women.americanheart.org*
- American Medical Women's Association: *www.amwa-doc.org*
- *JAMA* Women's Health Information Center: *www.ama-assn.org/special/womh/womh.htm*
- Johns Hopkins Intelihealth: *www.intelihealth.com* (click on "Women's health")
- Office on Women's Health (U.S. Department of Health & Human Services): *www.4women.gov/owh*
- Womens' Health Initiative: *www.nhlbi.nih.gov/whi*

Commonly used medical abbreviations

Here is a list of commonly used medical abbreviations. You may find this list helpful when you're using the flowcharts in this book.

AAA	abdominal aortic aneurysm		AROM	active range of motion; artificial rupture of membranes
ABC	airway, breathing, and circulation		ASA	acetylsalicylic acid (aspirin)
ABG	arterial blood gas		ASD	atrial septal defect
ACE	angiotensin-converting enzyme		AV	atrioventricular
ACLS	advanced cardiac life support		AVM	arteriovenous malformation
ACTH	adrenocorticotropic hormone		BBB	bundle-branch block
ADH	antidiuretic hormone		BCP	birth control pill
ADLs	activities of daily living		BE	barium enema
AED	automated external defibrillator		b.i.d.	two times per day
AFB	acid fast bacilli		BKA	below-knee amputation
AFIB	atrial fibrillation		BM	bowel movement
AIDS	acquired immunodeficiency syndrome		BMR	basal metabolic rate
AKA	above-knee amputation		BP	blood pressure
ALL	acute lymphocytic leukemia		BPH	benign prostatic hyperplasia
ALS	amyotrophic lateral sclerosis		BSA	body surface area
AMA	against medical advice		BSE	breast self-examination
ANA	antinuclear antibody		BUN	blood urea nitrogen
AP	anteroposterior; apical pulse		BW	birth weight
ARDS	acute respiratory distress syndrome		C	centigrade; Celsius
ARF	acute renal failure; acute respiratory failure		Ca	calcium

CABG	coronary artery bypass graft	DM	diabetes mellitus
CAD	coronary artery disease	DNA	deoxyribonucleic acid
CAPD	continuous ambulatory peritoneal dialysis	DNR	do not resuscitate
CAVH	continuous arteriovenous hemofiltration	DOA	date of admission; dead on arrival
CBC	complete blood count	DOB	date of birth
CC	chief complaint	DPT	diphtheria, pertussis, and tetanus
CCU	coronary care unit	*DSM-IV*	*Diagnostic and Statistical Manual of Mental Disorders,* 4th ed.
CDC	Centers for Disease Control and Prevention	DTR	deep tendon reflex
CEA	carcinoembryonic antigen	DVT	deep vein thrombosis
CF	cystic fibrosis	D_5W	dextrose 5% in water
CK	creatine kinase	DX	diagnosis
CMV	cytomegalovirus	ECF	extended care facility; extracellular fluid
CNS	central nervous system	ECG	electrocardiogram
COPD	chronic obstructive pulmonary disease	ECMO	extracorporeal membrane oxygenator
CP	cerebral palsy	ECT	electroconvulsive therapy
CPAP	continuous positive airway pressure	ED	emergency department
CPP	cerebral perfusion pressure	EDC	estimated date of confinement
CPR	cardiopulmonary resuscitation	EDD	estimated date of delivery
C&S	culture and sensitivity	EEG	electroencephalogram
CSF	cerebrospinal fluid	EENT	eyes, ears, nose, and throat
CT	computed tomography	EF	ejection fraction
CV	cardiovascular	ELISA	enzyme-linked immunosorbent assay
CVP	central venous pressure	EMG	electromyogram
CXR	chest X-ray	EMS	emergency medical services
DC	direct current	ENT	ear, nose, and throat
DHEA	dehydroepiandrosterone	EOM	extraocular movements
DIC	disseminated intravascular coagulation	ER	emergency room; expiratory reserve
DJD	degenerative joint disease	ERCP	endoscopic retrograde cholangiopancreatography
DKA	diabetic ketoacidosis	ERV	expiratory reserve volume

ESR	erythrocyte sedimentation rate		Hb	hemoglobin
ETOH	ethanol (ethyl alcohol)		HBIG	hepatitis B immunoglobulin
F	Fahrenheit		HBsAg	hepatitis B surface antigen
FBS	fasting blood sugar		HCG	human chorionic gonadotropin
FDA	Food and Drug Administration		HCT	hematocrit
FEF	forced expiratory flow		HEENT	head, ears, eyes, nose and throat
FEV	forced expiratory volume		Hg	mercury
FFP	fresh frozen plasma		H/H	hemoglobin and hematocrit
FH	family history		HHA	home health aide
FHR	fetal heart rate		HHNS	hyperosmolar hyperglycemic nonketotic syndrome
FRC	functional residual capacity		HIV	human immunodeficiency virus
FSH	follicle-stimulating hormone		HLA	human leukocyte antigen
FSP	fibin split products		HMO	health maintenance organization
F/U	follow-up		H_2O	water
FUO	fever of unknown origin		H_2O_2	hydrogen peroxide
FVC	forced vital capacity		HOB	head of bed
G	gravida		HPI	history of present illness
g	gram		h.s.	hour of sleep
GB	gallbladder		HSV	herpes simplex virus
GBS	gallbladder series		IABP	intra-aortic balloon pump
GERD	gastroesophageal reflux disease		ICD	implantable cardioverter-defibrillator
GFR	glomerular filtration rate		ICP	intracranial pressure
GI	gastrointestinal		ICU	intensive care unit
GP	general practitioner		I&D	incision and drainage
gr	grain		I.M.	intramuscular
gtt	drop		I&O	intake and output
GU	genitourinary		IOP	intraocular pressure
GVHD	graft-versus-host disease		IPPB	intermittent positive-pressure breathing
GYN	gynecology		IU	international unit

IUD	intrauterine device	mEq	milliequivalent
I.V.	intravenous	Mg	magnesium
IVP	intravenous pyelography	mg	milligram
JVD	jugular vein distention	MI	myocardial infarction
K	potassium	MIBG	meta-iodobenzylguanidine
KCl	potassium chloride	ml	milliliter
kg	kilogram	MRA	magnetic resonance angiography
KUB	kidneys, ureters, and bladder (X-ray)	MRI	magnetic resonance imaging
KVO	keep vein open	MS	multiple sclerosis; mitral stenosis
L	left, liter	Na	sodium
LDH	lactate dehydrogenase	N/A	not applicable
LDL	low-density lipoprotein	NaCl	sodium chloride
LE	lower extremity	NAD	no acute distress
LFT	liver function tests	NAS	no added salt
LH	luteinizing hormone	NG	nasogastric
LLL	left lower lobe	NICU	neonatal intensive care unit
LLQ	left lower quadrant	NKA	no known allergies
LMP	last menstrual period	NMR	nuclear magnetic resonance
LOC	level of consciousness	NPO	nothing by mouth
LP	lumbar puncture	NSAID	nonsteroidal anti-inflammatory drug
LUE	left upper extremity	NSR	normal sinus rhythm
LUL	left upper lobe	NWB	non-weight bearing
LUQ	left upper quadrant	OB	obstetrics
LVEDP	left ventricular end-diastolic pressure	o.d.	daily
LVH	left ventricular hypertrophy	OOB	out of bed
MAO	monoamine oxidase	OPV	oral polio vaccine
MAP	mean arterial pressure	OR	operating room
mcg	microgram	ORIF	open reduction internal fixation
MCL	midclavicular line	OT	occupational therapy

OTC	over the counter	RA	right atrium; right arm; renal artery
P	pulse	RAI	radioactive iodine
PAT	paroxysmal atrial tachycardia	RAP	right atrial pressure
PAWP	pulmonary artery wedge pressure	RBBB	right bundle-branch block
PCA	patient-controlled analgesia	RBC	red blood cell
PCI	percutaneous coronary intervention	REM	rapid eye movement
PDA	patent ductus arteriosus	Rh	Rhesus factor
PE	physical examination	RICE	rest, ice, compression, elevation
PERRLA	pupils equal, round, react to light and accommodation	RLE	right lower extremity
PET	positron-emission tomography	RLL	right lower lobe
PFT	pulmonary function tests	RLQ	right lower quadrant
PICC	peripherally inserted central catheter	RML	right middle lobe
PID	pelvic inflammatory disease	ROM	range of motion
PIH	pregnancy-induced hypertension	RR	respiratory rate
PKU	phenylketonuria	R/T	related to
PMI	point of maximal impulse	RUL	right upper lobe
PMS	premenstrual syndrome	RUQ	right upper quadrant
P.O.	by mouth	Rx	prescription, treatment, or therapy
PRBC	packed red blood cells	S.C.	subcutaneous
p.r.n.	as needed	SG	specific gravity
PROM	passive range of motion	SIDS	sudden infant death syndrome
PSA	prostate-specific antigen	S.L.	sublingual
PT	prothrombin time	SLE	systemic lupus erythematosus
PTCA	percutaneous transluminal coronary angioplasty	SNF	skilled nursing facility
PTT	partial thromboplastin time	SOB	shortness of breath
PVC	premature ventricular contraction	SSE	soapsuds enema
PVD	peripheral vascular disease	SSRI	selective-serotonin reuptake inhibitors
q.h.	every hour	STD	sexually transmitted disease
q.o.d.	every other day	STS	serologic test for syphilis

SVD	spontaneous vaginal delivery		VD	venereal disease
T_3	triiodothyronine		VDRL	Venereal Disease Research Laboratory (test)
T_4	thyroxine		VF	ventricular fibrillation
TAH	total abdominal hysterectomy		VO	verbal order
TB	tuberculosis		$\dot{V}/\dot{Q}$	ventilation-perfusion
Tc	technetium		VSD	ventricular septal defect
TCA	tricyclic antidepressants		VT	ventricular tachycardia
TEE	transesophageal echocardiogram		V_T	tidal volume
TENS	transcutaneous electrical nerve stimulation		WBC	white blood cell
TIA	transient ischemic attack		WNL	within normal limits
TIBC	total iron-binding capacity		WPW	Wolff-Parkinson-White (syndrome)
t.i.d.	three times per day			
TMJ	temporomandibular joint			
T.O.	telephone order			
TPN	total parenteral nutrition			
TPR	temperature, pulse, and respirations			
TSH	thyroid stimulating hormone			
TUR	transurethral resection			
TURP	transurethral resection of the prostate			
TX	treatment			
U	unit			
UA	urinalysis			
UE	upper extremity			
URI	upper respiratory infection			
USP	*United States Pharmacopeia*			
UTI	urinary tract infection			
UV	ultraviolet			
VAD	vascular access device; ventricular assist device			
VC	vital capacity			

Selected references

American Heart Association. *Guidelines for Cardiopulmonary Resuscitation and Emergency Cardiovascular Care.* Dallas: American Heart Association, 2000.

Apple, S., and Lindsay, J. *Principles & Practice of Interventional Cardiology.* Baltimore: Lippincott Williams & Wilkins, 2000.

Bartlett, J.G. *2002 Pocket Book of Infectious Disease Therapy,* 11th ed. Baltimore: Lippincott Williams & Wilkins, 2002.

Bartlett, J.G. *Management of Respiratory Tract Infections,* 3rd ed. Baltimore: Lippincott Williams & Wilkins, 2001.

Bickley, L.S., and Szilagyi, P.G. *Bates' Guide to Physical Examination and History Taking,* 8th ed. Philadelphia: Lippincott Williams & Wilkins, 2003.

Braunwald, E., et al., eds. *Harrison's Principles of Internal Medicine,* 15th ed. New York: McGraw-Hill Book Co., 2001.

Bullock, B.L., and Henze, R.L. *Focus on Pathophysiology.* Philadelphia: Lippincott Williams & Wilkins, 2000.

Burroughs, A., and Leifer, G. *Maternity Nursing: An Introductory Text,* 8th ed. Philadelphia: W.B. Saunders Co., 2001.

Busse, W.W., et al. "Pathology of Severe Asthma." *Journal of Allergy and Clinical Immunology* 106(6):1033-42, December 2000.

Copel, L.C. *Nurse's Clinical Guide: Psychiatric and Mental Health Care,* 2nd ed. Springhouse, Pa.: Springhouse Corp., 2000.

DeVita, V., et al., eds. *Cancer: Principles and Practice of Oncology.* Philadelphia: Lippincott Williams & Wilkins, 2001.

Diagnostic and Statistical Manual of Mental Disorders, Fourth Edition, Text Revision. Washington, D.C.: American Psychiatric Association, 2000.

Diagnostics: An A-to-Z Nursing Guide to Laboratory Tests & Diagnostic Procedures. Springhouse, Pa.: Springhouse Corp., 2001.

Diseases, 2nd ed. Philadelphia: Lippincott Williams & Wilkins, 2002.

ECG Cards, 3rd ed. Springhouse, Pa.: Springhouse Corp., 2000.

ECG Interpretation Made Incredibly Easy, 2nd ed. Springhouse, Pa.: Springhouse Corp., 2002.

Elkin, M.K., et al. *Nursing Interventions and Clinical Skills,* 2nd ed. St. Louis: Mosby–Year Book, Inc., 2000.

Fleischer, A.B., Jr. *20 Common Problems in Dermatology.* New York: McGraw-Hill Book Co., 2000.

Fluids and Electrolytes Made Incredibly Easy, 2nd ed. Springhouse, Pa.: Springhouse Corp., 2002.

Fraunfelder, F.T., et al. *Current Ocular Therapy,* 5th ed. Philadelphia: W.B. Saunders Co., 2000.

Goldman, L., and Ausiello, D., eds. *Cecil Textbook of Medicine,* 22nd ed. Philadelphia: W.B. Saunders Co., 2004.

Grenvik, A., et al, eds. *Textbook of Critical Care,* 4th ed. Philadelphia: W.B. Saunders Co., 2000.

Handbook of Diagnostic Tests, 3rd ed. Philadelphia: Lippincott Williams & Wilkins, 2003.

Handbook of Geriatric Nursing Care, 2nd ed. Philadelphia: Lippincott Williams & Wilkins, 2003.

Handbook of Medical-Surgical Nursing, 3rd ed. Springhouse, Pa.: Springhouse Corp., 2002.

Harwood-Nuss, A., et al., eds. *The Clinical Practice of Emergency Medicine,* 3rd ed. Philadelphia: Lippincott Williams & Wilkins, 2001.

Hickey, J.V. *The Clinical Practice of Neurological and Neurosurgical Nursing,* 5th ed. Philadelphia: Lippincott Williams & Wilkins, 2002.

Humes, H.D., et al., eds. *Kelley's Textbook of Internal Medicine,* 4th ed. Philadelphia: Lippincott Williams & Wilkins, 2000.

Isaacs, A., ed. *Lippincott's Review Series: Mental Health and Psychiatric Nursing.* Philadelphia: Lippincott Williams & Wilkins, 2001.

Katz, D.L. *Nutrition in Clinical Practice: A Comprehensive, Evidence-based Manual for the Practitioner.* Philadelphia: Lippincott Williams & Wilkins, 2001.

Ketner, K. "Identifying the Adolescent at Risk" in *Summary of 23rd Annual California Coalition of Nurse Practitioners Educational Conference.* 2000.

Kirsner, J.B., ed. *Inflammatory Bowel Disease,* 5th ed. Philadelphia: W.B. Saunders Co., 2000.

Koopman, W., ed. *Arthritis and Allied Conditions: A Textbook of Rheumatology,* 14th ed. Philadelphia: Lippincott Williams & Wilkins, 2001.

Lahita, R., et al., eds. *Textbook of Autoimmune Diseases.* Philadelphia: Lippincott Williams & Wilkins, 2000.

Lewis, S.M., et al., eds. *Medical-Surgical Nursing: Assessment and Management of Clinical Problems,* 5th ed. St. Louis: Mosby–Year Book, 2003.

Maas, M., et al. *Nursing Care of Older Adults: Diagnoses, Outcomes, and Interventions.* St. Louis: Mosby–Year Book, Inc., 2001.

Mahan, L.K., and Escott-Stump, S. *Krause's Food, Nutrition, and Diet Therapy,* 10th ed. Philadelphia: W.B. Saunders Co., 2000.

Oman, K.S., et al. *Emergency Nursing Secrets.* Philadelphia: Hanley & Belfus, 2001.

Pillitteri, A., et al. *Maternal and Child Health Nursing: Care of the Childbearing and Childrearing Family,* 4th ed. Philadelphia: Lippincott Williams & Wilkins, 2002.

Rakel, R.E., ed. *Conn's Current Therapy, 2003.* Philadelphia: W.B. Saunders Co., 2003.

Smeltzer, S., and Bare, B., eds. *Brunner & Suddarth's Textbook of Medical-Surgical Nursing,* 10th ed. Philadelphia: Lippincott Williams & Wilkins, 2004.

Smith, R., et al. "American Cancer Society Guidelines for Early Detection of Cancer" *CA-A Journal for Clinicians* 50:34-49, 2000.

Stone, D.R., and Gorbach, S.L. *Atlas of Infectious Diseases.* Philadelphia: W.B. Saunders Co., 2000.

Thiedke, C., and Rosenfeld, J.A. *Women's Health.* Philadelphia: Lippincott Williams & Wilkins, 2000.

Tierney, L.M., et al., eds. *Current Medical Diagnosis and Treatment 2003.* Stamford, Conn.: Appleton & Lange, 2003.

Tintinalli, J., et al, eds. *Emergency Medicine: A Comprehensive Study Guide,* 6th ed. New York: McGraw-Hill Book Co., 2004.

White, G.M., and Cox, N.H. *Diseases of the Skin: A Color Atlas and Text.* St. Louis: Mosby–Year Book, Inc., 2000.

Index

A

Abdominal aortic aneurysm
  abdominal mass and, 5i
  abdominal pain and, 7i
  abdominal rigidity and, 11i
  back pain and, 49i
  bruits and, 77i
Abdominal distention, 2, 3i
Abdominal mass, 4, 5i
Abdominal pain, 6, 7i, 8i, 9i
Abdominal rigidity, 10, 11i
Acne vulgaris
  papular rash and, 299i
  pustular rash and, 341i
Acoustic neuroma
  absent corneal reflex and, 99i
  tinnitus and, 385i
  vertigo and, 403i
Acquired immunodeficiency syndrome
  anorexia and, 23i
  chills and, 89i
  lymphadenopathy and, 241i
Acromegaly, hirsutism and, 211i
Acute angle-closure glaucoma. *See*
  Glaucoma.
Acute tubular necrosis
  anuria and, 27i
  oliguria and, 287i
  polyuria and, 317i
Adams-Stokes syndrome, Cheyne-
  Stokes respirations and, 87i
Adenofibroma, breast nodule and, 67i
Adenomyosis, dysmenorrhea and, 133i
Adhesive capsulitis, arm pain and, 37i
Adrenal carcinoma, gynecomastia and,
  189i. *See also* Adrenocortical
  carcinoma, hirsutism and.
Adrenal crisis, level of consciousness
  decrease and, 237i

Adrenal insufficiency. *See also* Adrenocortical insufficiency.
  excessive weight loss and, 415i
  orthostatic hypotension and, 291i
Adrenal tumor, amenorrhea and, 17i
Adrenocortical carcinoma, hirsutism
  and, 211i. *See also* Adrenal carcinoma, gynecomastia and.
Adrenocortical hypofunction. *See*
  Adrenocortical insufficiency.
Adrenocortical insufficiency. *See also*
  Adrenal insufficiency.
  anorexia and, 23i
  fatigue and, 165i
  hyperpigmentation and, 217i
Adult respiratory distress syndrome
  anxiety and, 29i
  rhonchi and, 355i
Affective disorder, depression and, 117i
Agitation, 12, 13i
AIDS. *See* Acquired immunodeficiency
  syndrome.
Airway obstruction
  apnea and, 33i
  nasal flaring and, 267i
  stertorous respirations and, 349i
Alcoholic cerebellar degeneration,
  dysarthria and, 131i
Alcoholism, anorexia and, 23i
Alcohol withdrawal
  agitation and, 13i
  generalized seizures and, 364i
  tremors and, 389i
Allergic conjunctivitis
  conjunctival injection and, 95i
  eye discharge and, 159i
  photophobia and, 307i
Allergic reaction, facial edema and, 149i

Allergic rhinitis
  facial edema and, 149i
  nasal obstruction and, 269i
  throat pain and, 381i
Alopecia, 14, 15i
  patterns of, 14i
Alopecia areata, alopecia and, 15i
ALS. *See* Amyotrophic lateral sclerosis.
Alzheimer's disease
  amnesia and, 19i
  apraxia and, 35i
  dystonia and, 143i
  myoclonus and, 265i
Amenorrhea, 16, 17i
Amnesia, 18, 19i
Amyloidosis, orthostatic hypotension
  and, 291i
Amyotrophic lateral sclerosis
  abnormal deep tendon reflexes
    and, 115i
  dysarthria and, 131i
  fasciculations and, 163i
  gag reflex abnormalities and, 175i
  muscle atrophy and, 255i
  muscle flaccidity and, 257i
  muscle spasms and, 259i
  muscle weakness and, 261i
  spasticity and, 259i
Anal fissure
  hematochezia and, 199i
  rectal pain and, 345i
Analgesia, 20, 21i
  testing for, 302
Anaphylactic shock, anxiety and, 29i
Anaphylaxis
  stridor and, 373i
  wheezing and, 417i

---

i refers to an illustration; t refers to a table.

Anemia. *See also* Aplastic anemia *and*
  Pernicious anemia, Romberg's
  sign and.
 bounding pulse and, 327i
 fatigue and, 165i
 muscle weakness and, 261i
 pallor and, 295i
Angina pectoris
 anxiety and, 29i
 chest pain and, 83i
 jaw pain and, 229i
Ankylosing spondylitis
 back pain and, 49i
 neck pain and, 273i
Anorectal fissure, hematochezia
  and, 199i
Anorectal fistula, rectal pain and, 345i
Anorexia, 22, 23i
Anorexia nervosa
 abnormal breath and, 73i
 amenorrhea and, 17i
 anorexia and, 23i
 excessive weight loss and, 415i
 oligomenorrhea and, 285i
Anosmia, 24, 25i
Anterior cerebral artery occlusion,
  anosmia and, 25i
Anterior cord syndrome, analgesia
  and, 21i
Anuria, 26, 27i
Anxiety, 28, 29i
 chest pain and, 85i
 polyphagia and, 315i
 tachycardia and, 377i
Anxiety attack
 clammy skin and, 367i
 palpitations and, 297i
Aortic aneurysm
 absent or weak pulse and, 325i
 mottled skin and, 368i
Aortic arch syndrome
 absent or weak pulse and, 325i
 syncope and, 375i
Aortic insufficiency
 abnormal pulse pressure and, 329i
 atrial gallop and, 181i
 bounding pulse and, 327i
 murmurs and, 253i
 pulsus bisferiens and, 331i
 ventricular gallop and, 181i
Aortic regurgitation. *See* Aortic insufficiency.

Aortic stenosis
 abnormal pulse pressure and, 329i
 murmurs and, 253i
 pulsus bisferiens and, 331i
Aphasia, 30, 31i
 types of, 30t
Aplastic anemia
 epistaxis and, 153i
 gum bleeding and, 185i
Apnea, 32, 33i
Appendicitis
 abdominal pain and, 7i
 anorexia and, 23i
 nausea and, 271i
 vomiting and, 411i
Apraxia, 34, 35i
Areolar gland abscess
 breast nodule and, 67i
 breast pain and, 69i
Arm pain, 36, 37i, 38i, 39i
Arnold-Chiari syndrome, opisthotonos
  and, 289i
Arrhythmia, sinus, 424i
Arterial insufficiency, alopecia and, 15i
Arterial occlusion
 absent or weak pulse and, 325i
 intermittent claudication and, 225i
 mottled skin and, 368i
 pallor and, 295i
 paresthesia and, 303i
Arterial occlusive disease, pallor
  and, 295i
Arteriosclerosis, abnormal pulse pressure and, 329i
Arteriosclerotic occlusive disease
 cyanosis and, 109i
 intermittent claudication and, 225i
Arthritis
 arm pain and, 37i, 38i, 39i
 Brudzinski's sign and, 75i
Asbestosis, pleural friction rub and, 311i
Asterixis, 40, 41i
 recognizing, 40i
Asthma
 anxiety and, 29i
 barrel chest and, 51i
 dyspnea and, 141i
 grunting respirations and, 347i
 nasal flaring and, 267i
 tachypnea and, 379i
 wheezing and, 417i
Asystole, 429i

Ataxia, 42, 43i
Atelectasis
 shallow respirations and, 348i
 tracheal deviation and, 387i
Atherosclerosis
 blood pressure increase and, 57i
 tinnitus and, 385i
Athetosis, 44, 45i
Atopic dermatitis, erythema and, 155i
Atrial contraction, premature, 425i
Atrial fibrillation, 426i
Atrial flutter, 426i
Atrial tachycardia, paroxysmal, 425i
Atrioventricular block, 427i
Atrophic vaginitis
 dyspareunia and, 135i
 postmenopausal vaginal bleeding
  and, 399i
Autonomic hyperreflexia, diaphoresis
  and, 119i
AV block. *See* Atrioventricular block.

B

Babinski's reflex, 46, 46i, 47i
Back pain, 48, 49i
Bacterial conjunctivitis
 conjunctival injection and, 95i
 eye discharge and, 159i
 photophobia and, 307i
 visual blurring and, 409i
Bacterial vaginosis, vaginal discharge
  and, 401i
Barrel chest, 50, 51i
 recognizing, 50i
Basilar skull fracture
 otorrhea and, 293i
 rhinorrhea and, 353i
Bell's palsy
 absent corneal reflex and, 99i
 drooling and, 129i
Benign positional vertigo, vertigo
  and, 403i
Benign prostatic hyperplasia
 bladder distention and, 53i
 nocturia and, 277i
 urinary frequency and, 391i
 urinary hesitancy and, 393i
 urinary incontinence and, 395i
Biliary disease, pruritus and, 321i
Bladder calculus
 urinary incontinence and, 395i
 urinary urgency and, 397i

---

i refers to an illustration; t refers to a table

442   INDEX

i refers to an illustration; t refers to a table.

i refers to an illustration; t refers to a table.

---

i refers to an illustration; t refers to a table.

i refers to an illustration; t refers to a table.

Hypomagnesemia
abnormal deep tendon reflexes
and, 115i
depression and, 117i
Hypomelanosis, hypopigmentation
and, 219i
Hyponatremia
depression and, 117i
orthostatic hypotension and, 291i
Hypoparathyroidism, depression
and, 117i
Hypophosphatemia, depression
and, 117i
Hypopigmentation, 218, 219i
Hypotension. *See* Blood pressure
decrease.
Hypothermia, bradycardia and, 63i
Hypothyroidism
alopecia and, 15i
bradycardia and, 63i
depression and, 117i
excessive weight gain and, 413i
menorrhagia and, 247i
muscle atrophy and, 255i
oligomenorrhea and, 285i
thyroid enlargement and, 383i
Hypovolemic shock
blood pressure decrease and, 55i
mottled skin and, 368i
Hypoxemia, agitation and, 13i
Hypoxic encephalopathy, decerebrate
posture and, 111i

I

Immune complex dysfunction, fever
and, 169i
Impetigo
pustular rash and, 341i
recognizing, 340i
Impotence, 220, 221i
Infection, fever and, 169i. *See also*
specific type.
Inflammatory bowel syndrome, fecal
incontinence and, 167i
Inflammatory disorders, fever and, 169i
Influenza, chills and, 89i
Inner ear infection, dizziness and, 125i
Insect bites, papular rash and, 299i
Insect toxins, abdominal rigidity
and, 11i
Insomnia, 222, 223i
Intermittent claudication, 224, 225i

Interstitial lung disease
clubbing and, 91i
cough and, 102i
Intervertebral disk disorder, back pain
and, 49i
Intestinal obstruction. *See also* Bowel
obstruction *and* Mechanical
intestinal obstruction.
constipation and, 97i
diarrhea and, 121i
nausea and, 271i
Intracranial aneurysm, diplopia
and, 123i
Intracranial arteriovenous malformation, tinnitus and, 385i
Intracranial hemorrhage, headache
and, 193i
Intracranial hypertension
bradycardia and, 63i
bradypnea and, 65i
Intracranial pressure, increased
agitation and, 13i
Cheyne-Stokes respirations and, 87i
Intraductal papilloma, nipple discharge
and, 275i
Involuntary rigidity, recognizing, 10
Iodine deficiency, thyroid enlargement
and, 383i
Iritis, miosis and, 249i
Iron deficiency anemia, pica and, 309i
Irritable bowel syndrome
abdominal distention and, 3i
abdominal pain and, 8i
constipation and, 97i
nausea and, 271i

J

Jaundice, 226, 227i
classifying, 226
Jaw pain, 228, 229i
Jugular vein distention, 230, 231i
evaluating, 230
Junctional contractions, 426i
Junctional rhythm, 426i
Junctional tachycardia, 427i

K

Kernig's sign, 232, 233i
eliciting, 232i
Klinefelter's syndrome, gynecomastia
and, 189i

L

Laboratory test values, normal, 420-423
Labyrinthitis
nystagmus and, 281i
vertigo and, 403i
Lacrimal gland tumor, ptosis and, 323i
Lactose intolerance
diarrhea and, 121i
hyperactive bowel sounds and, 60i
Large-bowel cancer, diarrhea and, 121i
Laryngeal cancer, hoarseness and, 213i
Laryngitis, hoarseness and, 213i
Laryngotracheobronchitis
cough and, 101i
retractions and, 351i
stridor and, 373i
Lead poisoning, anosmia and, 25i
Leg pain, 234, 235i
causes of, 234
Leukemia
epistaxis and, 153i
gum swelling and, 187i
lymphadenopathy and, 241i
purpura and, 339i
Level of consciousness decrease, 236,
237i
Light flashes, 238, 239i
Limb circumference, measuring, 254i
Liver cancer, hepatomegaly and, 207i
Liver, percussing, 206i
Low blood pressure. *See* Blood pressure
decrease.
Lumbosacral sprain, back pain and, 49i
Lung cancer
cough and, 103i
hemoptysis and, 205i
Lymphadenopathy, 240, 241i
causes of, 240
Lymphoma
lymphadenopathy and, 241i
purpura and, 339i

M

Macular degeneration, scotoma
and, 359i
Malignancy, excessive weight loss
and, 415i
Malignant melanoma, hyperpigmentation and, 217i
Malingering disorder, bizarre gait
and, 177i

---

i refers to an illustration; t refers to a table.

i refers to an illustration; t refers to a table.

i refers to an illustration; t refers to a table.

i refers to an illustration; t refers to a table.

i refers to an illustration; t refers to a table.

i refers to an illustration; t refers to a table.